ECMO

Extracorporeal Cardiopulmonary Support in Critical Care

4th Edition

Gail Annich, M.D.

William Lynch, M.D.

Graeme MacLaren, M.D.

Jay Wilson, M.D.

Robert Bartlett, M.D.

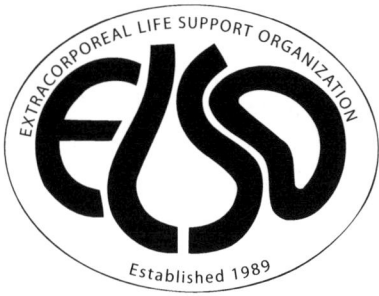

Senior Editors: Gail Annich, Graeme MacLaren
Editors: Robert Bartlett, William Lynch, Jay Wilson
Manuscript Editor: Cindy Cooke
Layout: Peter Rycus

Previous editions 1996, 2000, 2005

Printed in the United States of America

ISBN 978-0-9656756-4-2

Dedication

The 4th edition of the Red Book is dedicated to Billie Lou Short MD and P. Pearl O'Rourke MD. For 30 years Billie and Pearl have been leaders in neonatology and pediatrics, pioneers (now icons) in ECMO, and dear friends to the life support community and to each other. They organized the Children's Hospital National Medical Center Conference on ECMO in 1984, which is the oldest running ECMO meeting and beloved by all who have attended over the decades. Despite skepticism by the senior neonatal community of the time, they did the clinical research which brought neonatal ECMO from a suspicious curiosity to standard practice, saving thousands of healthy children in the process.

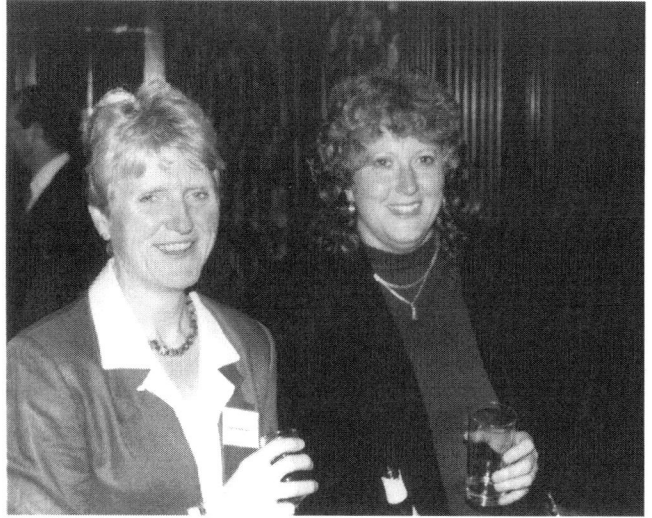

Billie Short has spent her entire career at Children's National Medical Center in Washington DC. She is currently Director of Neonatology in that hospital and the George Washington University Medical School. With her colleagues, she began the neonatal ECMO program at CNMC in 1984. This program has been at the forefront of clinical practice, education, and research in neonatal ECMO for decades. Billie pioneered the studies of brain injury and brain function in neonatal ECMO patients. With Penny Glass she has conducted and reported the definitive followup studies on ECMO patients over the years.

P. Pearl O'Rourke started the ECMO program at Children's Hospital Boston in 1986. She conducted the second prospective randomized trial of ECMO in neonatal respiratory failure, corroborating the results of the first trial. Pearl is a pediatric intensivist and moved from Boston to Seattle Children's Hospital in 1988, establishing the ECMO program in that hospital. During a year as assistant to Senator Edward Kennedy, she became expert in government healthcare policies. She is currently responsible for compliance and clinical research practices at Partners HealthCare in Boston (Massachusetts General Hospital, Brigham and Women's Hospital, and Children's Hospital Boston).

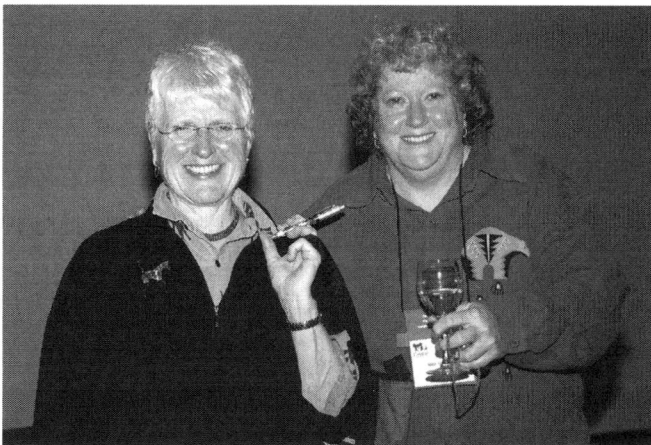

The editors and the ELSO Steering Committee are proud to recognize these fabulous clinician/researchers who have brought so much to pediatrics, intensive care, and thousands of patients.

Thank you Billie and Pearl!

List of Contributors

Patrick F. Allan MD
Lieutenant Colonel, US Air Force
Department of Pulmonary, Critical Care, and Sleep
Medicine
Wright-Patterson Medical Center
Wright-Patterson Air Force Base, OH

Christopher S.D. Almond MD MPH
Associate in Cardiology
Heart Failure and Transplant Services
Boston Children's Hospital
Assistant Professor of Pediatrics
Harvard Medical School, Boston, MA

Gail Annich MD MS FRCP(C)
Associate Professor Pediatric Critical Care
Medical Director of PICU
Director of Pediatric ECMO
Director of Pediatric CPR/RRT
C.S. Mott Children's Hospital
University of Michigan
Ann Arbor, MI

Matthias Arlt MD
Head of Cardiothoracic Anesthesia
Department of Anesthesia
University Hospital Regensburg
Airmedical Service Regensburg
Regensburg, Germany

Robert H Bartlett MD
Professor of Surgery, Emeritus
University of Michigan
Ann Arbor, MI

John Beça FCICM FRACP
Clinical Director, PICU
Starship Children's Hospital
Director of ECMO
Starship Children's Hospital and Auckland City
Hospital
Auckland, New Zealand

Desmond Bohn MB FRCPC
Department of Critical Care Medicine
The Hospital for Sick Children
Toronto, Canada

Susan L. Bratton MD MPH
Professor of Pediatrics
University of Utah Division of Pediatric Critical
Care Medicine
Primary Children's Medical
Center Salt Lake City, Utah

Patrick D Brophy MD
Associate Professor
Director Division of Pediatric Nephrology, Dialysis
and Transplantation
University of Iowa
University of Iowa Children's Hospital
Iowa City, IA

Kate L Brown MPH MRCPCH
Consultant Cardiac Intensive Care
Great Ormond Street Hospital for Children NHS
Trust
Honorary Senior Lecturer Institute of Child Health
University of London
London, United Kingdom

Holger Buchholz MD
Clinical Assistant Professor Division of Cardiac
Surgery
Director Pediatric Artificial Heart Program
Adult Artificial Heart Program
Pediatric Heart Failure Program
University of Alberta, Stollery Children's Hospital
and Mazankowski Alberta Heart Institute
Edmonton, Alberta, Canada

Warwick Butt FRACP FCICM
Director ICU
Royal Childens Hospital
Associate Professor Department of Paediatrics
University of Melbourne
Melbourne, Australia

Jeremy W. Cannon MD, SM, FACS
Director, Adult ECLS Program
Lieutenant Colonel, US Air Force
San Antonio Military Medical Center
San Antonio, TX

Robin Chapman RN
Corporate Quality
University of Michigan Health System

John Chuo MD
Assistant Professor of Pediatrics
Perelman School of Medicine, University of Penn-
sylvania
Neonatal Quality Informatics Officer
Children's Hospital of Philadelphia
Philadelphia, PA

Steven A. Conrad MD PhD FCCM
Medical Director, Extracorporeal Life Support
Program
Professor of Medicine, Pediatrics, and Emergency
Medicine
Louisiana State University Health Sciences Center
Shreveport, LA

David S. Cooper MD MPH
Associate Director, Cardiovascular Intensive Care
Unit
Director, Cardiac ECLS Program
Cincinnati Children's Hospital Medical Center
Assistant Professor of Pediatrics
University of Cincinnati College of Medicine
Cincinnati, Ohio, United Sates

Timothy T. Cornell MD
Assistant Professor
Division of Pediatric Critical Care
Department of Pediatrics and Communicable Dis-
eases
University of Michigan
Ann Arbor, MI

Marcelo Cypel MD MSc
Assistant Professor of Surgery
University of Toronto
Division of Thoracic Surgery
Toronto General Hospital
University Health Network

Heidi J. Dalton MD FCCM
Chief, Critical Care Medicine
Professor of Child Health
University of Arizona College of Medicine/Phoenix
Phoenix Children's Hospital
Phoenix, AZ

Björn Frenckner MD PhD
Professor of Pediatric Surgery
Astrid Lindgren Children's Hospital
Karolinska Institutet
Stockholm, Sweden

Gail M. Faulkner RGN RSCN
ECMO Co-ordinator
University Hospitals of Leicester NHS Trust
Glenfield Hospital
Leicester, United Kingdom

Richard Firmin MBBS FRCS
Glenfield Hospital
University of Leicester
Leicester, United Kingdom

Geoffrey M. Fleming MD FAAP
Medical Director Pediatric ECMO
Assistant Professor of Pediatrics
Division of Pediatric Critical Care
Vanderbilt University School of Medicine
Nashville, Tennessee

James D. Fortenberry MD FCCM FAAP
Pediatrician In Chief
Children's Healthcare of Atlanta
Professor of Pediatrics
Division of Pediatric Critical Care Medicine
Emory University School of Medicine
Atlanta, Georgia

Edward B. Goldman JD
Associate Professor of Obstetrics and Gynecology
Director of the Program in Sexual Rights and Reproductive Justice
University of Michigan

Jonathan Haft MD
Medical Director, Extracorporeal Life Support Program
Assistant Professor of Cardiac Surgery and Anesthesia
University of Michigan Health System
Ann Arbor, MI

William E. Harris CCP FPP
Chief Perfusionist
Ochsner Medical System
New Orleans, Louisiana

Chris Harvey MBBS FRCS
Glenfield Hospital
Leicester, United Kingdom

Michael H. Hines MD FACS
Professor of Pediatric Surgery, Cardiovascular
University of Texas Medical School at Houston
ECMO Director, Children's Memorial Hermann Hospital and
Memorial Hermann Hospital
Houston, Texas

Jennifer C. Hirsch MD MS
Assistant Professor of Surgery and Pediatrics
Surgical Director, Pediatric Cardiothoracic Intensive Care Unit
Mott Children's Hospital
University of Michigan
Ann Arbor, Michigan

Ronald B. Hirschl MD
Arnold G. Coran Professor
Head, Section of Pediatric Surgery
C.S. Mott Children's Hospital
University of Michigan
Ann Arbor, Michigan

Jeffrey P. Jacobs MD FACS FACC FCCP
Cardiovascular and Thoracic Surgeon
Surgical Director of Heart Transplantation and Extracorporeal Life Support Programs
All Children's Hospital
The Congenital Heart Institute of Florida (CHIF)
Clinical Professor
Department of Surgery
University of South Florida (USF)
Saint Petersburg and Tampa, Florida

Shaf Keshavjee MD MSc FRCSC FACS
Surgeon-in-Chief, James Wallace McCutcheon Chair in Surgery
Director, Toronto Lung Transplant Program
Professor, Division of Thoracic Surgery and Institute of Biomaterials and Biomedical Engineering
University of Toronto.
Toronto, Canada

Tracy K. Koogler MD
Associate Professor of Pediatrics
Assistant Director of the MacLean Center for Clinical Medical Ethics
University of Chicago

Kevin P. Lally MD MS
Professor and Chairman
Department of Pediatric Surgery
The University of Texas-Houston Medical School
Houston, Texas

John D. Lantos MD
Professor of Pediatrics, University of Missouri
Kansas City
Director, Children's Mercy Hospital Bioethics
Center
Kansas City, MO

Scott Lawson MS CCP
Chief Perfusionist, Director of Circulatory Support
Heart Institute
The Children's Hospital
Denver, Colorado

Laurance Lequier MD FRCPC
Director, ECLS Program
Stollery Children's Hospital
Associate Clinical Professor of Pediatrics
University of Alberta
Edmonton, Alberta Canada

Philip H. Letourneau MD
Surgical Research Fellow
Department of Surgery
The University of Texas-Houston Medical School
Houston, Texas

William R. Lynch MS MD
Associate Professor
Director of ECLS/ECMO
Department of Cardiothoracic Surgery
University of Iowa
Iowa City, Iowa

Graeme MacLaren MBBS FCICM FCCM
Director, Cardiothoracic Intensive Care
Assistant Professor of Surgery and Paediatrics
National University Health System
Singapore

M Patricia Massicotte MD Msc FRCPC MHSc
Director, Vascular Patency and Thrombosis Program
Stollery Children's Hospital
Professor of Pediatrics
University of Alberta
Edmonton, Alberta Canada

Inger Mossberg RN
Department of ECMO
Astrid Lindgren Children's Hospital
Karolinska Institutet
Stockholm, Sweden

Mark T Ogino MD
Chair, ELSO Logistics and Education Committee
Associate Professor of Clinical Pediatrics
Perelman School of Medicine, University of Pennsylvania
Children's Hospital of Philadelphia Newborn Care
Medical Director of Neonatology, Chester County
Hospital
Philadelphia, PA

Erik C. Osborn MD
Director, Adult ECLS Program
Lieutenant Colonel, US Army
Division of Pulmonary/Critical Care
Tripler Army Medical Center
Honolulu, HI

Kenneth "Palle" Palmer MD
Department of ECMO
Astrid Lindgren Children's Hospital
Karolinska Institutet
Stockholm, Sweden

Giles J Peek MD FRCS CTh FFICM
Director of Paediatric & Adult ECMO
Glenfield Hospital
Leicester, United Kingdom

Alois Philipp
Head Bioengineer
Department of Cardiothoracic Surgery
University Hospital Regensburg
Regensburg, Germany

Thomas Pranikoff MD FACS
Director, ECLS Program
Wake Forest Baptist Medical Center
Associate Professor of Surgery and Pediatrics
Wake Forest School of Medicine
Winston Salem, NC

Jeffrey D. Punch MD
Jeremiah and Claire Turcotte Professor of Transplantation Surgery
Chief, Section of Transplantation
Department of Surgery
University of Michigan
Ann Arbor, MI

Alvaro Rojas-Pena MD
Research Investigator – ECMO laboratory coordinator
Department of Surgery – Section of Transplantation
University of Michigan
Ann Arbor, MI

Peter T. Rycus MPH
Extracorporeal Life Support Organization
University of Michigan
Ann Arbor, MI

Joshua W. Salvin MD MPH
Instructor in Pediatrics
Harvard Medical School Assistant in Cardiology
Cardiac Intensive Care Unit Children's Hospital Boston
Boston, MA

Billie Lou Short MD
Chief, Division of Neonatology
Executive Director ECMO Program
Children's National Medical Center
Professor of Pediatrics
The George Washington University School of Medicine
Washington, DC

Jeffrey B. Sussmane MD MBA FCCM
Medical Director ECLS
Miami Children's Hospital
Miami, Florida

Denise M. Suttner MD
University of California at San Diego
Rady Children's Hospital
Clinical Professor of Pediatrics
San Diego, CA

Ravi R. Thiagarajan MBBS, MPH
Senior Associate in Cardiology
Cardiac Intensive Care Unit, Children's Hospital Boston
Associate Professor of Pediatrics
Harvard Medical School
Boston, MA

John M. Toomasian MS CCP
Extracorporeal Life Support Laboratory
University of Michigan Medical School
Ann Arbor, Michigan

Melissa M. Tyree MD
Director, Neonatal/Pediatric ECLS Program
Lieutenant Colonel, US Air Force
Division of Neonatology
Tripler Army Medical Center and
Hanuola ECMO Program, Kapiolani Medical Center for Women and Children
Honolulu, HI

Christina J. VanderPluym MD
Fellow, Heart Transplant/VADs
Children's Hospital Boston
Boston, MA

Shayan Vyas MD
Fellow Critical Care Medicine
Miami Children's Hospital
Miami, Florida

Jay M Wilson MD
Senior Associate in Surgery &
Director of Surgical Critical Care & ECMO
Childrens Hospital Boston
Associate Professor of Surgery Harvard Medical School
Boston, MA

Vamsi V. Yarlagadda MD
Instructor in Pediatrics, Harvard Medical School
Assistant in Cardiology, Cardiac Intensive Care Unit
Children's Hospital Boston
Boston, MA

Joseph B. Zwischenberger MD
Surgeon-In-Chief, UKHealthCare
Johnston-Wright Professor and Chairman
Department of Surgery
University of Kentucky

Preface to the 4th Edition

The ECMO "Red Book" has been the landmark reference for extracorporeal life support since the first edition was published in 1995 and there have been many developments in prolonged life support since the publication of the last edition in 2005. New devices are available which have improved the safety, simplicity, and management of ECMO so much that we refer to this new era as ECMO II. In ECMO II, patients can be cared for by a trained ECMO ICU nurse so that a small core team can manage many patients in several ICUs simultaneously. The chapters on devices, techniques, team training and economics reflect the impact of ECMO II.

ELSO first published guidelines for patient management in 2007, and this edition is based on the updated guidelines. ECMO was successful in the management of critically ill patients during the worldwide H1N1 influenza epidemic of 2009. This rekindled interest in ECMO amongst adult critical care practitioners and led to the rapid growth of ECMO in adult respiratory failure. Managing ECMO patients awake has progressed to extubation and ambulation on ECMO, first in lung transplant candidates, and recently in ARDS patients. This 4th edition of the "Red Book" reflects all of these changes and highlights the cutting-edge technology already in development.

In the spirit of academic collaboration, as with the previous editions, any of the figures, tables, or text not previously bound by copyright may be reproduced in scientific publications without further permission (conditional on the source being referenced). We would like to express our sincere appreciation to all of the experts from the ECMO community who have freely shared their time and knowledge to write this book.

Gail Annich
Graeme MacLaren

Table of Contents

1

The History and Development of Extracorporeal Support

Jim Fortenberry MD

"There is properly no history, only biography"

-Ralph Waldo Emerson

Biographical Beginnings: People

The development of extracorporeal support can rightfully be understood as the biographic collection of the men and women dedicated to the underlying effort to mimic or replace normal human body cardiopulmonary functions during an acute illness. First efforts to understand the idea of extracorporeal support could be traced to as early as 1693, when Jean Baptiste Denis performed experiments cross-transfusing the blood of a human with the "gentle humors of a lamb" to determine if living blood could be transmitted between two creatures (Figure 1-1). However, realistic efforts to provide extracorporeal support began around 1930 with the work of John Gibbon MD and his wife, Mary. Dr. Gibbon, driven by the death of a patient from a pulmonary embolus, developed a freestanding roller pump device for extracorporeal support. The initial device was the size of a spinet piano.[1] However, 16 years passed until the first human use of the device in the operating theater to assist repair of an atrial septal defect in 1953, in an 18 year old patient, Cecilia Bavolek (Figure 1-2). Shortly afterward in 1954, the esteemed cardiac surgeon C. Walton Lillehei MD per-formed cardiac surgery via cross circulation using a bubble oxygenator he invented with Richard DeWall (Figure 1-3). The remarkable chronicles of early extracorporeal development were captured by Dr. Lillehei in the first edition of the ELSO "Red Book."[2,3]

The next steps in the development of extracorporeal support were a testimony to the collaboration between biomedical engineers, physiologists, physicians, and surgeons to

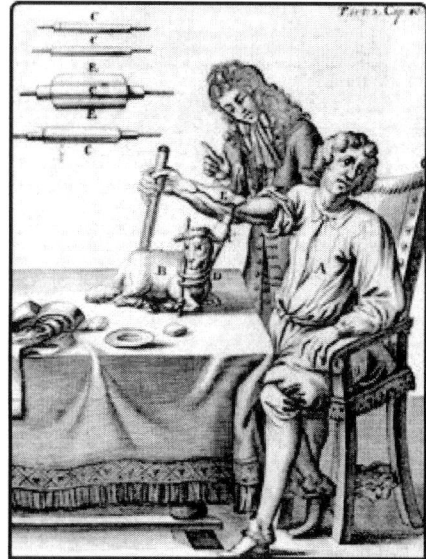

Figure 1-1. Woodcarving of experiments circa 1693 by Jean Baptiste Denis to drain human blood into a sheep.

1

create devices that could provide support for more extended time periods without massive hemolysis and plasma leakage. Early attempts in the operating room and the ICU for extracorporeal support were limited by the nature of available artificial lung devices and blood gas interfaces. Bubble oxygenators did not create an interface between blood and gas, producing hemolysis within hours. Ongoing advances in use of extracorporeal support would have been impossible without developments in technology by other innovators such as Drs. Theodor Kolobow, Drinker, and Bartlett. One early discovery that revolutionized the artificial lung was the synthesis of silicone rubber in 1957 by Kammermeyer,[4] which was found to be strong enough to withstand hydrostatic pressure and yet be permeable to gas transfer. Development of a spiral coil silicone membrane oxygenator provided a device for prolonged bypass support to allow recovery outside of the operating room.[5,6] The use of the silicone membrane oxygenator led to the use of the term extracorporeal membrane oxygenation (ECMO).

The benefits of extracorporeal support during a procedure and recovery postoperatively in children with congenital heart disease encouraged physicians to attempt its use. Baffes et al.[7] first reported the use of extracorporeal support for surgery itself, followed by experiences from other centers. Indications in these patients were often related to low cardiac output due to ventricular failure or pulmonary vasospastic crisis following surgical repair of complex heart lesions.

Efforts became devoted to extending extracorporeal support outside of the operating theater. Dr. JD Hill reported on the first prolonged extracorporeal circuit use outside of the operating room in 1972.[8] Hill cannulated a 24 year old male with post-traumatic acute respiratory distress syndrome and provided support with a Bramson membrane lung. The patient, a victim of a motorcycle accident who sustained a ruptured aorta, received venoarterial support for 75 hours with subsequent decannulation and survival. Adult ECMO support efforts continued, although survival was low.

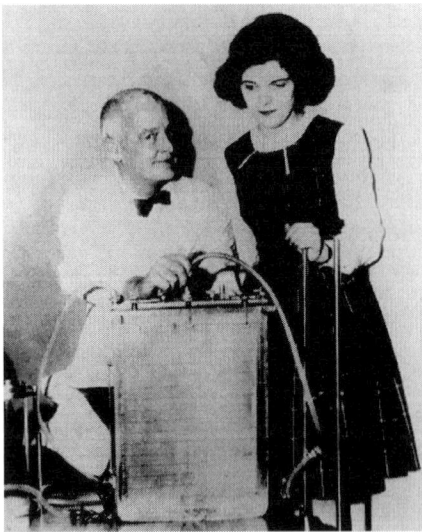

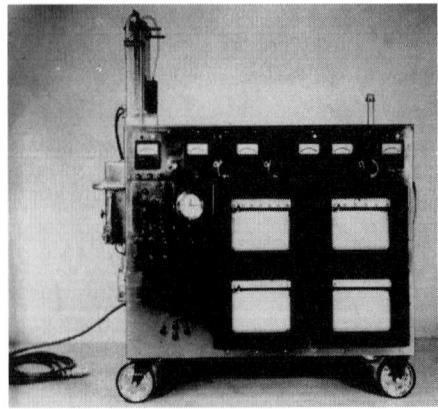

Figure 1-2. John H. Gibbon MD and patient Cecilia Bavolek, who underwent the landmark repair in 1953 of an atrial septal defect utilizing an extracorporeal circuit. The two pose before the Plexiglas-covered "lung" ten years after the procedure. Right: original device, approximately the size of a spinet piano (source: Jefferson University Archives).

At the same time, a remarkable collaboration was occurring between engineering researchers and adult surgeon Dr. Robert Bartlett (Figure 1-4), who can be characterized as the father of modern extracorporeal support. His pioneering work advanced the clinical use of extracorporeal technology both from bench and operating room to the bedside. In addition, Bartlett was the first to utilize extracorporeal support for neonates and children. In 1972, Dr. Bartlett successfully provided ECMO support to a two year old boy following a Mustard procedure for correction of transposition of the great vessels with subsequent cardiac failure. The patient underwent ECMO support for 36 hours until recovery.[9]

In 1975, Bartlett made a therapeutic decision that brought this burgeoning technology to neonates with primary respiratory conditions. Faced with a newborn infant dying from meconium aspiration pneumonia and resultant pulmonary hypertension, Bartlett and colleagues brought an ECMO oxygenator to the NICU bedside from the laboratory and sought consent from the infant's mother, who had de-

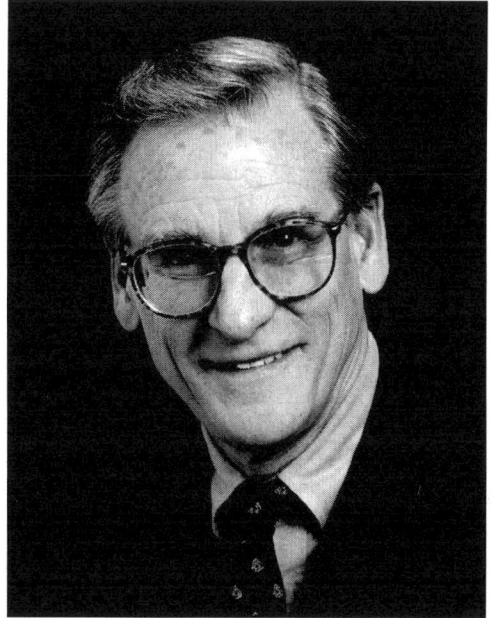

Figure 1-4. Dr. Robert H. Bartlett

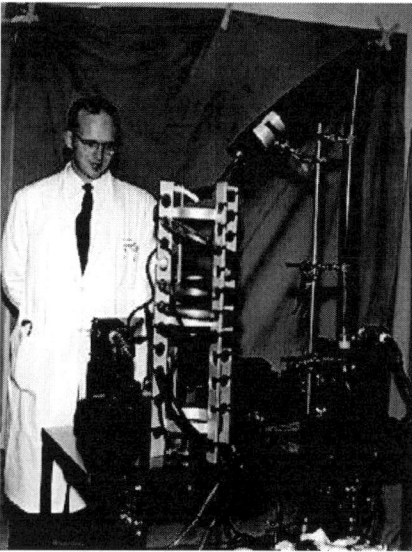

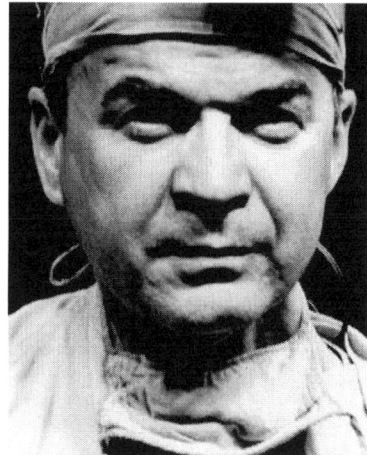

Figure 1-3. Bubble oxygenator invented and first use in 1954. Left: Inventor Richard DeWall with device. Right: Dr. C. Walton Lillehei, cardiovascular surgeon and innovator in cardiopulmonary bypass.

3

livered her after crossing the Mexican border into Orange County, California. She signed and then disappeared, leaving her baby behind. The nursing staff named the child Esperanza, Spanish for "hope."[10] She received ECMO support for 72 hours, and then was decannulated with recovery and a subsequent normal life.[11,12] Bartlett continued to treat neonates and helped drive growing successful use in neonates around the world. Published reports showed increasing improvements in outcomes, increasing survival rates 75% for neonatal diseases previously associated with only 10% survival.[13]

With growing interest, experience, and early publications reporting success, the medical community sought randomized, controlled trial (RCT) evidence of the benefits of neonatal extracorporeal support over standard therapies. Dr. Bartlett and colleagues at the University of Michigan initiated an ECMO RCT with an intriguing statistical twist to give preference to a therapy which appeared superior. Their "randomized play the winner" approach began with randomization but gave increased randomization preference based on the success or failure of the previous patient. During the study, the first patient receiving ECMO, survived. The next patient, randomized to standard care, died. Increased randomization preference went to ECMO, and the next ten patients all receiving ECMO, survived (P = .0000001). The study[14] was published in 1985 to significant controversy and discussion, including concern that control patients did not undergo informed consent. The findings however encouraged growing use of ECMO support in neonates.

A second effort to prospectively assess the effects of ECMO took advantage of ECMO and standard therapy being provided in separate intensive care units. Dr. Pearl O'Rourke, a pediatric critical care physician at Boston Children's Hospital (Figure 1-5), led a two phase RCT. The study design included a phase one approach with a traditional 50/50 randomization of patients until one arm had four deaths,

followed by a phase two utilizing an adaptive design to favor the "winner" of the first phase. Overall, 19/20 (97%) of ECMO patients survived compared to 60% of control patients.[15] The study, published in 1989, again brought great controversy in the medical community and the media.[16,17] Ironically, the outcry from many medical professionals and the lay press was that randomization to standard therapy without ECMO was unethical, implying a loss of equipoise and subtly demonstrating recognition of the benefits of ECMO.

The long-desired RCT evidence for outcome benefit in neonatal ECMO for persistent pulmonary hypertension was provided by a study performed in the United Kingdom from 1993 to 1995[18] that remains to date the largest randomized trial for ECMO use. The study, authored by Dr. Firmin and colleagues, enrolled 55 centers and took advantage of the country's regionalized medical and ECMO system, with randomization either to stay in the referral center for standard therapy or transfer to the regional ECMO center. A significant survival difference (60% in ECMO patients vs. 40% with standard therapy; NNT 3-4) supported the superiority of ECMO in neonatal respiratory failure, and etched its value in stone.

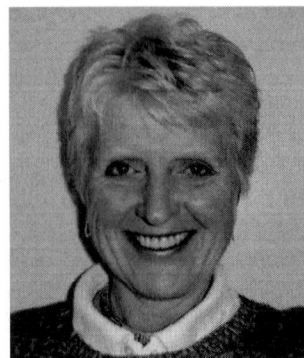

Figure 1-5. Dr. Pearl O'Rourke

Propagation of ECMO

Even absent the elusive "perfect" trial, support for, and use of ECMO in neonates grew globally. Neonatal ECMO served as a role model for rapid propagation of medical technology for treatment of disease, and served as a demonstration model in a National Institutes of Health workshop for diffusion of technology in 1990 (Figure 1-6), outlining the meteoric rise from concept to clinically accepted, if still controversial, therapy. The NIH workshop chair, Dr. Anne Lennarson-Greer, noted, "The diffusion of an innovation is a highly social process. The spread of even a simple technology ... is characterized by many interpersonal contacts and differentiated social roles."

The concept of rapid technology diffusion as a social enterprise aptly described ECMO. Dissemination of information for ECMO accelerated with the development of meetings and networks dedicated to ECMO issues. Multiple centers sprung up nationally and internationally, often with movement of physicians and staff to develop a new center, and always with collaboration from the experienced centers. For instance, in 1983 only three institutions regularly performing ECMO (Medical College of Virginia, University of Michigan, and University of Pittsburgh) were represented at one of the meetings. By 1986, nineteen institutions provided ECMO support to neonates.[20] A voluntary alliance of these active centers emerged. In 1989, a steering committee formed (Table 1-1 and Figure 1-7) and created the bylaws to form the Extracorporeal Life Support Organization (ELSO). The purpose of ELSO was to pool common data on ECMO use, compare outcomes, and exchange ideas for optimal use of ECMO support.

ELSO meetings attracted representatives from all institutions from the small number of institutions performing ECMO to present their experience. The growing interest in ECMO led to the development of a week-long meeting totally dedicated to ECMO directed by Dr. Billie Short and sponsored by DC Children's National Medical Center. Attendance was broadened by a growing international community experience. The community of international ECMO

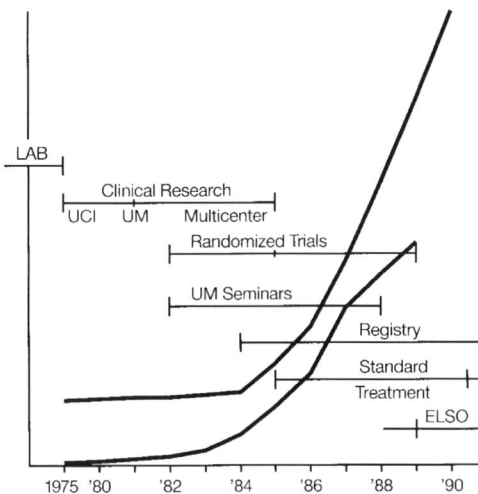

Figure 1-6. Graphic representation of development and propagation of ECMO, from NIH Report of the Workshop on Diffusion of ECMO Technology, 1993.

Table 1-1. Charter Members of First Extracorporeal Life Support Organization Steering Committee, 1989

Members	Location
Robert Bartlett	Ann Arbor, MI
William Kanto	Augusta, GA
Fred Ryckman	Cincinnati, OH
Larry Cook	Louisville, KY
Martin Keszler	Washington, DC
Billie Lou Short	Washington, DC
P. Pearl O'Rourke	Seattle, WA
J. Devn Cornish	San Diego, CA
Charles Stolar	New York, NY
Michael Klein	Detroit, MI
Phyllis McClelland	Ann Arbor, MI
Sandy Snedecor	Ann Arbor, MI

experience also grew with the first European symposium on extracorporeal lung support in Paris in 1991. This meeting was associated with the foundation of the European Extracorporeal Life Support Organization (EESO). In 1994, the international ECMO conference represented the first combined meeting of ELSO and EESO.

ELSO became the epicenter for the development of thought and definition of the operation of an ECMO center and guidelines which could be utilized by a growing number of centers. In addition, it became the steering organization for future randomized trial work. Awards for ELSO Centers of Excellence were developed to provide center recognition around ELSO recommendations.

Key efforts of ELSO were the publication of manuals and textbooks to help codify approaches to ECLS care. The need for a collated text of ECMO knowledge was recognized and two members of the steering committee, Drs. Robert Arensman and Devn Cornish, edited the first textbook in 1993. The first Red Book was published in 1995 and now has entered its fourth edition as a collaboration of experts in the ECMO community.

A critical element of propagation of ECMO technology was the development of a standardized international patient database to track results and provide evaluation of indications and outcomes in a large population, a huge improvement over traditional small case series

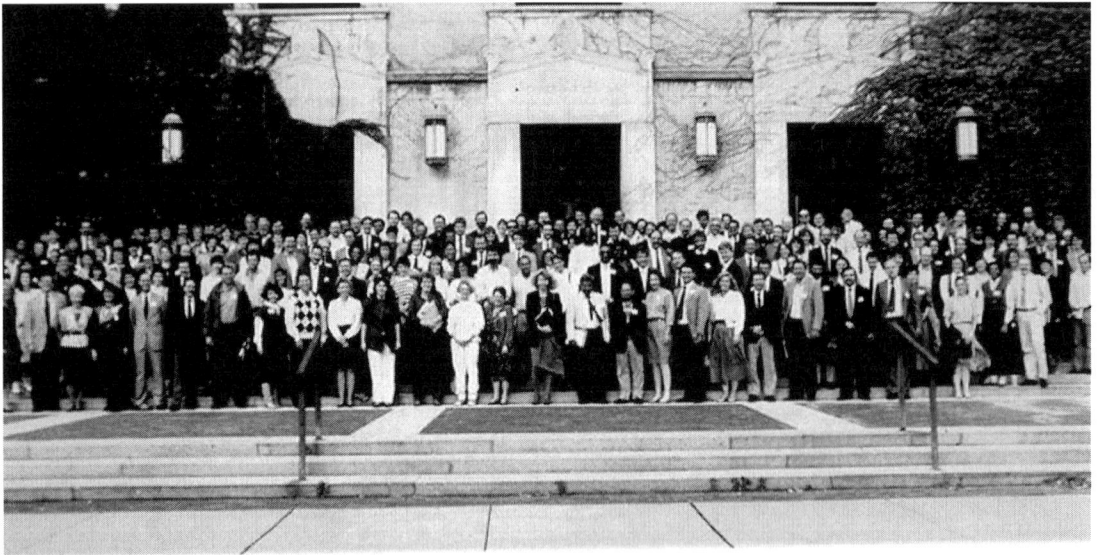

EXTRACORPOREAL LIFE SUPPORT ORGANIZATION
Charter Meeting

October 1-3, 1989   **Ann Arbor, Michigan**

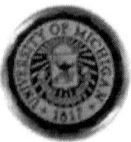

Figure 1-7. Attendees at Charter Meeting of the Extracorporeal Life Support Organization, October 1989.

experience.[20] This early registry, which transitioned into the ELSO Registry, allowed for participating institutions to collate and compare outcomes with the national and international centers. International ELSO Registry involvement grew from handful of centers in 1989 to 218 participating centers in 2011. To date in 2011, the registry database has captured over 48,000 patients and provided data for hundreds of publications and countless queries for centers seeking experience around ECMO use in a specific condition. Use of neonatal ECMO (from the ELSO Registry) peaked in 1992 at 1,516 cases. The development of additional new therapies such as inhaled nitric oxide, however, led to a decline in the numbers of patients requiring ECMO, to current levels half of the peak.

The annual ELSO meeting served as an opportunity to share neonatal ECMO data, and increasing pediatric and adult cardiorespiratory ECMO experience. Efforts to use ECMO for pediatric cardiac and respiratory failure increased with the success of neonatal ECMO and its availability in growing numbers of centers. A variety of case series suggested efficacy of ECMO in pediatric respiratory failure.[21,22] However, the relatively low numbers of pediatric patients suitable for ECMO across the country precluded a definitive trial. A multicenter RCT was attempted in the 1990s by Fackler and Heulitt, but was stopped due to enrollment difficulties, and lower than expected mortality in the study population.[23] In the absence of a RCT the most significant supporting data available to clinicians have been a case-control study performed by Green and colleagues[24] that demonstrated improved outcomes associated with use of ECMO. In particular, patients in the 50th to 75th percentile mortality risk group receiving ECMO had significantly lower mortality than matched control patients with standard therapy.

Perseverance: Adult ECMO Experience

Since the initial development of extracorporeal support for pulmonary embolus by Dr Gibbon, clinicians have sought to utilize the benefits of ECMO to allow recovery in adult respiratory failure. However, the road to acceptance of the benefits of ECMO in adults has been a slow one. Interestingly, the first attempt at an ECMO RCT was an adult trial directed by Zapol et al. and supported by the NIH comparing venoarterial (VA) ECMO to standard therapy for severe respiratory failure.[25] The study, while well intentioned, was hampered by a variety of factors including the choice of moribund patients for study entry, the use of multiple centers in which ECMO had not been performed prior to the trial and the utilization of VA support in patients potentially requiring only respiratory support. The study demonstrated very poor survival (approximately 10%) in both groups and led to reluctance to employ ECMO for adults for many years. A later adult RCT in 1994[2] randomized patients with ARDS to receive either extracorporeal CO_2 removal with VA support vs. standard therapy utilizing a computerized protocol for ventilator management. The study, again, showed no difference in outcomes. Concerns included the lack of experience with extracorporeal use in some centers as well as the very high blood loss associated in study patients. Despite these disappointing studies, physicians such as Dr. Luciano Gattinoni[27] and Dr. Bartlett persevered in its use in adults, reporting significant survival improvement compared to historical controls.

Perseverance of effort in adults led to develop another RCT for ECMO support in adult respiratory failure, the CESAR trial led by Dr. Giles Peek and colleagues. This UK study took advantage of the regionalized ECMO approach which had allowed the success of the neonatal UK trial, and also utilized the venovenous approach to ECMO in respiratory failure with its inherent advantages. Patients were randomized to either remain at a standard treatment center or be transferred to a regional ECMO center. Patients receiving care at the ECMO center demonstrated significantly improved intact survival compared to standard center treatment. The study results drew increased interest again in ECMO use for adults. These findings, published in 2009[28] also coincided with the worldwide H1N1 pandemic, with increasing use of ECMO for affected adults with encouraging findings.[29]

The growing use of ECMO nationally and internationally has been documented in the ELSO registry (Figure 1-8). Continued areas of growth include pediatric and adult respiratory failure, and pediatric cardiac failure. Pediatric cardiac failure use has grown in association with the proliferation of cardiac centers providing ECMO support and aggressive intervention in neonates with congenital heart disease. While a pediatric respiratory failure RCT to date has not been achieved, the encouraging results of the neonatal and adult trials suggest that likely ECMO benefits in pediatric patients could be "sandwiched" between those of the neonatal and adult patient groups.

In summary, the development of extracorporeal support has demonstrated the power of:

- People with a passion for patients
- Partnership between medicine and technology
- Propagation of research to the bedside
- Perseverance in seeking evidence of benefit

The next chapter in the development of extracorporeal support will likely include even more exciting steps, but it will certainly gain from those who set the stage.

"The future is unknowable, but the past should give us hope"

– Sir Winston Churchill

Centers by Year

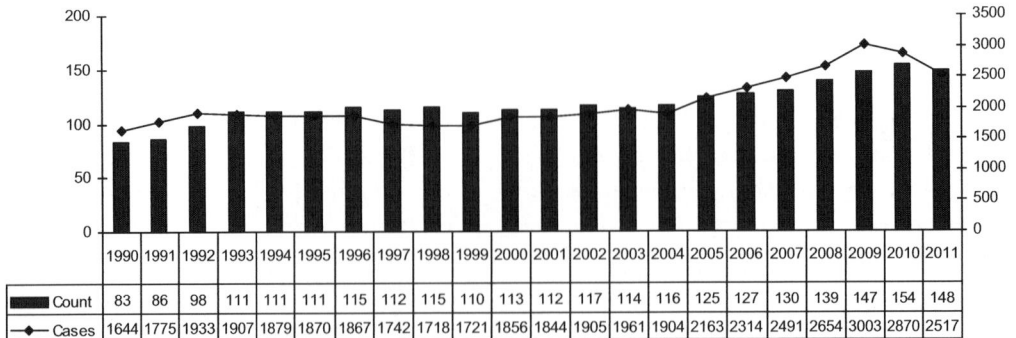

	1990	1991	1992	1993	1994	1995	1996	1997	1998	1999	2000	2001	2002	2003	2004	2005	2006	2007	2008	2009	2010	2011
Count	83	86	98	111	111	111	115	112	115	110	113	112	117	114	116	125	127	130	139	147	154	148
Cases	1644	1775	1933	1907	1879	1870	1867	1742	1718	1721	1856	1844	1905	1961	1904	2163	2314	2491	2654	3003	2870	2517

Figure 1-8. ELSO Registry statistics to 2011.

8

References

1. Jefferson Medical College Archives.
2. Lillehei CW: History of the development of extracorporeal circulation in Arensman RM, Cornish JD, eds. Extracorporeal Life Support in Critical Care (1ˢᵗ edition), Boston: Blackwell Publications, 1993.
3. Kanto WP, Shapiro MB: The development of prolonged extracorporeal circulation in Zwischenberger JB, Bartlett RH, eds. ECMO: Extracorporeal Cardiopulmonary Support in Critical Care, Ann Arbor, MI: ELSO, 1995.
4. Kammermeyer K. Silicone rubber as a selective barrier. Ind Eng Chem 1957;49:1685.
5. Kolobow T, Zapol W, Pierce JE et al. Partial extracorporeal gas exchange in alert newborn lambs with a membrane artificial lung perfused via an AV shunt for periods up to 96 hours. Trans ASAIO 1968; 14:238.
6. Bartlett RH, Isherwood J, Moss RA, Olszewski WL, Polet H, Drinkes P. A toroidal flow membrane oxygenator: four day partial bypass in dogs. Surg Forum; 1969;20:152-3.
7. Baffes TG, Fridman JL, Bicoff JP, Whitehill JL. Extracorporeal circulation for support of palliative cardiac surgery in infants. Ann Thorac Surg 1970;10:354-63.
8. Hill JD, O'Brien TG, Murray JJ et al. extracorporeal oxygenation for acute post-traumatic respiratory failure (shock-lung syndrome): use of the Bramson Membrane Lung. N Engl J Med 1972;286:629-34.
9. Bartlett RH, Gazzaniga AB, Fong SW, Jefferies MR, Roohk HV, Haiduc N. Extracorporeal membrane oxygenator support for cardiopulmonary failure. Experience in 28 cases. J Thorac Cardiovc Surg 1977;73:375-86.
10. Bartlett RH. Esperanza. Trans ASAIO 1985;31:723-35.
11. Bartlett RH. Artificial organs: basic science meets critical care. J Am Coll Surg 2003;196:171-9.
12. Wolfson PJ. The development and use of extracorporeal membrane oxygenation in neonates. Ann Thorac Surg 2003;76:S224-9
13. Bartlett RH. Extracorporeal life support in the management of severe respiratory failure. Clin Chest Med 2000;21:555-61.
14. Barlett RH, Roloff DW, Cornell RG, et al. Extracorporeal circulation in neonatal respiratory failure: a prospective randomized study. Pediatrics 1985;76:479-86.
15. O'Rourke PP, Crone RK, Vacanti JP, et al. Extracorporeal membrane oxygenation and conventional medical therapy in neonates with persistent pulmonary hypertension of th newborn: a prospective randomized study. Pediatrics 1989;84:957-963.
16. Knox RA. A Harvard study on newborns draws fire. Boston globe, August 7, 1989:25.
17. Marwick C. NIH Research Risks Office reprimands hospital institutional review board. JAMA 1990;263:2420.
18. UK Collaborative ECMO Trial Group. UK collaborative randomized trial of neonatal extracorporeal membrane oxygenation. Lancet 1996;348:75-82.
19. Wright L, Ed. Report of the Workshop on Diffusion of ECMO Technology; National Institutes of Health, 1993
20. Custer JR, Bartlett RH. Recent research in extracorporeal life support for respiratory failure. ASAIO J 1992;38:754-71.
21. Moler FW, Palmisano J, Custer JR. Extracorporeal life support for pediatric respiratory failure: predictors of survival from 220 patients. Crit Care Med 1993;21:1604-11.
22. Pettignano R, Fortenberry JD, Heard M, Labuz M, Kesser KC, Tanner AJ, Wagoner SF, Heggen J. Primary use of the venovenous approach for extracorporeal membrane oxygenation in pediatric acute respiratory failure. Pediatr Crit Care Med 2003; 4:291-8.
23. Fackler J, Bohn D, Green T, Heulitt, M, Hirshl R, Klein M, Martin L, Newth K, Nichols D, Steinhart C,Ware J. ECMO for

9

ARDS; stopping a RCT. Am J Resp Crit Care Med 1997; 155:A504.

24. Green TP, Timmons OD, Fackler JC, et al. The impact of extracorporeal membrane oxygenation on survival in pediatric patients with acute respiratory failure. Pediatric Critical Care Study Group. Crit Care Med 1996;24:323-9.

25. Zapol WM, Snider MT, Hill JD et al. Extracorporeal membrane oxygenation in severe acute respiratory failure. A randomized prospective study. JAMA 1979;242:2193-6.

26. Morris AH, Wallace CJ, Menlove RL, et al. Randomized clinical trial of pressure-controlled inverse ratio ventilation and extracorporeal CO2 removal for adult respiratory distress syndrome. Am J Resp Crit Care Med 1994;149:295-305.

27. Gattinoni L, Pesenti A, Bombino M et al. Role of extracorporeal oxygenation in adult respiratory distress syndrome management. New Horiz 1993;1:603-12.

28. Peek GJ, Mugford M, Tiruvoipati R et al. Efficacy and economic assessment of conventional ventilatory support versus extracorporeal membrane oxygenation for severe adult respiratory failure (CESAR): a multicentre randomised controlled trial. Lancet 2009;374:1351-63.

29. Davies A, ANZIC ECMO Investigators et al. Extracorporeal Membrane Oxygenation for 2009 Influenza A(H1N1) Acute Respiratory Distress Syndrome H1N1 JAMA 2009: 304:1888-95.

2

Physiology of Extracorporeal Life Support

Robert H. Bartlett MD

Physiology of Extracorporeal Life Support

Management of extracorporeal life support is the ultimate in applied physiologic care of critically ill patients. A thorough understanding of respiratory, hemodynamic, metabolic, renal, and coagulation pathophysiology is a prerequisite for the management of these patients. In this chapter we will review physiologic and pathophysiologic principles which are central to the management of extracorporeal life support. The principles are the same whether applied to newborn infants, children, or adults. Although use of these principles has resulted in improved technology and improved management over the last three decades, the physiologic principles remain the same as those presented in previous publications on this topic.[1,2] The principles of physiology and pathophysiology presented in this chapter are discussed in much more detail in "Critical Care Physiology" by this author.[3]

Extracorporeal life support is achieved by draining venous blood, removing carbon dioxide (CO_2) and adding oxygen (O_2) through an artificial lung, and returning the blood to the circulation via a vein (venovenous) or artery (venoarterial). When used in the venovenous (VV) mode the artificial lung is in series with the native lungs and replaces part or all of native lung function. When used in the venoarterial (VA) mode the artificial lung is in parallel with

the native lungs, and replaces part or all of both heart and lung function.

Normal physiology

Oxygen kinetics: The integration of metabolism, hemodynamics, and respiration

The fire of life: Normal values for oxygen consumption and delivery in adults are shown in Figure 2-1. Oxygen consumption (VO_2) is

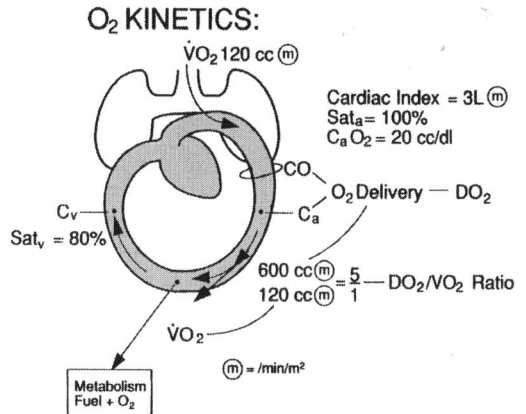

Figure 2-1. Oxygen delivery (DO_2) is normally 5x oxygen consumption (VO_2). The oxygen content of arterial blood (CaO_2) is 20 cc/dL when normal blood is fully saturated with oxygen (Sat_a). Removal of 20% of the oxygenated arterial blood results in a venous oxygen content (Cv) of 80% which corresponds to a venous saturation (Sat_v) of 80%.

controlled by tissue metabolism and is thus decreased by rest, paralysis, and hypothermia and increased during muscular activity, infection, hyperthermia, and increased levels of catecholamine and thyroid hormones. The metabolic rate is defined as the VO_2, or calculations based on the VO_2 (the volume of oxygen consumed multiplied by 5 cal/L estimates the energy expenditure expressed in calories). The values for VO_2 in normal resting humans is 5-8 cc/kg/min in newborn infants, 4-6 cc/kg/min in children, and 3-5 cc/kg/min in adults. The basal metabolic rate is controlled by the hypothalamus. The metabolic rate is independent of the substrates for metabolism (oxygen and foodstuffs), until the availability of those substrates is very low. The amount of oxygen absorbed across the lung in the process of pulmonary gas exchange is exactly equal to the amount of oxygen consumed by peripheral tissues during metabolism (the Fick principle) regardless of the status of pulmonary function. Hence, VO_2 can be measured at the airway or calculated as the product of arterial venous oxygen content difference times cardiac output (the Fick equation). Some of the relevant values and calculations are shown in Table 2-1.

Oxygen is present in the blood as both oxygen dissolved in plasma and as oxygen bound to hemoglobin in red cells. The amount of oxygen in blood is measured as oxyhemoglobin saturation (as a percentage of maximum), the partial pressure of oxygen dissolved in plasma (PO_2 in mmHg), and the total amount of oxygen is described as the oxygen content in cc of oxygen per deciliter of blood. The oxygen content is rarely measured directly for clinical applications and we are accustomed to describing blood oxygenation in terms of PaO_2 or hemoglobin saturation. However, oxygen content is the most important measurement in the physiologic management of critically ill patients. The relationship of PaO_2, saturation and oxygen content is described in Figure 2-2. Typical values for venous and arterial blood at different levels of hemoglobin are identified. Notice that there is more oxygen in normal blood with a PO_2 of 40 than in anemic blood with a PO_2 of 100.

Oxygen uptake in the normal lung

How does oxygen get into blood? It is worth considering this question to understand the pathophysiology of lung failure, and understand

Table 2-1. Normal values for the variables in oxygen kinetics. Measurements which are not related to body size (gases in blood for example) are the same for any patient, but variables related to body size (oxygen delivery and consumption for example) must be normalized to body size expressed as weight or surface area.

Definitions & Formulas		Normal
CaO_2	Oxygen content, arterial	20 cc/dl
CvO_2	Oxygen content, venous	16 cc/dl
$AVDO_2$	Arteriovenous oxygen difference	4 cc/dl
DO_2	Oxygen delivery	600 cc/min/m^2
VO_2	Oxygen consumption	120 cc/min/m^2
VCO_2	CO_2 produced	100 cc/min/m^2
REE	Resting energy expenditure	25 cal/kg/d

Oxygen Content = (Hbgm/dl X %sat X 1.36 cc/gm) + (pO$_2$ X .003 ccO$_2$/mmHg/dl)

Oxygen Delivery = CaO$_2$ X cardiac index

Fick's Axiom: O$_2$ consumed via lung = O$_2$ consumed in metabolism

CaO$_2$ or CvO2 = Oxygen Content = ccO$_2$/dl = O$_2$ bound to Hb + O$_2$ dissolved

     O$_2$ bound to Hb = Hb gm/dl x % sat x 1.36 ccO$_2$/gm

     O$_2$ dissolved = pO$_2$ x .003 ccO$_2$/mmHg/dl

AVDO$_2$ = CaO$_2$ - C$_V$O2

how artificial lungs simulate normal physiology. The physical chemistry that goes on in the capillaries of the lung is elegantly simple. The partial pressure of oxygen in inhaled air is 150 mmHg, and the PO_2 in venous blood is 40 mmHg. They are separated by a membrane only two flat cells thick which is freely permeable to respiratory gases. The membrane is a short tube 10 μ in diameter, so red cells have to pass through one at a time. At rest each red cell is in the capillary for one second. During that time oxygen passes from the alveolar air into the blood plasma in response to the concentration gradient. Oxygen dissolved in the plasma is immediately bound to hemoglobin in the red cells. Oxyhemoglobin saturation reaches 100% (at PO_2 90 mmHg) in 0.25 seconds. During the six seconds of a single respiratory cycle, the PO_2 in alveolar air falls from 150 to 90, and then refreshed during the next inspiration. These reactions are so efficient that the arterial blood will be fully saturated with a PO_2 90 even if the blood passes through the capillary much faster (higher cardiac output), or if the inlet hemoglobin is only 50% saturated (hypermetabolism). The net result is that the amount of oxygen absorbed across the lung is exactly equal to the amount of oxygen consumed in metabolism.

Hemodynamics

The normal cardiac output is a balance of the force and volume of each cardiac contraction, heart rate, and the resistance to flow in the arterial circulation. These factors are regulated in turn by ventricular filling pressure (blood volume), vascular tone, and blood viscosity (hematocrit). The reflexes which maintain systemic oxygen delivery minute-to-minute are effected by changes in cardiac output. During exercise, cardiac output increases because epinephrine is secreted and vascular resistance falls. During hypoxemia, chemoreceptors trigger an increase in heart rate. During anemia, cardiac output increases because of the decrease in blood viscosity. During hypovolemia, catecholamines mediate increased rate and contraction and increased vasomotor tone. All of these reflexes interact to maintain systemic oxygen delivery at five times consumption. When the heart fails, we assist these reflexes with control of blood volume, vasoactive drugs, or mechanical devices.

Systemic Oxygen Delivery (DO₂)

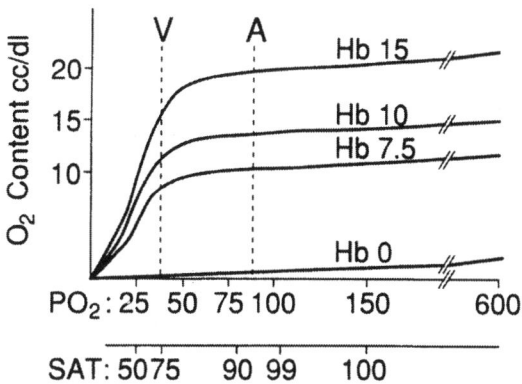

Figure 2-2. The relationships between PO_2 saturation and oxygen content in venous and arterial blood. Normal arterial blood (hemiglobin 15 gr/dL) has an oxygen content of 20 cc/dL and normal venous blood has an oxygen content of 15 cc/dL. Corresponding contents for degrees of anemia are shown in the other isobars. Notice that the saturation and PO_2 is the same for normal and anemic blood. The most important number for study of respiratory physiology in extracorporeal support is the oxygen content.

DO_2 is the amount of oxygen delivered to peripheral tissues each minute, or the product of arterial oxygen content times cardiac output. Oxygen delivery is controlled by cardiac output, hemoglobin concentration, hemoglobin saturation, and dissolved oxygen, in that order. The normal value for DO_2 is four to five times VO_2 regardless of patient size. The normal relationship between DO_2 and VO_2 is shown in Figure 2-3. The normal ratio is 5:1, and when

13

VO_2 changes secondary to variations in metabolism, DO_2 readjusts by increasing or decreasing cardiac output to maintain the normal ratio. A unique aspect of cardiorespiratory homeostasis is the tendency to maintain systemic oxygen delivery at the normal level. In anemia, the cardiac output will increase until DO_2 is normalized. For example, the best treatment for a ventilated patient who is hypoxic, anemic, tachycardic, hypotensive, and hypermetabolic is usually red cell transfusion (rather than using high doses of inotropic drugs or increasing FiO_2).

If systemic oxygen delivery is moderately decreased (e.g., by decreasing cardiac output), there is no change in oxygen consumption, so the amount of oxygen extracted from each deciliter of arterial blood is greater. This results in decreased oxygen saturation of venous blood (SvO_2). SvO_2 measures the ratio of $DO_2:VO_2$. If DO_2 is severely decreased, there is not enough oxygen to meet metabolic demands and an-aerobic metabolism occurs leading to metabolic acidosis and shock. In practice, this situation occurs when the DO_2/VO_2 ratio is less than 2:1. Between this critical point at a DO_2/VO_2 ratio of 2:1 and the normal ratio of 5:1, decreased delivery is compensated for by increased extraction, maintaining normal hemodynamic and metabolic stability. Since mixed venous blood oxyhemoglobin saturation reflects this ratio exactly, it is the most important monitor for managing critically ill patients. If the arterial blood is fully saturated the venous saturation decreases proportionate to the amount of oxygen extracted from arterial blood. Thus if the oxygen extraction ratio is 20% the venous saturation will be 80%; if the oxygen extraction ratio is 33% the venous saturation will be 67%, etc. The levels of venous saturation corresponding to various $DO_2:VO_2$ ratios are identified in Figure 2-3. The same relationships hold when VO_2 is increased. In a septic patient VO_2 may be as high as twice normal, and DO_2 increases to maintain the ratio at 5:1. This is why septic patients are described as "hyperdynamic." These relationships are shown in Figure 2-4.

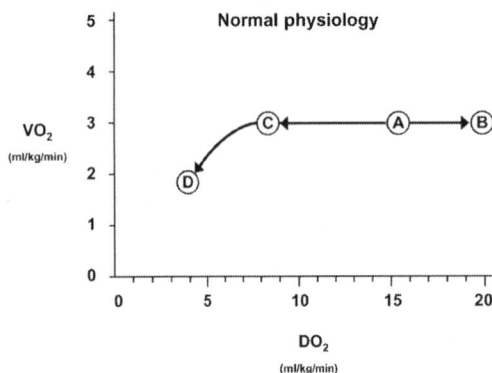

Figure 2-3. The normal relationships between oxygen consumption and oxygen delivery. Oxygen consumption (VO_2) stays constant at resting conditions. Oxygen delivery is normally 5x consumption (circle A) at stable oxygen consumption if oxygen delivery is increased (circle B) there is no change in consumption. If oxygen delivery is decreased (from circle A to circle C) oxygen consumption is unchanged, but when oxygen delivery drops below that point oxygen consumption becomes delivery dependent and decreases (circle D).

Carbon Dioxide Production and Excretion

The amount of CO_2 produced during systemic metabolism each minute (VCO_2) is approximately equal to the amount of oxygen consumed. The ratio of CO_2 production to oxygen consumption is known as the respiratory quotient, and depending on the energy substrate it varies from 0.7 for fat to 0.8 for protein to 1.0 for carbohydrate. Under normal conditions the rate and depth of breathing are controlled to maintain the arterial PCO_2 at 40 mmHg. Even a slight increase in metabolically produced CO_2 will result in a proportionate increase in alveolar ventilation, just enough to increase CO_2 excretion so that the arterial PCO_2 will remain at 40. Unlike systemic oxygen delivery, CO_2 excretion is not affected by hemoglobin or blood flow but is very sensitive to changes in ventilation.

14

For this reason, and because CO_2 excretion is much more efficient than oxygenation in the lung, CO_2 removal can be maintained at normal levels by hyperventilation, even during severe lung dysfunction.

Pathophysiology of cardiac and pulmonary failure.

We manage critically ill patients based on an understanding of normal metabolism, oxygen kinetics, and hemodynamics. Normal resting physiologic function of vital organs is about four times the requirements for basal function. In other words there is reserve of organ function four times that required for normal activity. Metabolism and organ function are adequate for normal life when kidney, liver, or intestine functions at 25% of resting normal. The same is true for heart and lung function, but we are all dependent on those organs minute-to-minute, not day-to-day. The pathophysiology and management of lung and heart failure are described in detail in chapters 3 and 4. The overall goal of management is to keep DO_2 at least twice VO_2, and preferably five times VO_2. ECLS is indicated when other treatment modalities cannot do this, or when the treatment required is itself contributing to organ failure.

Normal Physiology of ECLS:

Modes of vascular access and perfusion:

In venoarterial bypass, the functions of both heart and lungs are replaced by artificial organs, either totally or partially. During partial VA bypass, perfusate blood mixes in the aorta with left ventricular blood which has traversed the lungs. Hence, the content of O_2 and CO_2 in the patient's arterial blood represents a combination of blood from these two sources, and the total systemic blood flow is the sum of the extracorporeal flow plus the amount of blood passing through the heart and lungs. Venoarterial access is shown in Figure 2-5.

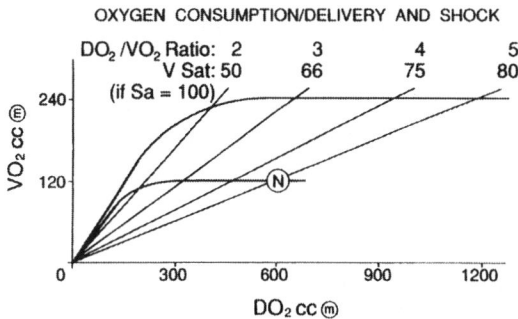

Figure 2-4. The normal relationships between oxygen consumption and delivery described in Figure 2-3 are shown as the normal isobar (circle N). If the metabolic rate increases (VO_2) because of exercise or sepsis homeostatic mechanisms increase oxygen delivery to restore the normal ratio of delivery to consumption to 5:1. This corresponds to a venous blood saturation of 80% if the arterial saturation is 100%.

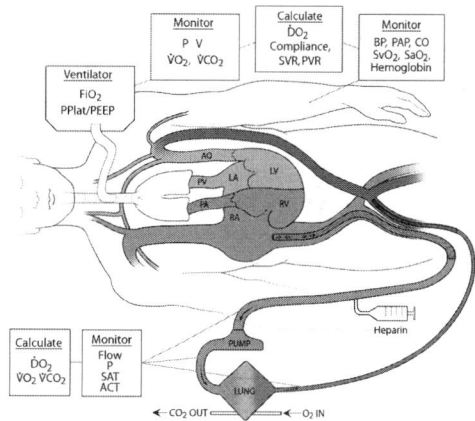

Figure 2-5. Venoarterial access via the femoral vessels. Venous blood drains from the inferior vena cava and is pumped through the membrane lung and returned to the right femoral artery. The amount of flow determines how far toward the aortic root the arterial perfusion will go. In partial VA bypass some blood passes through the lungs and enters the left atrium and left ventricle and mixes with the perfusate blood in the aorta. The variables which we monitor and calculate are used to regulate both the extracorporeal circuit and the mechanical ventilator.

In <u>venovenous bypass</u>, the perfusate blood is returned to the venous circulation and mixes with venous blood coming from the systemic organs, raising the oxygen content and lowering CO_2 content in right atrial blood. Some of this mixed blood may be returned to the extracorporeal circuit ("recirculation") and some of it passes into the right ventricle, the lungs, and into the systemic circulation. Since the volume of blood removed is exactly equal to the volume of blood re-infused, there is no net effect on central venous pressure, right or left ventricle filling, or hemodynamics. The content of oxygen and CO_2 in the patient's arterial blood represents that of right ventricle blood modified by any remaining pulmonary function that might exist. Systemic blood flow is the native cardiac output and is unrelated to the extracorporeal flow. Venovenous access is shown in Figure 2-6.

<u>Arteriovenous</u> (AV) extracorporeal circulation is commonly used in intermittent hemodialysis but not in continuous renal replacement therapy or for cardiac support. On the contrary, it places additional volume work on the heart. The AV route can be used for gas exchange provided the arterial blood is desaturated and the cardiovascular system can tolerate the arteriovenous fistula with a large enough flow to achieve adequate gas exchange. This is, after all, the mechanism of gas exchange in the placenta and fetus. Because of the blood flow requirements for gas exchange support, the arteriovenous route is not a reasonable approach to provide total extracorporeal respiratory support, except when the patient can tolerate a large arteriovenous shunt and increase in cardiac output (such as a premature infant). However, AV flow through a membrane lung can provide CO_2 excretion, decreasing the need for mechanical ventilation.[4]

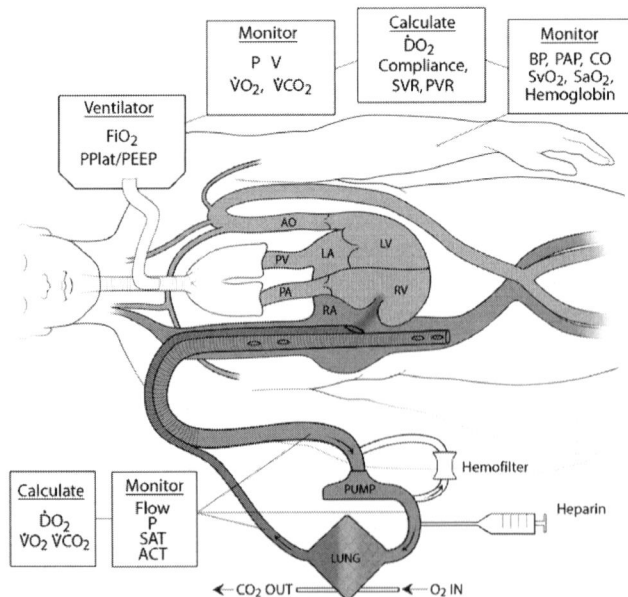

Figure 2-6. Venovenous access. Venous blood is drained from the superior and inferior vena cava and pumped through the membrane lung and back into the right atrium. The variables which we monitor and calculate are used to control the mechanical ventilator and the extracorporeal circuit. Notice that there is no direct arterial infusion, so the systemic oxygenation will reflect the mixture of some venous blood with the ECMO return blood. This mixture passes through the native lungs. If there is no native lung function the arterial saturation will be less than 95%.

VA ECLS Compared to CPB

Much has been written about the physiology and pathophysiology of total VA bypass for cardiac surgery.[5] While the principles of gas exchange and blood flow are the same, there are several important differences between the conduct of ECLS and bypass in the operating room. Some of the more important differences are summarized in Figure 2-7. Because the sole purpose of operating room cardiopulmonary bypass (CPB) is to permit operations on the heart, total venoarterial bypass is always used. Because there is stagnation of blood in the pulmonary circulation, some chambers of the heart, and parts of the extracorporeal circuit, total anticoagulation is required, achieved by giving a large dose of heparin to make the whole blood clotting time infinitely long. This anticoagulation, coupled with uncontrolled blood flow into the operative field from the coronary sinus, bronchial veins, arterioluminal vessels, and thebesian veins, results in continuous bleeding which is managed by aspiration and filtration of the shed blood with return to the venous reservoir (cardiotomy suction or autotransfusion). To minimize this bleeding into the field, and to minimize any risks associated with high blood flow, it is common practice to manage systemic perfusion at abnormally low levels of blood flow ($2\text{-}2.4$ $L/min/m^2$) and abnormally low hematocrit (typically 20%). This combination of low blood flow and low hematocrit leads to very low systemic oxygen delivery, which could result in oxygen debt and metabolic acidosis, except that total body hypothermia is usually implemented, maintaining the ratio of delivery to consumption in the normal range of 5:1. Therefore a very efficient heat exchanger and a large water bath are required for cardiopulmonary bypass for heart surgery.

It is always possible to inadvertently aspirate large amounts of air into the venous catheters and it is convenient to rapidly raise or lower the entire blood volume of the patient at times during cardiac operations. Therefore a large venous reservoir is included in the venous drainage line, both to trap aspirated air and to allow frequent variations in intracorporeal versus extracorporeal blood volume. Because the blood is totally anticoagulated, blood does not clot in this large reservoir. It is common practice during cardiac surgery to arrest the heart to permit a still operating field, and to clamp the aorta above the coronary ostia but below the perfusion catheter to minimize coronary blood flow for the purpose of allowing operations directly on the coronary vessels and to minimize coronary sinus flow during operations on the right side of the heart. Because the myocardium is without blood flow during aortic cross clamping, various techniques must be employed to minimize ischemic damage to the myocardium. This has resulted in an entire sub-science and literature related to myocardial perfusion and protection during VA bypass for cardiac surgery. The cornerstone of all these techniques is direct myocardial hypothermia achieved by a combination of topical cooling and cold coronary perfusate. Because the aorta is cross clamped and the heart is arrested during most cardiac operations, bronchial and thebesian blood flow will cause gradual filling and eventually over-distention of the left

	OR CPB	ICU ECLS/ECMO
Venous reservoir	Yes	No
Heparin (ACT	↑ Dose (>600)	Titrated (120-180)
Autotransfusion	Yes	No
Hypothermia	Yes	No
Hemolysis	Yes	No
Anemia	Yes	No
Arterial filter	Yes	No
Venous drainage	Right atrium	Right atrium
Pump control	Perfusion/Reservoir	Perfusionist/Servo-control
Gas exchange	Membrane Lung	Membrane Lung
Heat exchanger	Yes	Yes
Monitors	SvO$_2$, pressure	SvO$_2$, pressure

Figure 2-7. Comparison of the important differences and similarities between operating room cardiopulmonary bypass and extracorporeal and prolonged extracorporeal support in the ICU.

atrium and left ventricle. Left unchecked, this over-distention damages the endocardium and myocardium, so that some system of left-sided venting of this blood is a necessary component of cardiopulmonary bypass for cardiac surgery.

In contrast, extracorporeal life support uses partial rather than total cardiopulmonary bypass, achieved by extrathoracic cannulation conducted at normothermia, normal blood flow and normal hematocrit, emphasizing normal systemic oxygen delivery to match metabolic needs. Heparinization is titrated to very low levels and bleeding should be an infrequent complication. The design of the extracorporeal circuit eliminates venous reservoirs, cardiotomy suction apparatus, and large heat exchangers. When there is some cardiac function, VA bypass for cardiac failure is managed at 80% support, allowing 20% of the venous return to be pumped by the failing native heart from right atrium to aorta to avoid left side overdistension and stagnation which leads to intracardiac thrombus formation. When there is no native cardiac function, the left side must be vented to avoid overdistension and intracardiac thrombosis is a potential problem. In venovenous bypass the entire circulation is totally dependent on unassisted myocardial function.

Aside from these differences in perfusion technology, the entire approach to management of extracorporeal circulation is quite different when comparing CPB to ECLS. Cardiopulmonary bypass is conducted in the operating room with the sole intention of operating upon the heart. There is an appropriate sense of urgency to minimize the time on bypass. Complications, including myocardial damage, renal failure, liver failure, hemolysis, and abnormal bleeding, increase proportionate to the amount of time on bypass. Unlimited amounts of bleeding in the operating field are tolerated and managed by autotransfusion, with the realization that the effect of heparin will be reversed by protamine at the end of the procedure. An hour or two of rewarming and attempts to come off bypass is considered an exceedingly long and tedious interval. Often large doses of catecholamines are given to encourage a sluggish heart simply in order to come off bypass. If the patient cannot be weaned off bypass in a few hours all hope is considered lost unless a mechanical support system can be instituted. The patient is anesthetized and paralyzed and it is impossible to directly evaluate neurologic function. Everyone caring for the patient from the surgeon to the circulating nurse measures success or failure in hours.

In contrast, ECLS is managed in the ICU by a team expecting days or weeks of continuous care. The patient is maintained awake or awakened at regular intervals to evaluate neurologic function. Feeding, ventilation, antibiotic management, and renal function are all-important aspects of ECLS care. The use of inotropic or vasoactive drugs and high ventilator settings is minimal, and weaning from bypass may proceed over a period of hours or days. The patient commonly lacks heart, lung, or renal function for days, and futility is conceded only after many days of vital organ failure.

Blood flow (hemodynamics):

During extracorporeal support we use blood flow to support both cardiac and pulmonary function so it is essential to understand the possibilities and limitations of blood flow.

Tubing and Cannulas

Blood flow through the extracorporeal circuit is limited by the size of the venous drainage cannula. Resistance to blood flow varies directly with the length of the cannula and inversely with the fourth power of the radius of the cannula. Consequently the shortest and largest internal diameter cannula that can be placed in the right atrium will allow the highest rate of extracorporeal blood flow. The superior vena cava allows the most direct access to the right atrium, and the right internal jugular vein usually has a large diameter. A cannula placed in the right internal jugular vein will usually permit venous drainage equivalent to the normal resting cardiac output of patients of all ages and sizes. Blood drains through the venous tubing to a pump that provides pressure that directs the blood through the membrane lung and back into the patient. There is significant resistance to flow through the membrane lung and across the reinfusion cannula, so the pressure on the arterial side of the circuit increases with increasing blood flow. In practice, the pump is set to deliver the desired flow and the post-pump pressure is simply monitored. Pressures as high as 300 mmHg are safe, although the higher the pressure, the higher the likelihood of blood leaks or circuit disruption. Pressure/flow characteristics of cannulas and tubing can be described by the "M" number,[6,7] as shown in Figures 2-8 and 2-9.

Pumps

Some measures must be taken to assure that the pump does not apply excessive suction to the venous catheter. There are three reasons for this: 1) negative pressure (over 600 mmHg) will cause cavitation (bubble formation) which causes hemolysis, 2) the right atrium and vena cava may become sucked into the catheter, causing endothelial damage, and 3) negative pressure anywhere in the system always increases the risk of air entrainment and air embolism. In cardiac surgery, these problems are avoided by including a large blood reservoir into which the venous line drains; air bubbles float to the top. A large reservoir is unacceptable for ECLS because the stagnant blood may thrombose and because the extracorporeal circuit must be maintained essentially at a constant volume.

Occlusive **roller pumps** could generate direct suction on the venous catheter. In practice, this problem is avoided by the inclusion of a small collapsible bladder positioned at the lowest point of the venous line. The bladder (or a transducer directly in the venous line) is attached to an electrical switch that slows or stops the roller pump whenever the pump suction results in negative pressure, then restarts the pump instantly when the filling pressure exceeds the pump suction (i.e., the venous drainage flow exceeds the pump flow). The "suction" on the venous cannula is the siphon created by the distance from the patient to the floor (typically 100-150 cmH$_2$O). Whenever the bladder collapses

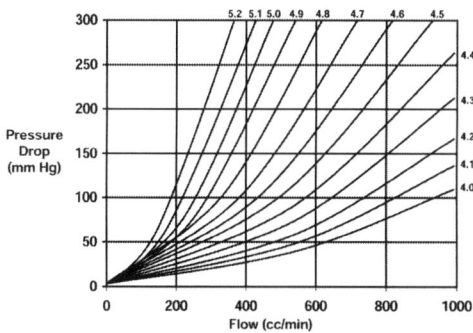

Figure 2-8. Pressure flow characteristics of several cannulas used for infants and children. The pressure flow characteristics must be known for each cannula, and are not described by the circumference (French size) or length.

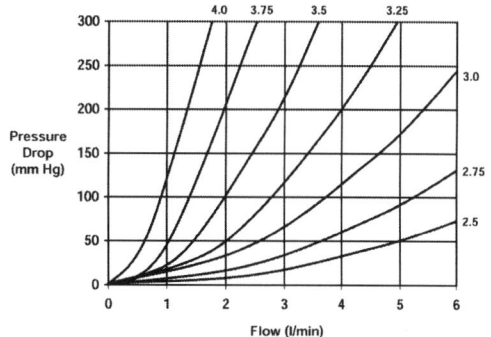

Figure 2-9. Pressure flow characteristics for cannulas for adult sized patients.

(or the transducer senses negative pressure) and the pump stops, the suction effect of the siphon between the patient and the level of the bladder stops, avoiding any continuing suction on the right atrium. Also, because the pump motor is slowed or turned off whenever the bladder is collapsed, the pump cannot generate excessive negative pressure in the blood between the pump and the bladder (which would cause cavitation and hemolysis). Thus this bladder and electrical switching mechanism provides servo regulation and some measure of safety for prolonged perfusion with a roller pump. The pump is adjusted to provide the desired level of gas exchange or cardiac support. As long as the venous drainage is adequate, suction pressure is acceptable and the desired flow is delivered. If venous drainage is impeded for any reason (e.g., hypovolemia, pneumothorax, kinking of the venous catheter), the pump stops and an alarm sounds. Flow resumes as soon as venous drainage is reestablished.

Early in the course of extracorporeal circulation, the operator increases the flow to the point at which the pump is stopped by servo regulation, thus identifying the physical limitation of venous drainage for the system. This flow rate is usually considerably greater than the flow actually required for extracorporeal support. However, if maximal flow through the system is inadequate after optimizing volume status another venous catheter must be added to gain more flow. The problems with roller pumps are: a sizable heavy motor is required, the tubing can wear or rupture in the pump head, and there is no limit to infusion pressure so there is always a risk of blowout.

Centrifugal pumps, in which a spinning rotor generates flow and pressure, should be ideal for prolonged extracorporeal circulation. Unlike roller pumps, the motor can be light and small, the components do not wear out, and the perfusion pressure is limited by the RPM, so blow out is rare. The problems are: stagnation and heating in the pump head leading to

thrombus, and cavitation and hemolysis when the inlet line is occluded. When centrifugal pumps are used for cardiac surgery the pump attaches directly to the venous reservoir and servo regulation is provided by level sensing or by the pump operator. In ECLS the pump inlet line is attached directly to the venous cannula. Many times a day, the venous drainage may be transiently but completely occluded (e.g., during coughing, hypovolemia, or kinking, manifested as "chattering" of the venous line). When the venous line is occluded the rotor keeps spinning, evacuating blood from the pump head creating a vacuum in the pump head which causes cavitation and hemolysis. This happens in a second (milliseconds at high RPM), so no servo regulation system is fast enough to prevent cavitation. The problem can be minimized by incorporating a collapsible bladder in the venous line to act as a mini reservoir,[8] or by servo regulating pump RPM based on inlet pressure sensing[9] which prevents continuing suction when the line is occluded for more than a few seconds. In practice centers that use centrifugal pumps limit the RPM to about 3000, and turn the flow down whenever the venous line is chattering. Stagnation and thrombus formation are essentially eliminated when the rotor is designed with a hole in the center.

Pneumatic and peristaltic pumps avoid many of these problems and have been used for ECLS. Pumps are described in more detail in chapter 8.

From the foregoing discussion, it can be seen that both building and monitoring the ECLS circuit requires knowledge of the pressure, flow, and resistance characteristics of each of the blood conduit components. Although these relationships can be calculated for straight tubes of known diameters, most access catheters have irregular diameters and side holes which require individual characterization. Our group described a standard system for describing pressure flow relationships in blood access devices, which we have called the M number.[6,7] If the

M number for a specific catheter is known, the pressure and flow over the full range of use can be determined from a nomogram (Figures 2-8 and 2-9). Cannulas are discussed in detail in chapter 9.

Non-Pulsatile Flow

The effect of venoarterial bypass on systemic perfusion is reflected in the pulse contour and pulse pressure. The extracorporeal pump creates a flow that is essentially non-pulsatile. Consequently, as more blood is routed through the extracorporeal circuit, the systemic arterial pulse contour becomes flatter, then intermittent, then is stopped altogether when total bypass is reached. At total bypass the left ventricle gradually distends with bronchial and thebesian flow and ejects when it is full, leading to an occasional pulsatile beat (Figure 2-10). In practice, it is unusual to reach total bypass for any sustained period with extrathoracic cannulation as long as there is cardiac function. Typically, venoarterial ECLS is run at about 80% of resting normal cardiac output, which allows 20% or more of the blood to pass through the lungs and left heart resulting in a diminished but discernible pulse contour. As long as total blood flow is adequate, the presence of a pulse contour is not important physiologically.[10,11,12] The discussion over pulsatile and non-pulsatile flow has been the subject of many research reports over the last three decades. The results of some of the more important studies are summarized in Figure 2-11. As long as total blood flow to the patient or experimental animal is on the high/normal side (typically > 100 cc/kg/min) there is no difference between pulsatile and non-pulsatile perfusion. Similarly if total blood flow is very low (typically < 40 cc/kg/min), inadequate oxygen delivery, shock, anaerobic metabolism, and acidosis occur with any type of perfusion. At low but barely adequate blood flow, the effects of hypoperfusion and acidosis are somewhat ameliorated by pulsatile flow. The reason is that non-pulsatile flow results in greater stimulation of the aortic and carotid sinus pressor sensors resulting in greater release of endogenous catecholamines with deleterious effects on the microcirculation. During ECLS all of the management effort is placed on maintaining normal or excessive systemic oxygen delivery, therefore non-pulsatile perfusion does not have any deleterious effects. In

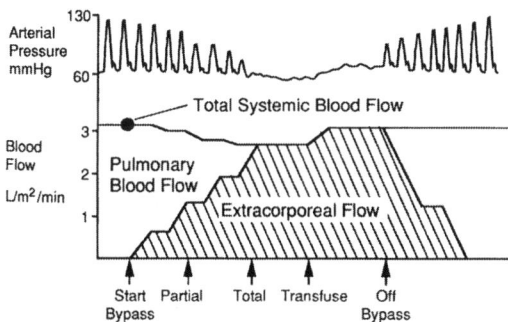

Figure 2-10. Systemic pressure, pulmonary artery flow, and total flow during partial and total venoarterial bypass.

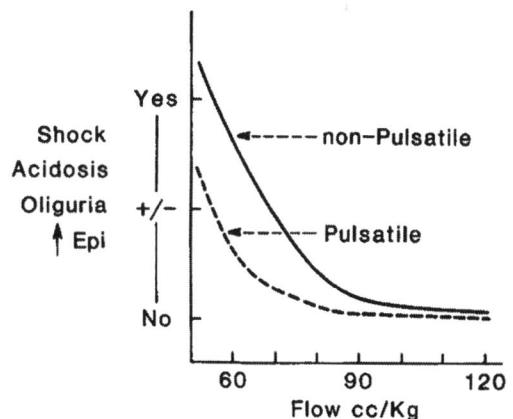

Figure 2-11. At normal total body blood flow over 90 cc/kg there is essentially no difference between pulsatile and nonpulsatile flow. At lower flows pulsatility minimizes the extent of shock, acidosis, and oliguria.

fact non-pulsatile perfusion can be maintained for months as long as total blood flow is adequate.[11,12] The kidney is the organ most sensitive to non-pulsatile flow, and the moderate anti-diuresis which occurs from non-pulsatile flow stimulating the juxtaglomerular apparatus can usually be overcome with small doses of diuretics.

Left Ventricle Function

As mentioned earlier in this discussion, draining blood from the left atrium and left ventricle is an essential part of cardiopulmonary bypass in the operating room. As long as the left ventricle is ejecting adequately, left-sided venting is not an issue during VA ECLS. If ECLS is being used for cardiac support, or if the preceding period of hypoxemia has resulted in myocardial stun with severe malfunction, the left side of the circulation can be become overdistended by bronchial and thebesian venous drainage directly into the left atrium and ventricle, resulting in cardiac damage and pulmonary edema. When this occurs (or more importantly before this occurs) some type of left side decompression must be instituted. To avoid LV distention it is important to maintain left ventricular function and ejection during partial

VA bypass. If myocardial failure does not allow ejection against the head of pressure generated by VA bypass, arterial resistance should be decreased by vasodilatation, or left-sided venting should be promptly undertaken. The left side can be vented by thoracotomy and direct cannulation of the left atrium or ventricle, or by transseptal atriotomy creating a small atrial septal defect in the catheterization laboratory. Another approach used in the laboratory by Kolobow is catheterization of the pulmonary artery by a small catheter to allow retrograde decompression into the right atrium.[13]

Hemodynamics with Venovenous Access

Venovenous bypass has no direct effect on hemodynamics, although the reduction in intrathoracic pressure from lowering positive-pressure ventilation after initiating VV ECMO may improve cardiac preload, reduce pulmonary vascular resistance, and improve right ventricular function. Blood is drained from and returned to the venous circulation at the same rate because the extracorporeal circuit is non-compliant. This is true whether venovenous bypass is achieved with two separate cannulas or with a single double lumen catheter.

Gas Exchange in Extracorporeal Life Support

Oxygen Delivery

During ECLS, oxygen delivery is controlled by the combination of blood oxygenation in the membrane lung, flow through the extracorporeal circuit, oxygen uptake through the native lung, and cardiac output through the native heart.

Blood oxygenation in the membrane lung is a function of the geometry, the thickness of the blood film, mixing created by secondary flows, the membrane material and thickness, the FiO_2, the residence time of red cells in the gas

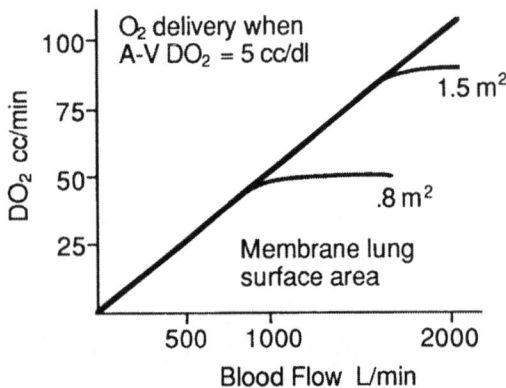

Figure 2-12. The concept of rated flow. Two oxygenators of different size and therefore different rated flow are compared. See the text for details.

exchange area, the hemoglobin concentration, and the inlet saturation (the latter two defining the oxygen uptake capacity of each deciliter of blood). All of these factors are included in a single descriptor of membrane lung function called "rated flow."[14] Rated flow is the amount of normal venous blood that can be raised from 75% to 95% oxyhemoglobin saturation in a given time period. This concept is illustrated in Figure 2-12. In this example, data for two membrane lungs are shown. The geometry of membrane Lung A is such that the rated flow is 1000 cc/min, corresponding to an actual oxygen transfer of 50 cc/min. The rated flow for Lung B is 1800 cc/min. We use this information to plan which membrane lung to use for ECLS, and to evaluate membrane lung performance during perfusion.

As long as the extracorporeal blood flow is less than the rated flow of the membrane lung and the venous saturation is 70%, the blood leaving the lung will be fully saturated and the amount of systemic oxygen delivery via the extracorporeal circuit will be controlled by blood flow and the oxygen uptake capacity. The amount of oxygen that can be taken up in each deciliter equals gmHb/dL x unsaturated fraction x 1.36 cc/gm. When the outlet blood is 100% saturated, the uptake capacity is the same as the A-VDO$_2$. If the hemoglobin concentration is low or the venous blood saturation is high, the amount of oxygen that can be taken up in the membrane lung is decreased. We can compensate for decreased oxygen-binding capacity by increasing blood flow. Conversely, we can achieve oxygen delivery at low blood flow by increasing oxygen-binding capacity, minimizing recirculation, and increasing hematocrit.

The resulting systemic PO$_2$ and systemic oxygen delivery are a function of oxygen delivery through the extracorporeal circuit and through the native heart and lung. In planning the size of the circuit and extracorporeal flow rate, it is assumed that there will be no gas exchange across the native lung. With this as-

sumption, in <u>venovenous bypass</u>, the arterial PO$_2$ and saturation will be identical to the values in the mixed venous (RV or PA) blood. Because of the nature of venovenous bypass, this saturation will never be higher than 95%, and typically will be closer to 80% saturation with a PO$_2$ of approximately 40 mmHG. Consequently, it is common for a patient on venovenous ECLS to be cyanotic and hypoxic. Systemic oxygen delivery is perfectly adequate as long as there is a compensatory increase in cardiac output. Improvement in native lung function results in increasing arterial oxygenation, and the amount of native lung function during VV bypass can be identified as the difference between venous to arterial saturation.

In <u>venoarterial bypass</u>, the interpretation of arterial blood gases is more complicated. The perfusate blood is typically 100% saturated with a PO$_2$ of 500 mmHg. When the lung is not functioning, the left ventricular ejected blood is identical to right atrial blood, typically with a saturation of 75% and a PO$_2$ of 35.

Oxygen supplied by the extracorporeal circuit

Membrane lung oxygenation is described in Figure 2-13. The amount of O$_2$ supplied to the

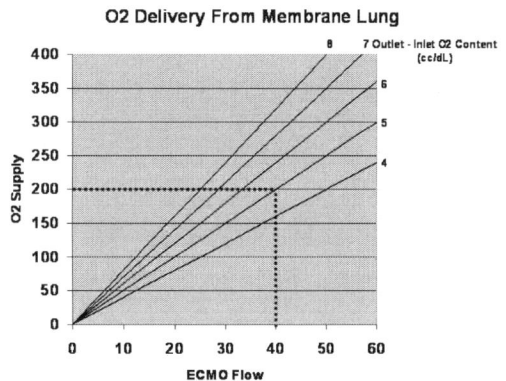

Figure 2-13. The amount of oxygen delivered from the membrane lung is calculated by subtracting the inlet oxygen content from the outlet oxygen content. These relationships over a range of outlet/inlet content differences and flows are shown in this nomogram.

patient by the extracorporeal circuit (ECC) is the membrane lung outlet-inlet O_2 content (cc/dL) times the flow in dL. For example, if the out-in O_2 content difference is 5 cc/dL and flow is 4 L/min, 200 cc of O_2 is supplied per minute (dotted line). If the patient's O_2 requirement is 220 cc/ min, circuit O_2 supply will be inadequate and SvO_2 will drop. When SvO_2 (i.e., the inlet saturation) drops at the same flow, the out-in content will increase (to 6 cc/cL for example) and O_2 supplied at 4 L/min is 250 cc/min. We can measure the mixed venous sat on VA and estimate it on VV.

Calculations based on mixing two flows

On ECMO we know the ECC flow, the saturation and content of the membrane lung inlet and outlet, and the arterial saturation and content. By measuring the saturation or content of the mixture of two blood flows with different saturations, if we know the flow and saturation of one, and if we know or estimate the saturation of the other, we can calculate that flow. In ECMO, part of the venous return is routed to the membrane lung and perfused into the patient. The remaining venous return

passes through the right atrium and mixes with the ECC perfusate flow in the right ventricle (in VV) or in the aorta (VA). The cardiac output is the sum of the two flows. These calculations use saturation, but O_2 content could be used (and is actually better). These calculations are presented in Figure 2-14 and incorporated into a nomogram in Figure 2-15.

CO_2 Removal

The amount of CO_2 eliminated in extracorporeal circulation is a function of membrane lung geometry, material, surface area, blood PCO_2, and, to a lesser extent, blood flow and membrane lung ventilating gas flow (commonly called "sweep" flow). The ventilating gas usually contains no CO_2, so the gradient for CO_2 transfer is the difference between the blood PCO_2 and zero (when the gas flow rate is high). As the PCO_2 drops during the passage of blood through the membrane lung, the gradient decreases, therefore CO_2 excretion is less at the blood outlet end of the device than at the inlet end. Consequently, the amount of CO_2 transfer is relatively independent of blood flow and only moderately dependent on inlet PCO_2,

Calculating cardiac output on ECMO
(mixing blood flow A and blood flowB
with same Hb but different O2Sat)

$$SO2_{A+B} = SO2_A \times \left[\frac{FlowA}{FlowA+B}\right] + SO2_B \times \left[\frac{FlowB}{FlowA+B}\right]$$

FlowA = ECC flow, FlowB= other venous return
Flow A + B = cardiac output

$$Y = a\left[\frac{Q}{x}\right] + b\left[\frac{x-Q}{x}\right] \quad xy = aQ + bx - bQ$$

$$x\ (y-b) = aQ - bQ$$

$$\text{Cardiac output} = \text{ECC Flow} \times \left[\frac{S_{ECC} - S_{venous}}{S_{arterial} - S_{venous}}\right]$$

Figure 2-14. During extracorporeal support blood from the circuit (A) is mixed with venous return blood which does not pass through the ECMO circuit (flow B). The total blood flow (cardiac output) is A+B. On ECMO we know the extracorporeal flow A, the saturation and content of the membrane lung inlet and outlet, and the arterial saturation and content. We can use this information to calculate the cardiac output using the saturation numbers in the equation described above.

with the major determinant of CO_2 elimination being total surface area and flow rate of the sweep gas. This is illustrated in Figure 2-9. Characteristics of removal of CO_2 for a typical membrane lung at different levels of PCO_2 are shown over a range of blood flows. Notice that the capacity for CO_2 removal is considerably greater than the capacity for oxygen uptake at the rated flow (see Figure 2-4). For any silicone rubber or microporous membrane oxygenator, CO_2 clearance will always be more efficient than oxygenation when the oxygenator is well ventilated and functioning properly.

The extracorporeal circuit is generally designed to supply total oxygen requirements. For this reason, the membrane lung will be capable of removing an excess of CO_2. Increasing sweep flow and the total surface area of the membrane lung in the extracorporeal circuit can selectively increase carbon dioxide transfer but not oxygen delivery

Following the rationale described above for oxygen delivery, assuming that there is no gas exchange across the native lung, the arterial PCO_2 will be the same as mixed venous PCO_2 in <u>venovenous</u> bypass; it will be a function of mixing perfusate and cardiac output blood in <u>venoarterial</u> bypass. However, because of the efficiency of extracorporeal CO_2 removal, the systemic PCO_2 can be "set" at any level by matching the membrane lung surface area and gas flow with systemic production of CO_2. In

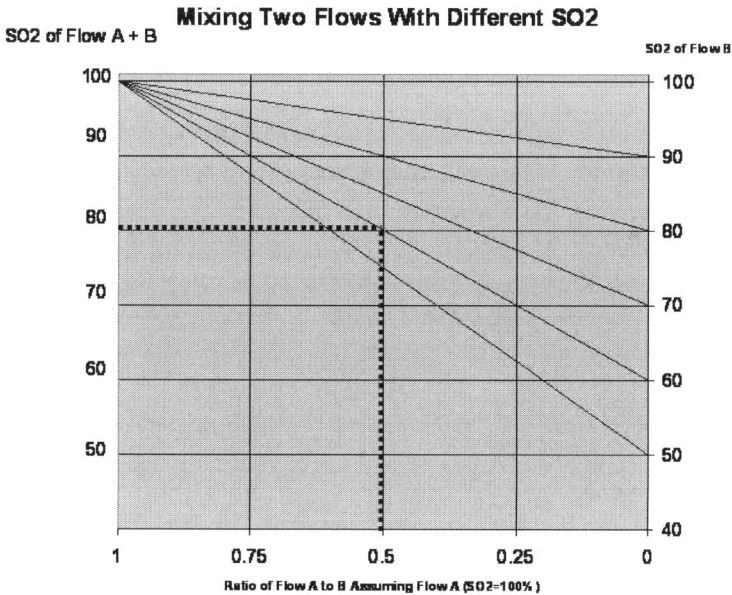

Figure 2-15. The calculations described in Figure 2.14 are combined into a nomogram in this figure. This assumes the saturation of blood leaving the membrane lung (flow A) is 100%. With that assumption this diagram allows determination of the ratio between the extracorporeal flow A and the unoxygenated venous return (flow B). If we know the patient arterial saturation (SO_2 of flow A + B), and we know the venous blood saturation (SO_2 of flow B) we can determine the ratio between flow A and flow B. Since we know flow A we can calculate flow B hence flow A + B. The saturation of venous return blood in venoarterial bypass is the same as the oxygenated inlet. In venovenous bypass the effective recirculation must be taken into account.

practice, the system is over-designed for CO_2 removal, and if bypass is run to supply total oxygen requirements, CO_2 removal will be excessive, resulting in significant respiratory alkalosis. This situation may be controlled by adding CO_2 to the sweep gas, thus decreasing the gradient and decreasing the amount of CO_2 transfer.

If the native lung can supply some oxygen absorption and the intent of extracorporeal circulation is primarily CO_2 removal, this can be accomplished with venovenous access and relatively low blood flow (ECCO$_2$R).[15]

Physiologic Principles in the Management of Extracorporeal Life Support

Based on an understanding of the physiology of extracorporeal circulation and of the pathophysiology of the patient's primary disease, it is obvious that the goal of extracorporeal life support is to maintain systemic oxygen delivery and CO_2 removal in the proper proportion to systemic metabolism. This is achieved at low ventilator or inotropic drug settings which could not otherwise be tolerated. This process should eliminate any further ventilator-induced lung injury and improve systemic perfusion, allowing time for the native lung or heart to recover from the acute illness.

Planning and Priming the Circuit

Although total support may never be necessary, the circuit must be planned with total support in mind. The tubing, connectors, and pump must be capable of adequate blood flow (typically 100 cc/kg/min for newborn infants, 75 cc/kg/min for children, and 50 cc/kg/min for adults). If venovenous access is used for respiratory support, these estimates of blood flow should be increased by 20%, since higher blood flow will be required for adequate oxygenation because of recirculation. The venous access catheter should be large enough to deliver this amount of blood flow at 100 cm of siphon, and the arterial or reinfusion catheter should be large enough to permit this level of blood flow at line pressures less than 300 mmHg proximal to the membrane lung. The membrane lung must have a rated flow higher than the maximal anticipated blood flow. Membrane lungs made from microporous materials are more efficient than the solid silicone rubber membrane lung, easier to prime, easier to manufacture, and have lower bedside pressure drop. The disadvantage to microporous membrane lungs is that plasma leakage can occur through the micropores in unpredictable fashion. This problem is addressed by coating the fibers with a very thin skin of gas permeable membrane (so called "solid" hollow fibers). This prevents plasma leakage, but there are still micro holes which can entrain air if the blood side pressure is less than ambient pressure. Various types of membrane lungs and their function are discussed in detail in the chapter on devices.

Once the circuit components have been selected and assembled in sterile fashion, the system is ready for priming. The system can be filled with CO_2 gas to displace any nitrogen which would form bubbles. Then a saline clear prime is used to displace the CO_2. The system is de-bubbled during circulation through a priming reservoir. A small amount of albumin can be added to decrease subsequent fibrinogen adsorption during initial blood exposure. In newborn infants this clear prime is usually displaced with one adult unit of packed red blood cells to maintain the hematocrit in the normal range during the initiation of ECLS. The blood is recirculated through the priming reservoir until the temperature is 37° C and the electrolytes and blood gases are near normal. Then the circuit is ready for connection to the patient. In older children and adults (and, in fact, in neonates in emergency circumstances) ECLS is usually initiated with a clear crystalloid and albumin prime. Once this solution is evenly mixed with the patient's blood, significant dilution of platelets, proteins, and red cells invariably occurs. Red cell transfusion is necessary to return the hematocrit to normal levels. It is important to be sure that the ionized calcium in the prime is the normal range,[16] otherwise acute severe myocardial depression and even cardiac arrest can follow the initiation of ECLS.

Cannulation

Cannulas are selected based on the size required for total support. If the vessels are not large enough to accommodate the cannulas, two venous or arterial cannulation sites may be required.

If venovenous access is used for respiratory support, perfusate blood is returned to a second vein or a double-lumen cannula. The femoral vein and a jugular vein are catheterized for 2-vein VV access. In 2-vein cannulation, recirculation is minimized when drainage is from the inferior vena cava and reinfusion is into the right atrium.[17] Double-lumen cannulas have more recirculation and the infusion lumen is small, requiring high pressure at high flow. The advantage is that only one vein is used for cannulation.[18]

When femoral VA access is used for cardiac support, infusion blood mixes with left ventricular outlet blood in the aorta. If the native lungs are failing, LV outflow blood is poorly oxygenated, resulting in differential flow with poor oxygenation to the head and good oxygenation to the feet (often called the Harlequin syndrome). The management of this situation is discussed in chapter 21.

Monitoring

ECLS requires several monitors in addition to patient vital signs, blood gases, and ventilator settings. Blood flow is monitored continuously with a flow meter or by counting rotations per minute on the roller pump. Although routinely used, this method of measuring flow can be grossly in error if the rollers are not occlusive or if the tubing is not round. Pressure should be monitored on the arterial side of the circuit, preferably before the membrane lung. An increasing pressure gradient across the membrane lung suggests thrombosis. The expected post-oxygenator pressure should be predicted for any given flow based on the M number of the return cannula. If the pressures are higher than expected, the arterial line or cannula is kinked or occluded. The most important parameter is continuous monitoring of mixed venous saturation. This can be measured by placing an Oximetrix® fiberoptic catheter through a Touhy Borst adapter into the venous line, or by a direct monitor on the line. Since venous drainage blood represents a mixture of blood from the superior vena cava, the inferior vena cava, and the coronary sinus, the SvO_2 is an accurate representation of the DO_2:VO_2 ratio during venoarterial bypass. With VA access, as long as the SvO_2 is in the range of 75% and all aspects of perfusion are going well, it is not necessary to measure systemic or circuit blood gases more frequently than approximately every 12 hours. If the system includes a transcutaneous oximeter and an on-line pCO_2 monitor, sampling of blood for gas analysis is rarely necessary. During venovenous bypass, the mixed venous saturation can be elevated because of recirculation. When SvO_2 is combined with transcutaneous oximetry in a patient on VV bypass, the adequacy of extracorporeal support and the amount of lung function can be assessed simultaneously. Measurement of end tidal CO_2 at the airway is another helpful monitor of native lung function. During the early days of an ECLS run, end tidal CO_2 may be 5 mmHg or less. As functioning lung units resume ventilation or as pulmonary blood flow to ventilated units increases, end tidal CO_2 will increase. When end tidal CO_2 is near normal (over 35 mmHg), a trial of weaning should be considered.

Managing the Patient on ECLS

The blood flow is set at a level that will provide total O_2 and CO_2 exchange, and mechanical ventilation is reduced to minimal or lung rest settings. Patient arterial blood gases are checked and continuous monitors are calibrated. Thereafter, venous saturation is maintained at the desired level by increasing or decreasing extracorporeal blood flow. $PaCO_2$ is maintained at about 40 mmHg by adjusting the flow rate and composition of sweep gas. Systemic blood pressure is maintained at the desired level by adjusting blood volume.

During ECLS, hemoglobin is maintained between 14 and 15 gm%. We are in an era when many intensivists consider the risks of blood transfusion to be greater than the risks of profound anemia. Equally compelling is the argument that the risks of physiologic and pharmacologic compensation for anemia are greater than the risks of transfusion. In ECLS there is no argument. The system depends on oxygen delivery determined by flow through the artificial lung. If the blood is anemic, higher flow is required to achieve the desired level of oxygen delivery. Since flow is limited by the resistance in the venous cannula, excessive suction may be required to increase flow, or an additional venous cannula may be required. Higher pump speed causes more damage to the cells and platelets, and increases the risk of blow out. Flow also depends on blood volume; to achieve higher blood volume and increase flow, there is a tendency to give more clear fluid which contributes to anemia and systemic edema. Even one of these risks is much greater than the hazards of transfusion, so proper use of the artificial lung mandates a normal hemoglobin level (14 to 15 gm%).

Platelet count is maintained at greater than 75,000 x10^9/L and activated clotting time is maintained no higher than 200 seconds. A major decrease in venous saturation with no change in the other settings is usually caused by an increase in metabolic rate, which may be transient (during crying or seizures) or sustained. A sustained increase in metabolic rate can be matched by an increase in blood flow or can be treated with sedation, paralysis, and/or hypothermia. A major increase in venous saturation with no change in other settings is usually caused by a decrease in metabolic rate or the onset of native lung function. Hypovolemia, catheter kinking or malposition, pneumothorax, or pericardial tamponade may cause a sudden decrease in venous drainage. A gradual decrease in systemic oxygenation or an increase in $PaCO_2$ may be a sign of deteriorating membrane lung function. Membrane lung function is assessed by measuring oxygen and CO_2 transfer and comparing the results to the expected transfer at that level of blood flow and CO_2 gradient. If the membrane lung is deteriorating, a new lung should be inserted. This is rarely necessary.

The Native Lung During ECLS

When ECLS is used solely for cardiac support, the lung may remain in normal condition throughout the time on bypass, including x-ray appearance and physiologic function. Since cardiac support always involves VA bypass, this normal native lung function is masked by a very extensive ventilation-perfusion mismatch in which low-normal levels of ventilation are grossly excessive compared to the amount of blood actually flowing through the pulmonary capillaries. This gives the impression of huge dead space ventilation which is reflected in low end tidal CO_2. If this VQ mismatch is treated by decreasing mechanical ventilation to very low levels of pressure then eventually alveolar collapse may occur. For this reason it is best to maintain the end expiratory pressure at 10-15 cmH$_2$O throughout VA ECLS for cardiac support, carefully limiting inspiratory plateau airway pressure to <30 cmH$_2$O. This may result in small tidal volumes which can be maintained at a low ventilatory rate. Even with these settings, excess CO_2 elimination may occur, and it is often necessary to incorporate carbon dioxide into the sweep gas during VA bypass when lung function is normal. The ideal approach is to extubate the patient and encourage spontaneous breathing by keeping the membrane lung outlet PCO_2 around 40. The fact that lung appearance and function remain normal during VA bypass for cardiac support is ample evidence that there is little or no direct effect of ECLS on lung capillary permeability or lung function.

However, there is usually some degree of lung abnormality and respiratory failure, ranging from mild cardiogenic pulmonary edema when ECLS is used for cardiac support to total and severe lung dysfunction when ECLS is used for respiratory support. In this situation, as soon as the preexisting high airway pressure is decreased, the small airways and alveoli that were held open by excessive distending pressures often collapse, leading to the x-ray picture of major consolidation and congestion ("white out"), and the physiologic picture of little or no gas exchange through the native lung. This is true on both venovenous and venoarterial modes of support. This period of no native lung function makes the patient entirely dependent on the extracorporeal circuit, and this is a precarious time during management of ECLS. If ECLS is discontinued, even for a minute to two, profound hypoxemia and cardiac arrest result. For this reason a set of backup ventilator settings is posted to be used in the event that ECLS is interrupted. Typically these settings are 100% oxygen, peak airway pressure 40 cmH_2O, PEEP 10 cmH_2O, rate 20-30. However, if the lung is totally consolidated, no amount of air delivered into the airway will recruit lung fast enough to sustain life in this phase, so great attention is devoted to avoiding this possible complication. One way of minimizing the total consolidation is to maintain mean airway pressure in the range of 10-20 cmH_2O. This approach, originally proposed for neonates by Keszler,[19] minimizes the risk of total consolidation, improves the safety

factor during the early days of ECLS, and appears to shorten the entire course on ECLS in newborn infants. Conventional methods of managing the severely injured lung including prone positioning, postural drainage, maintenance at dry weight, full nutrition, and bronchoscopy as needed are continued in the ECLS patient.

Pulmonary vascular resistance is an important indicator of the prognosis for lung recovery. Even though hypoxic vasoconstriction is at its maximum in the totally consolidated lung, pulmonary vascular resistance is only slightly elevated. Of course this is only significant during venovenous bypass because the full cardiac output is passing through the pulmonary circulation as well as the systemic circulation. For this reason, even if cardiac output is not directly measured, a comparison of mean systemic artery pressure to mean pulmonary artery pressure affords a direct comparison of the relationship between systemic and pulmonary vascular resistance. Normally the systemic vascular resistance is 25 $mmHg/L/m^2$ and the normal pulmonary vascular resistance is 3 $mmHg/L/m^2$ (corresponding to a mean pulmonary artery pressure 20 mmHg, wedge pressure 10 mmHg, and cardiac index 3 $L/m^2/min$). During total lung consolidation the pulmonary artery pressure may rise from 3-6 Wood units (mean PAP as high as 30) and may be sustained at this level for several days. If progressive lung destruction and fibrosis occurs, eventually this fibrosis obliterates the pulmonary capillary bed and pulmonary vascular resistance rises to systemic levels. When this occurs, right ventricular failure occurs and it is virtually impossible to resuscitate the heart in these circumstances, even on full venovenous bypass. For all these reasons, following the ratio between pulmonary and systemic mean blood pressure during ECLS has become a very valuable indicator of the likelihood of lung recovery.

During prolonged uncomplicated ECLS, function of other vital organs is maintained at normal levels. Specifically kidney, liver, host defenses, brain, and gut functions are normal as long as the primary disease does not affect physiology of these organs. Function of these organs, and changes associated with disease and with ECLS are discussed in detail in other chapters in this book.

Weaning and Decannulation

Indicators of lung recovery include increasing PaO_2 or decreasing $PaCO_2$ without changing ventilator or ECLS settings, increased VO_2 or VCO_2 measured via the airway, increasing compliance, and a clearing chest x-ray. Indicators of cardiac recovery include increasing SvO_2 with no change in VO_2 or other parameters, increasing pulse contour, and improving contractility detected by echocardiography.

When native lung or cardiac function improves, extracorporeal flow is gradually decreased, allowing the native lung to carry more of the load. When 70 to 80% of the gas exchange is occurring via the native lung (i.e., the extracorporeal flow rate is 20 to 30% of the initial flow rate), the patient should be tried off bypass at moderate ventilator settings. In veno-arterial bypass the tubing leading to the patient is clamped, permitting continuing circulation through a bridge. If gas exchange and perfusion are adequate, the catheters can be removed, usually after another period of low flow bypass, to be sure that lung function will be maintained. In venovenous bypass, a trial off bypass consists of capping off gas flow to the membrane lung but continuing extracorporeal flow. With this arrangement, the venous saturation monitor becomes a useful guide to the adequacy of systemic oxygen delivery during the trial.

Using these simple physiologic principles of management, extracorporeal circulation can be maintained in the absence of pulmonary function for weeks.

References

1. Bartlett, RH: "Physiology of Extracorporeal Life Support", in: ECMO: Extracorporeal Cardiopulmonary Support in Critical Care, Second edition, JB Zwischenberger et al,editors. Extracorporeal Life Support Organization, 41-66, 2000.
2. Bartlett RH. Physiology of ECLS. Chapter 2 in ECMO: Extracorporeal Cardiopulmonary Support in Critical Care, Third edition, van Meurs K et al, editors. Extracorporeal Life Support Organization, 5-27, 2005.
3. Bartlett RH. Critical Care Physiology. University of Michigan Faculty Reprint Series. Scholarly Publications Office Ann Arbor, Mi 2010.www.lib.umich.edu/mpublishing.
4. Zwischenberger JB, Alpard SK, Conrad SA, Johnigan RH, Bidani A. Arteriovenous carbon dioxide removal: development and impact on ventilator management and survival during severe respiratory failure. Perfusion 14:299-310, 1999.
5. Bartlett RH and Delius RE: "Physiology and Pathophysiology of Extracorporeal Circulation," In: 3rd Edition of Techniques in Extracorporeal Circulation, Kay (editor), Butterworths, London, 8-32, 1992.
6. Montoya JP, Merz SI, Bartlett RH. A standardized system for describing flow/pressure relationships in vascular access devices. Trans ASAIO 37:4-8, 1991.
7. Delius RE, Montoya JP, Merz SI, McKenzie J, Snedecor S, Bove EL, Bartlett RH: A new method for describing the performance of cardiac surgery cannulas. Ann Thorac Surg 53:278-81, 1992.
8. Tamari Y, Lee-Sensiba K, Leonard EF, et al: The effects of pressure and flow on hemolysis caused by Bio-Medicus centrifugal pumps and roller pumps. Guidelines for choosing a blood pump. J Thor Cardiovasc Surg 106:997-1007, 1993.
9. Pedersen TH, Videm V, Svenning JL, et al. Extracorporeal membrane oxygenation

using a centrifugal pump and a servo regulator to prevent negative inlet pressure. Ann Thoracic Surgery 63:1330-1338, 1997.

10. Tominaga R, Smith WA, Massiello A, et al: Chronic non-pulsatile blood flow. J Thorac Cardiovasc Surg 108:907-12, 1994.

11. Bernstein EF, Cosentino LC, Reich S, et al: A compact low hemolysis non-thrombogenic system for nonthoracotomy prolonged left ventricular bypass. Trans ASAIO 20:643, 1974.

12. Golding LAR, Murakami H, Harasaki H, et al: Chronic non-pulsatile blood flow. ASAIO J 28:81-85, 1982.

13. Kolobow T, Rossi F, Borellim M, Foti G. Long term closed chest partial and total cardiopulmonary bypass by peripheral cannulation for severe right and/or left ventricular failure including ventricular fibrillation. Trans ASAIO 34:485-489, 1988.

14. Galletti PM, Richardson PD, Snider MT. A standardized method for defining the overall gas transfer performance of artificial lungs. Trans ASAIO 18:359, 1972.

15. Pesenti A, Gattinoni L, Kolobow T, Damia G. Extracorporeal circulation in adult respiratory failure. Trans ASAIO 34:43-47, 1988.

16. Melliones JN, Moler FW, Custer JR, et al: Hemodynamic instability after the initiation of extracorporeal membrane oxygenation: Role of ionized calcium. Crit. Care Med 19:1247-1251, 1991.

17. Rich PB, Awad SS, Crotti S, Hirschl RB, Bartlett RH, Schreiner RJ: A prospective comparison of atrio-femoral and femoro-atrial flow in adult veno-venous extracorporeal life support. J Thorac Cardiovasc Surg 116:628-32, 1998.

18. Wang D, Zhou X, Liu X, Sidor B, Lynch J, Zwischenberger JB. Wang-Zwische double lumen cannula-toward a percutaneous and ambulatory paracorporeal artificial lung. ASAIO J. Nov-Dec;54(6):606-11, 2008.

19. Keszler M, Subramanian KNS, Smith YA, et al: Pulmonary management during extracorporeal membrane oxygenation. Crit Care Med. 17:495-500, 1989.

3

Cardiac Failure: Principles and Physiology

Ravi R. Thiagarajan MBBS MPH, Vamsi Yarlagadda MD, Susan L. Bratton MD MPH

Introduction

Cardiac failure occurs when the cardiovascular system is unable to provide the oxygen and nutrients required to meet the metabolic needs of the tissues.[1,2] Congestive heart failure, a clinical manifestation of cardiac dysfunction, is one of the leading causes of hospital admission, resource use, and health care expenditure in adult patients with heart disease. Causes of congestive heart failure include diseases that: 1) decrease systolic myocardial contractility (e.g., myocarditis or ischemic heart disease) or create diastolic dysfunction of the heart, 2) increase volume load to the heart (e.g., congenital heart disease resulting in a large left to right shunt), 3) increase pressure load to the heart (e.g., severe aortic stenosis), and 4) vascular disease in the systemic or pulmonary vascular beds that increase the resistive workload to the heart.[1] Many compensatory mechanisms in the human body exist that help maintain cardiac output when myocardial diseases result in decreased myocardial function. When these compensatory mechanisms are overcome and cardiac output and organ perfusion can no longer be maintained, decompensated cardiac failure clinically recognized as cardiogenic shock occurs. Cardiogenic shock is a common indication for admission to the intensive care unit for both adults and children.

When conventional medical or surgical supportive measures fail to improve cardiac function the use of mechanical circulatory support is a final option. Extracorporeal membrane oxygenation (ECMO) has been used to support cardiovascular and respiratory function in adults and children with shock unresponsive to conventional medical therapies for treatment of shock. A knowledge of the physiological mechanisms underlying acute and chronic cardiovascular dysfunction are essential to the successful management of patients with cardiovascular dysfunction especially those needing mechanical circulatory support with ECMO. This chapter describes the physiology of cardiac failure, the body's compensatory mechanisms, and the physiological principles necessary for management of patients with cardiac failure requiring ECMO.

Determinants of cardiac output

Cardiac output is determined by both myocardial and vascular function.[1,2] Blood pressure is a crude and insensitive indicator but frequently used to assess cardiac function. Determinants of cardiac output can be stated as:

Cardiac output = Stroke volume x Heart Rate.

Cardiac output can be augmented by increase in either Stroke Volume (SV) and/or heart rate. In neonates stroke volume is relatively fixed, and changes in cardiac output are primarily caused by changes in heart rate. The determinants of SV are complex as it is determined by preload and afterload conditions imposed on the ventricle, and the contractile function of the myocardium. We will briefly review the role of preload, afterload, and contractile function as determinants of stroke volume. For the purpose of this discussion, we will consider the ventricle as a single unit with an inflow and outflow rather than consider the combination of the right and left ventricle with their associated interactions.

Preload

Preload is the same as the end diastolic ventricular volume (EDV). When the EDV is increased, stroke volume (SV) and the pressure generated by the ventricle increases. This is because increasing diastolic muscle stretch by EDV results in increased force of myocardial contraction (Frank-Starling's law).[1-3] The relationship of EDV and SV is linear. However the more easily measured surrogate of EDV, end-diastolic pressure (EDP), does not increase in linear fashion when EDV increases because EDP for any given EDV is determined by the compliance of the ventricle. In myocardial disease, ventricular compliance is often decreased, and EDP is higher for a given EDV. Furthermore, SV may not increase after an incremental increase in EDP and may actually decrease because the increase in EDP decreases preload by decreasing venous return and myocardial contractility as explained below.

Venous return to the heart is determined by circulating blood volume, the pressure in the venous system (mean systemic filling pressure), and the downstream or atrial pressure as shown below:

Venous return = Mean systemic venous pressure – Atrial pressure

An increase in atrial pressure can decrease venous return to the heart by decreasing this pressure gradient. The atrial pressure is generally the same as ventricular EDP in the absence of atrio-ventricular valve obstruction. When contractility remains constant, preload augmentation from volume administration, increases venous return by increasing mean systemic venous pressure, resulting in increased EDV, SV, and cardiac output. However, the increase in EDV may also result in increased EDP. As previously stated, EDP for a given EDV is determined by ventricular compliance. Thus, if the ventricle is non-compliant, as is frequent in myocardial disease, then increased volume results in an exaggerated increase in EDP. Increased EDP along with a decrease in venous return can decrease coronary perfusion pressure (arterial diastolic pressure–EDP) leading to myocardial ischemia and loss of myocardial contractility. Together these factors can explain the deterioration in myocardial contractility and decreased cardiac output with increasing EDP. Although preload or venous return augment stroke volume and cardiac output in the heart with normal contractile function, the effect of preload augmentation on stroke volume and cardiac output in cardiac failure may be blunted, and in some instances can be dangerous.

Afterload

Afterload is the workload imposed by any factor that resists ejection of blood from the ventricle.[1] Several factors determine afterload: 1) vascular impedance and ejection pressure which are determined by the elastance of the great vessels and resistance imposed by the smaller vessels, 2) wall stress applied to the ventricle, and 3) inertia or mass of blood within the ventricle. Both vascular resistance and wall stress play major roles in determining ventricular afterload. The concept of wall stress as explained by Laplace's law is shown below:

Wall stress = (pressure x radius)/2 x thickness

Pressure, is the transmural (TM) pressure applied to the ventricle and is determined by intraluminal (EDP) and extraluminal (pericardial or intra-thoracic) pressure as shown below:

TM = Intraluminal – Extraluminal Pressure.

During inspiration, extraluminal pressure decreases and afterload increases by increase in TM pressure. Use of positive end-expiratory pressure (PEEP) increases extraluminal pressure and decreases wall stress and afterload to the ventricle by decreasing TM pressure. The radius of the ventricle may be increased by increased end-diastolic volume resulting in increased wall stress to the heart. Increased wall stress may result in decreased contractility by increasing the myocardial oxygen demand as well as decreasing coronary blood flow.

When afterload is increased pressure generated (force of contractility) has to increase to maintain flow. The relationship between resistance and flow is shown by below (Ohm's law):

Resistance = Perfusion Pressure x Flow

In other words, the effect of increased afterload to the ventricle results in the need for increased systolic pressure generation for aortic valve opening to maintain cardiac output. Thus the force of myocardial contraction has to increase to maintain stroke volume and cardiac output. When the heart function is normal, increases in contractility can often compensate for increased afterload, thus maintaining stroke volume and cardiac output. However, the effect of increased afterload on diseased myocardium with poor contractile function is a further decrease in stroke volume and cardiac output. Thus increased systemic vascular resistance mediated by the endothelium, baroreceptors, and many humoral agents in response to low cardiac output in patients with cardiac failure as a compensatory mechanism to preserve vital organ (brain, kidneys, heart) blood flow and

perfusion may increase the resistive workload of the heart. Although important for survival, increased afterload from vasoconstriction is eventually detrimental to cardiac function and recovery, and thus modification of vasomotor tone is an important component of therapeutic management of cardiac failure.

Contractility

The contractile function of the heart is determined by preload, afterload, and contractile health of the myocardium. Changes in preload and afterload may lead to changes in myocardial contractility to cause changes in cardiac output. Changes in preload are thought to alter cardiac output more than do changes in afterload.

Compensated and Decompensated Cardiac Failure

Several compensatory mechanisms present in the cardiovascular system are acutely triggered to restore cardiac output when it is decreased as a result of diminished ventricular function. When ventricular function decreases, stroke volume for a given preload decreases.[1,2] Cardiac output is maintained by an increase in heart rate. As cardiac failure progresses, sympathetic stimulation results in release of adrenomedullary catecholamines, aldosterone production, renin-angiotensin, and vasopressin release that result in salt and water retention, and arteriolar vasoconstriction. Salt and water retention increases preload and venous return. Vasoconstriction can also cause preload augmentation by increasing mean systemic venous pressure. Vasoconstriction also results in preservation of end-organ function by redirecting blood flow away from the skin and muscle towards vital organs such as the brain, heart, and kidney as previously stated, although important for preservation of vital organ function and survival, vasoconstriction increases the resistive workload posed to the heart, eventually impeding cardiac output and function. Furthermore, increased mean systemic venous pressure from salt and water retention can result in transudation of fluid from the vein into the tissue causing edema, and decreased arteriovenous (AV) pressure gradients across organ beds from increased means systemic venous pressure can decrease end-organ perfusion and result in end-organ ischemia and decreased function.

If the patient remains compensated, myocardial hypertrophy can occur to augment cardiac output and decrease wall stress. However, because myocardial blood flow is not increased, ischemia and loss of contractility ensue. Chronic sympathetic stimulation results in decreased myocardial response to catecholamines by down regulation and desensitization of beta-receptors. Patients with compensated cardiac failure may be fully compensated at rest but remain intolerant to exercise or illness because of their inability to increase cardiac output to meet the increased demands for oxygen delivery.

When the compensatory mechanisms fail, inadequate delivery of oxygen and nutrients to tissues and organs causes decompensated heart failure and shock. If the cardiovascular system remains unsupported, metabolic acidosis, end-organ dysfunction and death may result. Management of cardiac failure and shock includes augmentation of myocardial performance by administration of inotropes for contractility, diuresis to remove excess fluid overload, afterload reduction to enhance myocardial performance, and correction of conditions exacerbating cardiac failure. Mechanical circulatory assistance with ECMO or ventricular assist devices (VAD) may be required when other supportive therapies fail to palliate cardiovascular function.

Cardiac Function on ECMO

The use of ECMO to support the circulation in patients with cardiac failure may help restore end-organ perfusion and provide myocardial rest.[4] For purposes of this discussion, we will consider both the right and the left heart together and support with venoarterial (VA) ECMO. Drainage of blood from the circulation into the ECMO circuit results in decreased right atrial (RA) and central venous pressure (CVP). As a result, decreased right ventricular (RV) ejection into the lungs decreases pulmonary venous return to the left atrium (LA) and can decrease left ventricular (LV) EDV and EDP. This "unloading" of the LV provides myocardial rest and the decrease in LVEDP may promote coronary blood flow to the myocardium and thus recovery. Return of blood into the aorta in VA ECMO can raise systolic and diastolic blood pressure and improve both end-organ and coronary perfusion. Decreased preload to the LV and RV decreases contractile function of both ventricles and reduces stroke volume because of decreased EDV and EDP.[5]

Animal experiments have shown that decreases in cardiac contractility during VA ECMO are primarily due to decreased preload and not to loss of intrinsic myocardial contractile function.[6] Similarly observation of cardiac performance in infants with persistent pulmonary hypertension of the newborn (PPHN) with normal pre-ECMO cardiac function have shown that decrease in contractility and ejection fraction during VA ECMO in these infants was due to decrease in preload rather than myocardial dysfunction.[5] The load dependent decrease in ventricular contractile function is transient, and return of myocardial contractile function is usual within 72 hours after onset on VA ECMO. Similar observational studies have not been conducted in patients with cardiac failure to clearly understand the effects of ventricular unloading on the contractile function of the ventricle. We can speculate that a similar decrease in contractility with unloading the ventricle occurs in patients with cardiac failure at the onset of ECMO, and that the decrease in contractility may occur at lower ECMO flow rates (i.e., higher EDV and EDP) because of the dependence of the diseased myocardium on higher preload for contractility. The flipside is that we can speculate a decrease in EDP and EDV may improve coronary perfusion, decrease excessive myocardial stretch, and the decrease in work load posed to the ventricle may promote myocardial performance and contractility. It is possible these effects vary among patients supported with ECMO for cardiac failure based on the severity of myocardial disease. Furthermore, reduction of central venous pressure by drainage of blood into the ECMO circuit reduces venous pressure and improves end-organ perfusion and function by increasing the arteriovenous gradient encouraging blood flow and perfusion into end-organs. Interpretation of myocardial contractility for patients supported with ECMO should take into account preload conditions at which time the data is obtained because contractility can be altered by filling conditions making assessment of cardiac function error prone. Finally, return of arterial pulsation (or contractile function) during ECMO support for patients supported for cardiac failure is a sign of myocardial recovery and the timing of such recovery has been shown to be associated with survival.[7]

Afterload to the heart is increased in patients supported with VA ECMO from many causes including vasoconstriction from compensatory sympathetic activated to preserve cardiac output because of decreased cardiac output from cardiac failure prior to onset of ECMO and increased mean arterial pressure due to blood flow into to the aorta from the arterial limb of the ECMO circuit.[4] The increase in mean arterial blood pressure increases the ejection pressure needed for aortic valve opening. If the systolic pressure generated by the left ventricle (LV) is inadequate to open the aortic valve, loss of native ejection occurs, arterial pulsations decrease, and retention of blood in the LV will result in increased LV EDV and EDP. In addition, return of blood flow from the bronchial circulation to the left atrium and LV may further increase left ventricular EDV and EDP. These effects combine to cause LV dilation, increased LV EDP and left atrial hypertension. The increased LV EDP can compromise coronary blood flow, cause ischemia, and impair myocardial recovery. Furthermore, left atrial hypertension can cause pulmonary edema, pulmonary hemorrhage, and impair gas exchange in the lungs. Left atrial hypertension must be relieved expeditiously by left heart decompression achieved either by surgical or trans-catheter decompression of the left atrium.

Martin et al. have shown that infants with PPHN and normal cardiac function supported with VA ECMO, have decrease in contractile function related to decreased preload rather than increase afterload.[8] Similar published reports describing the influence of afterload on myocardial contractility in patients receiving VA ECMO support with cardiac failure are not available. Hence the importance of afterload on the failing heart supported with VA ECMO is not known. However, reducing afterload during VA ECMO support in patients with myocardial dysfunction may promote LV ejection that can reduce LVEDP and relief from the deleterious effects of LA hypertension and can reduce the compensatory pre-ECMO cardiac failure mediated vasoconstriction decreasing the resistive workload of the ventricle that may promote myocardial recovery and weaning.

When LV function is not severely compromised in patients supported with ECMO, coronary blood flow is primarily from native cardiac output ejected from the LV. Animal studies show that during VA ECMO, hypoxemic cardiac output (partial pressure of oxygen $25 - 40$ mmHg) is associated with decreased LV function.[9] Thus in patients with preserved ventricular ejection, it is important to oxygenate blood ejected to the lungs and returning to the left side by provision of adequate ventilation to preserve myocardial oxygenation and function.

Summary

VA ECMO in patients with decompensated heart failure can help "unload" the left ventricle, promote coronary blood flow, decrease myocardial stretch, and promote myocardial recovery. Decrease in preload during VA ECMO is primarily responsible for a transient decrease in myocardial function. Although afterload is increased, it is not thought to affect myocardial performance, however it may be important to decrease afterload in patients with cardiac failure supported on ECMO to decrease resistive workload on the myocardium to facilitate recovery and weaning from ECMO. The load dependent decrease in contractility is often transient and recovery of myocardial function is seen in most instances. Interpretation of studies aimed at assessing contractile function of the heart for patients supported with ECMO should take into account the preload conditions at the time of data collection.

References

1. Epstein D, Wetzel RC. Cardiovascular Physiology and Shock. In: Nichols DG, Ungerleider RM, Spevak PJ, Greeley W, J., Cameron DE, Lappe DG, Wetzel RC, eds. Critical Heart Disease in Infants and Children. Second ed. Philadelphia, Pa: Mosby; 2006:17 - 72.

2. Guyton AC, Hall JE. Cardiac Failure. Textbook of Medical Physiology. Eleventh ed. Philadephia, PA: Elsevier Inc; 2006:258 - 265.

3. Guyton AC, Hall JE. Heart Muscle; The Heart as a Pump and Function of the Heart Valves. Textbook of Medical Physiology. Eleventh ed. Philadelphia, PA: Elsevier Inc; 2006:103 - 114.

4. Fuhrman BP, Hernan LJ, Rotta AT, Heard CM, Rosenkranz ER. Pathophysiology of cardiac extracorporeal membrane oxygenation. Artif Organs. 1999;23(11):966-969.

5. Martin GR, Short BL. Doppler echocardiographic evaluation of cardiac performance in infants on prolonged extracorporeal membrane oxygenation. Am J Cardiol. 1988;62(13):929-934.

6. Shen I, Levy FH, Vocelka CR, O'Rourke PP, Duncan BW, Thomas R, Verrier ED. Effect of extracorporeal membrane oxygenation on left ventricular function of swine. Ann Thorac Surg. 2001;71(3):862-867.

7. Duncan BW, Hraska V, Jonas RA, Wessel DL, Del Nido PJ, Laussen PC, Mayer JE, Lapierre RA, Wilson JM. Mechanical circulatory support in children with cardiac disease. J Thorac Cardiovasc Surg. 1999;117(3):529-542.

8. Martin GR, Chauvin L, Short BL. Effects of hydralazine on cardiac performance in infants receiving extracorporeal membrane oxygenation. J Pediatr. 1991;118(6):944-948.

9. Shen I, Levy FH, Benak AM, Rothnie CL, O'Rourke PP, Duncan BW, Verrier ED. Left ventricular dysfunction during extracorporeal membrane oxygenation in a hypoxemic swine model. Ann Thorac Surg. 2001;71(3):868-871.

4

Acute Hypoxic Respiratory Failure in Children

Desmond Bohn MB FRCPC

Introduction

The management of acute respiratory failure has changed radically since mechanically assisted ventilation using negative pressure was first introduced in the 1930s. Although these devices were remarkably effective in the treatment of diseases associated with weakness or paralysis of the respiratory muscles (pump failure), they were not effective in diseases involving the pulmonary parenchyma (lung failure). The demonstration that positive pressure ventilation was effective for the treatment of acute respiratory failure was first demonstrated 40 years ago during the poliomyelitis epidemic in Europe and Scandinavia when patients were tracheostomized and manually ventilated with gases delivered by a simple anesthetic circuit.[1] This in turn led to the development of the first mechanical positive pressure ventilators by Engstrom in Scandinavia and Emerson in North America and ushered in the era of intensive care medicine. The succeeding interval has seen major technological advances in ventilator design without a dramatic improvement in the survival of the pulmonary disease processes they were designed to treat. We are now in an era where we have a variety of choices for ventilator and adjunctive management strategies for the treatment of acute hypoxic respiratory failure (AHRF) in both adults and children.

While many of these have not improved survival perhaps the most important advance is that we now recognize the reality that, when it comes to dealing with patients with the type of parenchymal lung disease typified by diffuse atelectasis and hypoxemia, positive pressure ventilation (PPV) is as likely to be part of the problem as well as the solution. One of the basic principles adopted in PPV in the past 40 years is that we should attempt to mimic normal physiology and this has governed our choice of ventilator settings until comparatively recently. This decreed that the objective was to achieve normocarbia and normoxia with increased tidal volumes when necessary. While this strategy is fundamentally sound and without hazard in the normal lung, the same does not necessarily apply in the diseased lung. With the increasing realization of the importance of ventilator induced lung injury, alternative ventilation strategies are being explored in the management of AHRF which are based more on the recognition that the ventilation strategy needs to be adapted to the underlying pathophysiology of the lung rather than slavishly following the principle of mimicking normal physiology. This new approach demands that we rethink some of the traditional teaching about normal respiratory physiology and concentrate on understanding the underlying pathophysiology of this type of lung disease as well as being aware of the increasing evidence for secondary lung injury produced by mechanical ventilation.

The Pathophysiology of Acute Lung Injury

For the purposes of this review we will ignore acute respiratory failure caused by neuromuscular or central nervous system diseases which come under the broad heading of failure of respiratory "pump," are typified by elevations in $PaCO_2$, minimal if any intrapulmonary shunting, and are easily managed with conventional ventilation settings. We will concentrate on diseases that produce acute "lung failure" which are typically associated with diffuse atelectasis, permeability edema, low lung compliance, and intrapulmonary shunting. We shall use as our paradigm the Acute Respiratory Distress Syndrome (ARDS), following the European/North American Consensus Conference definition of four quadrant infiltrates on chest x-ray, absence of cardiac failure and a PaO_2/FiO_2 ratio <200.[2]

In the non-diseased state the total cardiac output passes through the pulmonary capillaries which are either juxtaposed to the alveoli (intra-alveolar) or contained within the interstitial space (extra-alveolar) with minimal leakage of fluid. This is because in the normal state the junctions between the capillary endothelial cells are only slightly permeable to fluid flux while they are impermeable to protein and solutes. The small amount of fluid that leaks into the interstitial space is reabsorbed by the lymphatics. The epithelial lining is impermeable to both fluid and solutes. This normal state of affairs can be perturbed by inhalational injury to the epithelial lining (aspiration, smoke inhalation, etc.) or by systemic diseases that damage the integrity of the endothelial (sepsis, trauma, embolism, etc.) which results in a number of pathological changes within the lung. Any of these insults can activate neutrophils and cause them to migrate to the lung where they attach to the endothelium and open the tight junctions resulting in leakage of fluid and protein, initially into the interstitial space and subsequently into the alveolus. The leakage of this fibrin-containing proteinaceous material results in inhibition of surfactant activity and in the formation of hyaline membranes around the alveolar lining. Epithelial injury results in damage to the surfactant-producing type 2 cells. There is frequent plugging of the pulmonary microcirculation with platelet thrombi and this, together with the release of thromboxane, produces a rise in pulmonary vascular resistance and pulmonary hypertension. This phase of ARDS is frequently referred to as the exudative phase. The gradual leakage of fluid into the interstitial space causes the lung to lose some of its elasticity, the earliest symptom being tachypnea as functional residual capacity (FRC) falls and the lung becomes stiffer. The initial blood gas abnormality is characteristically hypoxemia and hypocarbia, the $PaCO_2$ only rising above normal later in the illness as respiratory muscle fatigue sets in. A second proliferative phase of ARDS follows which is characterized by fibroblast infiltration into the interstitial space and the laying down of fibrous tissue, the harbinger of the development of chronic lung disease. At this stage there is gross destruction of air spaces, dilatation of terminal bronchi, leading eventually to a honeycomb appearance to the lung. In the 1970s pathologists frequently referred to this constellation of findings as "respirator lung." Clinicians argued that mechanical ventilation allowed time for the full expression of the underlying disease and that these lesions had little to do with the ventilator. The only damage that was unequivocally due to the ventilator was the constellation of air leak syndromes known collectively as barotrauma. Anything else was attributed to oxygen toxicity. In reality it is difficult for a pathologist looking down a microscope at a section of lung tissue to define where the primary lung disease stops and ventilator induced injury begins.

The Evolution of Positive Pressure Ventilation and PEEP in the Management of ARDS

Since the early days of the use of mechanical ventilation, it has been recognized that positive pressure respiration does not mimic normal breathing. If this were so, patients with normal lungs could be ventilated on FiO_2 of 0.21 at the same tidal volumes and respiratory rates seen in spontaneous breathing. It was Bendixen[3] in 1963 who showed that during general anesthesia, mechanical ventilation in patients with normal lungs was associated with a fall in PaO_2 and a rise in $PaCO_2$. He ascribed this change to the development of atelectasis due to the loss of the normal intermittent "sighing" present in the unanesthetized spontaneously breathing human. He proposed the use of an intermittent large tidal volume breath or "sigh" to overcome this problem which then became a design feature of ventilators of that period. It was not until a decade later that Froese and Bryan[4] showed that the major cause of atelectasis with the induction of anesthesia and muscle relaxation was a loss in lung volume due to the cephalad movement of the diaphragm. To compensate for this physiological aberration we have resorted to increasing the inspired oxygen concentration and delivered tidal volumes to well in excess of those used in spontaneous respiration. However in diseased lungs, what seemed like a medical imperative, i.e., to normalize blood gases in patients with diffusely atelectatic, low compliant lung disease by using ever larger tidal volumes, rarely resulted in survival. It wasn't until the 1970s that it was first shown that by maintaining a positive end-expiratory pressure (PEEP) oxygenation could be improved. Ashbaugh[5] in the original report of patients with ARDS showed that PEEP was effective in ventilated patients while Gregory[6] went on to show that a similar strategy could be used successfully in spontaneously breathing newborn infants with hyaline membrane disease. During the succeeding 20 years the use of positive pressure ventilation with PEEP has proved successful in improving oxygenation in both ARDS and infant respiratory distress syndrome (IRDS). The question is how much PEEP should be applied, given the potentially negative effect on hemodynamics. This was addressed in the classic paper by Suter and Fairley in 1975.[7] They applied incremental increases in PEEP while measuring cardiac output, oxygen delivery, and lung compliance. They coined the term "best PEEP," which was the level at which the improvement in oxygenation and lung compliance was matched by the least adverse effect on cardiac output. This varied from 0-15 cmH_2O, the magnitude of the PEEP depending on the severity of the loss of lung compliance. Further increase in PEEP above the optimal level resulted in decrease in both compliance and oxygen transport.

One of the major difficulties in setting a PEEP level or indeed any ventilatory parameter in ARDS is the heterogeneity of the disease process. This became strikingly clear with the advent of thoracic CT scans. In ARDS the disease looks diffuse on the plain film, but on the CT scan there are frequently a collection of densities in the dependent parts of the lung, with the nondependent lung looking more or less normal.[8,9] Furthermore, these densities, which presumably represent atelectatic or flooded units, are mobile as their location can change with posture. It is clear that the pressures required to open the dependent regions of the lung may overdistend the nondependent regions. Although the application of PEEP is consistently associated with improved oxygenation in ARDS, the recognition that mortality from oxygenation failure has not been reduced significantly in the past twenty years despite major improvements in ventilator technology has led to a search of alternate rescue therapy in an attempt to improve oxygenation in the situation where the lung is already damaged from a combination of underlying disease and ventilator therapy. In order to critically evaluate whether these innovations represent a useful option in ARDS we must discuss the role that positive pressure ventilation plays in the development of acute lung injury.

Ventilation Induced Lung Injury: Experimental Models of Genesis and Prevention

The term barotrauma was originally the most commonly used term to described damage to the lung from the ventilator and is usually understood to refer to a constellation of air leak syndromes, the incidence of which rises almost linearly with the peak pressure. We need another word for barotrauma, as this merely reflects the end stage of the more subtle but equally serious epithelial and endothelial injury leading to pulmonary edema and protein leak induced by mechanical ventilation and high inspired oxygen levels. The first clear study of the problem was a classic paper by Webb and Tierney.[10] Rats with normal lungs were mechanically ventilated with room air for a target period of one hour. Those ventilated at pressures of 45/0 cmH_2O developed severe hypoxemia, decreased compliance and died with post mortem evidence of extensive alveolar and perivascular edema. Those ventilated at 30/0 cmH_2O had reasonable gas exchange, no change in compliance, and all survived. Animals ventilated at 14/0 cmH_2O showed no abnormality. Thus a clear dose/response was established for the induction of lung injury. Since then there have been numerous animal studies which have shown high airway pressures used in normal lungs can result in a pattern of lung injury indistinguishable from the human form of ARDS.[11-16] Cyclical lung distention delivered by positive-pressure ventilation (PPV) with peak inspiratory pressures of 30 cmH_2O or above can produce permeability edema and pathological changes which are similar to ARDS and the consequences of this can be at least partially prevented by PEEP. Given the fact that patients with this type of lung disease require positive intrathoracic pressure to reverse their hypoxemia, these studies would

suggest that the ideal strategy to prevent ongoing injury would be to prevent lung overdistention by limiting the peak inspiratory pressure while maintaining a lung volume with sufficient PEEP to prevent alveolar derecruitment. There are several experimental studies comparing the degree of injury using low tidal volume/high PEEP with low PEEP/high tidal volume ventilation, high PEEP and low PEEP strategies.[17-19] This led to the development of the concept of the inflection point on the pressure volume curve, below which rapid derecruitment and lung collapse occurred during the expiratory phase of positive pressure ventilation (Figure 4-1). The application of PEEP above the inflection point should, in theory, prevent this.

Apart from direct injury to the lung tissue, there are important remote effects due to cytokine release associated with PPV. There are now experimental data which shows that lung overdistention *per se* results in the release of cytokines which may be responsible for multiorgan injury and dysfunction.[20] Although very high airway pressures were used in this animal model the investigators demonstrate a protective effect with the use of PEEP. Finally, it should be pointed out that the important variable is not airway pressure but transpulmonary pressure--that is the difference in pressure between the alveolus and the pleural space (it should be noted that mouth pressure does not necessarily equal alveolar pressure because of flow resistive pressure drops in the small airways). In instances where intra-abdominal pressure is high or the chest wall is stiff, higher than usual airway pressures may be required to achieve adequate alveolar ventilation without this necessarily being injurious to the lung.

Pulmonary Oxygen Toxicity

Although most of the attention has been focused on positive pressure in the development of secondary lung injury, high inspired oxygen concentrations also play an important role.

There are many published studies of animal primate models showing that prolonged exposure to high inspired oxygen concentrations results in proliferation of type II epithelial cells and increased endothelial permeability.[21-30] In human disease it is obviously difficult to separate what is the primary disease process from the effects of exposure of the injured lung to high oxygen concentrations. However a study on normal humans showed that breathing an FiO_2 of 0.95 for 17 hours resulted in an increase in the albumin concentration in BAL fluid, demonstrating the development of a permeability edema.[31] In light of this it would seem logical that an essential part of any ventilation strategy in patients with acute lung injury would include measures to minimize high oxygen concentrations using measures to recruit and retain lung volume.

Epidemiology and Markers of Acute Lung Injury

The term 'acute respiratory distress syndrome' was first coined by Ashbaugh[5] in an article in Lancet in 1967 which described the acute onset of tachypnea, hypoxemia and loss of compliance in 11 previously healthy adults and one child, seven of whom died. At autopsy all had diffuse atelectasis, alveolar hemorrhage and edema together with hyaline membrane formation. The similarity to the lungs of premature infants with hyaline membrane disease prompted the authors to call it the Adult Respiratory Distress Syndrome. Among the treatments described as being "therapeutic trials of apparent value" was positive end-expiratory pressure. In the succeeding almost 40 years a large body of literature has been amassed on

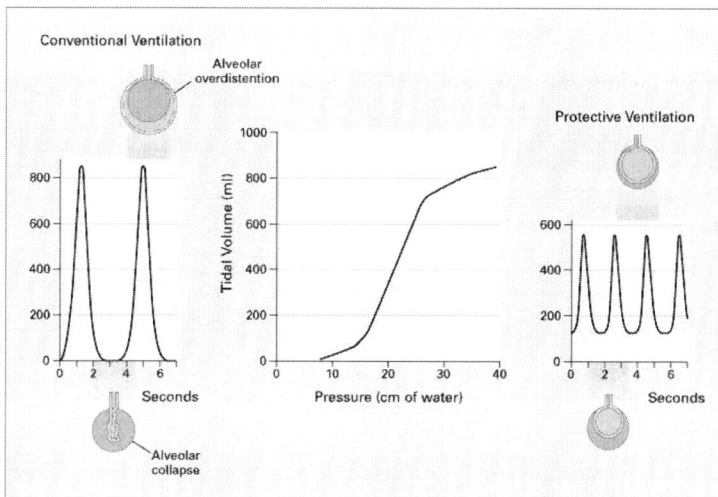

Figure 4-1. Tidal volumes and pressure volume curve representing tradition and lung protective ventilation strategies in a 70 kg adult. The upper and lower inflection points on the pressure volume curve are 14 and 26 cmH_2O (center panel). The use of a traditional tidal volume of 12 mls/kg and no PEEP (left panel) results in alveolar over distention when pressure exceeds the upper inflection point and alveolar collapse at end expiration as end expiratory lung volume falls below the lower inflection point.. The pressure limited ventilation strategy using 6 mls/kg (right panel) prevents over distention at the open inflection point and PEEP 2 cmH_2O above the lower inflection point prevents alveolar collapse at end volume. From Tobin MJ. Advances in mechanical ventilation. N Engl J Med 2001; 344:1986. Reproduced with permission.

the topic which reports mortality rates of as low as 30% and as high as 80%. Since ARDS is a syndrome rather than a disease entity, mortality may be significantly influenced by the underlying disease process. Patients with sepsis and immunodeficiency tend to have higher mortality rates. Gattonini[32] has divided ARDS into pulmonary and extra-pulmonary causes and shown different responses to the mechanical effects of PEEP. In adult studies the overall mortality in large cohort studies has been approximately 60%,[33-39] whereas in the control arm of several controlled trials the mortality has been lower, in the range of 40-50%.[40-44] This difference can be partly accounted for by the large number of patients excluded in several of these studies. Factors that have been shown to influence survival include the development of multiorgan failure, use of low PEEP, increasing FiO_2 requirements, and ventilation with high tidal volumes.[34-36, 40, 44]

Epidemiological data on ARDS/ALI in pediatric ARDS is harder to come by. Data from studies on children requiring mechanical ventilation published in the 1980s and 1990s suggested that the mortality was similar to adult ARDS.[45-48] However more recently published studies in an era where there has been an increasing focus on ventilation-induced lung injury has shown that the mortality is in the range of 20-30% (see Table 4-1).[49-57] Attempts have been made to predict outcome in order to select patients for alternative ventilation strategies, including ECMO, using either physiological scoring systems or measures of the severity of the oxygenation defect.

In hypoxic newborns the Oxygenation Index (OI) has proved to be a reasonably robust predictor of mortality and is widely accepted as indicator for the initiation of ECMO. In the older child where oxygenation failure is frequently part of multiorgan failure the OI was thought to

Table 4-1. Published studies of predictors of outcome in acute hypoxic respiratory failure in children.

Study Design	Year	Inclusion Criteria	Patient Numbers	Mortality
Rivera[25]	1990	FiO_2 0.9 PIP > 25 cmH$_2$O	42	55%
Timmons[27]	1991	FiO_2 0.5 PEEP > 6 cmH$_2$O	44	75%
Tamburro[26]	1991	FiO_2 0.6 PaO$_2$ < 60 mmHg	37	46%
Davis[24]	1993	Lung Injury Score > 2.5	60	60%
Timmons[34]	1995	$FiO_2 \geq 0.5$ PEEP ≥ 6 cmH$_2$O x 12 hrs	470	43%
Fackler[29]	1997	$FiO_2 \geq 0.5$ PEEP ≥ 6 cmH$_2$O x 12 hrs	161	20%
Peters[31]	1998	PaO$_2$/FiO$_2$ < 200	110	22%
Dahlem[28]	2003	P/F <300	44	27%
Trachsel[30]	2005	$FiO_2 \geq 0.5$ PEEP ≥ 6 cmH$_2$O x 12 hrs	131	27%
Flori[32]	2005	P/F <300	328	22%

be less reliable. In the multicenter retrospective study of outcomes in 470 ventilated patients in the 1990s, an era before lung protective ventilation was widely adopted, included those treated with ECMO and high frequency oscillatory ventilation (HFOV). This showed that the combination of the OI, PIP, PEEP, age, FiO_2, and PRISM score were the best predictors of outcome.[58] A subsequent publication using these data that analyzed the outcome in severe AHRF in ECMO-eligible patients suggested that the use of ECMO resulted in improved survival.[59] This formed the basis for the design of a prospective multicenter randomized controlled trial (RCT) comparing ECMO with a pressure-limited lung protective ventilation strategy. This study was terminated after enrolling 406 patients when it was found that the mortality in the ECMO eligible patients was only 18% compared to the predicted rate of 40%.[50]

Two more recent studies have confirmed the relationship between outcome, measured by mortality and duration of ventilation using the severity of the oxygenation defect (OI and PaO_2/FiO_2) as well as nonpulmonary organ dysfunction.[51,53] The difference in mortality between adult and pediatric studies may be accounted for the fact that many of the children who would fit ARDS/ALI criteria have single system lung disease similar to AHRF in newborns. This is especially true in the first two years of life which raises the question as to whether these patients should be classified as acute hypoxic respiratory failure (AHRF) rather than ARDS.[53,60] Where ECMO fits in the treatment algorithm for children with isolated pulmonary failure in an era of lung protective ventilation strategies remains to be determined and can only be judged on a case-by-case basis.

The Development of a Lung Protective Ventilation Strategy

Tidal Volume Limitation

The traditional, or perhaps the historical, approach to mechanical ventilation has been one targeted on the objective of a normal PaO_2 and $PaCO_2$ and the accepted practice has been to use tidal volumes of 10-15 ml/kg to achieve this. With the increasing recognition that these volumes can injure the already damaged lung has come the realization that ventilation with reduced tidal volume with a pressure limited target rather than $PaCO_2$ may be a safer option. The origin of this revolutionary approach can be traced back to a landmark paper by Darioli and Perret[61] published in 1984 entitled "Mechanical controlled hypoventilation in status asthmaticus." In it they described a series of adult patients ventilated using the volume control mode but with tidal volumes of 8-12 mls/kg, a low inspiratory flow rate and a rate of 6-10 cycles/min. They set the maximum PIP at 50 cmH$_2$O. If this was exceeded with the initial settings the tidal volume was reduced further and the $PaCO_2$ allowed to rise. All patients survived, the duration of ventilation was short (<3 days) and this in an era where 10-20% mortality was the norm for ventilation support in severe status asthmaticus. What was even more important was that they enunciated the principle that normocarbia should not be the objective in this situation as the measures required to achieve it are potentially harmful if not lethal. They defined the objective to be correction of hypoxemia while ignoring hypercarbia up to the level of 90 mmHg.

The next important study that served to support this position was the paper published in 1990 by Hickling.[62] He hypothesized that simply reducing the tidal volume and allowing the CO_2 to rise would be equally effective in preventing the ventilation induced lung injury.

This revolutionary concept was put to the test in 50 patients with ARDS as defined by a Lung Injury Score of >2.5 and a PaO_2/FiO_2 ratio of <150. The ventilation strategy used was SIMV volume controlled ventilation with the target of a PIP of less than 30 cmH_2O when this could be easily achieved and always less than 40 cmH_2O with a tidal volume of as low as 5 mls/kg if necessary. In many instances this resulted in significant degrees of hypercarbia but no attempt was made to correct this. The oxygenation strategy was increasing levels of PEEP with the objective of reducing the FiO_2 to <0.6. Patients were allowed to breathe spontaneously. Severity of illness data, defined using the Apache II Score, was collected. The remarkable result was that the hospital mortality in this series was 16% compared with a predicted mortality of 39%. Despite criticism that this was retrospective data and did not conform to the gold standard of proof by a randomized controlled clinical trial, no single study has done more to influence ventilation practices in the past 20 years. Both these studies have used the volume control mode with limitation of tidal volume as a method of reducing the PIP. The alternative option as a method of preventing volume distention of the injured lung is to use the pressure control mode with limitation of the PIP. It has been suggested that this may be preferable for, as well as allowing for a decelerating gas flow pattern, it guarantees that the preset PIP will not be exceeded. This has led to a renewed interest from adult intensivists in a mode of ventilation that was abandoned 30 years ago except in neonatal AHRF. In fact, the credit for the development of this permissive hypercapnia approach really belongs to Wung[63] who advocated it in the management of persistent pulmonary hypertension of the newborn (PPHN) in 1985.

Based on the accumulated experimental data from animals (and limited human experience) a pressure-limited permissive hypercapnia strategy would seem to make sense as long as we accept that hypercarbia *per se*, while not desirable, is not intrinsically harmful. While few would argue that modest elevations of $PaCO_2$ in the range of 50 mmHg are of concern, levels of >100 mmHg cause great anxiety to a generation of critical care physicians trained to strict adherence to the physiological norm.

What then is the basis for these concerns and how do we weigh them up against the potential for doing harm by continuing the practice of ventilating to a normal $PaCO_2$? Acute elevations in CO_2 result in the rapid development of an intracellular acidosis. A rising hydrogen ion concentration produces an increase in pulmonary vascular resistance and in cerebral blood flow, which may be harmful in cerebral injury or pulmonary hypertension. Apart from this there is little evidence that pH levels as low as 7.2 have any adverse effect on myocardial performance or tissue oxygen delivery, while hypocapnia has the opposite effects.[64,65] Indeed, experimental evidence would suggest the contrary. In animal models of ischemia reperfusion of the lung and sepsis hypocapnia has been shown to worsen while hypercarbia and acidosis has been shown to attenuate the injury.[66-71] In the clinical situation, as long as the kidneys are working patients can compensate for pH levels that drop as low as 7.1 with effective renal bicarbonate retention. In both the permissive hypercapnia series reported above, there was very effective renal compensation and in neither was bicarbonate used to correct a respiratory acidosis. In Hickling's study $PaCO_2$s of over 100 mmHg were permitted with pHs dropping as low as 7.1 without the administration of bicarbonate. The remarkably improved survival would suggest that acidosis had little adverse effect on myocardial performance. There is also evidence in children that very high (>200 mmHg) levels of $PaCO_2$ are not associated with adverse consequences, as long as oxygenation is maintained.[72]

If we accept that pressure-limited ventilation with low tidal volumes and permissive hypercapnia is unlikely to be harmful and is at least as effective as pressure control in ARDS, do we have any evidence to prove that it may in fact lower mortality? Although the retrospective studies published to date suggest that this is true, there are now several published prospective studies in adults comparing this approach with a standard ventilation technique. Amato[40] in a randomized controlled clinical trial in adult patients with ARDS compared a standard volume control mode with a ventilation strategy that used a low tidal volume combined with PEEP level set above the inflection point in order to reduce the FiO_2 to <0.5. They were able to demonstrate improved survival to ICU discharge in the lung protective group. Although on the face of it this result would suggest that tidal volume limitation will reduce mortality in ARDS, one has to be cautious in interpreting this as the definitive study given the fact that the tidal volumes (10-15 ml/kg) used in the conventional arm of this study resulted in $PaCO_2$ levels of 35-38 mmHg, which would not be in keeping with current conventional practice. Three other randomized controlled trials also failed to demonstrate a beneficial effect using tidal volume limitation in ARDS patients but none used the aggressive lung recruitment strategies advocated by Amato.[41-43] However, building on the observations made in the experimental study of Tremblay,[20] which demonstrated the release of cytokines associated with lung distention, Ranieri demonstrated a reduction in mediators of injury in a randomized trial of a low-stretch versus conventional tidal volume ventilation in adults with ARDS, with a trend towards improved survival.[73]

The definitive study in heightening awareness of the issue of ventilation-induced lung injury in ARDS was the ARDSNet randomized trial of 6 ml/kg versus 12 ml/kg tidal volume.[44] Eight hundred patients were randomized and the results showed a relative risk reduction in mortality of 22% in the low tidal volume group. Although this is a landmark study in ARDS it cannot be assumed that 6 ml/kg tidal volume

should be adopted as the universal standard ventilator setting for all patients. In the first instance a large number of patients were screened for study entry but not included. Secondly, it has subsequently been pointed out that a significant number of patients in the 12 ml/kg arm of the study actually had their tidal volumes increased following randomization,[74] which begs the question as to whether at least part of the outcome difference was due to injurious ventilation in that group rather than a protective effect of 6 ml/kg. Clearly it would be unwise to assume that 6 ml/kg tidal volume represents a standard that should be adopted for all patients with ARDS.[75] Rather, the study should be interpreted as showing that high tidal volume ventilation contributes to mortality in ARDS and that tidal volume reduction with hypercarbia is safe and may improve outcome. A further analysis of the ARDSNet data addressed the commonly held belief that plateau pressure levels of 30-35 $cmsH_2O$ are "safe" in ARDS patients.[76] The authors were unable to find any data to support this belief while at the same time not suggesting that tidal volume should be reduced to <6 ml/kg.

There have been no RCTs of tidal volume limitation in children with ARDS, nor are there likely to be. Two studies are worthy of comment though. Albuali[55] in a retrospective review examined ventilation practices in two different eras; 1988-1992 compared with 2000-2004. In the first era the average tidal volume was 10 ml/kg versus 8 ml/kg in the second. This was associated with a reduction in mortality from 39% to 21% and an increase in ventilator-free days. Furthermore, they were able to demonstrate a relationship between increased tidal volume and mortality. Erickson,[56] on the other hand, in a prospective data collection in all ventilated children with ALI over a one year period in PICUs in Australia and New Zealand, demonstrated the opposite. In their series increased tidal volume was associated with reduced mortality. This result is difficult to interpret because the 35% mortality for ALI and 44% for ARDS in their series is considerably higher than other published pediatric series.[53,54,77] Expert opinion recommendations for the ventilation of children with ARDS/ALI include avoiding tidal volume of >10 ml/kg and keeping plateau pressures to less than 30 cmH$_2$O.[57,78]

Lung Recruitment: The High PEEP "Open Lung" Strategy

In the first published tidal volume-reduction ventilation trial by Amato, part of the explanation for the improved survival was ascribed to an aggressive lung recruitment strategy using high levels of PEEP to prevent the secondary injury caused by opening and closing of collapsed terminal lung units during the respiratory cycle as illustrated in Figure 4-1. There have been three further large multicentre RCTS that have addressed this issue. The first from the ARDSNet comparing a high lung volume recruitment strategy with low PEEP was closed before target enrollment without showing a survival benefit.[79] Two further large RCTs (>700 patients) compared high versus moderate levels of PEEP where a tidal volume of 6 ml/kg was used in both arms of the study.[80,81] Neither showed a survival benefit but there was an increase in ventilator-free days and organ dysfunction with the high PEEP strategy. A recently published systematic review of the topic which included studies on ARDS and ALI concluded that high PEEP improved survival only in the group of adult patients with ARDS. There are no similar published studies in children.

Algorithm for a Lung Protective Ventilation Strategy in ARF

The following is an outline of a lung protective strategy for the management of patients with severe oxygenation failure who constitute a group with a potential for high mortality. The definition is based on data from pediatric patients which suggests that the requirement for FiO$_2$ ≥ 0.5 and a PEEP ≥ 6 cmH$_2$O for more than 12 hours predicts a mortality of 40%.[58] It has as its basis the prevention of lung overdistention by the use of low tidal volumes and PEEP, together with the objective of reducing FiO$_2$ to the lowest level compatible with adequate oxygenation. A balance has to be struck between what would be *desirable* in all situations (low PIP and low FiO$_2$) and what would be *tolerable* in situations of severe lung disease in order not to aggravate the lung injury. This approach clearly separates ventilation (CO$_2$ elimination) dictated by PIP and ventilator rate from oxygenation which is determined by PEEP and FiO$_2$. The basis for this protocol is as follows:

Ventilation:
Desirable Objective PIP ≤ 30 cmH$_2$O normal pH or compensated respiratory acidosis (pH > 7.2)
Tolerance PIP ≤ 35 cmH$_2$O pH 7.10

Oxygenation:
Desirable Objective FiO$_2$ ≤ 0.5 SaO$_2$ 90%
Tolerance SaO$_2$ 85%

The strategy to achieve this would be by:
1. Pressure-limited ventilation to a maximum PIP of 35 cmH$_2$O.
2. Ignore hypercarbia and target the pH rather than the PaCO$_2$ with the objective of a compensated respiratory acidosis (pH > 7.2) but a tolerance for a pH as low as 7.10.
3. Increase the PEEP to a level that enables reduction of FiO$_2$ < 0.5, compatible with a saturation of 90% (PaO$_2$ 60 mmHg).

Ventilation Strategy

Ventilation (CO$_2$ elimination) is controlled by PIP and respiratory rate. The objective is to limit PIP to a maximum of 35 cmH$_2$O, ignoring the PaCO$_2$ as long as there was an appropriate pH compensation (pH > 7.20). Patients are to be managed with a pressure-limited mode (pressure control or pressure-limited volume control). The initial pressure setting objective is no higher than 30 cmH$_2$O with a ventilation rate of 20-40 per minute, depending on age. If the first blood gas shows an uncompensated respiratory acidosis (pH <7.20) on two consecutive readings two hours apart, the PIP is increased to 35 cmH$_2$O. Once the target PIP of 35 cmH$_2$O is reached, the pH and PaO$_2$ is measured. If the pH is > 7.20 at or below the target PIP, the pressure is reduced to the target PIP of 30 cmH$_2$O regardless of PaCO$_2$ level. If the pH falls below 7.20 on PIP 35 cmH$_2$O, the respiratory rate may be increased

by 5 per minute. If this fails to restore the pH to > 7.20, 2 mmol/kg of intravenous bicarbonate may be given. If the pH is consistently < 7.20 at a PIP of 35 cmH$_2$O, consider increasing the tolerance to pH 7.10 rather than increasing the PIP. See Figure 4-2.

Oxygenation Strategy

The principal determinants of PaO$_2$ in mechanically ventilated patients with acute respiratory failure are FiO$_2$ and PEEP. The combination of PEEP and inspiratory time dictate the mean airway pressure (MAP). As high inspired

VENTILATION ALGORITHM

OBJECTIVE: pH >7.20 PIP ≤30 cmH2O
TOLERANCE: pH >7.10 PIP <35 cm H20

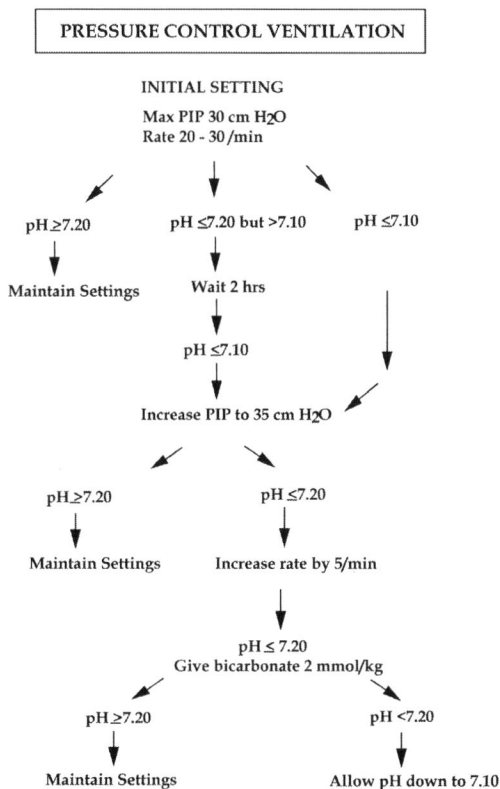

PRESSURE CONTROL VENTILATION

INITIAL SETTING
Max PIP 30 cm H2O
Rate 20 - 30 /min

| pH ≥7.20 | pH ≤7.20 but >7.10 | pH ≤7.10 |

Maintain Settings   Wait 2 hrs

pH ≤7.10

Increase PIP to 35 cm H2O

| pH ≥7.20 | pH ≤7.20 |

Maintain Settings   Increase rate by 5/min

pH ≤ 7.20
Give bicarbonate 2 mmol/kg

| pH ≥7.20 | pH <7.20 |

Maintain Settings   Allow pH down to 7.10

Figure 4-2. Ventilation Algorithm for the minimization of lung injury during positive pressure ventilation

oxygen concentrations have been identified as producing secondary lung injury, the objective is to use the lowest FiO_2 consistent with a PaO_2 > 55 mmHg or an arterial saturation > 90%. To guarantee full oxygenation and adequate saturation at the outset of the study, the FiO_2 is set at 0.8 initially together with a minimum PEEP of 6 cmH_2O. The FiO_2 is then reduced in increments of 0.05 as long as the PaO_2 remains above 55 mmHg or the saturation remains above 90% the objective of FiO_2 of <0.5. If the FiO_2 cannot be reduced to this level without PaO_2 dropping to less than 55 mmHg or the saturation to < 90%, the FiO_2 is maintained at the lowest level while

PEEP is added in increments of 2 cmH_2O until PaO_2 increases to above 55 mmHg. PEEP will continue to be added in increments of 2 cmH_2O while the FiO_2 is reduced to a maximum of 0.5. PEEP up to a level of 20 cmH_2O is used. If the PaO_2 cannot be maintained above 55 mmHg or the saturation above 90% by the addition of the maximum level of PEEP (20 cmH_2O), FiO_2 may be increased in increments of 0.05 until a target PaO_2 and saturation are reached. If an FiO_2 of > 0.70 is required then consideration should be given to tolerating an SaO_2 of 85 - 90%. See Figure 4-3.

OXYGENATION ALGORITHM

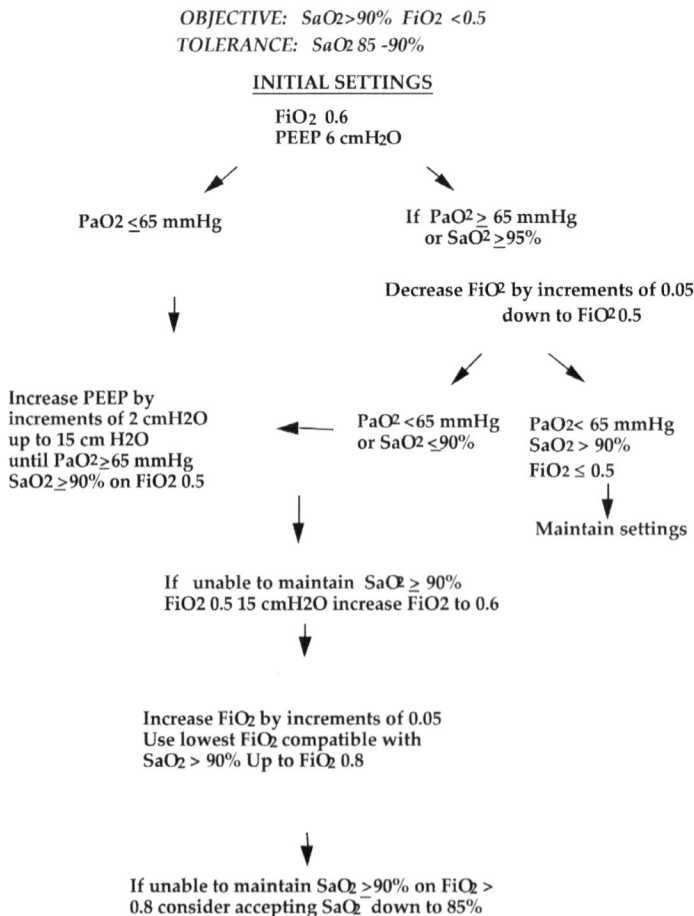

Figure 4-3. Oxygenation Algorithm for the minimization of oxygen toxicity and lung injury during positive pressure ventilation.

Alternative Ventilation Strategies for ARDS

The alternative ventilation strategies for the treatment of ARDS include those that use standard tidal volumes and rates but vary the inspiratory time (prolonged I:E ratio), those that use reduced PIP and tidal volume while maintaining a normal $PaCO_2$ by either ventilating dead space (high frequency ventilation), reducing the dead space (intratracheal pulmonary ventilation), or allowing the $PaCO_2$ to rise (pressure limited ventilation - permissive hypercapnia). In addition to these there are adjuncts to mechanical ventilation (surfactant and nitric oxide) as well as providing PPV by mask (noninvasive ventilation). Finally, one can eliminate the secondary injury altogether by removing the ventilator altogether and providing extracorporeal oxygenation. The characteristics of these various alternative strategies are summarized in Table 4-2. The more commonly used ventilation strategies will be discussed in detail.

High Frequency Ventilation

The concept that tidal volume could be reduced while maintaining minute ventilation with rapid rates was first introduced in the 1970s as a ventilatory support technique used during surgical procedures involving the upper airway, which were made more feasible by having a relatively motionless surgical field. This was subsequently redesigned as a support mode in the management of patients with acute respiratory failure as a way of mitigating the effects of pulmonary barotrauma and proved particularly useful in the management of patients with bronchopleural fistula. There are various forms

Table 4-2. Modes of ventilation.

Ventilation Mode	Flow	Airway Pressure	Main Features	Disadvantages
Volume Control (VC)	Variable according to rate of gas flow. Commonly rapid constant with plateau but can be decelerating at slow gas flow	Compliance & resistance dependent. Gradual rise to peak followed by plateau	Guaranteed minute volume	Not leak compensated High airway pressures in severe lung disease
Pressure Control (PC)	Decelerating	Square wave Preset pressure	More even distribution of gas flow. Leak compensated	Varying TV & MV according to compliance
Pressure Control Inverse Ratio Ventilation (PC-IRV)	Decelerating	Square wave	Lower PIP	Auto-PEEP Cardiovascular compromise
Pressure Regulated Volume Control	Decelerating	Square wave	Lowest airway pressure with guaranteed minute volume	PIP can vary below preset level
Pressure Limited Ventilation	Decelerating	Square wave	Low tidal volume Reduced secondary injury	Hypercapnia
Intratracheal Pulmonary Ventilation (ITPV)	High constant gas flow		Reduced dead space	High gas flow can lead humidifier "blow out"
Airway Release Ventilation (ARV)	High constant gas flow	CPAP with intermittent release	Spontaneous respiration	Useful only in mild lung injury
High Frequency Ventilation	High constant gas flow	Sustained MAP	Very low TV Reduced secondary injury	Underestimation of MAP and less than ideal humidity on HFJV

of high frequency ventilation now being used in clinical medicine, the characteristics of which are summarized in Table 4-3. This review will concentrate on the two most commonly used in clinical medicine, namely High Frequency Oscillatory Ventilation (HFOV) and High Frequency Jet Ventilation (HFJV). Both have been used to treat patients with IRDS and ARDS with the objective of minimizing lung injury by using small tidal volume ventilation while maintaining oxygenation using a high open lung volume strategy.

There is little rationale for considering HFV as just "another ventilator" which happens to operate at faster rates and lower airway pressures than conventional ventilators, without a clear understanding of the situations where these features may be a considerable advantage in patient management. There are several situations where a case can be made for considering using HFV in preference to conventional mechanical ventilation (CMV):

1. to improve oxygenation by recruiting lung volume while avoiding cyclical lung distention with high PIPs (the "open lung" strategy),
2. achieving more effective CO_2 elimination in situations where this may be particularly important, e.g., persistent pulmonary hypertension of the newborn (PPHN),
3. minimizing the effect of secondary or therapy induced lung injury in situa-

tions of diffuse parenchymal lung disease with hypoxia,
4. to minimize the effect on cardiovascular function by reducing airway pressures,
5. to improve operating conditions in certain procedures on the airway and lung.

High Frequency Oscillatory Ventilation (HFOV)

The discovery that a high frequency sine wave was capable of moving CO_2 out of the lung was first made serendipitously during experiments in paralyzed animals designed to measure thoracic impedance. Following this original observation the same technique was shown to produce excellent gas exchange in normal animals using tidal volumes well below dead space.[82] The principle that oxygen would diffuse down a concentration gradient had been well established 20 years before when it was shown that arterial oxygen saturation could be maintained over periods of apnea as long as 20 minutes if a high flow of gas was delivered directly into the airway. This technique, known as apneic oxygenation, was used to advantage during anesthesia for laryngeal surgery where oxygen and volatile agents at high flows were delivered via a catheter placed through the vocal cords. The technique was limited in duration by the inevitable rise in $PaCO_2$ (3-6 mmHg/min) that occurred with apnea. However, it was noted that some CO_2 elimination would occur due to

Table 4-3. Various forms of high frequency ventilation for acute hypoxic respiratory failure.

Type	Rate	Expiratory Phase	Application
High Frequency Positive Pressure Ventilation (HFPPV)	60-120/min	Passive	Surgical procedures, IRDS, ARDS
High Frequency Oscillatory Ventilation (HFOV)	60-900/min	Active	IRDS, ARDS in children
High Frequency Jet Ventilation (HFJV)	60-300/min	Passive	IRDS, ARDS

the washout of dead space and that improved the nearer the catheter was placed to the carina. It was also demonstrated that cardiac contraction enhanced the diffusion of CO_2 up the trachea towards the carina, a phenomenon referred to as cardiogenic mixing. The application of the high frequency sine wave to the airway solved the problem of hypercarbia by further enhancing the diffusion of CO_2 due to extremely efficient mixing of gases within the lung. Although the delta P (difference between peak and end expiratory pressures) is high when measured at the peak of the airway in this system, this does not reflect alveolar pressure, which is much lower. Although there is some bulk flow, this is insufficient for alveolar ventilation and the enhanced gas exchange is accounted for by accelerated diffusion. The first oscillators used to demonstrate this were either adapted from a loudspeaker design or engineering prototypes using a piston within a cylinder driven by a high speed electric motor at speeds of up to 25 Hz. The original animal experiments were performed at 15 Hz (900/min) with fresh gas flows in the circuit of up to 10-15 liters/min with attempts to use an expiratory valve in the circuits.

Following the development of those pioneering prototypes, HFOV has progressed from being a physiological curiosity to an alternative mode of ventilation with potential advantages in the management of AHRF. In this type of lung disease the conventional ventilator cycle not only produces a convective flow of gas to sweep CO_2 out of the lung, but it has to produce a pressure within the lung in excess of alveolar "opening pressure" in order to achieve oxygen exchange. In the low compliant, atelectatic lung, such as is seen in acute lung injury, airway pressure during the expiratory phase of the respiratory cycle falls below closing pressure, unless high levels of positive end expiratory pressure (PEEP) are used. It is this constant opening and closing of terminal airway units under high pressure which results in further injury to the already damaged lung. HFOV offers an entirely differ-

ent ventilation strategy for dealing with this form of lung disease. In the first instance high volume cycling is not necessary to eliminate CO_2 as numerous studies attest to the excellent $PaCO_2$ control with HFOV. Increasing airway pressure by adjusting fresh gas flow can then be used as a device to raise MAP above alveolar opening pressure and maintain lung volume at that level, where the small airway pressure swings around the mean will be less injurious to the lung by avoiding the continual cycle of inflation and collapse of terminal lung units.

There have now been a large number of prospective RCTs comparing HFOV with conventional ventilation in preterm infants[83-89] as well as rescue studies in term infants.[90,91] These have shown that HFOV is an effective form of ventilation which may reduce the incidence of chronic lung disease and the need for ECMO without having impact on survival. This is perhaps not surprising in an era where the widespread use of surfactant replacement therapy has been associated with a dramatic reduction in mortality.

The use of HFOV has extended outside the newborn period with the demonstration of its efficacy as a rescue therapy for older children (up to 35 kg) with ARF complicated by pulmonary barotrauma.[92] This was followed by a randomized controlled clinical trial of CMV and HFOV in children outside the newborn period with hypoxemia despite high mean airway pressures or airleak.[93] The study was a randomized crossover design and the HFOV strategy used the open lung approach with a MAP setting 5 cmH_2O above that used on conventional ventilation. However, the conventional ventilation mode did define a lung protective strategy. The survival was higher in the HFOV group when the numbers of patients who were randomized into that arm and did not cross, together with patients who were crossed over from CMV to HFOV, were taken into account. However, this was a small study (n=58) and it would be difficult to show an outcome benefit in a study of this size. Also there was a prolonged period of time on conventional mechanical ventilation before randomization which makes this more of a rescue study than a true evaluation of two different ventilation strategies. In contrast to this an RCT of early intervention with HFOV in adults with ARDS showed a definite trend to lower mortality in patients randomized to HFOV although the study was underpowered so this did not reach statistical significance.[94] The study design included pressure-limited, permissive hypercapnia in the conventional arm and a lung recruitment strategy used with HFOV.

Despite a high level of evidence that the use of HFOV influences outcome in pediatric patients with ARDS it has been widely adopted as an effective rescue strategy.[95] There is also the recognition that it needs to be combined with a lung recruitment strategy that requires the use of high mean airway pressures to open up the lung and that this should be used as a method of improving oxygenation and decreasing the FiO_2. Therefore the strategy requires that the initial MAP settings be 2-5 cmH_2O above that used on the conventional ventilator and that this should be incrementally increased until there are signs of lung recruitment as evidenced by the ability to reduce the FiO_2 while maintaining the same or improved SaO_2. This can be confirmed radiologically by being able to count 9 or more posterior ribs. Mean airway pressures of 35 cmH_2O or higher are frequently required to achieve this and can be tolerated as long as hemodynamic instability does not occur.

Prone Position Ventilation

There is now recognition that the standard supine position for nursing the critically ill patient may be less than ideal in patients with AHRF. Froese and Bryan showed over twenty years ago that during positive pressure ventilation there was a cephalad movement of the dorsal part of the diaphragm and loss of lung volume in people with normal lungs ventilated in the supine position[4] and Bryan advocated ventilating in the prone position.[96] With positive pressure ventilation in the supine position there is preferential perfusion of dependent lung regions and CT images of patients with ARDS have shown that this is the most prominent area for hemorrhage and edema formation.[8,9] Several studies have now described the practice of turning hypoxic patients with ARDS/ALI to the prone position with improvement in oxygenation and decreases in intrapulmonary shunt, although this finding is not universal.[97] The proposed mechanisms for this improvement are increased FRC, change in regional diaphragm motion, redistribution of blood flow to less injured lung units and improved secretion clearance. Studies of experimental lung injury have shown that when turning to the prone position preferential perfusion does not shift to the ventral part of the lung and that edema is more uniformly distributed along the gravitational axis. There was also no change in FRC or regional diaphragm movement. The explanation for the decreased shunting seen with the prone position seems to be that the gravitational distribution of pleural pressure is much more uniform in the prone position. In the supine position the gravitational forces result in pleural pressure becoming positive in the dependent lung regions and dorsal lung units being below closing volume. This finding suggests that transpulmonary pressure may not exceed airway pressure in this region resulting in lung collapse. The gravitational pleural pressure differences in the thorax are much less in the prone position resulting in less of the lung being below closing volume and decreased shunt.

The clinical and physiological studies seem to suggest that there may be a benefit in terms of gas exchange from changing from the supine to the prone position when ventilating patients with hypoxemia due to ARDS.[98-104] Translating this into an outcome benefit has proved more challenging. In the largest study in adults where patients with a P/F ratio were randomized to prone position ventilation for 6 or more hours out of 24 there was no difference in outcome although there was a consistent and reproducible improvement in oxygenation.[105] However, a subgroup analysis showed that there was a significant reduction in mortality (20 versus 40%) in those patients with the worst oxygenation defect (P/F <82). This potential to improve the outcome in the most severely hypoxemic patients was confirmed in a recently published meta-analysis of ten RCTs. This concluded that there was a survival benefit in the most severely hypoxemic patients (PaO$_2$/FiO$_2$ <100 mmHg).[106]

Studies in children with ARDS or AHRF are relatively few. Prospective case series demonstrate a high response rate in terms of improvement in oxygenation[107-109] and Kornecki[110] found a similar effect in a small randomized trial. An RCT of prone positioning in children with ALI in which patients were ventilated in the prone position for 20 hours each day compared with supine position showed no benefit on survival.[77] However, the clinical studies would suggest that prone position ventilation, while not benefiting all patients, should be included in the algorithm for the management of patients with severe hypoxemia.

Adjuncts to Positive Pressure Ventilation

Surfactant Replacement Therapy

Surfactant deficiency as the cause of AHRF in premature newborn infants was first described over 30 years ago. The lack of surfactant causes an increase in surface tension forces at alveolar level and the diffusely atelectatic lung that is so typically seen in this disease. If these surface tension forces are reduced with the administration of surfactant, then the tendency for these alveoli to collapse will be reduced and ventilation can be applied at lower peak airway pressures. With the development of naturally occurring and synthetic surfactants

this has now become a reality. Few therapies in the treatment of AHRF in any age group have undergone such extensive study as surfactant replacement therapy in IRDS. There are now over 30 published RCTs of either synthetic or naturally occurring surfactant given at the time of delivery or shortly thereafter. These have been reviewed in a meta-analysis by Jobe[111] which concluded that surfactant replacement therapy has reduced the mortality in premature infants with IRDS. As well as this, most controlled trials have been able to demonstrate a reduction in other complications associated with prematurity, such as pneumothorax, intraventricular hemorrhage, and patent ductus arteriosus The data on the incidence of bronchopulmonary dysplasia is less convincing. Some studies have shown a reduction in the incidence while others have not. Be that as it may, surfactant replacement therapy remains one of the few unqualified success stories in the treatment of neonates with AHRF over the past 20 years.

The place of surfactant replacement therapy outside the newborn is less clear. Since the first descriptions of ARDS in the 1960s it has been recognized that there were surfactant abnormalities in the lungs of these patients without clear evidence of deficiency. There is abundant experimental and clinical evidence to show that surfactant is inactivated in ARDS, probably secondary to the protein leak into the alveolus. Samples of broncho-alveolar lavage fluid taken from adult patients with ARDS and postmortem lung lavage studies in patients who died with ARDS have shown changes in the surfactant protein and phospholipid concentration and altered surface tension behavior of the fluid.[112] Although the administration of surfactant can be shown to improve oxygenation and compliance in experimental models of ARDS, showing benefit in humans with ARDS has proved more problematic. An RCT of nebulized Exosurf in adult patients with sepsis-induced ARDS demonstrated no benefit.[113] Although this result was disappointing, it may be premature to dismiss surfactant replacement therapy as ineffective. Not all surfactants are equally efficacious and the synthetic varieties which do not have any of the surfactant proteins (A, B, or C) may be less than ideal in this situation. A prospective randomized controlled open label trial of bovine surfactant in adult patients with ARDS patients showed superior gas exchange and improved survival in the surfactant treated patients.[114] However, a larger prospective RCT of recombinant surfactant replacement therapy in ARDS showed no benefit.[115]

The situation is somewhat more promising in children. Case series and randomized studies suggest that some patients with AHRF may see an improvement in oxygenation with surfactant replacement therapy.[116-118] In a recent RCT of a natural surfactant containing both proteins B and C (Calfactant) Wilson found that mortality was lower in those patients receiving surfactant (19 vs 36%) without any difference in ventilator free days, which was the primary end point of the study.[54] The greatest difference in mortality was seen in those patients who were less than 12 months of age. This again underscores that the epidemiology of ARDS/ALI in this age group is more likely to be single system lung disease where lung specific therapy is likely to have the greatest impact on outcome. Dramatic responses to surfactant replacement therapy have been reported in immuno-suppressed children with pneumocystis pneumonitis.[116,117,119] However, there is no clear evidence to support its routine use in children with ARDS. As well as being a very expensive therapy, its use is not without risk.

Inhaled Nitric Oxide (iNO)

Few therapies in critical care medicine in the past 20 years have generated the interest and enthusiasm surrounding the medical use of inhaled nitric oxide. Since the first experiments in the 1970s which described the vital role played by the intact endothelium in inducing vascular

dilatation and the subsequent identification of NO as endothelial derived relaxing factor there has been rapid progression through experimental studies which have demonstrated that inhaled NO is a highly selective pulmonary vasodilator to its introduction into clinical medicine. It has now become evident that nitric oxide is a biologically important compound with ubiquitous actions that involve multiple organ systems. Nitric oxide is synthetized from L-arginine by the enzyme nitric oxide synthetase (NOS). NO is then diffused rapidly from the endothelial cell into the vascular smooth muscle where it stimulates guanylate cyclase to produce cyclic guanosine monophosphate (CGMP), a potent vasodilator. The systemic nitrodilators currently in clinical use work by a similar mechanism but their pulmonary vasodilator effects cannot be separated from the systemic. In the case of iNO the vasodilator properties are confined to the pulmonary circulation because the marked affinity of NO for the heme moiety of hemoglobin results in its rapid binding and inactivation as soon as it crosses the alveolar capillary membrane. Nitric oxide is a very unstable molecule which reacts with oxygen to form higher oxides of nitrogen, the most toxic of which is nitrogen dioxide. The speed of this reaction is proportional to both the concentration of oxygen and the duration of exposure and is greatly enhanced by high inspired oxygen concentrations.

The initial animal experiments on NO demonstrated its remarkable ability to selectively dilate the pulmonary vascular bed after pulmonary vasoconstriction had been induced by either inhalation of a hypoxic gas mixture or the infusion of the potent vasoconstrictor thromboxane. In these studies there seemed to be a dose dependent vasodilator effect as the inhaled concentration was increased from 10 up to 80 ppm.

There has also been increasing experience in the use of iNO as part of the ventilatory management of both pediatric and adult patients with ARDS. In this situation pulmonary hypertension is secondary to the inflammatory mediated release of pulmonary vasoconstrictors, the development of pulmonary microthrombi, and areas of local ventilation-perfusion mismatch, rather than being the primary pathophysiological disturbance. Again the published studies represent experience of its use as rescue therapy in non-controlled clinical trials, often as an adjunct to other alternative ventilation therapies. Most of these show a pulmonary vasodilator effect with a fall in pulmonary vascular resistance in the range of 20-30% and an improvement in oxygenation secondary to an improvement in ventilation-perfusion matching.[120-126] Although the introduction of iNO frequently allows for adjustment of ventilator settings to levels of airway pressure and inspired oxygen less associated with secondary lung injury it remains to be seen whether there will be a reduction in mortality in syndrome that is associated with multiple organ failure and where hypoxemia is frequently not the mode of death. There are also concerns about the safety of adding iNO in situations where sepsis is frequently the underlying etiology, given the fact that septic shock has been shown to be associated with the overproduction of endogenous NO. The conversion of nitric oxide to peroxynitrite, which has been shown to damage type 2 alveolar epithelial cells, is also potentially hazardous in the already injured lung.[127]

There are now at least six published RCTs of inhaled nitric oxide in adult patients with ARDS.[128-133] While most have shown an improvement in oxygenation in a significant number of patients, this is frequently not sustained and none has shown a benefit in terms of increased survival. The most recent randomized 385 patients with hypoxemia and P/F <250 to receive either 5ppm iNO or placebo gas, having excluded patients with sepsis and multi-organ failure.[131] There was no difference in outcome as measured by survival and time off assisted ventilation. Randomized studies and case series in pediatric patients with AHRF have reached

similar conclusions.[120-123,134-136] Having said this iNO may still have a place in the treatment algorithm for severe hypoxemia because there are a small minority of patients that demonstrate a dramatic improvement in oxygenation. Perhaps the most effective way of delivery of this gas is to use it in combination with HFOV. Studies in both adults and children suggest that this technique of lung recruitment allows for more effective delivery of iNO at alveolar level than with conventional ventilation.[137,138] A summary of the published literature would support a short trial of iNO in severe hypoxemia which would be discontinued unless such a response is seen, bearing in mind that the therapy is expensive and not without potential harmful effects. Aside from this there clearly is no benefit from the routine use of iNO in this patient population.[139,140]

NonInvasive Ventilation

One of the most important innovations in mechanical ventilation in the past ten years has been the widespread use of noninvasive ventilation (NIV) in acute respiratory failure. First introduced into clinical medicine as CPAP by Gregory[6] in 1971 for the management of lung disease of prematurity it has only been reintroduced into the management of older children and adults with acute respiratory failure relatively recently.[141-146] The potential advantages include avoidance of endotracheal intubation together with the need to use sedating and paralyzing drugs and the reduction in the incidence of sinusitis, sepsis and nosocomial pneumonia. In patients with heart failure NIV also has a beneficial effect on cardiac function by decreasing left ventricular afterload.[147] There have been a number of randomized trials in adults comparing early use of NIV in acutely ill patients with AHRF to standard care, which usually consists of oxygen by face mask or endotracheal intubation and positive pressure ventilation. The results of these have been somewhat conflicting. Most show improvement in oxygenation with the use of NIV but in terms of intubation rates, duration of ICU stay and mortality some suggest benefit and others are neutral.[148-150] Studies of the use of NIV in the management of adult patients who fail extubation show that it does not decrease the need for reintubation.[151,152] However, there seems to be a more clearly demonstrated benefit in immunocompromised patients and those with malignancies where case series and randomized trials have shown that early intervention improves outcome.[148,153-155] A summary of the accumulated experience with NIV in ICU patients would indicate that early intervention in patients who are tachypneic and hypoxemic before they develop hypercarbia and multiorgan dysfunction increases the likelihood for the avoidance of intubation and a potential outcome benefit.[143,146,156]

There is far less published pediatric experience with NIV, which mostly consists of case series but there is an accumulating experience which would suggest that in selected patients its early use may avoid the need for intubation.[144,157-161]

Extra-Pulmonary Therapies in ARDS

Steroids and Fluids

Since ARDS is a multiorgan syndrome rather than a lung specific disease it stands to reason that there are a number of non-pulmonary interventions that may have an important impact on outcome. Meduri and colleagues have published a number of nonrandomized clinical studies of the use of steroids in the late "proliferative" phase of ARDS.[162] Patients are typically beyond the first week of their illness and are characterized by signs of an inflammatory phase with fever, elevated white cell counts and evidence of fibroblast infiltration on lung biopsy. In a randomized, placebo-controlled trial Meduri showed improved survival and a reduced incidence of organ dysfunction in a

study of only 26 patients.[163] This finding has to be interpreted with some caution because it has not been confirmed in a much larger multicenter study and the routine use of steroids cannot be recommended in patients with ARDS.[164]

One of the features of ARDS in any age group is the increased degree of endothelial permeability that leads to the leakage of protein rich fluid into the alveolar space leading to atelectasis. A standard approach to this problem has been fluid restriction and the use of diuretic therapy to "dry out" the lung. Clinical studies in adults have suggested that this approach may improve oxygenation without there being any measurable impact on survival.[165,166] Martin, in a randomized trial of patients who were hypoproteinemic, has shown that the combination of albumin and Lasix improves gas exchange and fluid balance.[167] The potential flaw associated with this is of sacrificing non-pulmonary organ function in order to achieve a better PaO_2. If the net effect is volume contraction, reduced cardiac output and decreased tissue oxygen delivery there is no net gain for the patient. Furthermore, the overenthusiastic use of diuretics and fluid restriction may push patients into renal failure which would have a major impact on outcome. A large RCT of conservative versus liberal fluid management strategy in adult patients with ALI showed no difference in mortality but reduced number of days on mechanical ventilation.[168] Therefore the issue of the "wet" lung versus the "dry" lung is still unresolved.

Acute Hypoxic Respiratory Failure – A Treatment Algorithm Based on Assessment of Severity and Indications for ECMO

Although the mortality of AHRF in children is approximately half that in adults, there are still groups of patients where the outcome is poor. These include patients with immunosuppression and suspected sepsis who frequently have multisystem organ dysfunction where the mode of death may not be hypoxemia.

However changes in ventilation strategies can have a significant impact on survival which has seen the survival in bone marrow transplant patients increase from 10 to over 40% in some series.[169-177] This leads to a reconsideration of whether ECMO is indicated for this patient group.[178] A second group with a very poor prognosis are infants with pertussis and pulmonary hypertension where ECMO has been particularly unsuccessful.[179-183] Implementation of a ventilation algorithm based on the severity of the oxygenation defect should guide decision making as to when to implement a change in ventilation strategy. Both the OI and the P/F ratio have been shown to be predictive of outcome and success in extubation in pediatric studies of AHRF.[51,53] Therefore a rising OI or a falling P/F ratio should be used to track the severity of the oxygenation defect and trigger the next step in the ventilation algorithm similar to the one described by Ullrich for adults with ARDS.[184] A similar protocol for pediatric patients would include the early use of NIV, pressure limited ventilation with high PEEP, HFOV, prone position ventilation, iNO, surfactant replacement therapy, and the consideration of ECMO where the patient remains hypoxemic with an OI that is rising. Also cooling febrile, hypoxemic patients in order to decrease oxygen consumption can be an effective strategy.[185]

The place of ECMO in the management algorithm of AHRF of children outside the newborn period is difficult to define. Outcome figures based on the ELSO Registry figures suggest an overall survival of around 40-50%, with single institution survival as high as 70-80%.[186-189] The problem with interpreting these sorts of data is that they are center-specific and do not account for widely different ventilation practices. While there is no debate that ECMO can be life saving therapy, the difficulty lies in what constitutes oxygenation failure in an era of various alternative ventilation strategies. The data on ventilator-induced lung injury suggests that sometimes the patient is being rescued from the therapy rather than the disease. The most successful ECMO outcomes will be in those patients with single system lung disease and the worst will be in those with hypoxia and multiple organ failure.

Summary

This review of pediatric AHRF has as its premise the frequently overlooked fact that ventilators do not cure lung disease, in fact they do the opposite. For too long mechanical ventilation has been guided by normal lung physiology with escalations in volume and pressure to achieve "normal" blood gases. We must now recognize that this approach may be inherently harmful and that the ventilator strategy in these patients must be adapted to match the underlying pathophysiology of the lung. Limitation of airway pressure and allowing some degree of hypercarbia is already paying dividends in improved survival in the management of status asthmaticus where mortality rates in the 1970s were 25-50% in patients requiring ventilation. In ARDS the "open lung" strategy with prevention of overdistention would seem to have the most to offer. This is particularly true in HFOV where the early application of an aggressive volume recruitment strategy followed by a reduction of mean airway pressure can be highly effective.

Determining improvement in outcome with changing ventilation practice will prove more difficult as it is a syndrome with a multiplicity of causes rather than a single disease entity. Non-conventional ventilation techniques probably have the most to offer patients with hypoxia due to single system pulmonary failure whilst those with immunosuppression and multiple organ dysfunction would be expected to benefit least. Given the multiplicity of therapies now available, there is a need for large well designed multicenter studies in children to determine what are truly effective and at what stage in the disease process they should be introduced.

References

1. Lassen HCA. A preliminary report on the 1952 epidemic of poliomyelitis in Copenhagen with special reference to the treatment of acute respiratory insufficiency. Lancet. 1953;1:37-41.

2. Bernard GR, Artigas A, Brigham KL, Carlet J, Falke K, Hudson L, et al. The American-European Consensus Conference on ARDS. American Journal of Respirology & Critical Care Medicine. 1994;149:818-24.

3. Bendixen HH, Hedley-Whyte J, Laver MB. Impaired oxygenation in surgical patients during general anaesthesia with controlled ventilation. N Engl J Med. 1963;269:991-6.

4. Froese A, Bryan AC. Effects of anaesthesia and paralysis on diaphragmatic mechanics in man. Anesthesiology. 1974;41:242-55.

5. Ashbaugh DG, Bigelow DB, Petty TL, Levine BE. Acute respiratory distress in adults. Lancet. 1967 Aug 12;2(7511):319-23.

6. Gregory GA, Kitterman JA, Phibbs RH, Tooley WH, Hamiliton WK. Treatment of the idiopathic respiratory-distress syndrome with continuous positive airway pressure. N Engl J Med. 1971;284:1333-9.

7. Suter PM, Fairley HB, Isenberg MD. Optimum end expiratory airway pressure in patients with acute pulmonary failure. New England Journal of Medicine. 1975;292:284.

8. Gattinoni L, Pelosi P, Vitale G, Presenti A, D'Andrea L, Mascheroni D. Body position changes redistribute lung computed-tomographic density in patients with acute respiratory failure. Anesthesiology. 1991;74:15-23.

9. Gattinoni L, Pesenti A, Bombino M, Baglioni S, Rivolta M, Rossi F, et al. Relationships between lung computed tomographic density, gas exchange, and PEEP in acute respiratory failure. Anesthesiology. 1988;69:824-32.

10. Webb HH, Tierney DF. Experimental pulmonary edema due to intermittent positive pressure ventilation with high inflation pressures. Protection by positive end-expiratory pressure. Am Rev Respir Dis. 1974;110:556-65.

11. Dreyfuss D, Basset G, Soler P, Saumon G. Intermittent positive pressure hyperventilation with high inflation pressures produces pulmonary microvascular injury in rats. Am Rev Respir Dis. 1985; 132: 880-4.

12. Kolobow T, Moretti MP, Fumagalli R, Mascheroni D, Prato P, Chen V, et al. Severe impairment in lung function induced by high peak airway pressure during mechanical ventilation. Am Rev Respir Dis. 1987;135:312-31.

13. Tsuno K, Prato P, Kolobow T. Acute lung injury from mechanical ventilation atmoderately high airway pressures. J Appl Physiol. 1990;69:956-61.

14. Dreyfuss D, Soler P, Basset G, Saumon G. High inflation pulmonary edema: effects of high airway pressure, high tidal volume and positive end-expiratory pressure. Am Rev Respir Dis. 1988;137:1159-64.

15. Hernandez LA, Coker PJ, May S, Thompson AL, Parker JC. Mechanical ventilation increases microvascular permeability in oleic acid-injured lungs. J Appl Physiol. 1990 Dec;69(6):2057-61.

16. Hernandez LA, Peevy KJ, Moise AA, Parker JC. Chest wall restriction limits high airway pressure-induced lung injury in young rabbits. J App Physiol. 1989; 66: 2364-8.

17. Corbridge TC, Wood LDH, Crawford GP, Chudoba MJ, Yanos J, Sznajder JI. Adverse effects of large tidal volume

and low PEEP in canine acid aspiration. American Review of Respiratory Disease. 1990;142(2):311-5.

18. Sandhar BK, Niblett DJ, Argiras EP, Dunnill MS, Sykes MK. Effects of positive end expiratory pressure on hyaline membrane formation in a rabbit model of the neonatal respiratory distress syndrome. Intensive Care Med. 1988;14:538-46.

19. Muscedere JG, Mullen JB, Gan K, Slutsky AS. Tidal ventilation at low airway pressures can augment lung injury. Am J Respir Crit Care Med. 1994;149(5):1327-34.

20. Tremblay L, Valenza F, Ribeiro S, Li J, Slutsky A. Injurious ventilatory strategies increase cytokines and c-fos m-RNA expression in an isolated rat lung model. Journal of Clinical Investigation. 1997;99(5):944-52.

21. Coalson JJ. Experimental models of bronchopulmonary dysplasia. Biol Neonate. 1997;71 Suppl 1:35-8.

22. Coalson JJ, King RJ, Winter VT, Prihoda TJ, Anzueto AR, Peters JI, et al. O2- and pneumonia-induced lung injury. I. Pathological and morphometric studies. J Appl Physiol. 1989 Jul;67(1):346-56.

23. Coalson JJ, Kuehl TJ, Prihoda TJ, deLemos RA. Diffuse alveolar damage in the evolution of bronchopulmonary dysplasia in the baboon. Pediatr Res. 1988 Sep;24(3):357-66.

24. Crapo JD, Hayatdavoudi G, Knapp MJ, Fracica PJ, Wolfe WG, Piantadosi CA. Progressive alveolar septal injury in primates exposed to 60% oxygen for 14 days. Am J Physiol. 1994 Dec;267(6 Pt 1):L797-806.

25. de los Santos R, Coalson JJ, Holcomb JR, Johanson WG, Jr. Hyperoxia exposure in mechanically ventilated primates with and without previous lung injury. Exp Lung Res. 1985;9(3-4):255-75.

26. de los Santos R, Seidenfeld JJ, Anzueto A, Collins JF, Coalson JJ, Johanson WG, Jr., et al. One hundred percent oxygen lung injury in adult baboons. Am Rev Respir Dis. 1987 Sep;136(3):657-61.

27. Delemos RA, Coalson JJ, Gerstmann DR, Kuehl TJ, Null DM, Jr. Oxygen toxicity in the premature baboon with hyaline membrane disease. Am Rev Respir Dis. 1987;136(3):677-82.

28. Fracica PJ, Knapp MJ, Piantadosi CA, Takeda K, Fulkerson WJ, Coleman RE, et al. Responses of baboons to prolonged hyperoxia: physiology and qualitative pathology. J Appl Physiol. 1991 Dec;71(6):2352-62.

29. Sackner MA, Landa J, Hirsch J, Zapata A. Pulmonary effects of oxygen breathing. A 6-hour study in normal men. Ann Intern Med. 1975 Jan;82(1):40-3.

30. Yusa T, Crapo JD, Freeman BA. Hyperoxia enhances lung and liver nuclear superoxide generation. Biochim Biophys Acta. 1984 Apr 10;798(2):167-74.

31. Davis WB, Rennard SI, Bitterman PB, Crystal RG. Pulmonary oxygen toxicity. Early reversible changes in human alveolar structures induced by hyperoxia. N Engl J Med. 1983 Oct 13;309(15):878-83.

32. Gattinoni L, Pelosi P, Suter PM, Pedoto A, Vercesi P, Lissoni A. Acute respiratory distress syndrome caused by pulmonary and extrapulmonary disease. Different syndromes? Am J Respir Crit Care Med. 1998;158(1):3-11.

33. Doyle RL, Szaflarski N, Modin GW, Wiener-Kronish JP, Matthay MA. Identification of patients with acute lung injury. Predictors of mortality. Am J Respir Crit Care Med. 1995 Dec;152(6 Pt 1):1818-24.

34. Estenssoro E, Dubin A, Laffaire E, Canales H, Saenz G, Moseinco M, et al. Incidence, clinical course, and outcome

in 217 patients with acute respiratory distress syndrome. Crit Care Med. 2002 Nov;30(11):2450-6.

35. Ferguson ND, Frutos-Vivar F, Esteban A, Anzueto A, Alia I, Brower RG, et al. Airway pressures, tidal volumes, and mortality in patients with acute respiratory distress syndrome. Crit Care Med. 2005 Jan;33(1):21-30.

36. Monchi M, Bellenfant F, Cariou A, Joly LM, Thebert D, Laurent I, et al. Early predictive factors of survival in the acute respiratory distress syndrome. A multivariate analysis. Am J Respir Crit Care Med. 1998 Oct;158(4):1076-81.

37. Roupie E, Lepage E, Wysocki M, Fagon JY, Chastre J, Dreyfuss D, et al. Prevalence, etiologies and outcome of the acute respiratory distress syndrome among hypoxemic ventilated patients. SRLF Collaborative Group on Mechanical Ventilation. Societe de Reanimation de Langue Francaise. Intensive Care Med. 1999 Sep;25(9):920-9.

38. Suchyta MR, Clemmer TP, Elliott CG, Orme JF, Jr., Weaver LK. The adult respiratory distress syndrome. A report of survival and modifying factors. Chest. 1992 Apr;101(4):1074-9.

39. Zilberberg MD, Epstein SK. Acute lung injury in the medical ICU: comorbid conditions, age, etiology, and hospital outcome. Am J Respir Crit Care Med. 1998 Apr;157(4 Pt 1):1159-64.

40. Amato MBP, Barbas CSV, Medeiros DM, Magaldi RB, Schettino G, Lorenzi-Filho G, et al. Effect of a protective-ventilation strategy on mortality in the acute respiratory distress syndrome. N Engl J Med. 1998;338(6):347-54.

41. Brochard L, Roudot-Thoraval F, Roupie E, Delclaux C, Chastre J, Fernandez-Mondejar E, et al. Tidal volume reduction for prevention of ventilator-induced lung injury in acute respiratory distress

syndrome. The Multicenter Trail Group on Tidal Volume reduction in ARDS. Am J Respir Crit Care Med. 1998 Dec;158(6):1831-8.

42. Brower RG, Shanholtz CB, Fessler HE, Shade DM, White P, Jr., Wiener CM, et al. Prospective, randomized, controlled clinical trial comparing traditional versus reduced tidal volume ventilation in acute respiratory distress syndrome patients [see comments]. Crit Care Med. 1999;27(8):1492-8.

43. Stewart TE, Meade MO, Cook DJ, Granton JT, Hodder RV, Lapinsky SE, et al. Evaluation of a ventilation strategy to prevent barotrauma in patients at high risk for acute respiratory distress syndrome. Pressure- and Volume-Limited Ventilation Strategy Group. N Engl J Med. 1998;338(6):355-61.

44. Ventilation with lower tidal volumes as compared with traditional tidal volumes for acute lung injury and the acute respiratory distress syndrome. The Acute Respiratory Distress Syndrome Network. N Engl J Med. 2000 May 4;342(18):1301-8.

45. Davis SL, Furman DP, Costarino AT. Adult respiratory distress syndrome in children: Associated disease, clinical course, and predictors of death. J Pediatr. 1993;123:35-45.

46. Rivera RA, Butt W, Shann F. Predictors of mortality in children with respiratory failure: possible indications for ECMO. Anaesthesia & Intensive Care. 1990;18:385-9.

47. Tamburro RF, Bugnitz MC, Stidham GL. Alveolar-arterial oxygen gradient as a predictor of outcome in patients with nonneonatal pediatric respiratory failure. Journal of Pediatrics. 1991;119:935-8.

48. Timmons OD, Dean JM, Vernon DD. Mortality rates and prognostic variables

in children with adult respiratory distress syndrome. J Pediatr. 1991;119:896-9.

49. Dahlem P, van Aalderen WM, Hamaker ME, Dijkgraaf MG, Bos AP. Incidence and short-term outcome of acute lung injury in mechanically ventilated children. Eur Respir J. 2003 Dec;22(6):980-5.

50. Fackler JC, Bohn D, Green TP, Heulitt M, Hirshl R, Klein M, et al. ECMO for ARDS; stopping a RCT. Am J Respir Crit Care Med. 1997;155(A504).

51. Flori HR, Glidden DV, Rutherford GW, Matthay MA. Pediatric acute lung injury: prospective evaluation of risk factors associated with mortality. Am J Respir Crit Care Med. 2005 May 1;171(9):995-1001.

52. Peters MJ, Tasker RC, Kiff KM, Yates R, Hatch DJ. Acute hypoxemic respiratory failure in children: case mix and the utility of respiratory severity indices. Intensive Care Med. 1998 Jul;24(7):699-705.

53. Trachsel D, McCrindle BW, Nakagawa S, Bohn DJ. Oxygenation Index Predicts Outcome in Children with Acute Hypoxemic Respiratory Failure. Am J Respir Crit Care Med. 2005;172(2):206-11.

54. Willson DF, Thomas NJ, Markovitz BP, Bauman LA, DiCarlo JV, Pon S, et al. Effect of exogenous surfactant (calfactant) in pediatric acute lung injury: a randomized controlled trial. Jama. 2005 Jan 26;293(4):470-6.

55. Albuali WH, Singh RN, Fraser DD, Seabrook JA, Kavanagh BP, Parshuram CS, et al. Have changes in ventilation practice improved outcome in children with acute lung injury? Pediatr Crit Care Med. 2007 Jul;8(4):324-30.

56. Erickson S, Schibler A, Numa A, Nuthall G, Yung M, Pascoe E, et al. Acute lung injury in pediatric intensive care in Australia and New Zealand: a prospective, multicenter, observational study. Pediatr Crit Care Med. 2007 Jul;8(4):317-23.

57. Randolph AG. Management of acute lung injury and acute respiratory distress syndrome in children. Crit Care Med. 2009 Aug;37(8):2448-54.

58. Timmons OD, Havens PL, Fackler JC. Predicting death in pediatric patients with acute respiratory failure. Pediatric Critical Care Study Group. Extracorporeal Life Support Organization. Chest. 1995;108(3):789-97.

59. Green TP, Timmons OD, Fackler JC, Moler FW, Thompson AE, Sweeney MF. The impact of extracorporeal membrane oxygenation on survival in pediatric patients with acute respiratory failure. Pediatric Critical Care Study Group. Crit Care Med. 1996;24(2):323-9.

60. Sokol J, Jacobs SE, Bohn D. Inhaled nitric oxide for acute hypoxemic respiratory failure in children and adults (Cochrane Review). Cochrane Database Syst Rev. 2003(1):CD002787.

61. Darioli R, Perret C. Mechanical controlled hypoventilation in status asthmaticus. Am Rev Respir Dis. 1984;129(3):385-7.

62. Hickling KG, Henderson SJ, Jackson R. Low mortality associated with low volume pressure limited ventilation with permissive hypercapnia in severe adult respiratory distress syndrome. Intensive Care Med. 1990;16(6):372-7.

63. Wung JT, James LS, Kilchevsky E, James E. Management of infants with severe respiratory failure and persistence of the fetal circulation, without hyperventilation. Pediatrics. 1985 Oct;76(4):488-94.

64. Laffey JG, Kavanagh BP. Carbon dioxide and the critically ill--too little of a good thing? Lancet. 1999 Oct 9;354(9186):1283-6.

65. Laffey JG, Kavanagh BP. Hypocapnia. N Engl J Med. 2002 Jul 4;347(1):43-53.

66. Shibata K, Cregg N, Engelberts D, Takeuchi A, Fedorko L, Kavanagh BP. Hypercapnic acidosis may attenuate acute lung injury by inhibition of endogenous xanthine oxidase. Am J Respir Crit Care Med. 1998 Nov;158(5 Pt 1):1578-84.

67. Laffey JG, Engelberts D, Duggan M, Veldhuizen R, Lewis JF, Kavanagh BP. Carbon dioxide attenuates pulmonary impairment resulting from hyperventilation. Crit Care Med. 2003 Nov;31(11):2634-40.

68. Laffey JG, Engelberts D, Kavanagh BP. Injurious effects of hypocapnic alkalosis in the isolated lung. Am J Respir Crit Care Med. 2000 Aug;162(2 Pt 1):399-405.

69. Laffey JG, Engelberts D, Kavanagh BP. Buffering hypercapnic acidosis worsens acute lung injury. Am J Respir Crit Care Med. 2000 Jan;161(1):141-6.

70. Laffey JG, Jankov RP, Engelberts D, Tanswell AK, Post M, Lindsay T, et al. Effects of therapeutic hypercapnia on mesenteric ischemia-reperfusion injury. Am J Respir Crit Care Med. 2003 Dec 1;168(11):1383-90.

71. Laffey JG, Tanaka M, Engelberts D, Luo X, Yuan S, Tanswell AK, et al. Therapeutic hypercapnia reduces pulmonary and systemic injury following in vivo lung reperfusion. Am J Respir Crit Care Med. 2000 Dec;162(6):2287-94.

72. Goldstein B, Shannon DC, Todres ID. Supercarbia in children: Clinical course and outcome. Crit Care Med. 1990;18:166-8.

73. Ranieri VM, Suter PM, Tortorella C, De Tullio R, Dayer JM, Brienza A, et al. Effect of mechanical ventilation on inflammatory mediators in patients with acute respiratory distress syndrome: a randomized controlled trial. Jama. 1999 Jul 7;282(1):54-61.

74. Eichacker PQ, Gerstenberger EP, Banks SM, Cui X, Natanson C. Meta-analysis of acute lung injury and acute respiratory distress syndrome trials testing low tidal volumes. Am J Respir Crit Care Med. 2002 Dec 1;166(11):1510-4.

75. Parshuram CS, Kavanagh BP. Positive clinical trials: understand the control group before implementing the result. Am J Respir Crit Care Med. 2004 Aug 1;170(3):223-6.

76. Hager DN, Krishnan JA, Hayden DL, Brower RG. Tidal volume reduction in patients with acute lung injury when plateau pressures are not high. Am J Respir Crit Care Med. 2005 Nov 15;172(10):1241-5.

77. Curley MA, Hibberd PL, Fineman LD, Wypij D, Shih MC, Thompson JE, et al. Effect of prone positioning on clinical outcomes in children with acute lung injury: a randomized controlled trial. JAMA. 2005 Jul 13;294(2):229-37.

78. Kissoon N, Rimensberger PC, Bohn D. Ventilation strategies and adjunctive therapy in severe lung disease. Pediatr Clin North Am. 2008 Jun;55(3):709-33, xii.

79. Brower RG, Lanken PN, MacIntyre N, Matthay MA, Morris A, Ancukiewicz M, et al. Higher versus lower positive end-expiratory pressures in patients with the acute respiratory distress syndrome. N Engl J Med. 2004 Jul 22;351(4):327-36.

80. Meade MO, Cook DJ, Guyatt GH, Slutsky AS, Arabi YM, Cooper DJ, et al. Ventilation strategy using low tidal volumes, recruitment maneuvers, and high positive end-expiratory pressure for acute lung injury and acute respiratory distress syndrome: a randomized controlled trial. Jama. 2008 Feb 13;299(6):637-45.

81. Mercat A, Richard JC, Vielle B, Jaber S, Osman D, Diehl JL, et al. Positive end-expiratory pressure setting in adults with acute lung injury and acute respiratory distress syndrome: a randomized controlled trial. Jama. 2008 Feb 13;299(6):646-55.

82. Bohn DJ, Miyasaka K, Marchak BE, Thompson WK, Froese AB, Bryan AC. Ventilation by high-frequency oscillation. J Appl Physiol. 1980 Apr;48(4):710-6.

83. Clark RH, Gerstmann DR, Null DM, deLemos RA. Prospective randomised comparison of high-frequency oscillatory and conventional ventilation in respiratory distress syndrome. Pediatrics. 1992;89:5-12.

84. Gerstmann DR, Minton SD, Stoddard RA, Meredith KS, Monaco F, Bertrand JM, et al. The provo multicenter early high-frequency oscillatory ventilation trial: improved pulmonary and clinical outcome in respiratory distress syndrome. Pediatrics. 1996;98:1044-57.

85. HIFI Study Group. High-frequency oscillatory ventilation compared with conventional mechanical ventilation in the treatment of respiratory failure in preterm infants. N Engl J Med. 1989;320(2):88-93.

86. HiFO Study Group. Randomised study of high-frequency oscillatory ventilation in infants with severe respiratory distress syndrome. J Pediatr. 1993;122:609-19.

87. Ogawa Y, Miyasaka K, Kawano T, Imura S, Inukai K, Okuyama K, et al. A multicenter randomized trial of high frequency oscillatory ventilation as compared with conventional mechanical ventilation in preterm infants with respiratory failure. Early Hum Dev. 1993;32(1):1-10.

88. Rettwitz-Volk W, Veldman A, Roth B, Vierzig A, Kachel W, Varnholt V, et al. A prospective, randomized, multicenter trial of high-frequency oscillatory ventilation compared with conventional ventilation in preterm infants with respiratory distress syndrome receiving surfactant. J Pediatr. 1998;132(2):249-54.

89. Kinsella JP, Truog WE, Walsh WF, Goldberg RN, Bancalari E, Mayock DE, et al. Randomized, multicenter trial of inhaled nitric oxide and high-frequency oscillatory ventilation in severe, persistent pulmonary hypertension of the newborn. J Pediatr. 1997 Jul;131(1 Pt 1):55-62.

90. Clark RH. High-frequency ventilation in acute pediatric respiratory failure. Chest. 1994;105(3):652-3.

91. Carter JM, Gerstmann DR, Clark RH, Snyder G, Cornish JD, Null DM, et al. High-frequency oscillatory ventilation and extracorporeal membrane oxygenation for the treatment of acute neonatal respiratory failure. Pediatrics. 1990;85:159-64.

92. Arnold JH, Truog RD, Thompson JE, Fackler JC. High-frequency oscillatory ventilation in pediatric respiratory failure. Crit Care Med. 1993 Feb;21(2):272-8.

93. Arnold JH, Hanson JH, Toro-Figuero LO, Gutierrez J, Berens RJ, Anglin DL. Prospective, randomized comparison of high-frequency oscillatory ventilation and conventional mechanical ventilation in pediatric respiratory failure [see comments]. Crit Care Med. 1994;22(10):1530-9.

94. Derdak S, Mehta S, Stewart TE, Smith T, Rogers M, Buchman TG, et al. High-frequency oscillatory ventilation for acute respiratory distress syndrome in adults: a randomized, controlled trial. Am J Respir Crit Care Med. 2002 Sep 15;166(6):801-8.

95. Arnold JH, Anas NG, Luckett P, Cheifetz IM, Reyes G, Newth CJ, et al.

High-frequency oscillatory ventilation in pediatric respiratory failure: a multicenter experience. Crit Care Med. 2000;28(12):3913-9.

96. Bryan AC. Conference on the scientific basis of respiratory therapy. Pulmonary physiotherapy in the pediatric age group. Comments of a devil's advocate. Am Rev Respir Dis. 1974;110:143-4.

97. Albert RK, Leasa D, Sanderson M, Robertson HT, Hlastala MP. The prone position improves arterial oxygenation and reduces shunt in oleic-acid-induced acute lung injury. Am Rev Respir Dis. 1987;135:628-33.

98. Blanch L, Mancebo J, Perez M, Martinez M, Mas A, Betbese AJ, et al. Short-term effects of prone position in critically ill patients with acute respiratory distress syndrome. Intensive Care Med. 1997;23(10):1033-9.

99. Chatte G, Sab JM, Dubois JM, Sirodot M, Gaussorgues P, Robert D. Prone position in mechanically ventilated patients with severe acute respiratory failure. Am J Respir Crit Care Med. 1997;155(2):473-8.

100. Douglas WW, Rehder K, Beynen FM, Sessler AD, Marsh HM. Improved oxygenation in patients with acute respiratory failure: the prone position. Am Rev Respir Dis. 1977;115(4):559-66.

101. Fridrich P, Krafft P, Hochleuthner H, Mauritz W. The effects of long-term prone positioning in patients with trauma- induced adult respiratory distress syndrome. Anesth Analg. 1996;83(6):1206-11.

102. Jolliet P, Bulpa P, Chevrolet JC. Effects of the prone position on gas exchange and hemodynamics in severe acute respiratory distress syndrome [see comments]. Crit Care Med. 1998;26(12):1977-85.

103. Langer M, Mascheroni D, Marcolin R, Gattinoni L. The prone position in ARDS patients: a clinical study. Chest. 1988;94(1):103-7.

104. Pappert D, Rossaint R, Slama K, Gruning T, Falke KJ. Influence of positioning on ventilation-perfusion relationships. in severe adult respiratory distress syndrome. Chest. 1994;106(5):1511-6.

105. Gattinoni L, Tognoni G, Pesenti A, Taccone P, Mascheroni D, Labarta V, et al. Effect of prone positioning on the survival of patients with acute respiratory failure. N Engl J Med. 2001 Aug 23;345(8):568-73.

106. Sud S, Friedrich JO, Taccone P, Polli F, Adhikari NK, Latini R, et al. Prone ventilation reduces mortality in patients with acute respiratory failure and severe hypoxemia: systematic review and meta-analysis. Intensive Care Med. 2010 Apr;36(4):585-99.

107. Casado-Flores J, Martinez de Azagra A, Ruiz-Lopez MJ, Ruiz M, Serrano A. Pediatric ARDS: effect of supine-prone postural changes on oxygenation. Intensive Care Med. 2002 Dec;28(12):1792-6.

108. Curley MA, Thompson JE, Arnold JH. The effects of early and repeated prone positioning in pediatric patients with acute lung injury. Chest. 2000 Jul;118(1):156-63.

109. Murdoch IA, Storman MO. Improved arterial oxygenation in children with the adult respiratory distress syndrome: the prone position. Acta Paediatr. 1994;83(10):1043-6.

110. Kornecki A, Frndova H, Coates AL, Shemie SD. A randomized trial of prolonged prone positioning in children with acute respiratory failure. Chest. 2001 Jan;119(1):211-8.

111. Jobe AH. Pulmonary surfactant therapy. N Engl J Med. 1993;328(12):861-8.

112. Gregory TJ, Longmore WJ, Moxley MA, Whitsett JA, Reed CR, Fowler AAd, et al. Surfactant chemical composition and biophysical activity in acute respiratory distress syndrome. J Clin Invest. 1991;88(6):1976-81.

113. Anzueto A, Baughman RP, Guntupalli KK, Weg JG, Wiedemann HP, Raventos AA, et al. Aerosolized surfactant in adults with sepsis-induced acute respiratory distress syndrome. Exosurf Acute Respiratory Distress Syndrome Sepsis Study Group. N Engl J Med. 1996;334(22):1417-21.

114. Gregory TJ, Steinberg KP, Spragg R, Gadek JE, Hyers TM, Longmore WJ, et al. Bovine surfactant therapy for patients with acute respiratory distress syndrome. Am J Respir Crit Care Med. 1997;155(4):1309-15.

115. Spragg RG, Lewis JF, Walmrath HD, Johannigman J, Bellingan G, Laterre PF, et al. Effect of recombinant surfactant protein C-based surfactant on the acute respiratory distress syndrome. N Engl J Med. 2004 Aug 26;351(9):884-92.

116. Creery WD, Hashmi A, Hutchison JS, Singh RN. Surfactant therapy improves pulmonary function in infants with Pneumocystis carinii pneumonia and acquired immunodeficiency syndrome. Pediatr Pulmonol. 1997 Nov;24(5):370-3.

117. Herting E, Moller O, Schiffmann JH, Robertson B. Surfactant improves oxygenation in infants and children with pneumonia and acute respiratory distress syndrome. Acta Paediatr. 2002;91(11):1174-8.

118. Moller JC, Schaible T, Roll C, Schiffmann JH, Bindl L, Schrod L, et al. Treatment with bovine surfactant in severe acute respiratory distress syndrome in children: a randomized multi-center study. Intensive Care Med. 2003 Mar;29(3):437-46.

119. Marriage SC, Underhill H, Nadel S. Use of natural surfactant in an HIV-infected infant with Pneumocystis carinii pneumonia. Intensive Care Med. 1996 Jun;22(6):611-2.

120. Abman SH, Griebel JL, Parker DK, Schmidt JM, Swanton D, Kinsella JP. Acute effects of inhaled nitric oxide in children with severe hypoxemic respiratory failure. J Pediatr. 1994 Jun;124(6):881-8.

121. Day RW, Allen EM, Witte MK. A randomised, controlled study of the 1-hour and 24-hour effects of inhaled nitric oxide therapy in children with acute hypoxemic respiratory failure. Chest. 1997;112(5):1324-31.

122. Day RW, Guarin M, Lynch JM, Vernon DD, Dean JM. Inhaled nitric oxide in children with severe lung disease: results of acute and prolonged therapy with two concentrations. Crit Care Med. 1996;24:215-21.

123. Nakagawa TA, Morris A, Gomez RJ, Johnston SJ, Sharkey PT, Zaritsky AL. Dose response to inhaled nitric oxide in pediatric patients with pulmonary hypertension and acute respiratory distress syndrome. J Pediatr. 1997;131:63-9.

124. Goldman AP, Haworth SG, Macrae DJ. Does inhaled nitric oxide suppress endogenous nitric oxide production? J Thorac Cardiovasc Surg. 1996 Aug;112(2):541-2.

125. Rossaint R, Falke KJ, Lopez F, Slama K, Pison U, Zapol WM. Inhaled nitric oxide for the adult respiratory distress syndrome. N Engl J Med. 1993;328(6):399-405.

126. Rossaint R, Gerlach H, Schmidt-Ruhnke H, al e. Efficacy of inhaled nitric oxide in patients with severe ARDS. Chest. 1995;107:1107-15.

127. Haddad IY, Gyorgy P, Hu P, Galliani C, Beckman JS, Matalon S. Quantification of nitrotyrosine levels in lung sections of patients and animals with acute lung injury. J Clin Invest. 1994;94:2407-13.

128. Dellinger RP, Zimmerman JL, Taylor RW, Straube RC, Hauser DL, Criner GJ, et al. Effects of inhaled nitric oxide in patients with acute respiratory distress syndrome: results of a randomized phase II trial. Inhaled Nitric Oxide in ARDS Study Group. Crit Care Med. 1998;26(1):15-23.

129. Lundin S, Mang H, Smithies M, Stenqvist O, Frostell C. Inhalation of nitric oxide in acute lung injury: results of a European multicentre study. The European Study Group of Inhaled Nitric Oxide. Intensive Care Med. 1999 Sep;25(9):911-9.

130. Michael JR, Barton RG, Saffle JR, Mone M, Markewitz BA, Hillier K, et al. Inhaled nitric oxide versus conventional therapy: effect on oxygenation in ARDS. Am J Respir Crit Care Med. 1998 May;157(5 Pt 1):1372-80.

131. Taylor RW, Zimmerman JL, Dellinger RP, Straube RC, Criner GJ, Davis K, Jr., et al. Low-dose inhaled nitric oxide in patients with acute lung injury: a randomized controlled trial. Jama. 2004 Apr 7;291(13):1603-9.

132. Troncy E, Collet JP, Shapiro S, Guimond JG, Blair L, Ducruet T, et al. Inhaled nitric oxide in acute respiratory distress syndrome: a pilot randomized controlled study. Am J Respir Crit Care Med. 1998;157:1483-8.

133. Meade MO, Granton JT, Matte-Martyn A, McRae K, Weaver B, Cripps P, et al. A randomized trial of inhaled nitric oxide to prevent ischemia-reperfusion injury after lung transplantation. Am J Respir Crit Care Med. 2003 Jun 1;167(11):1483-9.

134. Demirakca S, Dotsch J, Knothe C, Magsaam J, Reiter HL, Bauer J, et al. Inhaled nitric oxide in neonatal and pediatric acute respiratory distress syndrome: dose response, prolonged inhalation, and weaning. Crit Care Med. 1996 Nov;24(11):1913-9.

135. Goldman AP, Tasker RC, Hosiasson S, Henrichsen T, Macrae DJ. Early response to inhaled nitric oxide and its relationship to outcome in children with severe hypoxemic respiratory failure. Chest. 1997 Sep;112(3):752-8.

136. Dobyns EL, Cornfield DN, Anas NG, Fortenberry JD, Tasker RC, Lynch A, et al. Multicenter randomized controlled trial of the effects of inhaled nitric oxide therapy on gas exchange in children with acute hypoxemic respiratory failure. J Pediatr. 1999 Apr;134(4):406-12.

137. Dobyns EL, Anas NG, Fortenberry JD, Deshpande J, Cornfield DN, Tasker RC, et al. Interactive effects of high-frequency oscillatory ventilation and inhaled nitric oxide in acute hypoxemic respiratory failure in pediatrics. Crit Care Med. 2002 Nov;30(11):2425-9.

138. Mehta S, MacDonald R, Hallett DC, Lapinsky SE, Aubin M, Stewart TE. Acute oxygenation response to inhaled nitric oxide when combined with high-frequency oscillatory ventilation in adults with acute respiratory distress syndrome. Crit Care Med. 2003 Feb;31(2):383-9.

139. Sokol J, Jacobs SE, Bohn D. Inhaled nitric oxide for acute hypoxic respiratory failure in children and adults: a meta-analysis. Anesth Analg. 2003 Oct;97(4):989-98.

140. Adhikari N, Granton JT. Inhaled nitric oxide for acute lung injury: no place for NO? Jama. 2004 Apr 7;291(13):1629-31.

141. Abou-Shala N, Meduri U. Noninvasive mechanical ventilation in patients with

acute respiratory failure. Crit Care Med. 1996 Apr;24(4):705-15.

142. Antonelli M, Pennisi MA, Conti G. New advances in the use of noninvasive ventilation for acute hypoxaemic respiratory failure. Eur Respir J Suppl. 2003 Aug;42:65s-71s.

143. Brochard L. Mechanical ventilation: invasive versus noninvasive. Eur Respir J Suppl. 2003 Nov;47:31s-7s.

144. Fortenberry JD. Noninvasive ventilation in children with respiratory failure. Crit Care Med. 1998;26(12):2095-6.

145. Teague WG. Noninvasive ventilation in the pediatric intensive care unit for children with acute respiratory failure. Pediatr Pulmonol. 2003 Jun;35(6):418-26.

146. Wysocki M, Antonelli M. Noninvasive mechanical ventilation in acute hypoxaemic respiratory failure. Eur Respir J. 2001 Jul;18(1):209-20.

147. Bradley TD. Continuous positive airway pressure for congestive heart failure. Cmaj. 2000;162(4):535-6.

148. Antonelli M, Conti G, Bufi M, Costa MG, Lappa A, Rocco M, et al. Noninvasive ventilation for treatment of acute respiratory failure in patients undergoing solid organ transplantation: a randomized trial. Jama. 2000 Jan 12;283(2):235-41.

149. Delclaux C, L'Her E, Alberti C, Mancebo J, Abroug F, Conti G, et al. Treatment of acute hypoxemic nonhypercapnic respiratory insufficiency with continuous positive airway pressure delivered by a face mask: A randomized controlled trial. Jama. 2000;284(18):2352-60.

150. Ferrer M, Esquinas A, Leon M, Gonzalez G, Alarcon A, Torres A. Noninvasive ventilation in severe hypoxemic respiratory failure: a randomized clinical trial. Am J Respir Crit Care Med. 2003 Dec 15;168(12):1438-44.

151. Esteban A, Frutos-Vivar F, Ferguson ND, Arabi Y, Apezteguia C, Gonzalez M, et al. Noninvasive positive-pressure ventilation for respiratory failure after extubation. N Engl J Med. 2004 Jun 10;350(24):2452-60.

152. Keenan SP, Powers C, McCormack DG, Block G. Noninvasive positive-pressure ventilation for postextubation respiratory distress: a randomized controlled trial. Jama. 2002 Jun 26;287(24):3238-44.

153. Conti G, Marino P, Cogliati A, Dell'Utri D, Lappa A, Rosa G, et al. Noninvasive ventilation for the treatment of acute respiratory failure in patients with hematologic malignancies: a pilot study. Intensive Care Med. 1998;24(12):1283-8.

154. Hilbert G, Gruson D, Vargas F, Valentino R, Gbikpi-Benissan G, Dupon M, et al. Noninvasive ventilation in immunosuppressed patients with pulmonary infiltrates, fever, and acute respiratory failure. N Engl J Med. 2001 Feb 15;344(7):481-7.

155. Meert AP, Close L, Hardy M, Berghmans T, Markiewicz E, Sculier JP. Noninvasive ventilation: application to the cancer patient admitted in the intensive care unit. Support Care Cancer. 2003 Jan;11(1):56-9.

156. Liesching T, Kwok H, Hill NS. Acute applications of noninvasive positive pressure ventilation. Chest. 2003 Aug;124(2):699-713.

157. Akingbola OA, Hopkins RL. Pediatric noninvasive positive pressure ventilation. Pediatr Crit Care Med. 2001 Apr;2(2):164-9.

158. Akingbola OA, Simakajornboon N, Hadley Jr EF, Hopkins RL. Noninvasive positive-pressure ventilation in pediatric status asthmaticus. Pediatr Crit Care Med. 2002 Apr;3(2):181-4.

159. Cheifetz IM. Invasive and noninvasive pediatric mechanical ventilation. Respir Care. 2003 Apr;48(4):442-53; discussion 53-8.

160. Fortenberry JD, Del Toro J, Jefferson LS, Evey L, Haase D. Management of pediatric acute hypoxemic respiratory insufficiency with bilevel positive pressure (BiPAP) nasal mask ventilation. Chest. 1995 Oct;108(4):1059-64.

161. Essouri S, Chevret L, Durand P, Haas V, Fauroux B, Devictor D. Noninvasive positive pressure ventilation: five years of experience in a pediatric intensive care unit. Pediatr Crit Care Med. 2006 Jul;7(4):329-34.

162. Meduri GU, Chinn AJ, Leeper KV, Wunderink RG, Tolley E, Winer-Muram HT, et al. Corticosteroid rescue treatment of progressive fibroproliferation in late ARDS. Patterns of response and predictors of outcome. Chest. 1994;105(5):1516-27.

163. Meduri GU, Headley AS, Golden E, Carson SJ, Umberger RA, Kelso T, et al. Effect of prolonged methylprednisolone therapy in unresolving acute respiratory distress syndrome. JAMA. 1998;280:159-65.

164. Steinberg KP, Hudson LD, Goodman RB, Hough CL, Lanken PN, Hyzy R, et al. Efficacy and safety of corticosteroids for persistent acute respiratory distress syndrome. N Engl J Med. 2006 Apr 20;354(16):1671-84.

165. Mitchell JP, Schuller D, Calandrino FS, Schuster DP. Improved outcome based on fluid management in critically ill patients requiring pulmonary artery catheterization. Am Rev Respir Dis. 1992;145(5):990-8.

166. Schuster DP. The case for and against fluid restriction and occlusion pressure reduction in adult respiratory distress syndrome. New Horiz 1993. 1993;1(4):478-88.

167. Martin GS, Mangialardi RJ, Wheeler AP, Dupont WD, Morris JA, Bernard GR. Albumin and furosemide therapy in hypoproteinemic patients with acute lung injury. Crit Care Med. 2002 Oct;30(10):2175-82.

168. Wiedemann HP, Wheeler AP, Bernard GR, Thompson BT, Hayden D, deBoisblanc B, et al. Comparison of two fluid-management strategies in acute lung injury. N Engl J Med. 2006 Jun 15;354(24):2564-75.

169. Ben-Abraham R, Paret G, Cohen R, Szold O, Cividalli G, Toren A, et al. Diffuse alveolar hemorrhage following allogeneic bone marrow transplantation in children. Chest. 2003 Aug;124(2):660-4.

170. Diaz de Heredia C, Moreno A, Olive T, Iglesias J, Ortega JJ. Role of the intensive care unit in children undergoing bone marrow transplantation with life-threatening complications. Bone Marrow Transplant. 1999 Jul;24(2):163-8.

171. Feickert HJ, Schepers AK, Rodeck B, Geerlings H, Hoyer PF. Incidence, impact on survival, and risk factors for multi-organ system failure in children following liver transplantation. Pediatr Transplant. 2001 Aug;5(4):266-73.

172. Hagen SA, Craig DM, Martin PL, Plumer DD, Gentile MA, Schulman SR, et al. Mechanically ventilated pediatric stem cell transplant recipients: effect of cord blood transplant and organ dysfunction on outcome. Pediatr Crit Care Med. 2003 Apr;4(2):206-13.

173. Hayes C, Lush RJ, Cornish JM, Foot AM, Henderson J, Jenkins I, et al. The outcome of children requiring admission to an intensive care unit following bone marrow transplantation. Br J Haematol. 1998 Aug;102(3):666-70.

174. Keenan HT, Bratton SL, Martin LD, Crawford SW, Weiss NS. Outcome of children who require mechanical ventilatory support after bone marrow transplantation. Crit Care Med. 2000 Mar;28(3):830-5.

175. Lamas A, Otheo E, Ros P, Vazquez JL, Maldonado MS, Munoz A, et al. Prognosis of child recipients of hematopoietic stem cell transplantation requiring intensive care. Intensive Care Med. 2003 Jan;29(1):91-6.

176. Rossi R, Shemie SD, Calderwood S. Prognosis of pediatric bone marrow transplant recipients requiring mechanical ventilation. Crit Care Med. 1999 Jun;27(6):1181-6.

177. Warwick AB, Mertens AC, Shu XO, Ramsay NK, Neglia JP. Outcomes following mechanical ventilation in children undergoing bone marrow transplantation. Bone Marrow Transplant. 1998 Oct;22(8):787-94.

178. Leahey AM, Bunin NJ, Schears GJ, Smith CA, Flake AW, Sullivan KE. Successful use of extracorporeal membrane oxygenation (ECMO) during BMT for SCID. Bone Marrow Transplant. 1998 Apr;21(8):839-40.

179. Halasa NB, Barr FE, Johnson JE, Edwards KM. Fatal pulmonary hypertension associated with pertussis in infants: does extracorporeal membrane oxygenation have a role? Pediatrics. 2003 Dec;112(6 Pt 1):1274-8.

180. Pooboni S, Roberts N, Westrope C, Jenkins DR, Killer H, Pandya HC, et al. Extracorporeal life support in pertussis. Pediatr Pulmonol. 2003 Oct;36(4):310-5.

181. Skladal D, Horak E, Fruhwirth M, Maurer H, Simma B. Successful treatment of ARDS and severe pulmonary hypertension in a child with Bordetella pertussis infection. Wien Klin Wochenschr. 2004 Nov 30;116(21-22):760-2.

182. Sreenan CD, Osiovich H. Neonatal pertussis requiring extracorporeal membrane oxygenation. Pediatr Surg Int. 2001 Mar;17(2-3):201-3.

183. Williams GD, Numa A, Sokol J, Tobias V, Duffy BJ. ECLS in pertussis: does it have a role? Intensive Care Med. 1998 Oct;24(10):1089-92.

184. Ullrich R, Lorber C, Roder G, Urak G, Faryniak B, Sladen RN, et al. Controlled airway pressure therapy, nitric oxide inhalation, prone position, and extracorporeal membrane oxygenation (ECMO) as components of an integrated approach to ARDS. Anesthesiology. 1999 Dec;91(6):1577-86.

185. Manthous CA, Hall JB, Olson D, Singh M, Chatila W, Pohlman A, et al. Effect of cooling on oxygen consumption in febrile critically ill patients. Am J Respir Crit Care Med. 1995 Jan;151(1):10-4.

186. Moler FW, Custer JR, Bartlett RH, Palmisano JM, Akingbola O, Taylor RP, et al. Extracorporeal life support for severe pediatric respiratory failure: an updated experience 1991-1993. J Pediatr. 1994;124(6):875-80.

187. Vats A, Pettignano R, Culler S, Wright J. Cost of extracorporeal life support in pediatric patients with acute respiratory failure. Crit Care Med. 1998 Sep;26(9):1587-92.

188. Weber TR, Kountzman B. Extracorporeal membrane oxygenation for nonneonatal pulmonary and multiple-organ failure. J Pediatr Surg. 1998;33(11):1605-9.

189. Swaniker F, Kolla S, Moler F, Custer J, Grams R, Barlett R, et al. Extracorporeal life support outcome for 128 pediatric patients with respiratory failure. J Pediatr Surg. 2000;35(2):197-202.

5

Blood Biomaterial Surface Interaction During ECLS

Gail M. Annich MD MS FRCP(C), Timothy T. Cornell MD, M. Patricia. Massicotte MD, Laurance L. Lequier MD

Introduction

Current extracorporeal life support (ECLS) applications have evolved from the early days of cardiopulmonary bypass (CPB), first successfully applied more than a half century ago. There have been many challenges bringing extracorporeal perfusion from the operating room and into the intensive care unit. CPB caused an acute inflammatory response and was fraught with problems related to coagulation, bleeding, and other organ dysfunction, and therefore was not considered to be a technology appropriate for long term circulatory or respiratory support. Significant advancements in the materials, components, and techniques of ECLS have been realized over the past 50 years. However, the inability to completely control the interaction between blood and the biomaterials of the extracorporeal circuitry and the subsequent inflammatory and coagulation reactions results in these same challenges to the use of ECLS today and going forward.

Although likened to CPB, ECLS differs significantly from open heart surgery or ventricular assist devices (VADs). The two main differences are the duration of the extracorporeal support and the amount of blood exposed to non-endothelial surfaces per unit of time. CPB for cardiac surgery continuously exposes the entire circulating blood volume to the wound and a significant area of the artificial biomaterial circuitry for a few hours or less. Large amounts of anticoagulation are required to prevent clotting, and essentially all elements in the blood are activated during this time. VADs expose circulating blood to a relatively small area of the artificial surface. Initially, the amount of blood exposed to the wound varies; however, once the device is placed, the wound blood is not circulated and the non-endothelial surface area of exposure is small. ECLS systems expose part of the blood volume to a large surface area of artificial biomaterial circuitry, but little to no wound blood is circulated, unless the patient has had recent cardiac surgery. Therefore, some anticoagulation is necessary to prevent clotting within the extracorporeal circuit, but less than that required in CPB because the stimulus to blood component activation is less. The basic mechanisms of blood protein and cellular activation during different applications of extracorporeal perfusion are identical, but the intensity of these reactions will vary depending upon the duration of the stimuli, the type of anticoagulants, patient variability, and type of artificial circuitry. Activation refers to conversion of blood zymogens to active enzymes, expression of blood cellular receptors, initiation of cell signaling, and release of vasoactive and cytotoxic substances.

Spontaneous bleeding and thrombosis are rare events in children and young adults. The negatively charged membranes of the vascular endothelium maintain the fluidity of blood via a complex interaction between plasma proteins and platelets. This normal physiologic hemostasis is disturbed when blood comes into contact with any non-endothelial surface. During ECLS, there is continuous contact between circulating blood and the foreign surface of the extracorporeal circuit. The hemostatic balance is shifted to hypercoagulability with patients and extracorporeal circuits and components at risk for thrombosis. In order to regain the loss of hemostatic balance and prevent thrombosis, administration of antithrombotic therapy is necessary. The most widely used antithrombotic therapy for the provision of ECLS is the anticoagulant, unfractionated heparin (UNFH). Unfortunately, the use of UNFH can result in bleeding in the systemic circulation and despite its use, clotting in the extracorporeal circuit. The bleeding and thrombosis that occur regularly

during the course of ECLS can ultimately result in significant clinical complications, including death. This chapter will discuss normal hemostasis, physiologic differences in hemostasis in children as compared to adults (developmental hemostasis), and the effect of the blood/biomaterial interaction during ECLS on normal hemostasis and inflammatory response.

Normal Hemostasis

Normal physiologic hemostasis is dependent upon maintaining a fine balance between thrombosis and hemorrhage. Coagulation and fibrinolysis are the two pathways responsible for hemostasis. These pathways are comprised of a number of protein components which when activated by a stimulus, interact with red blood cells and platelets and result in thrombus formation (coagulation) and/or thrombus degradation (fibrinolysis).

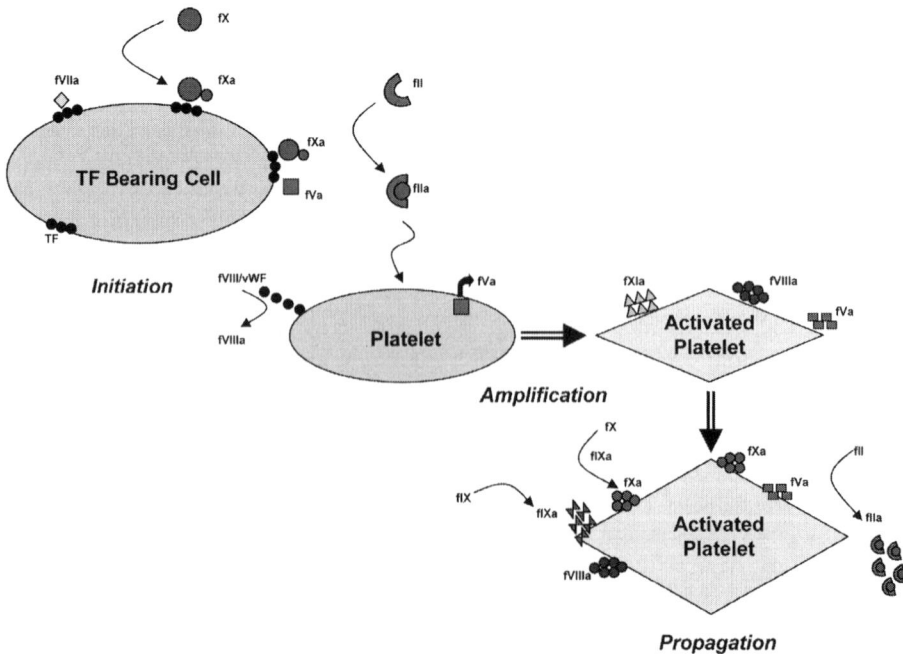

Figure 5-1. Cell-based coagulation occurs on different cell surfaces in three overlapping steps: initiation, amplification, and propagation.

Activation of the Coagulation Pathway

The classic 'coagulation cascade' model of hemostasis described a series of reactions involving activation of various factors along extrinsic and intrinsic pathways. According to this model, stimulation of either the extrinsic or intrinsic coagulation pathway led to a common pathway which resulted in the production of thrombin and subsequent formation of a stable fibrin clot. This 'coagulation cascade' model suggested that the coagulation factors themselves were responsible for controlling hemostasis, while various cells provided a phospholipid surface for the procoagulant reactions to occur. The cell-based model of hemostasis replaces the classic 'coagulation cascade' model, and proposes that cells play very active roles in controlling coagulation.[1] Cell-based coagulation takes place on different cell surfaces in three overlapping steps: initiation, amplification, and propagation (Figure 5-1).

The initiation phase occurs on a tissue factor-bearing cell or cellular fragments.[2] Tissue factor (TF) is expressed on a large number of cells including endothelial cells, vascular smooth muscle cells, and fibroblasts. TF antigen is also found circulating in peripheral blood, delivered to sites of vascular injury by neutrophils, monocytes, and macrophages. TF becomes available through a number of different mechanisms including: exposure on damaged vessel wall (surgery, trauma), through aberrant expression by activated monocytes or endothelial cells when stimulated by sepsis (various different organisms), or inflammation (cytokines). The activated factor VII-TF complex successively activates a number of coagulation proteins resulting in thrombin (fIIa) generation.

The small amount of thrombin generated in the initiation phase is essential for procoagulant progression to the amplification phase. In the amplification phase, platelets and co-factors (f) (fV, fVIII, fXI) are activated in order to prepare for more significant thrombin generation. During the propagation phase, fIXa, accelerated by fVIIIa, binds to activated platelets causing further fX activation. The complexing of fXa with fVa, to membrane surfaces leads to a burst of thrombin (fIIa) generation. This thrombin generation results in the cleavage of fibrinogen to fibrin monomers, which polymerize to consolidate the initial platelet plug into a stable fibrin clot.

Activation of the Fibrinolytic Pathway

The above cell-mediated coagulation is regulated continuously by the fibrinolytic pathway. The fibrinolytic pathway (constituent proteins: tissue plasminogen activator (tPA), tPA, and plasminogen) is activated when thrombin is generated. This regulation occurs in three phases as well: termination, elimination, and stabilization (Figure 5-2). Tissue factor pathway inhibitor (TFPI), along with protein C and S, antithrombin (AT), and α^2macroglobulin participate in the initial termination of coagulation and ultimately prevent formation of pathologic thrombi.

TFPI inhibits TF, fVIIa, and fXa, while AT inhibits thrombin, fIXa, fXa, fXIa, and the TF-VIIa complex. Protein S is a cofactor for protein C-mediated fVa and fVIIIa inhibition. Fibrin deposits are eliminated because fibrin attracts plasminogen and tissue plasminogen activator (tPA) which converts plasminogen to plasmin. The increasing plasmin concentrations cause thrombus degradation by digesting fibrin (fibrinolysis) into soluble fragments, including D-dimer. The fibrinolytic pathway is modulated by the inhibitor protein plasminogen activator inhibitor 1 (PAI-1) to prevent degradation of all thrombi, including important hemostatic plugs, which prevent hemorrhage. Stabilization of coagulation counteracts fibrinolysis through thrombin-activated fVIIIa, which converts loosely interlaced fibrin into a tightly knitted aggregate.

Developmental Hemostasis

The "balance" of hemostasis is maintained in infants and children despite very different levels of constituent proteins and inhibitors of coagulation (decreased factors XII, XI, X, IX, VII, II, and protein C and S and AT; increased α^2 macroglobulin) and fibrinolysis (decreased tPA, plasminogen and increased PAI-1) which approach adult levels at different developmental stages up to puberty. These normal physiologic differences in hemostasis are termed "developmental hemostasis."[3] Epidemiologic studies have demonstrated that infants and children have decreased venous thrombosis compared to adults which is a result of unique protective mechanisms (increased α^2 macroglobulin, decreased thrombin generation, and altered vessel wall properties). However, there are high risk cohorts of children with an increased incidence of thrombosis, including children who undergo ECLS.

Initiation of ECLS: Coagulation Pathway Activation and Inflammatory Response

When blood is exposed to the non-biologic surfaces of an extracorporeal circuit, a complex inflammatory response is initiated involving both the coagulation pathway and the inflammatory response pathway (Figure 5-3).[4] This complex response leads to capillary leak which can cause temporary dysfunction of every organ. In fact, the response to extracorporeal circulation is remarkably similar, clinically and biochemically, to that seen in the systemic inflammatory response syndrome (SIRS) and the acute respiratory distress syndrome (ARDS).[5] During ECLS, blood is circulated via a mechanical pump and is independent of physiological controls. This system is in parallel with the native heart. The native heart is responsive to physiologic controls but is only partially utilized, either because of disease or lack of inflow. Mechanisms that normally maintain physiologic

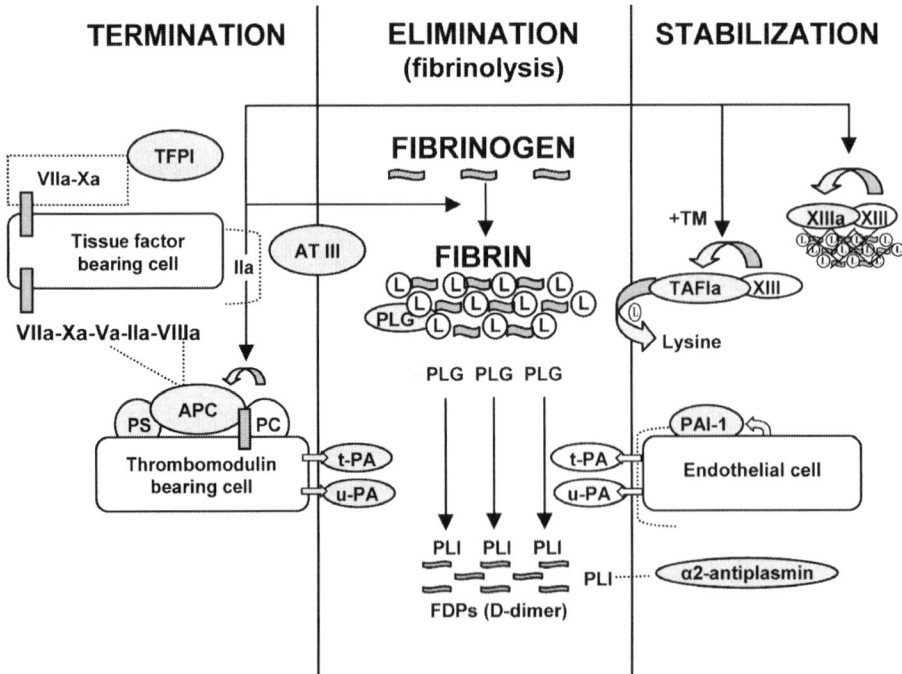

Figure 5-2. Regulation of the Fibrinolytic System: termination, elimination, and stabilization.

homeostasis are disrupted which results in increased acuity to the already physiologically compromised patient.

Pathophysiology of the blood surfaces interaction

Contact with synthetic, non-endothelial cell surfaces, shear stresses, turbulence, cavitation, and osmotic forces directly injure blood.[6] Plasma proteins and lipoproteins are progressively denatured during ECLS.[1,2] Protein denaturation increases plasma viscosity, produces macromolecules, decreases protein solubility, and increases protein reactive side groups. Plasma IgG, IgA, IgM, and albumin decrease more than expected from hemodilution.[7] Red blood cells (RBCs) develop reversible echinocytic changes, but some are also hemolyzed by shear forces and activated complement.[8,9] Roller pumps cause more hemolysis than centrifugal pumps, although with improved technology this is less

of an issue.[10] Platelets and white blood cells (WBCs) are also injured during perfusion, but the consequences of activation of these cells far outweigh the effects of direct injury. In addition, the effect of shear rate on platelets and other components of coagulation are also critically important. The higher the shear rate, the more platelet deposition and generation of fXa by augmentation of TF:VIIa complex. While at lower shear rates, there is less platelet deposition and more fibrin deposition.

Multiple blood cells and plasma protein systems are activated as part of a series of cellular and enzymatic reactions that occur during the initiation and maintenance of ECLS. The response involves the contact and complement systems, along with the activation of coagulation, fibrinolysis, and most cell lines including platelets, neutrophils, monocytes, lymphocytes, and endothelial cells.[11]

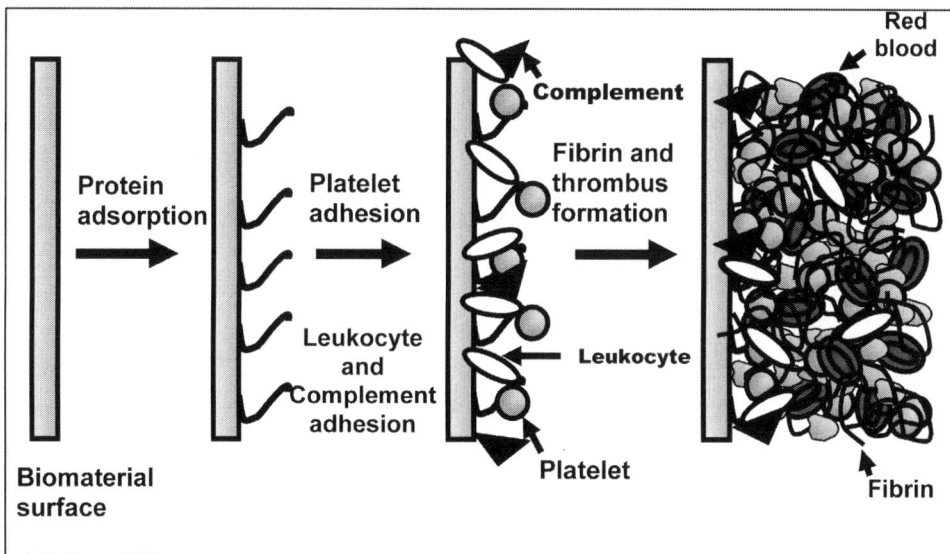

Figure 5-3. Simplistic representation of the blood-surface interaction during ECLS. This shows the components relevant to thrombosis and even though complement and leukocytes are considered to be involved with inflammation, they are also very relevant participants in thrombosis formation.

Platelets

Platelets are the mainstay for hemostasis and preservation of vascular wall integrity. Platelets respond to minimal stimulation and become activated when they encounter a thrombogenic stimulus such as injured endothelium, subendothelium, or artificial surfaces. Normal platelets participate in the balance of hemostasis through the following activities: activation, adhesion, secretion of active substances, and aggregation. Collagen exposure and von Willebrand Factor (vWF) released by the damaged blood vessel results in platelet adhesion. In high shear stress conditions (arteries and microvessels) high molecular weight vWF mediates platelet adhesion by binding to collagen and the non-activated platelet through the platelet receptor glycoprotein (GP) Ib-IX-V. GPIb and GPIIb-IIIa have the highest density on platelets and are important in the platelet surface interaction which occurs during ECLS. GPIb mediates the platelet interaction with VWF. The adherence of platelets via GPIb to adsorbed VWF is dependent upon shear stress, which is necessary to provide the conformational change in VWF which allows binding to occur.[12] In low shear stress conditions (large veins) platelet adhesion occurs through direct interaction via GP VI with collagen. Platelet secretion occurs from intracellular granule collections and results in a number of actions due to agents released including:

- Increasing platelet adhesion and aggregation (released: adenosine diphosphate, vWF, fibrinogen, and thrombospondin)
- Participation in coagulation (released: fV, fibrinogen)
- Increased vascular tone and contraction (released: serotonin)
- Increased cell proliferation and migration (released: platelet derived growth factor, PDGF).

- Fibrinogen binds to activated platelets through the receptor GPIIb-IIIa and acts as a bridge between platelets resulting in aggregation.

GPIIb-IIIa (CD41/CD61) is the dominant platelet receptor. Resting platelets with inactive GPIIb-IIIa have a low affinity for binding adsorbed fibrinogen. Once the platelet is activated and conformational shape change of the platelet occurs, the high-affinity binding site of GPIIb-IIIa is exposed and binding of soluble fibrinogen occurs, which in turn leads to platelet aggregation and platelet leukocyte aggregates by the crosslinking of 2 GPIIb-IIIa receptors or by the crosslinking of GPIIb-IIIa with Mac-1 on the leukocyte. These crosslinks are made by fibrinogen.

Platelet activation and adhesion, as described above, is known to occur during both CPB and ECLS, as well as with vascular access catheters and grafts. Both adherent platelets and platelet microparticles are procoagulant in nature, and therefore provide continual, ongoing stimulus for the above described physiologic platelet responses. It is known that during ECLS platelet adhesion and aggregate formation reduce the circulating platelet count; however, it should be noted that high consumption and formation of microemboli, rather than occlusive thrombi, can occur even in the event of minimal adhesion to the circuitry surface. As ECLS continues, adherent platelets detach, leaving fragments of platelet membrane behind; these will also detach and circulate. The circulating platelet pool during ECLS consists of decreased numbers of morphologically normal platelets, increased numbers of platelets at various stages of activation (e.g., pseudopod formation, degranulation, and membrane receptor loss), and new larger platelets released from the bone marrow. Bleeding times increase in the presence of structurally normal-appearing platelets,[13] and as ECLS continues beyond 24 hours, platelet consumption continues.

Leukocytes

Neutrophils, monocytes, and lymphocytes are the main groups of cells involved in the inflammatory responses during ECLS. Exposure of patient blood to the extracorporeal circuit results in activation of innate immunity. Circulating leukocytes, including peripheral blood mononuclear cells (PBMCs) are activated in part by tissue factor activation,[14] complement,[15] and endotoxin.[16] This activation releases numerous circulating pro-inflammatory cytokines (e.g., TNF-α and IL-1β) that activate circulating neutrophils facilitating their adhesion to the vascular surfaces of numerous organs.[17] The leukocyte activation also results in an array of potent oxygen metabolites and proteolytic enzymes being released. The material characteristics of the artificial surfaces modulate the absorption of proteins to the surface and therefore moderate the level of activation. Neutrophil counts decrease immediately after ECLS initiation because of dilution and recover slowly thereafter. The principal agonists for activating neutrophils during ECLS are kallikrein and C5a.[18] Both CPB and ECLS cause accumulation of activated neutrophils in pulmonary perivascular and interstitial tissue. This accumulation is associated with increased capillary permeability, interstitial edema, and large alveolar-arterial oxygen differences during and after perfusion.[19] During open heart surgery, monocytes are activated to express TF, in both the wound and extracorporeal circuit, but the activation in the circuit is delayed for several hours.[20] Extracorporeal perfusion decreases the total number of lymphocytes and specific subsets of lymphocytes, particularly B lymphocytes, natural killer cells, helper T-cells, and T-suppressor lymphocytes.[21] Lymphocyte counts usually recover within five days of weaning from ECLS; slower recovery is associated with a poor prognosis.[22]

This pro-inflammatory response has been thought to be responsible for the physiologic derangements observed early after the blood contacts the extracorporeal circuit. A compensatory, anti-inflammatory response syndrome (CARS) also exists that is aimed at countering the pro-inflammation.[23] While CARS is a necessary response, an exaggerated or dysregulated CARS response can impair immunity thus rendering a host susceptible to infection and infectious sequelae such as sepsis and multiple organ dysfunction syndrome (MODS).[24]

Endothelial cells

Endothelial cells maintain the fluidity of blood and the integrity of the vascular system. Endothelial cells produce prostacyclin, heparin sulfate, tPA, and TFPI, which help regulate the coagulation pathway. Endothelial cells produce protein S, which is a necessary cofactor for normal protein C function; protein C is a natural anticoagulant. Endothelial cells also produce vasoactive substances and cytokines such as nitric oxide (NO), prostacyclin, endothelin-1, IL-1, IL-6, and platelet activating factor (PAF) as well as inactive substances such as histamine, norepinephrine, and bradykinin.[25] Prostacyclin concentrations increase rapidly at the start of CPB and then begin to decrease.[26]

Complement

The alternative complement pathway, as opposed to the classic complement pathway, is primarily activated by ECLS as part of this pro-coagulant activation and inflammation.[27] The alternative pathway does not require antibody or immune complexes for activation. It is activated by foreign surfaces including microbial organisms or elements, particles, or biomaterial surfaces. Complement activation via the alternative pathway occurs spontaneously at a low rate, but a hydrolyzed C3 is formed, factor B becomes activated and then initiates the cleavage of C3 to form C3a and C3b. During ECLS or CPB, with a biomaterial surface to bind C3b covalently to its hydroxyl or amine groups, factor B and D binding occurs, and the alternative C3 convertase (C3bBb) is formed, creating a positive amplification loop.

Activation of the Coagulation System during ECLS

Within seconds of blood contact with the nonbiologic surface of the extracorporeal circuit, plasma proteins are adsorbed onto that surface to form a monolayer of bound proteins.[28] The physical and chemical composition of the polymer determines which proteins are most likely to adhere to that surface, which may not be the proteins of greatest concentration within the plasma. Adsorbed fXII and fibrinogen undergo conformational changes, triggering activation of the contact system. The contact system consists of four primary plasma proteins: fXII, prekallikrein, high molecular weight kininogen (HMWK), and C-1 inhibitor. FXIIa in the presence of HMWK activates fXI which initiates the activation of fIX in the presence of fVIIIa to produce the tenase complex.[29] The tenase complex binds fX to produce fXa. Activation of coagulation occurs through TF expression on activated cells (monocytes, macrophages, neutrophils, activated endothelial cells, smooth muscle cells, apoptotic cells), or cellular components (platelet microparticles or circulating vesicles). TF is a cell-bound glycoprotein expressed in the vascular subendothelium, and many other cells including activated monocytes.[30] TF complexes with fVII in conjunction with a phospholipid surface forming the TF:VIIa complex which in turn activates fX to Xa.[31] FXa facilitates the conversion of prothrombin to thrombin, and fibrinogen to fibrin as described in more detail earlier.

Platelets adhere to the surface of the extracorporeal circuit and become activated, which leads to platelet aggregation and further activation of the coagulation system. Platelet activation and consumption occurs upon initiation of ECLS such that platelet number and function decrease within the first hour of ECLS.[32] This platelet activation and consumption continues throughout the course of ECLS often requiring regular transfusions of platelets, and with the platelet activation neutrophils also become activated producing cytokines and further contributing to the inflammatory response to extracorporeal circulation.[33]

The fibrinolytic system has the important role of limiting the extent of clot formation and eventually dissolving it. The presence of circulating thrombin stimulates endothelial cells to produce tPA which participates in the cleavage of plasminogen to plasmin.[34] Plasmin lyses fibrin to dissolve clot and inhibits fibrinogen and factors V, VII, IX and XI. The cleavage reaction to form plasmin produces D-dimers, which have been shown to be elevated during the course of neonatal ECLS as a marker of ongoing fibrinolysis.[35] Evidence for early activation of both the contact and fibrinolytic systems has been demonstrated by peak concentrations of fXIIa and fibrin degradation products in neonates early after the initiation of ECLS.[36] Such significant activation of the coagulation system results in a pattern of consumptive coagulopathy with half of infants and children in one study having demonstrated deficiencies in both platelets and coagulation factors soon after the initiation of ECLS, even with the use of fresh frozen plasma (FFP) in the circuit priming volume.[37]

Despite the activity of plasmin and the fibrinolytic system described above, the use of an extracorporeal circuit results in continued activation of the coagulation system and generation of thrombin. Endogenous antithrombotic activity becomes overwhelmed and this necessitates the use of an exogenous anticoagulant to maintain the integrity of the extracorporeal circuit.

Activation of the Innate Immune System and Resultant Immune Dysregulation

Activation of the coagulation system and thrombin generation does not occur in isolation but in conjunction with the activation of the innate immune system. The initial activation of the components of the innate immune system by the ECLS circuit cumulatively contributes to the SIRS response that can clinically manifest as hemodynamic instability and capillary leak. Thus, depending on the degree of the innate immune response, a slight increase in hemodynamic support may be necessary following the first few hours after initiation of ECLS. The initial SIRS response is counterbalanced by a compensatory anti-inflammatory response (CARS) meant to reestablish homeostasis and reset the innate immune system. However, a prolonged CARS response may lead to an acquired immunosuppressed state placing the patient at risk for nosocomial infections.

Increased attention is being placed on understanding the immunology of this CARS phase. A key feature of this biologic response is the presence of "deactivated" monocyte.[38] This term has been used to describe monocytes that did not produce TNF-α to ex vivo endotoxin challenge in patients with septic shock as compared to the response in unaffected patients.[39,40] This deactivated state is also associated with a decrease in the cell surface MHC-II molecule, HLA-DR. In time, the term "immunoparalysis" was coined to refer to the combination of decreased *ex vivo* LPS responsiveness and HLA-DR expression (less than 30% normal).[41] The presence of these parameters following CPB has been preliminarily observed.[42,43] The one study investigating the impact of immunoparalysis following CPB in children examined HLA-DR expression in 82 children and showed that HLA-DR expression less than 60% 72 hours after CPB was predictive of the development of sepsis with an odds ratio of nearly 13.[43] Although the incidence of immunoparalysis while on ECLS is unknown, the potential for an acquired immunosuppressed state must be acknowledged and attention to proper antibiotic usage, adequate nutrition, and practices for the prevention of nosocomial infections are warranted.

The use of extracorporeal life support for critically ill patients who fail conventional therapies is becoming an important tool in critical care medicine. Understanding the normal function of the coagulation system and normal inflammatory response, and pairing this with the pathophysiology of the blood biomaterial interface are crucial to maintaining stability in these patients while being supported on ECLS. Ultimately mimicking the endothelium and obviating the need for systemic anticoagulation would significantly reduce the risks in this patient population.

References

1. Hoffman M. A cell-based model of coagulation and the role of factor VIIa. Blood Reviews. 2003;17:S1-S5.
2. Becker RC. Cell-Based Models of Coagulation: A Paradigm in Evolution. Journal of Thrombosis and Thrombolysis. 2005;20:65-68.
3. Male C, Johnston M, Sparling C, Brooker L, Andrew M, Massicotte P. The influence of developmental haemostasis on the laboratory diagnosis and management of haemostatic disorders during infancy and childhood. Clinics in Lab Med. 1999; 19:39-69.
4. Wan S, LeClerc JL, Vincent JL. Inflammatory response to cardiopulmonary bypass. Chest. 1997;112:676-692.
5. Peek GJ and Firmin RK. The inflammatory and Coagulative Response to Prolonged Extracorporeal Membrane Oxygenation. ASAIO J. 1999;45:250-263.
6. Leverett LB, Hellums JD, Alfrey CP, Lynch EC. Red blood cell damage by shear stress. Biophys J. 1972;12:257-273.
7. Clark RE, Beauchamp RA, Magrath RA, Brooks JD, Ferguson TB, Weldon CS. Comparison of bubble and membrane oxygenation in short and long perfusion. J Thorac Cardiovasc Surg. 1979;78:655-666.
8. Woodman RC, Harker LA. Bleeding complications associated with cardiopulmonary bypass. Blood. 1990;76:1680-1697.
9. Salama A, Hugo F, Heinrich D, et al. Deposition of terminal C5b-9 complement complexes on erythrocytes and leukocytes during cardiopulmonary bypass. N Eng J Med. 1988;318:408-414.
10. Kawahito K, Nose Y. Hemolysis in different centrifugal pumps. Artificial Organs. 1997;21:285-290.
11. Bowen FW, and Edmunds HL Jr. Coagulation, anticoagulation and the interaction of blood and artificial surfaces. In: Zwischen-berger JB, Steinhorn RH, Bartlett, RH, eds. ECMO: Extracorporeal cardiopulmonary support in critical care. 2nd Ed. Ann Arbor, Mich ELSO; 2000:67-96.
12. Gorbet MB, Sefton MV. Biomaterial-associated thrombosis: roles of coagulation factors complement, platelets and leukocytes. . 2004;25:5681-5703.
13. Anderson HL, Ciley RE, Zwischenberger JB, et al. Thrombocytopenia in neonates after extracorporeal membrane oxygenation. ASAIO Trans. 1986;32:534-537.
14. Shibamiya, A., et al., Formation of tissue factor-bearing leukocytes during and after cardiopulmonary bypass. Thromb Haemost, 2004. 92(1): p. 124-31.
15. Wan, S., J.L. LeClerc, and J.L. Vincent, Inflammatory response to cardiopulmonary bypass: mechanisms involved and possible therapeutic strategies. Chest, 1997. 112(3): p. 676-92.
16. Tsunooka, N., et al., Bacterial translocation secondary to small intestinal mucosal ischemia during cardiopulmonary bypass. Measurement by diamine oxidase and peptidoglycan. Eur J Cardiothorac Surg, 2004. 25(2): p. 275-80.
17. Levy, J.H. and K.A. Tanaka, Inflammatory response to cardiopulmonary bypass. Ann Thorac Surg, 2003. 75(2): p. S715-20.
18. El Habbal MH, Carter H, Smith L, Elliot MJ, Strobel S. Neutrophil activation in paediatric extracorporeal circuits: effect of circulation and temperature variation. Cardiovascular Research. 1995;29:102-107.
19. Ratliff NB, Young WG Jr, Hackel D, Mikat E, Wilson JW. Pulmonary injury secondary to extracorporeal circulation. An ultrastructural study. J Thorac Cardiovasc Surg. 1973; 65:425-432.
20. Barstad RM, Ovrum E, Ringdal MA, et al. Induction of monocyte tissue factor procoagulant activity during coronary artery bypass surgery is reduced with heparin-coated

extracorporeal circuit. Br J Haematol. 1996; 94:517-525.

21. DePalma L, Yu M, McIntosh CL, Swain JA, Davey RJ. Changes in lymphocyte subpopulations as a result of cardiopulmonary bypass. The effect of blood transfusion. J Thorac Cardiovasc Surg. 1991;101:240-244.

22. Kawahito K, Kobayashi E, Misawa Y, et al. Recovery from lymphocytopenia and prognosis after adult extracorporeal membrane oxygenation. Arch Surg. 1998;133:216-217.

23. Zimmerman, J.J., Congenital heart disease, cardiopulmonary bypass, systemic inflammatory response syndrome, compensatory anti-inflammatory response syndrome, and outcome: evolving understanding of critical care inflammation immunology. Crit Care Med, 2002. 30(5): p. 1178-9.

24. Mokart, D., et al., Early postoperative compensatory anti-inflammatory response syndrome is associated with septic complications after major surgical trauma in patients with cancer. Br J Surg, 2002. 89(11): p. 1450-6.

25. Vane JR, Anggard EE, Botting RM. Regulatory functions of the vascular endothelium. N Eng J Med. 1990; 323:27-36.

26. Faymonville ME, Deby-Dupont G, Larbuisson R, et al. Prostaglandin E2, prostacyclin, and thromboxane changes during nonpulsatile cardiopulmonary bypass in humans. J Thorac Cardiovasc Surg .1992;104:666.

27. ValhonartH, Swinford RD, Ingelfinger JR, et al. Rapid activation of the alternative pathway of complement by extracorporeal membrane oxygenation. ASAIO J. 1999;45:113-114.

28. Horbett TA. Principles underlying the role of adsorbed plasma proteins in blood interactions with foreign materials. Cardiovasc Pathol. 1993;2:137S.

29. Yeh T Jr., Kavarana MN. Cardiopulmonary bypass and the coagulation system. Progress Ped Cardiol. 2005;21:87-115.

30. Edgington TS, Mackman N, Brand K, et al. The structural biology of expression and function of tissue factor. Thromb Haemost. 1991;66:67-79.

31. Edmunds LH Jr., Colman RW. Thrombin during cardiopulmonary bypass. Ann Thorac Surg. 2006;82:2315-2322.

32. Robinson TM, Kickler TS, Walker LK, et al. Effect of extracorporeal membrane oxygenation on platelets in newborns. Crit Care Med. 1993;21:1029-1034.

33. Fortenberry JD, Bhardwaj V, Niemer P, et al. Neutrophil and cytokine activation with neonatal extracorporeal membrane oxygenation. J Pediatr. 1996;128:670-678.

34. Levin EG, Marzec U, Anderson J, et al. Thrombin stimulates tissue plasminogen activator from cultured human endothelial cells. J Clin Invest. 1984;74:1988-1995.

35. Urlesberger B, Zobel G, Zenz W, et al. Activation of the clotting system during extracorporeal membrane oxygenation in term newborn infants. J Pediatr. 1996;129:264-268.

36. Plotz FB, van Oeveren W, Bartlett RH, et al. Blood activation during neonatal extracorporeal life support. J Thorac Cardiovasc Surg. 1993;105:823-832.

37. McManus ML, Kevy SV, Bower LK, et al. Coagulation factor deficiencies during initiation of extracorporeal membrane oxygenation. J Pediatr. 1995;126:900-904.

38. Volk, H.D., et al., Alterations in function and phenotype of monocytes from patients with septic disease--predictive value and new therapeutic strategies. Behring Inst Mitt, 1991(88): p. 208-15.

39. Asadullah, K., et al., Very low monocytic HLA-DR expression indicates high risk of infection--immunomonitoring for patients after neurosurgery and patients during high dose steroid therapy. Eur J Emerg Med, 1995. 2(4): p. 184-90.

40. Volk, H.D., et al., Monocyte deactivation-rationale for a new therapeutic strategy in

sepsis. Intensive Care Med, 1996. 22 Suppl 4: p. S474-81.

41. Volk, H.D., P. Reinke, and W.D. Docke, Clinical aspects: from systemic inflammation to 'immunoparalysis'. Chem Immunol, 2000. 74: p. 162-77.

42. Hummel, M., et al., Monitoring of the cellular immune system in patients with biventricular assist devices awaiting cardiac transplantation. Clin Transplant, 1994. 8(1): p. 59-66.

43. Allen, M.L., et al., Early postoperative monocyte deactivation predicts systemic inflammation and prolonged stay in pediatric cardiac intensive care. Crit Care Med, 2002. 30(5): p. 1140-5.

6

The Registry of the Extracorporeal Life Support Organization

Steven A. Conrad MD PhD, Peter T. Rycus MPH

Introduction

The systematized collection and analysis of large databases is a powerful tool for the study of both common and uncommon population characteristics. Patient registries are collections of secondary patient data related to a specific condition or diagnosis, having had undergone a specific procedure, or based on some other topic of interest. Post-marketing drug surveillance,[1] coronary artery bypass grafting,[2] and chronic diseases such as diabetes, asthma, and congestive heart failure[3] are some examples where registries have contributed to improved understanding or changes in practice. Analysis of a registry for left ventricular assist devices has provided support for the efficacy and risk during post-marketing surveillance that was noted during earlier trials.[4]

The Extracorporeal Life Support Organization (ELSO), founded in 1989, maintains a registry of extracorporeal membrane oxygenation and related therapies that contains data collected since 1976. Over 140 active extracorporeal life support (ECLS) centers contribute to the registry which contained over 48,000 cases at the time of this writing. The cases submitted span all age groups from neonates to adults, and represent centers from over thirty countries around the globe.

In addition to documenting the growth and development of ECLS over the past 35 years, the ELSO Registry has served several important functions:

Longitudinal documentation of ECLS application

Extracorporeal life support is a technology-based therapy that evolves over time due to improvements in technology, patient care experience, pharmacology, and others. The registry provides the ability to track this information over time.

Quality improvement benchmarking

ELSO distributes semiannual international reports that summarize the cumulative experience in the registry to all centers, and individual center reports to each center. These reports support benchmarking a center's performance against the remaining active centers in a confidential manner.

Research database

ELSO has supported a large number of research publications that have used data extracted from the ELSO Registry. These publications have provided information that has improved the understanding of this technology and helped shaped its practice.

Patient care support

ECLS is used to support patients with a wide range of causative or coexisting conditions, some of which may be uncommon. The ability to query the Registry database for data related to these conditions, or to particular types of support devices, has permitted numerous centers to make better informed decisions in the care of their patients.

Regulatory device approval

The ELSO registry maintains information on the various devices used in extracorporeal support, and can provide comparative data for new device approval. Registry data has also been used to support the approval of long-term support devices including left ventricular assist devices.

History

The registry, initiated in 1988 and containing data from 1976, was implemented as four individual databases in the dBase format using Microsoft FoxPro: neonatal respiratory, pediatric respiratory, neonatal/pediatric cardiac, and adult respiratory databases. Each database had a different schema implemented as a single flat table. The databases were comprised largely of free text fields resulting in non-standardized data entry, higher data storage requirements, and inefficiencies in search and retrieval. The neonatal respiratory database collected the largest dataset, while the adult respiratory database held a minimal dataset.

This original database structure was successful in supporting ELSO centers in patient care and research. As the applications of ECLS have increased in both number and scope, the limitations of the database in its original struc-

ture became evident. A specific search, for example, would typically require a manual examination of free-text fields to detect alternate entries, followed by construction of a complex query which had to be executed across multiple tables. Searches often had to be repeated on the different databases and compiled manually.

To support the continued growth of the Registry, a re-engineering of the Registry database was undertaken in 1998. The goals and features of the new Registry include the following:

- Conversion from four databases to a single registry database structure to store all ECLS cases, eliminating the a-priori division into categories (above) for which a given case may not be mutually exclusively classified (i.e., a case with both cardiac and respiratory components)
- Restructuring from a single-table (flat-file) structure to a multi-table normalized data structure with established integrity rules
- Implementation of validation rules to reduce data entry errors
- Use of an extensible, industry-accepted database query language for all data access (Structured Query Language [SQL])
- Development of a single, uniform data entry form for all ECLS cases
- Elimination of all but a few essential free-text data fields to provide consistency of ECLS data through the use of predefined data categories and classifications
- Adoption of standardized hierarchical classification systems for diagnoses (ICD-9-CM) and surgical procedures current procedural terminology (CPT) to allow data retrieval based on any desired range of specificity

The first update to the Registry was conversion to a Microsoft Access database, with patient data stored in a back-end database and accessed through an Access front-end. The following year the database was migrated to Microsoft SQL

Server to provide for an increase in performance, reliability, and security. The traditional paper entry form was discontinued on implementation of the Microsoft Access database and was rewritten as a Microsoft Word electronic form. This electronic form was discontinued with the deployment of the online registry.

The web-based online registry application was put into production in 2011. The application affords a number of advantages over the existing format:

- Direct entry into the Registry database, including incremental data entry, allowing immediate inclusion in queries and reports.
- Full time global availability
- Access to all cases previously entered by a center, with the ability to search based on demographic data
- Enhanced data validation to improve data integrity
- Customization of data entry formats for various global cultures
- Unlimited inclusion of support records such as diagnoses, procedures, cannulations, complications, and infectious organisms which were previously limited by the data entry form
- Online lookup (with partial matching) of ICD-9 and CPT codes, eliminating need to independently acquire these codes prior to data entry

Anticipated future enhancements include advanced querying capability, report generation, and data importing from external databases.

Data Collection and Reporting

Registry Data Collection

The Registry includes data about patients undergoing ECLS with details on several aspects of ECLS support. Patient demographic information includes age, gender, and race. For neonates, information is collected about the delivery, such as birth weight, maternal age, Apgar scores, gestational age, and delivery type. If a CDH is present, details on this condition is collected.

Each patient can have one or more ECLS support runs. Data collected from each run includes diagnoses (standardized as ICD-9 codes), procedures (as CPT codes), infectious organisms with specimen type, pre-support information such as admission time, pre-support conditions, and therapies used to support the patient prior to ECLS. Pre-ECLS measurements including blood gases, ventilator settings, and hemodynamics are collected. Dates of support, support type and mode, cannulation details, and equipment used are included. An additional set of measurements of blood gases, ventilator settings, and hemodynamics are repeated at 24 hours post-initiation. Complications associated with the run are recorded using predefined categorized complications. Finally, outcome data such as discontinuation reason, organ failures, and discharge information are recorded.

Registry Addenda

The main Registry form contains general information about each ECLS run. In doing so, it lacks more specialized data which are important for some ECLS applications. In the use of ECLS for cardiac support, for example, specialized information includes descriptions of complex congenital cardiac abnormalities and specifics on cardiac surgical procedures. These data are unique to cardiac support, and no standardized classification systems adequately document such situations.

In 1998, ELSO initiated a cardiac addendum to the Registry for recording additional case-specific data related to use of ECLS following congenital heart disease surgery. Because of the relational structure of the re-engineered Registry, incorporation of the cardiac addendum data was accomplished without changes to the existing database structure. Additional data collection is performed through the use of addendum online forms, and includes ELSO-developed diagnosis and procedure codes, surgical procedure details, functional evaluation, and outcome.

In 2011, an addendum for capturing information on the use of ECLS for resuscitation (ECPR, extracorporeal CPR) was included with the online registry release. This addendum records resuscitation times, medications, equipment and priming information, return of spontaneous circulation (ROSC) times, and cooling details.

Registry Reports

Registry data are published in report form semiannually in two formats. An International Summary provides a Registry-wide report (Figure 6-1) that is distributed to all active centers. A second, center-specific report containing a subset of the data specific to a given center is also distributed to each respective center. Each report contains information on each of the major patient groups (neonatal respiratory, pediatric respiratory, adult respiratory, and cardiac). Information in each of these groups includes number of runs, diagnoses, support mode details, and complications.

Implementation

Database

The database supporting the registry is currently implemented in Microsoft SQL Server®, a relational database server running under Windows Server 2008. The database schema, summarized in Figure 6-2, is extensible with the ability to support additional addenda to the existing ECLS application, as well support for new applications related to ECLS.

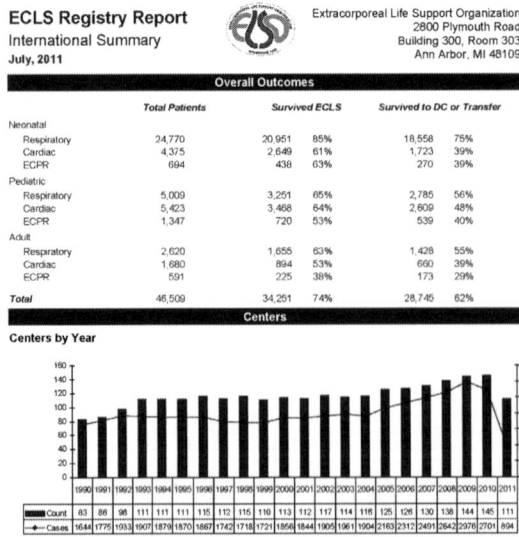

ECLS Registry Report
International Summary
July, 2011

Extracorporeal Life Support Organization
2800 Plymouth Road
Building 300, Room 303
Ann Arbor, MI 48109

Overall Outcomes

	Total Patients	Survived ECLS		Survived to DC or Transfer	
Neonatal					
Respiratory	24,770	20,951	85%	18,558	75%
Cardiac	4,375	2,649	61%	1,723	39%
ECPR	694	438	63%	270	39%
Pediatric					
Respiratory	5,009	3,251	65%	2,785	56%
Cardiac	5,423	3,468	64%	2,609	48%
ECPR	1,347	720	53%	539	40%
Adult					
Respiratory	2,620	1,655	63%	1,428	55%
Cardiac	1,680	894	53%	660	39%
ECPR	591	225	38%	173	29%
Total	46,509	34,251	74%	28,745	62%

Centers

Centers by Year

	1990	1991	1992	1993	1994	1995	1996	1997	1998	1999	2000	2001	2002	2003	2004	2005	2006	2007	2008	2009	2010	2011
Count	83	86	98	111	111	111	115	112	115	110	113	112	117	114	116	125	126	130	138	144	145	111
Cases	1644	1775	1933	1907	1879	1870	1867	1742	1718	1721	1856	1844	1905	1961	1904	2163	2312	2491	2642	2978	2701	894

Figure 6-1. Sample page from the ELSO International Summary. The International Summary has Registry-wide summary data that is distributed to all ECLS centers. No center-specific information is provided.

Online Application

Data entry is handled through a secure online web application (Figure 6-3 and Figure 6-4). After authentication, the user can access all previous cases and enter new cases. Data entry and modification are allowed on recently entered cases, but locked after a predetermined amount of time to prevent inadvertent changes to existing patients. All data entry fields are in the form of checkboxes and selection lists for streamlined data entry. Standardized codes such as ICD-9, CPT, and complication codes can be searched directly in the application.

Registry Data Summary

Data have been collected from 1976 to present from 185 centers globally, with 145 centers currently active and submitting cases. The number of centers continues to grow annually (Figure 6-5), and is expected to increase further due to the increased accessibility of the Registry as an online application. A summary of outcomes for all age groups and types of support is given in Table 6-1.

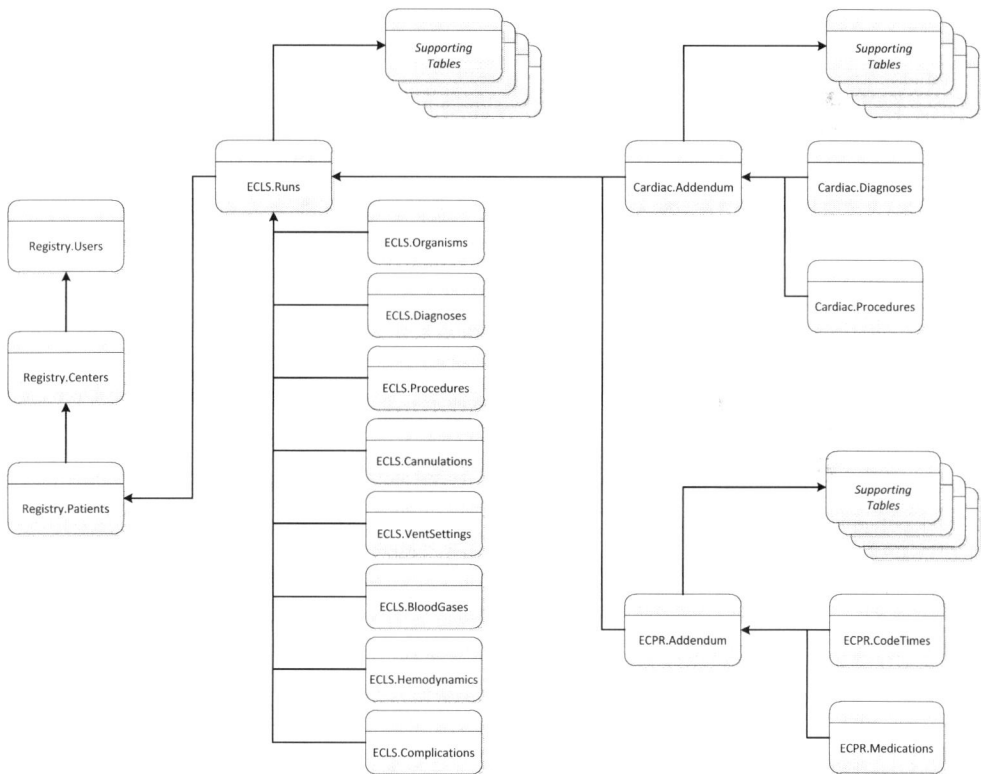

Figure 6-2. Abridged representation of the ELSO Registry database schema. This diagram shows the major tables in the database to demonstrate the principal relationships.

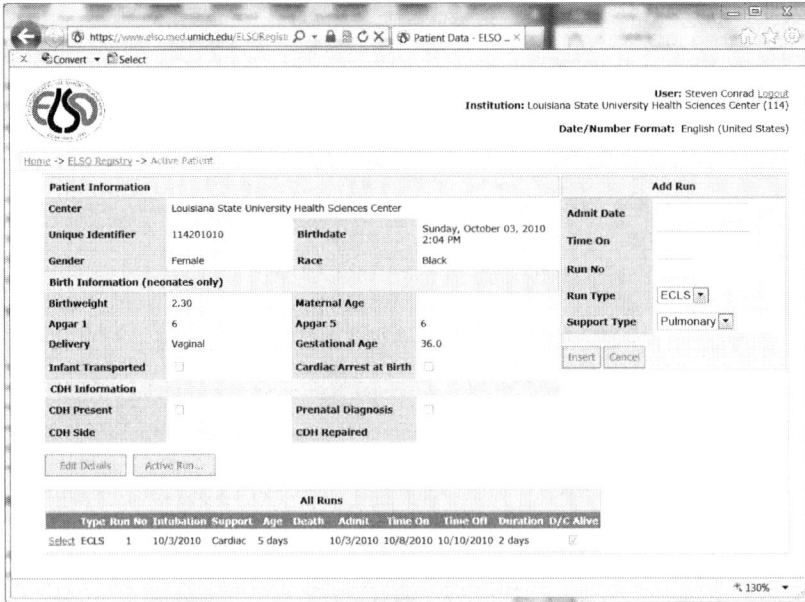

Figure 6-3. Sample page from the online application showing patient information.

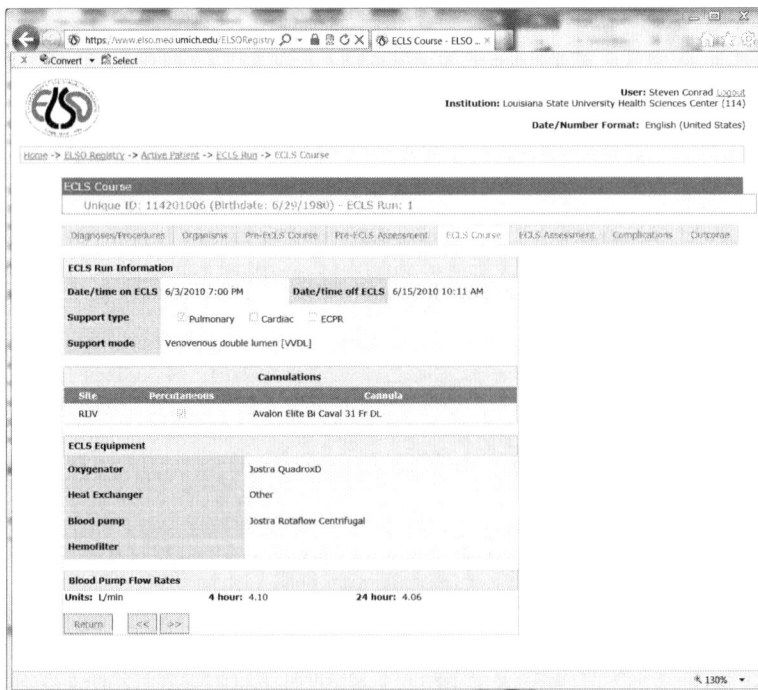

Figure 6-4. Sample page from the online application showing ECLS course data collection.

Table 6-1. Cumulative summary of procedure types and outcomes for the ELSO Registry as of July 2011.

	Total	Survived ECLS		Survived to Discharge	
Neonatal					
Respiratory	24,770	20,951	85%	18,558	75%
Cardiac	4,375	2,649	61%	1,723	39%
ECPR	694	438	63%	270	39%
Pediatric					
Respiratory	5,009	3,251	65%	2,785	56%
Cardiac	5,423	3,468	64%	2,609	48%
ECPR	1,347	720	53%	539	40%
Adult					
Respiratory	2,620	1,655	63%	1,428	55%
Cardiac	1,680	894	53%	660	39%
ECPR	591	225	38%	173	29%
Total	46,509	34,251	74%	28,745	62%

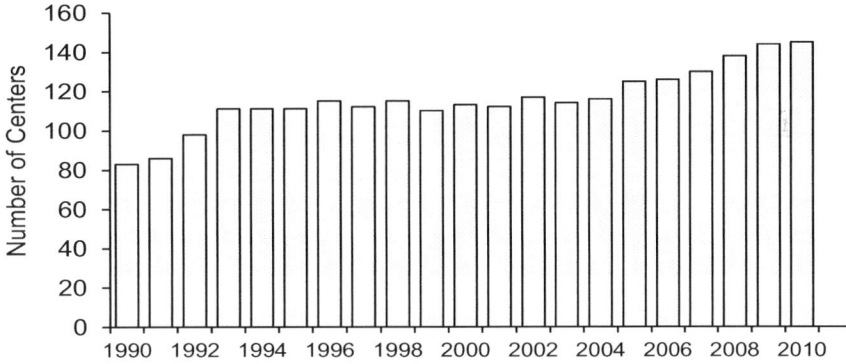

Figure 6-5. Graph of the growth of active centers participating in the ELSO Registry. As of 2010, there were 145 centers providing data to the Registry.

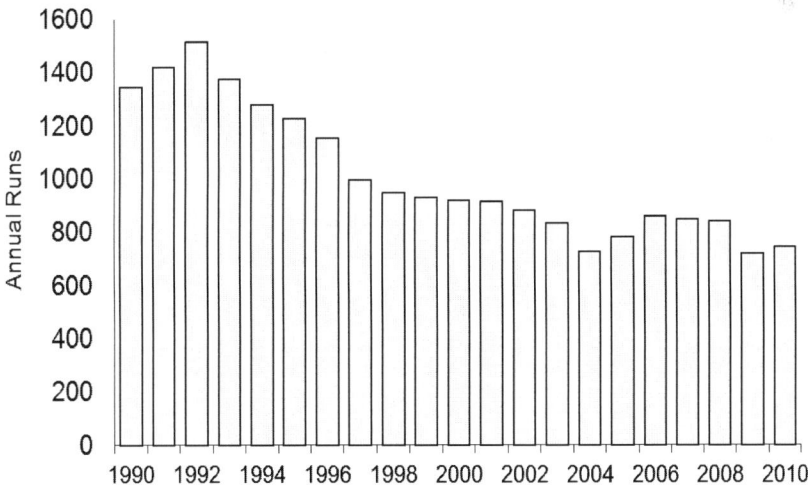

Figure 6-6. Graph showing the number of runs performed annually for neonatal respiratory support.

Neonatal

The number of neonatal respiratory support cases performed increased annually, peaking in 1992, then declining over the next several years before becoming stable in the recent several years (Figure 6-6). The cause of this decline most likely represents the application of alternative therapies which successfully averted the need for ECLS in many cases. The introduction of exogenous surfactant administration began in the early 1990s and has increased in frequency. Additionally, the availability of inhaled nitric oxide (iNO) for pulmonary artery vasodilatation combined with improvements in ventilator management, especially high frequency oscillatory ventilation (HFOV), are other new therapies which may have contributed to the reduced requirement for ECLS.

Survival rates and duration of support for the major neonatal diagnoses are given in Table 6-2. Cumulative survival rates are the highest for meconium aspiration syndrome (94%) and lowest for CDH (51%). Diagnosis-specific annual survival rates have not changed significantly over the past decade except for a slight decline in survival in patients supported for CDH (Figure 6-7).

Venovenous support is accepted to be the preferred mode of support for respiratory failure. However, venoarterial (VA) support remains the most common support mode for neonatal respiratory support, although the incidence of VA support is decreasing (Figure 6-8). Historically, >75% of patients have been supported in the VA configuration, but in 2010 this fell to <60%. The reason for the predominance of VA support may be attributable to large center experience with the mode, the coexistence of marked cardiac depression, or other reasons not captured by the Registry.

The Registry tracks a number of pre-defined complications, including both mechanical (equipment-related) and patient-related (Table 6-3). In general, complications are recorded if they require intervention or result directly in morbidity. Cerebral infarction and hemorrhage, serious patient-related complications, occurred in 7.5% and 7.0% of neonates, respectively. Hemorrhagic complications also occurred, including bleeding from cannulation sites (7.1%), other surgical sites (6.3%), and the GI tract (1.7%). Hemolysis (plasma hemoglobin >50 mg/dl) was reported in 10.9% of cases. The most common mechanical complications are clots in the circuit, with a 15.3% incidence. Tubing rupture occurred in 0.3% of cases, and oxygenator failure was reported in 6%.

Pediatric

The application of ECLS in pediatric respiratory support is expanding, with over 400 cases reported in 2009 (Figure 6-9). The lower value in 2010 most likely represents delayed reporting. The most common diagnoses leading to

Table 6-2. Registry cumulative summary of neonatal diagnoses with average and longest run times, and survival to hospital discharge.

	Total Cases	Avg Run Time (hours)	Longest Time (hours)	% Survival
MAS	7,814	131	1,327	94%
CDH	6,280	250	2,549	51%
PPHF/PFC	4,129	151	1,176	78%
Sepsis	2,646	140	1,200	75%
RDS	1,508	135	1,093	84%
Pneumonia	345	237	1,002	57%
Air leak	117	167	656	74%
Other	2,261	176	1,433	63%

Table 6-3. Representative complications in the neonatal respiratory support group.

Complication	Incidence (% reported)	Survival (%)
Mechanical		
Oxygenator failure	6.0	53
Pump malfunction	1.7	66
Raceway rupture	0.3	58
Cannula problems	11.7	67
Clots	15.3	67
Air in circuit	5.2	72
Patient-related		
Intracranial hemorrhage	7.0	44
Intracranial infarction	7.5	54
Seizures	10.7	62
Cannulation site bleeding	7.1	64
Surgical site bleeding	6.3	44
GI bleeding	1.7	45
Hemolysis	10.9	65
Pulmonary hemorrhage	4.5	43
Culture-proven infection	6.0	53
Hyperbilirubinemia	7.4	64

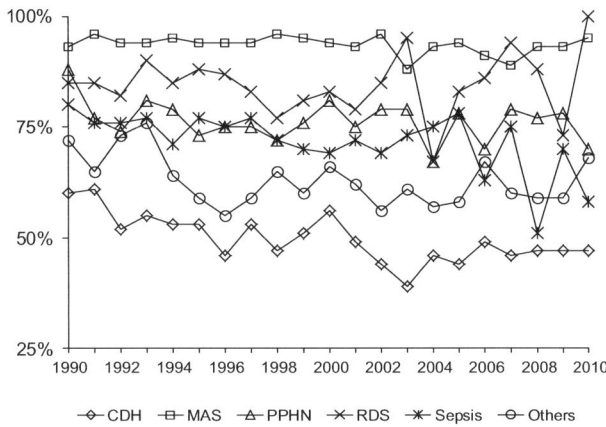

Figure 6-7. Graph showing the survival over the past two decades of neonates for the most common diagnoses. Legend: CDH – congenital diaphragmatic hernia, MAS – meconium aspiration syndrome, PPHN – persistent pulmonary hypertension of the newborn (persistent fetal circulation), and RDS – neonatal respiratory distress syndrome.

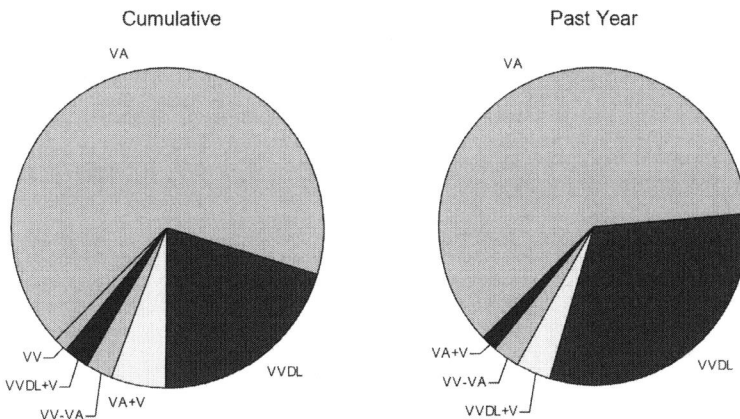

Figure 6-8. Graph showing cumulative modes of support (left) and modes of support used in the past year for neonatal respiratory failure. There has been an increase in the use of venovenous support, but venoarterial support remains the most common method.

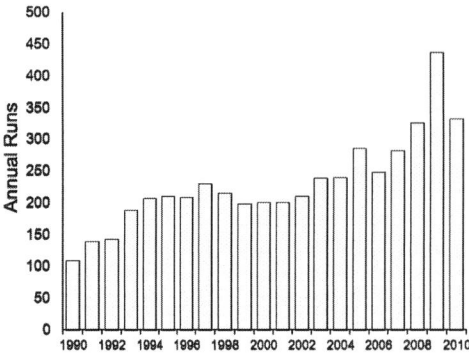

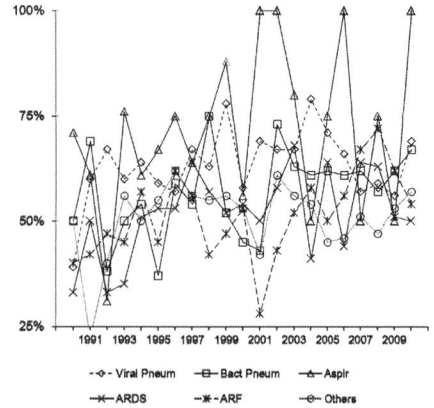

Figure 6-9. Graph showing the number of runs performed annually for pediatric respiratory support. The lower value in 2010 most likely represents delayed reporting.

Figure 6-10. Graph showing the survival over the past two decades of pediatric patients for the most common diagnoses. Legend: ARDS – acute respiratory distress syndrome, ARF – acute respiratory failure, other.

Table 6-4. Registry cumulative summary of pediatric diagnoses with average and longest run times, and survival to hospital discharge.

	Total Cases	Avg Run Time (hours)	Longest Time (hours)	% Survival
Viral pneumonia	1,014	321	1,372	63%
Bacterial pneumonia	550	284	1,411	58%
Aspiration pneumonia	206	270	2,437	67%
ARDS, post-op/trauma	123	249	935	59%
ARDS, other	411	310	2,026	53%
Other respiratory failure	861	250	1,483	51%
Other	1,903	219	2,968	52%

Table 6-5. Representative complications in the pediatric respiratory support group.

Complication	Incidence (% reported)	Survival (%)
Mechanical		
Oxygenator failure	13.0	43
Pump malfunction	2.5	47
Raceway rupture	0.8	59
Cannula problems	15.7	51
Clots	8.3	52
Air in circuit	3.8	49
Patient-related		
Intracranial hemorrhage	6.0	22
Intracranial infarction	3.8	35
Seizures	5.9	34
Cannulation site bleeding	16.3	51
Surgical site bleeding	14.4	46
GI bleeding	4.1	25
Hemolysis	9.9	43
Pulmonary hemorrhage	7.8	30
Culture-proven infection	18.2	47
Hyperbilirubinemia	4.7	28

the application of ECLS for respiratory support are provided in Table 6-4. Survival rates have been increasing over the past decade, from 30% survival prior to 1986, to presently over 50% (Figure 6-10). Pneumonia caused by various infectious etiologies continues to be the most common diagnosis with 61% survival. Pediatric acute respiratory distress syndrome (ARDS), primarily due to non-operative conditions or post-traumatic injury, has a 54% reported survival. Over 800 patients experienced a diverse set of other causes for acute respiratory failure (ARF) and had a 52% overall survival.

The most common mode of initial support for pediatric ECLS has traditionally been VA, but the use of VV is increasing, and is now about as common as VA (Figure 6-11). Since 1976, 30% overall of reported cases have been initiated on VV support, but in the past year, this has risen to >45%. The use of a double-lumen catheter for VV access is also increasing and is currently the predominant mode of VV access.

The profile of complications in the pediatric group differs from the neonatal in several aspects (Table 6-5). Non-intracranial bleeding complications are higher in the pediatric group than in the neonatal group, whereas intracranial bleeding is slightly lower. The latter is not un-expected given the immaturity of the neonatal brain. However, the development of intracranial hemorrhage is associated with a substantial drop in survival in the pediatric group. Clots and air in the circuit are less frequent, and equipment failure more frequent, in the pediatric group, possibly related to the higher circuit blood flows and longer duration of support. Hyperbilirubinemia is less frequent in the pediatric group but associated with a lower survival, since this finding in pediatric patients more likely represents multiple organ dysfunction. Culture-proven infections are more common in pediatrics, likely related to the longer duration of support.[5]

Adult

The most rapidly growing segment of ECLS is for support of severe respiratory failure in the adult (Figure 6-12). The number of adult cases remained small until 1994, most likely because earlier randomized, controlled trials suggested no significant benefit in this age group.[6,7] A consistent increase in the number of cases ensued, with a sharp doubling of the number of cases in 2009. The latter coincided with reports of use of ECLS in patients with severe H1N1 infection,[8] and the publication of the CESAR trial,[9] each

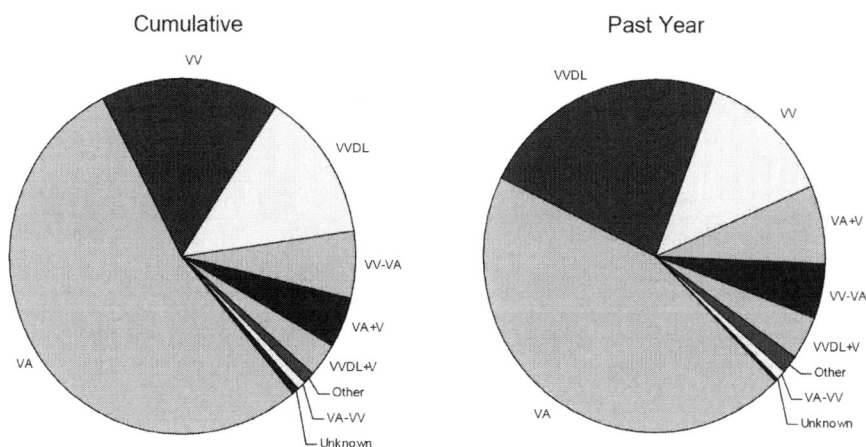

Figure 6-11. Graph showing cumulative modes of support (left) and modes of support used in the past year for pediatric respiratory failure. There has been an increase in the use of venovenous support, and this mode now comprises about half of support for respiratory failure.

raising global awareness of adult ECLS. Supported by improvements in technique, including experience with VV ECLS and percutaneous cannulation, recent experience has led to better results with fewer complications than previously reported.

Cumulative overall survival for all diagnoses is 55%, representing a slight improvement from previous years. Unlike the pediatric group, ARDS is the most common diagnosis leading to ECLS in adults, with survival rates of 51% for non-trauma or surgical etiologies, as well as for trauma or surgical-related ARDS (Table 6-6). The highest survival is seen with viral pneumonia (65%).

Venovenous access is the predominant mode of support in adults with severe acute respiratory failure, accounting for about 80% of initial modes as reported to the Registry in 2010 (Figure 6-13). The introduction of a dual lumen venovenous cannula for adult patients resulted in an adoption of this approach for VV support. In 2010 over 60% of VV cannulations were with the dual lumen cannula. The mode of support in adult ECLS was not recorded prior to 1998.

The complication profile for adults is similar to that of pediatrics (Table 6-7), except for a higher proportion of patients requiring inotropic agents for support (57% for adults vs. 38% for pediatrics). Cannulation site and surgical site

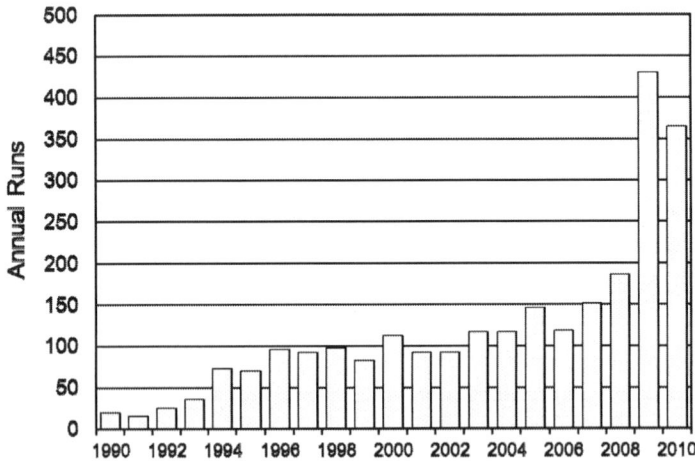

Figure 6-12. Graph showing the number of runs performed annually for adult respiratory support. The lower value in 2010 most likely represents delayed reporting.

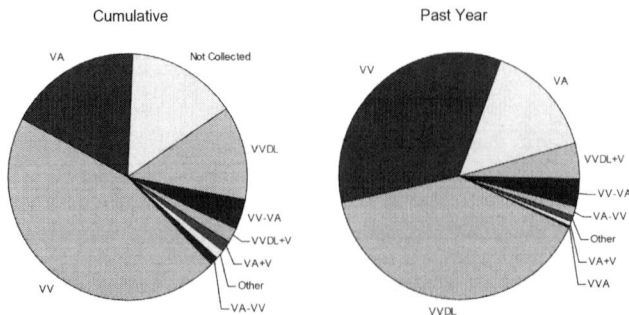

Figure 6-13. Graph showing cumulative modes of support (left) and modes of support used in the past year for adult respiratory failure. Venovenous support accounts for the majority of support modes, and the use of the dual lumen cannula has received widespread adoption, now comprising about 60% of VV cannulations.

bleeding occurred in 12% and 22%, respectively. GI bleeding was infrequent (5.3%). The infection rate was similar to that of pediatric patients (21%). Intracranial complications were less frequent than in pediatric patients, but survival was lower if they occurred.

Cardiac

The number of cases of ECLS for cardiac support reported to the ELSO Registry has shown a steady annual increase over the past decade (Figure 6-14 – Figure 6-17). Over 11,500 cases were reported to the ELSO Registry through 2010, with an overall survival of 44%. The majority are neonatal (38%) and pediatric patients (47%), with adults comprising the re-

mainder (15%). The adult group represents the most rapidly growing group, with the number of annual cases supported more than doubling between 2004 and 2010. The cumulative survival has remained relatively consistent over the past several years at about 44%.

Congenital defects in the perioperative period constitute the vast majority of cardiac diagnoses, with an overall survival of 39%. Cardiomyopathy, myocarditis, cardiogenic shock, and cardiac arrest account for most of the remaining diagnoses. Myocarditis is associated with a better survival than other diagnoses. Cardiac transplant support accounted for 4% of cases, postoperative support 78%, bridge to transplant 5%, and the remaining 13% were for non-postoperative cardiac support.

Table 6-6. Registry cumulative summary of adult diagnoses with average and longest run times, and survival to hospital discharge.

	Total Cases	Avg Run Time (hours)	Longest Time (hours)	% Survival
Viral pneumonia	110	275	1,357	65%
Bacterial pneumonia	459	234	1,585	59%
Aspiration pneumonia	66	207	1,663	61%
ARDS, post-op/trauma	220	233	1,326	53%
ARDS, other	392	299	5,014	48%
Other respiratory failure	149	245	1,317	56%
Other	1,297	202	3,018	53%

Table 6-7. Representative complications in the adult respiratory support group.

Complication	Incidence (% reported)	Survival (%)
Mechanical		
Oxygenator failure	17.0	45
Pump malfunction	2.5	35
Raceway rupture	0.3	25
Cannula problems	18.4	44
Clots	8.3	52
Air in circuit	1.8	56
Patient-related		
Intracranial hemorrhage	3.9	16
Intracranial infarction	2.2	21
Seizures	1.3	42
Cannulation site bleeding	18.2	52
Surgical site bleeding	18.2	42
GI bleeding	5.3	29
Hemolysis	7.0	36
Pulmonary hemorrhage	8.4	37
Culture-proven infection	21.8	44
Hyperbilirubinemia	8.6	33

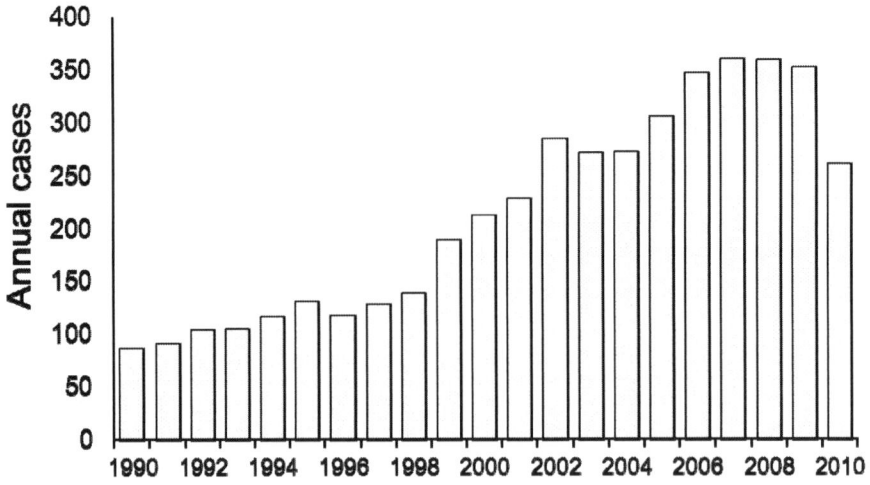

Figure 6-14. Graph showing the number of runs performed annually for neonatal cardiac surgery. The lower value in 2010 most likely represents delayed reporting.

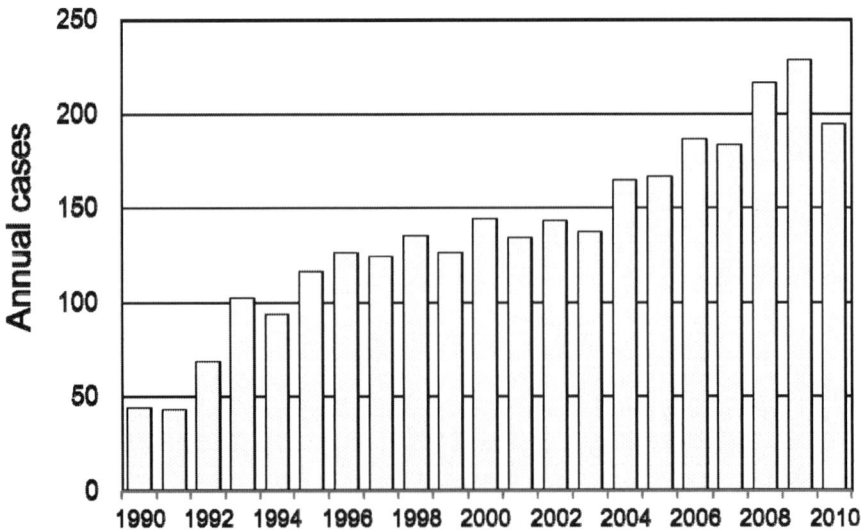

Figure 6-15. Graph showing the number of runs performed annually for infant (age 1 month to 1 year) cardiac surgery. The lower value in 2010 most likely represents delayed reporting.

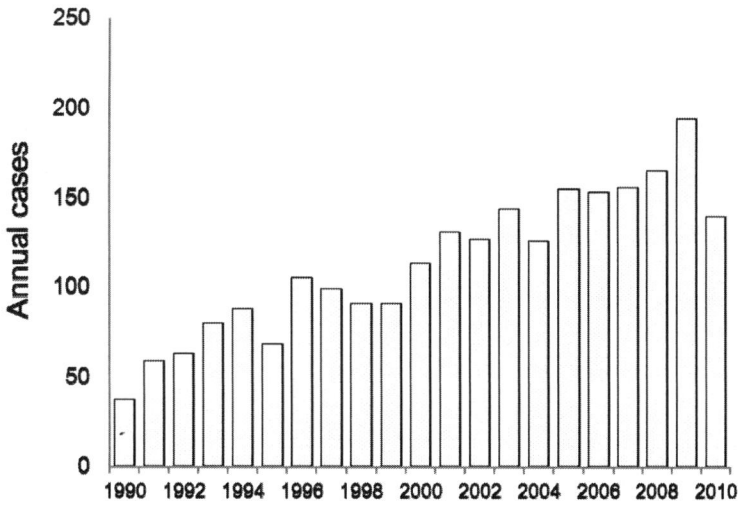

Figure 6-16. Graph showing the number of runs performed annually for pediatric (age 1 to 16 years) cardiac surgery. The lower value in 2010 most likely represents delayed reporting.

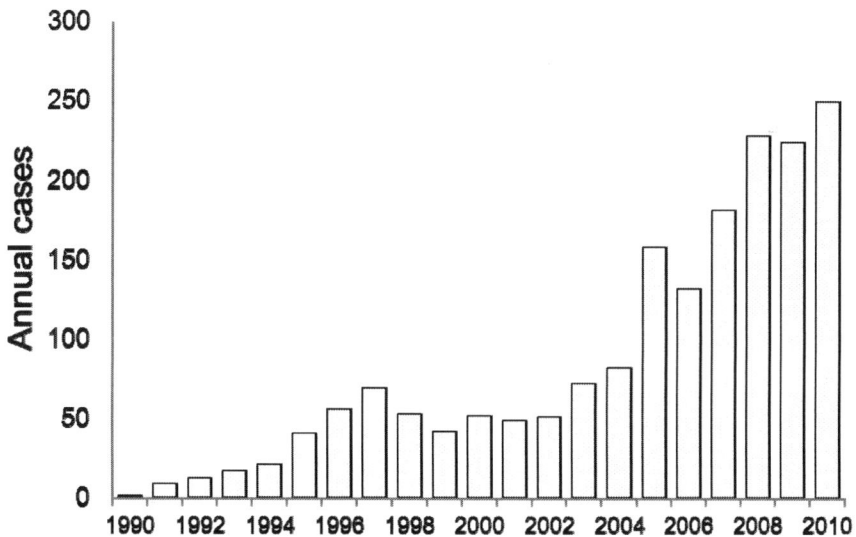

Figure 6-17. Graph showing the number of runs performed annually for adult (age over 16 years) cardiac surgery. The lower value in 2010 most likely represents delayed reporting.

The Registry contains data for the major groups of cardiac operations performed for the correction of left-to-right shunts, left-sided obstructive lesions, hypoplastic left heart syndrome, right-sided obstructive lesions, cyanotic heart disease with increased or decreased pulmonary blood flow, and unclassified lesions.

Surgical site bleeding was reported in 31% of patients. The most common complication was the requirement for inotropes, which were reported in 62% of all patients, but highest in adults (76%). Cardiac dysrhythmias occurred in 20%, and infectious complications in 11%. Renal dysfunction requiring intervention was reported in about 30%. Mechanical complications, including cannula problems, were not common.

Recent Trends

Extracorporeal life support techniques are dynamic, adapting to introduction in new technologies and practices. The use of percutaneous cannulation for venovenous support in acute respiratory failure is increasing (Figure 6-18), and now accounts for about a third of all VV cannulations. The use of centrifugal pumps is also increasing, coinciding with the increased availability of newer pump designs in markets such as the United States, as well as the introduction of newer plasma-resistant, efficient, low flow-resistant membrane lungs (Figure 6-19). These new membrane lung designs afford considerable advantages, and now account for the vast majority of membrane lungs used for extracorporeal support (Figure 6-20).

Summary

The ELSO Registry has arguably contributed to the successful growth of extracorporeal support by capturing the ECLS experience since its earliest clinical application. It remains an important and comprehensive database on the application and outcomes of ECLS for respiratory and cardiac failure in all age groups, and

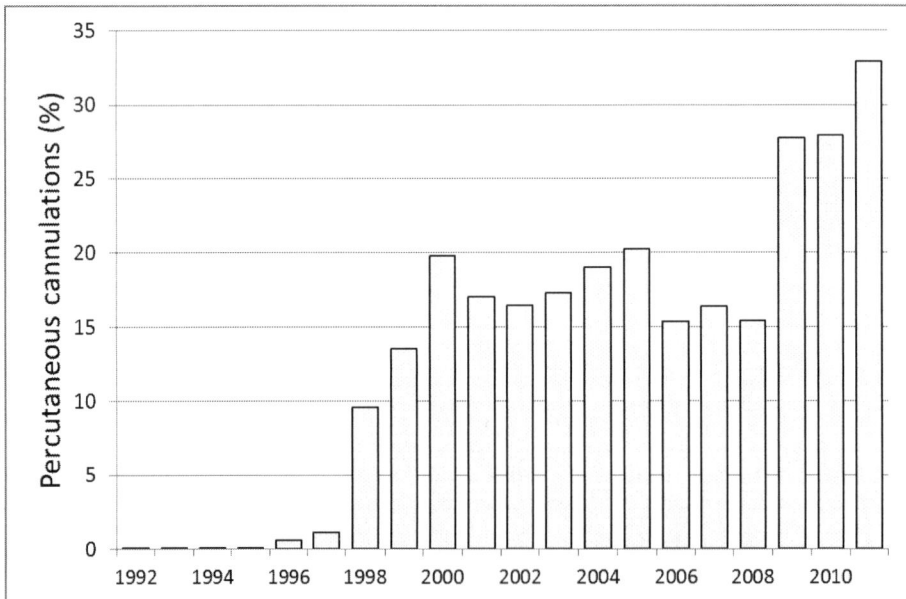

Figure 6-18. Graph showing the rising use of percutaneous cannulation for venovenous respiratory support over the past two decades.

is an important source of information for the clinical practice of ECLS and for support of academic contributions.

The ELSO Registry also contributes to quality improvement by providing center-specific data for benchmarking performance against the international experience. The online version recently introduced can make data available in a more timely fashion.

The Registry has a number of weaknesses in addition to its strengths. It can capture summary information, but cannot provide in-depth information which may be needed to support clinical practice. It is a voluntary registry, and therefore does not capture the full domestic, and

especially the international, experience. Even with well-defined data fields and instructions, the misinterpretation of fields can lead to errors in reporting and analysis, although the online form is designed to reduce errors and improve data integrity. Outcome data are very limited, as the Registry only captures basic outcome information.

The Registry now allows for the integration of specialized data collection projects without modifications to the database structure, such as the recent additions of addendum forms to capture data following ECLS for cardiac support and for the recently expanding extracorporeal CPR application.

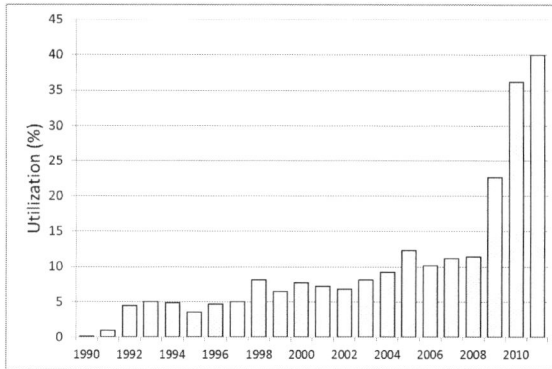

Figure 6-19. Graph showing the rising use of centrifugal pumps for extracorporeal support over the past two decades. The sharpest increases have occurred in the previous three years, coinciding with availability of newer centrifugal pump designs in markets such as the United States.

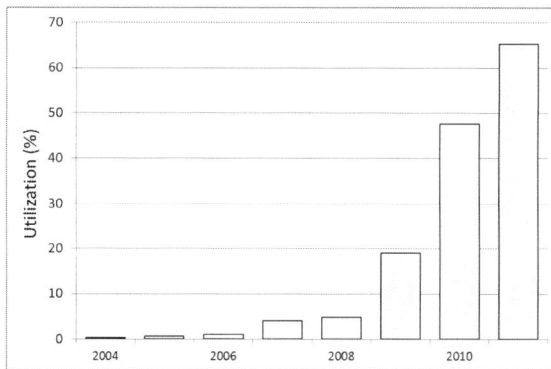

Figure 6-20. Graph showing the dramatic rise in use of plasma-resistant, low flow-resistance membrane lungs for extracorporeal support since their introduction. The sharpest increases have occurred in the previous three years, coinciding with availability of these devices in newer markets such as the United States, and now account for the majority of membrane lung types.

103

A number of trends have been identified. There is an increasing use of venovenous support for respiratory failure, an increasing use of newer technologies such as centrifugal pumps and plasma-resistant diffusion membranes, and of use of dual lumen cannulas in all age groups. Future enhancements that are now being considered for the online registry application include an addendum to capture details of renal replacement therapies, and the addition of physiological scoring systems.

References

1. McNeil, J.J., et al., The Value of Patient-Centred Registries in Phase IV Drug Surveillance. Pharmaceutical Medicine, 2010. 24(5): p. 281-288.
2. Hannan, E.L., et al., Long-Term Outcomes of Coronary-Artery Bypass Grafting versus Stent Implantation. New England Journal of Medicine, 2005. 352(21): p. 2174-2183.
3. Casalino, L., et al., External Incentives, Information Technology, and Organized Processes to Improve Health Care Quality for Patients With Chronic Diseases. JAMA: The Journal of the American Medical Association, 2003. 289(4): p. 434-441.
4. Starling, R.C., et al., Initial FDA Post-Approval Study INTERMACS Registry Results with a Continuous Flow Left Ventricular Assist Device as a Bridge to Heart Transplantation. Journal of cardiac failure, 2009. 15(6): p. S46.
5. Bizzarro, M.J., et al., Infections acquired during extracorporeal membrane oxygenation in neonates, children, and adults. Pediatr Crit Care Med, 2011. 12(3): p. 277-81.
6. Zapol, W.M., et al., Extracorporeal membrane oxygenation in severe acute respiratory failure. A randomized prospective study. JAMA, 1979. 242(20): p. 2193-6.
7. Morris, A.H., et al., Randomized clinical trial of pressure-controlled inverse ratio ventilation and extracorporeal CO2 removal for adult respiratory distress syndrome. Am J Respir Crit Care Med, 1994. 149(2 Pt 1): p. 295-305.
8. Davies, A., et al., Extracorporeal Membrane Oxygenation for 2009 Influenza A(H1N1) Acute Respiratory Distress Syndrome. JAMA, 2009. 302(17): p. 1888-95.
9. Peek, G.J., et al., Efficacy and economic assessment of conventional ventilatory support versus extracorporeal membrane oxygenation for severe adult respiratory failure (CESAR): a multicentre randomised controlled trial. Lancet, 2009. 374(9698): p. 1351-63.

7

Preface to Sections II-V

Gail M. Annich MD MS FRCP(C), Graeme MacLaren MBBS FCICM FCCM

Section II General Management and Outcomes:

This section of the 4th Edition is devoted to all aspects of ECLS circuitry, including the latest generation devices and their effects on critical illness physiology; details of vascular access both routine and elaborate; circuit anticoagulation; ECLS-related procedures; and general aspects of patient management such as infection, nutrition, fluid balance, sedation, and hypothermia. These chapters build on the ELSO guidelines for management of ECLS, which are published and regularly updated on the ELSO web site at www.elso.med.umich.edu. These guidelines describe useful and safe practice but are not intended as a universal standard of care. They are revised at regular intervals when new information, devices, medications, and techniques become available.

The original ELSO guidelines were published in 2007. However, since that time new pumps, new oxygenators, and safer, simpler circuits have become widely available. In addition, the advent of novel double lumen cannulas and access techniques have had wide-ranging effects on patient management and decreased some of the risks seen in venoarterial (VA) cannulation. The combination of routine surface coatings and smaller circuits with high blood flow has decreased the risk of circuit thrombosis. Easier extracorporeal management has led to easier patient care. Managing ECMO patients awake, extubated, and even ambulant is becoming progressively more common in some centers.

Section III Patient Specific Management and Outcomes:

This section of the 4th Edition is devoted to specific patient groups, categorized both by age and disease process. It is the hope of the editors that this section provides a reference to determine patient eligibility for ECLS while elaborating on how to manage these increasingly complex patients. There are dedicated chapters on neonatal, pediatric, and adult patients. Pediatric and adult patients are further classified into respiratory or cardiac failure. Congenital diaphragmatic hernia stands alone as a chapter, as does ECPR (ECLS support during cardiopulmonary resuscitation).

Section IV Other Uses for ECLS:

With the development of smaller, safer, and more robust systems, the potential indications for extracorporeal life support technology have exploded beyond isolated cardiac or respiratory failure. This section of the 4th Edition details such applications. The other extracorporeal technology chapters include pediatric VAD devices, plasmapheresis, and artificial lungs. In addition, chapters are specifically devoted to sepsis, organ support for transplantation, and catheterization laboratory procedures. A short discussion of the future of ECMO completes this section.

Section V Logistics and Legalities of ECLS:

This is the final section of the 4th Edition. Logistics encompasses the triage of patients to regional centers, transport of patients on ECLS, and details of how to run an ECLS program. A separate chapter is devoted to the regulations and legalities of ECLS as they apply to North American practice. The final chapter discusses relevant ethical issues surrounding ECLS, providing helpful insight into how to manage complex patients and make decisions about futility of care.

All of the chapters in this 4th Edition have been written by clinicians experienced in ECLS management and care. They provide a comprehensive reference for ECLS use across all patient populations.

8

The Circuit

John M. Toomasian MS CCP, D. Scott Lawson MS CCP, William E. Harris CCP

Introduction

The extracorporeal life support (ECLS) circuit is the set of disposable artificial organs and equipment that allow for mechanical support of the failing heart and/or lungs for days, weeks, or months at a time. The circuit must be designed to meet the expected metabolic demands of the patient including adequate oxygen (O_2) delivery and carbon dioxide (CO_2) removal. The circuit may also provide access for additional therapeutic modalities such as hemofiltration, continuous renal replacement therapy, and cardiovascular intervention. In short the circuit must be capable of mechanically supporting the patient, allowing the diseased organs time to recover. The circuit must be overseen and managed by an individual who is available at the bedside and trained in all aspects of troubleshooting and diagnosing any irregularities that could occur in the circuit. This chapter will focus on these fundamental components and how they are used to support the patient.

The traditional ECLS circuit consists of three primary components: gas exchange device, servo regulated blood pump, and heat exchanger. The circuit should be capable of maintaining the patient at normothermia, so a heat exchanger is part of the system. The heat exchanger is positioned distal to the gas exchange device or may be integrated with the gas exchange device.

The roller pump-bladder box circuit was popularized by Robert H. Bartlett and the team at the University of Michigan (Figure 8-1). As ECLS grew in the 1980s, this circuit has been modeled, copied, and described in detail by many centers throughout the world. This system has served as the model for newer ECLS

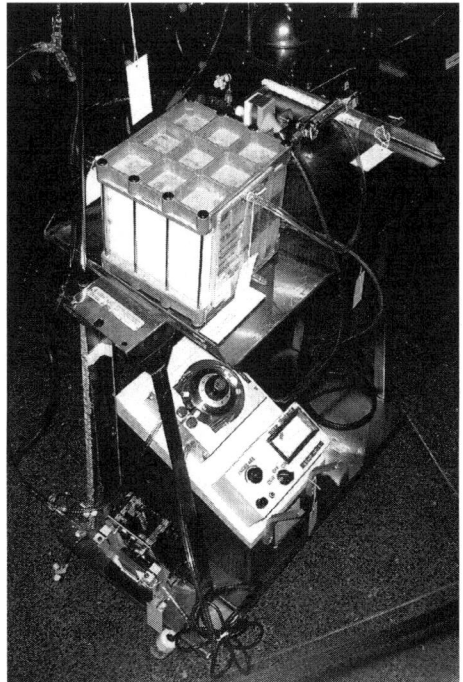

Figure 8-1. Original UC Irvine-University of Michigan ECMO circuit. Donated to Smithsonian Institution in 2004. Courtesy of John M. Toomasian.

circuit configurations and has been eloquently described in the first three editions of this textbook.[1-3] This chapter will also describe new devices with an emphasis on management guidelines established by the Extracorporeal Life Support Organization (ELSO). This circuit design provides a footprint for systems of the future which will satisfy performance standards while requiring less monitoring and maintenance.

The gold standard for gas exchange devices in ECLS has been the Kolobow silicone rubber membrane lung[4] which has been used for almost 50 years. The Kolobow lung has been manufactured and marketed by many companies and has served as the principle gas exchanger for the vast majority of extended ECLS cases through 2008. The device is available in a variety of sizes and configurations and has been very effective at exchanging O_2 and CO_2. The silicone membrane had a spiral wound configuration which resulted in a long blood path. The long blood path created high resistance to blood flow requiring a high pressure gradient. Priming was complex and time consuming. While some centers used early generation centrifugal pumps, the roller pump was typically required to generate the necessary pressure gradient, especially for long duration support. It was not uncommon to see an inlet/outlet pressure gradient exceeding 200 mmHg. Despite these few shortcomings, the Kolobow device has had an outstanding and reliable performance record of supporting gas exchange for days, weeks, or months.

The use of a roller pump offered another set of unique challenges. In the early days, venous return was gauged visually and pump adjustment to optimize drainage was done manually. This was tedious and required experience. If the pump flow exceeded the venous return, the positive blood displacement characteristics of the roller pump could entrain air into the circuit. To minimize this risk, a small compliant bladder was designed as a strategy to servo regulate the

pump speed. The pump would run when the bladder was filled with blood. When pump flow was greater than venous drainage, the bladder would collapse, tripping a switch that slowed or stopped pump flow. The system could also be servo regulated by measuring the pressure within both the arterial and venous lines and adjusting or modulating the pump flow down or off when the pressure parameter was exceeded.[5] Roller pumps still work remarkably well; however, there is the risk of a pump raceway rupture that could have a catastrophic end result. If standard polyvinylchloride (PVC) tubing is used in the raceway, it can withstand a 48-hour period of support without failure when properly occluded. Rupture resistant PVC tubing has been developed to serve as the raceway conduit in roller pumps. By altering the plasticizer content, the raceway tubing is made more durable and can tolerate the repetitive impact trauma induced by the occlusive roller pump. The use of rupture resistant PVC, or polyurethane tubing, can extend performance for several weeks,[6] but the risk of a raceway rupture is always a concern and requires a bedside specialist to monitor and troubleshoot.[7,8]

The use of first generation centrifugal pumps for ECLS was limited because of the high resistance of the Kolobow gas exchanger. The combination of early generation centrifugal pumps with the Kolobow lung often resulted in red cell destruction as suggested by high levels of plasma free hemoglobin.[9,10] Hemolysis was due to heat generated thrombus, stagnant blood flow zones in the pump head, excessive shear, and a high energy requirement to spin the pump head.

In the United States, many ECLS circuit components are used in an "off-label" application. All devices are approved for use by the FDA (US Food and Drug Administration). The majority of these components are manufactured for short term intraoperative use (six hours) during cardiopulmonary bypass (CPB). Off-label use experience has been gained by many centers and applied to select patient groups for extended periods of time. Governmental restrictions for device use vary by country. This chapter will describe the various components and how they might be used during long term ECLS. This chapter does not reflect any specific manufacturer's recommendations.

General principles of circuit design

The ECLS circuit must provide an adequate circulatory platform to mechanically support patients with compromised heart and/or lung function. This is accomplished by delivering blood through an artificial lung by a blood pump into the patient's vasculature. Vascular access and all related techniques and components for cannulation are described in Chapter 9. The circuit is made from different biomaterials and plastics that can induce circuit thrombosis, thus the patient and the circuit are anticoagulated. Chapter 11 deals with the techniques of anticoagulation. Each circuit can vary in its sophistication and complexity; however, each new level of complexity requires an additional need of a dedicated operator with the ability to troubleshoot and rectify problems that may result. Figure 8-2 shows a typical schematic of an ECLS circuit for an adult. It consists of a number of circuit access sites, monitoring sites, and tubing shunts, including an arteriovenous (AV) bridge. There will be variations of circuit design that are dependent on patient size, physiologic needs, and the institution's practice

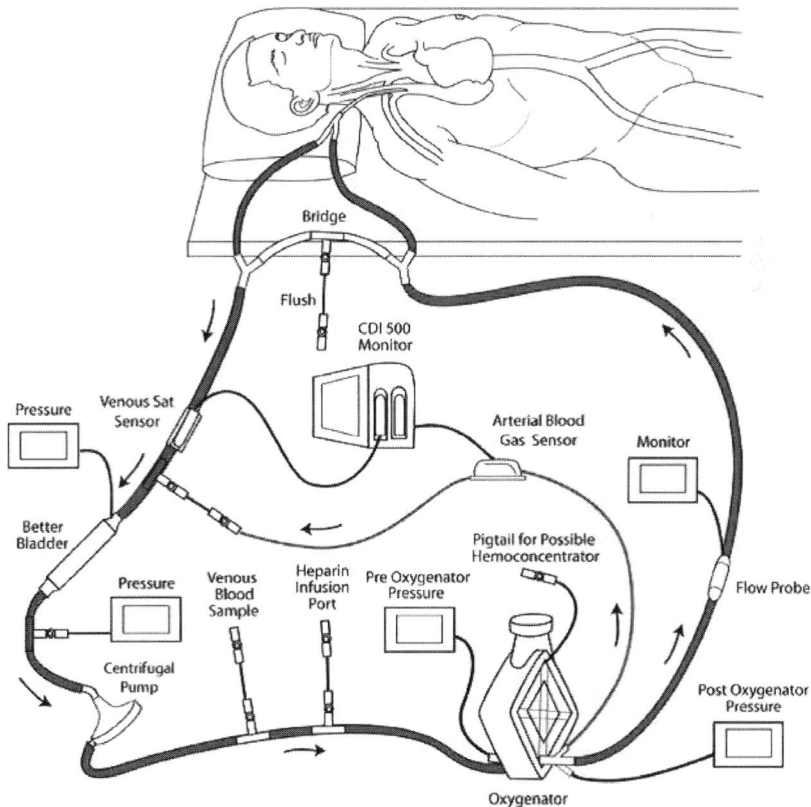

Figure 8-2. Extracorporeal Life Support Circuit, Courtesy of Ochsner Medical Center, New Orleans.

philosophy. A more simple circuit design may consist of only a centrifugal pump and gas exchanger with little or no peripheral access to the circuit (Figure 8-3).

When designing the circuit, a few simple rules should be considered. First, the shorter and simpler the circuit, the easier it is to manage. The tubing that connects the patient to the essential components of the circuit should not be lengthy, for the resistance increases as tubing length increases.[11] Streamlining the orientation and accessibility of components may reduce the mechanical stress and turbulence inflicted on the blood elements. Large volume circuits also expose the blood to additional foreign surface areas that may promote a larger inflammatory response and chance of thrombosis.[12] Large volume circuits increase the priming volume and the use of banked blood components, as well as colloid and crystalloid solutions. Large volume circuits have an increased area for heat loss. Ideally, the circuit should be designed as short as possible but adequate in length to allow for patient movement and transport. Smaller circuit volumes may decrease circuit induced capillary leakage and associated extravascular tissue edema.

By keeping the circuit simple, fewer potential circuit related problems should occur. Many circuits contain longer than required lengths of extra tubing, and an excessive number of stopcocks and connectors. Each connector causes turbulent blood flow, potential blood element damage, and areas of stagnation inducing clot formation. In addition, every luer site included as a site for circuit access is also a site to entrain air or leak blood. For instance, an inline temperature site is redundant if adequate temperature monitoring of the patient is possible by peripheral measures and if attention is made to the water recirculation unit that warms the heat exchanger. Straight connectors utilizing double luer access should be considered when possible, eliminating the Y-connectors often used with an AV bridge or a "diamond." The circuit is safer with fewer connections.

With simple design objectives, new circuit components are now being developed and introduced for clinical use. Gas exchange devices have been developed that maximize exterior hollow fiber technology with compressed surface polymers such as polymethylpentene (PMP). These materials are much more efficient in gas transfer and have a very low device blood path pressure gradient. Safer blood pumps, including new generation centrifugal pumps, are much more efficient than their predecessors and are easily coupled with a low resistance gas exchange device to provide the necessary support without the problems of hemolysis and mechanical failure. More sophisticated computer controlled servo regulated systems exist and in conjunction with more streamlined and improved cannula designs, many of the troubles observed with roller pumps and older gas exchangers have been significantly reduced. Biocompatible circuits also continue to make progress to reduce some of the deleterious effects of the circuit surfaces on blood elements.[13]

Criteria for selecting circuit components

Based on the guidelines adopted by the Extracorporeal Life Support Organization (ELSO), the ECLS circuit must be capable of providing

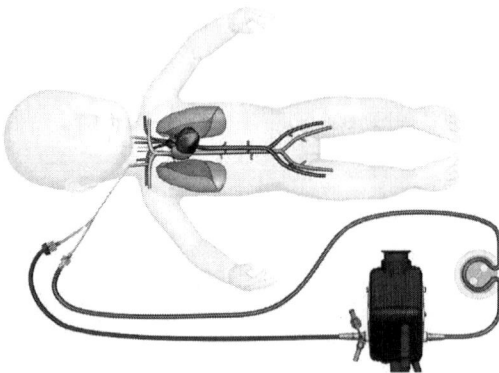

Figure 8-3. Simplified ECLS Circuit, courtesy of Maquet Cardiopulmonary.

total metabolic support for the patient, unless the intent is specifically partial support (i.e., CO_2 removal for asthma). Blood flow may be provided by one or more different flow modalities, each flow modality having specific indications.

Blood flow for cardiac support

Vascular access is venoarterial (VA) for cardiac support. Vascular access may be extrathoracic or intrathoracic. The various circuit components are selected to support a blood flow rate of 3.0 $L/m^2/min$. In general target flow rates are: 100cc/kg/min (neonates), 80cc/kg/min (pediatrics), and 60cc/kg/min (adults). Patients with single ventricle cardiac lesions may require higher flow rates.[14] The best measure of adequate systemic perfusion is a mixed venous saturation greater than 70%. This can be measured directly or noninvasively from the venous drainage line. Achieving the desired flow is determined by the vascular access site(s), drainage tubing diameter, cannula size(s), resistance, and pump properties.

Blood flow and gas exchange for respiratory failure

Vascular access can be either venoarterial or venovenous (VV). Venovenous is the mode of choice unless limited by patient anatomy. The gas exchange device and blood flow should be capable of oxygen delivery and CO_2 removal at least equal to the metabolic oxygen consumption of the patient. The normal oxygen delivery rates are: 6cc/kg/min (neonates), 4-5cc/kg/min (pediatrics), 3cc/kg/min (adults).[15] This usually equates to VV blood flow rates of 120ml/kg/min for neonates ranging downward to 60-80 ml/kg/min for adults. Oxygen delivery capability is determined by the blood flow rate, hemoglobin concentration, inlet hemoglobin saturation, and the gas exchange device's gas transfer properties. Carbon dioxide removal always exceeds

oxygen delivery when the circuit is planned for full support.

Blood flow and gas exchange for CO_2 removal only

If the circuit is planned for CO_2 removal only, vascular access can be venoarterial, venovenous, or arteriovenous. Venoarterial and venovenous modes will require a pump within the circuit. Arteriovenous mode has adequate pressure gradient to drive blood flow through a low resistant membrane device without the addition of a blood pump. Typical blood flow is approximately 25% of the cardiac output, which is sufficient to remove the CO_2 produced by metabolism (3-6cc/kg/min). Carbon dioxide removal is determined by the blood flow and the gas exchanger's sweep gas rate, the inlet pCO_2 and the gas exchange device's gas transfer properties.

Circuit components

The basic ECLS circuit includes: cannulas, conduit tubing, blood pump, gas exchange device, and heat exchanger. Some circuit components can be integrated (i.e., heat exchanger and artificial lung). The circuit becomes more complex with each additional component; such as an isolated heat exchanger, circuit shunts (i.e., bridges, recirculation lines), connector based oxygen saturation measurement systems, monitors, bubble detectors, and alarms. Added complexity may limit the operation of the circuit to a trained specialist.

Blood tubing

The tubing length and diameter will contribute to the resistance to blood flow. Tubing size is chosen to allow free venous drainage with minimal resistance. The blood flow through one meter of tubing at 100 mmHg pressure gradient for common internal diameter tubing (inches) is: 3/16": 1.2 L/min; ¼": 2.5 L/min; 3/8": 5L/min; ½":10L/min.[16]

The majority of conduit tubing is made from a formulation of polyvinylchloride mixed with a plasticizer. The amount of plasticizer determines the tubing's durometer or flexibility. Di-2(ethylhexyl) phthalate (DEHP) is a plasticizer widely used to make PVC flexible. It is present in a wide variety of hospital plastic products including bags for intravenous fluids, blood storage, and parental nutrition as well as products used during CPB, ECLS, and hemodialysis.

The FDA issued a public notification regarding exposure to DEHP.[17] Concerns exist over the release of DEHP from PVC products. The lipid content of the liquid the PVC is in contact with, the temperature, and the duration of contact affects the leaching of DEHP. Various adverse effects have been reported in laboratory animals, with the greatest concern being its effects on the male reproductive system.[18] The FDA concluded that there are possible health risks from DEHP exposure and concluded that non–DEHP containing substitute products should be used in male neonates, pregnant women, and peripubertal boys when available. The leaching of DEHP does occur in ECMO circuits but coated circuits decrease or eliminate DEHP leaching from pre-primed ECMO circuits.[19]

An arteriovenous "bridge" connecting the arterial and venous lines located close to the patient is another variation of the basic circuit (Figure 8-2). The bridge allows for the blood to be recirculated in situations in which the patient is removed from support. It has widely been used during venoarterial support, particularly for trialing periods off mechanical support, during weaning, or during an emergency. However, a bridge is not required during venovenous support. When clamped, the bridge is a stagnant area that can contribute to thrombosis. Periodically the bridge is opened and "flashed" allowing blood to shunt through the connection to reduce the incidence of clot formation in this stagnant area. Several studies have demonstrated the adverse effects of this practice.[20-22] In general, if a bridge is used, it should be maintained closed during most of the ECLS run, with a protocol for purging the bridge of stagnant blood when it is not in use. A bridge may be constructed from high flow stopcocks and ¼ inch tubing. This type of bridge has been a successful low flow shunt used in many centers.

Blood pumps

The blood pump should be able to provide the required blood flow for the patient, as described in the ELSO Guidelines. Pump options include: modified roller pump with inlet pressure control, centrifugal or axial rotary pump with inlet pressure control, or peristaltic pump. Each pump should be capable of adjusting for and addressing the following parameters.

Inlet pressure (suction pressure)

Inlet pressure is the pressure of the venous blood draining from the patient via the inlet line to the blood pump. With the pump's inlet line occluded, the suction (negative pressure) exerted by the pump should not exceed a negative 100-300 mmHg. As a function of pump speed, the inlet pressure can vary from a small positive pressure to a low subatmospheric pressure. However, significantly higher negative pressure (negative 750 mmHg or greater) can occur when the venous drainage is occluded.

When blood flow is exposed to extreme negative pressure, a phenomenon called outgassing or cavitation occurs.[23] Cavitation pulls the dissolved gasses in blood (oxygen, carbon dioxide) out of solution and causes the local red cells in that portion of tubing or pump head to hemolyze. Inlet pressure values in excess of negative 300 mmHg can be avoided by a servo controlled pressure sensor on the pump's inlet that slows the pump to minimize negative pressure exerted on the inlet line.[24] Alternatively, operating the pump at lower speed (typically measured in revolutions per minute; RPM) in order to minimize the negative pressure at the pump inlet is another strategy to decrease the risk of cavitation and associated hemolysis. Manual adjustment of the speed control may be required to minimize the pump RPMs that would avoid repeated line chatter, reoccurrence of an extreme negative pressure, and possible occurrences of cavitation. Ideally the inlet pressure to a centrifugal pump should be measured so that the pump speed can be adjusted for extremes in negative pressure.[25]

Outlet pressure (line pressure)

Outlet pressure refers to the pressure in the line exiting the pump head. When the pump's outlet line is occluded, the outlet pressure should not exceed 400 mmHg. Although pump generated pressures greater than 400 mmHg are not inherently hemolytic to red blood cells, a centrifugal pump's speed may significantly increase heat generation as a function of RPM. There is also concern for the integrity of blood tubing connectors when line pressure exceeds 400 mmHg. The ability for any pump to dissipate heat is an important factor and is inherent in its design. Outlet pressure can also be servo controlled to minimize the risk of generating an extreme positive pressure.

Hemolysis

The plasma hemoglobin should be < 15 mg/dL under most conditions.[26] If the plasma hemoglobin exceeds 50 mg/dL, the cause should be investigated. Causes may relate to intermittent venous line chattering, air-blood interface related to cardiac surgery, partial circuit or component thrombosis. Hemolysis can also be a consequence of water and blood mixing. This can happen if the integrity of the heat exchanger membrane has been violated.

Power failure

The pump should have a battery life capable of at least one hour of operation, and a system to manually crank the pump in the event of power failure. A backup system should be available if there is no method to manually hand crank the pump. The pump should alarm in situations where reverse flow may occur if power fails (i.e., arterial to venous in the VA mode).

Pump types

Roller pumps

A roller pump is a positive displacement pump capable of generating forward flow as a function of the tubing size and pump speed. Roller pumps must be constantly monitored and servo regulated to prevent excessive levels of negative inlet pressure or positive outlet pressure. Roller pumps have been fundamental in the conduct of CPB and ECLS. Roller pumps are advantageous when lower blood flows are utilized and blood flow management in 10-25cc increments is required. Although clinical complications related to roller pumps are rare, they do exist and can be dramatic upon occurrence.[27] Roller pumps are described in detail in the first three volumes of the ECMO Redbook.[1-3]

Centrifugal blood pumps

Centrifugal blood pumps were not commonly used during the first few decades of ECLS when the Kolobow silicone rubber membrane lung was the mainstay. The first centrifugal pump used off-label was the early generation Bio-Medicus pump. This pump used a disposable pumphead which consisted of a series of concentric cones that would spin, creating centrifugal force that directed blood forward to a dedicated outlet. A fixed shaft anchored the cones and a seal was incorporated within

113

the blood path resulting in a stagnant blood zone at the pumphead's base. A consequence of this design was localized heat generation. Heat was poorly dissipated and at high RPM, the heat generation and sheer stress resulted in hemolysis.[28-30]

Newer, more efficient designs of centrifugal pumps, along with the introduction of low resistance gas exchange devices, have allowed for safer use of these pumps.[31, 32] Many new designs have been introduced for CPB or ventricular assist support and show promise for extended use. These designs all vary but have incorporated a key design feature described by Mendler,[33] which is a hole within the pumphead. This hole allows blood to continually wash the area around the rotor, thus reducing or eliminating any stagnant area(s). This reduces the mechanically induced hemolysis that was observed in earlier centrifugal pump designs.[34]

Both magnetically driven and magnetically suspended centrifugal pumps are available for use in ECLS. As shown in Figures 8-4 and 8-5, magnetically driven pumpheads have a rotor that couples directly to a shaft or bearing. When connected to the drive motor, the magnetic attraction couples the disposable pumphead to the motor. As the motor spins, the pumphead spins according to the RPM generated by the pump motor. Localized heat is generated around the seal and sufficient washout around the seal occurs, minimizing heat-induced thrombosis. There is no direct contact between the motor and blood, for the blood is contained within the disposable pumphead. A flow meter is required to measure the blood flow rate exiting the pumphead.

A magnetically levitated pump contains no seals or bearings. The pump rotor is levitated within the disposable pumphead housing by a magnetic field so that when the motor is powered up, the resultant magnetic field aligns and maintains the rotor in a position in which there is no direct contact to any other part of the pumphead housing (Figure 8-6). When the pump is engaged the magnetic field fluctuates allowing the rotor to spin at the rate set by the control console. A flow meter is also required to measure the blood flow.

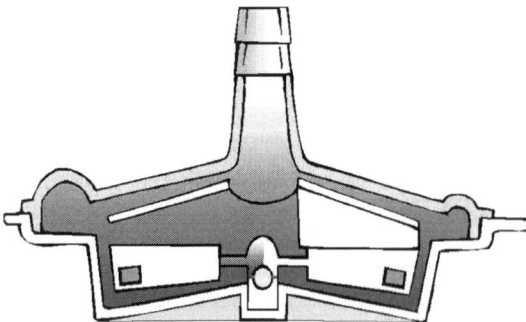

Figure 8-4. Cross sectional diagram of a magnetically driven pivot bearing centrifugal pump (Rotaflow).

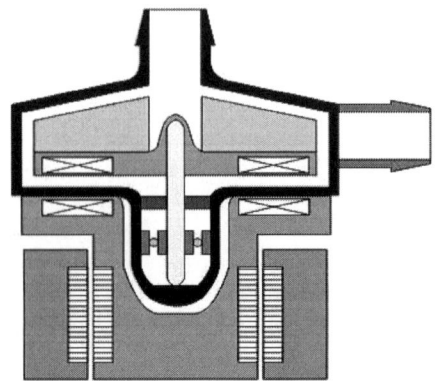

Figure 8-5. Cross sectional diagram of a magnetically coupled, shaft driven centrifugal pump.

Commercial centrifugal pumps

Table 8-1 summarizes certain performance specifications of many commercial centrifugal pumps. A description and synopsis of many centrifugal pumps including a description of their US regulatory status is also described.

Maquet Rotaflow (cleared for up to 6 hours of use by the US FDA for CPB, CE Mark)

The Rotaflow centrifugal pumphead features a low-friction one-point pivot bearing (sapphire ball & PE calotte) that supports a multi-finned impeller (Figure 8-7). The pumphead is controlled by a remote drive motor tethered to a control console. An ICU version of the system is available for ECLS that incorporates additional safety features that minimize inadvertent manipulation of the speed control or

Table 8-1. Kinetic Pump Specifications.

	Maquet Rotaflow	Sorin Revolution	Medtronic Affinity	Medtronic BPX-80	Medtronic BPX-50	Levitronix Centrimag	Levitronix Pedimag	Medos DP3
Static Volume (mL)	32	57	40	86	48	31	14	17
Maximum Flow (LPM)	10	8	10	10	1.5	10	1.5	8
Inlet Outlet Port Size (in.)	3/8	3/8	3/8	3/8	1/4	3/8	1/4	3/8

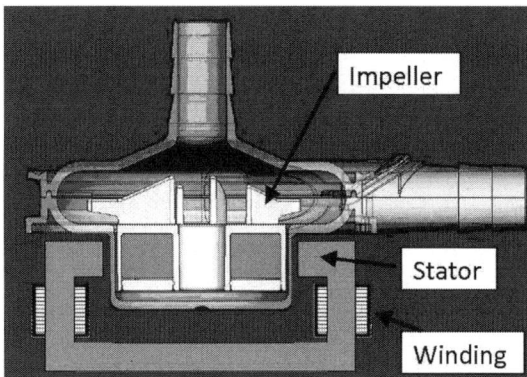

Figure 8-6. Cross section diagram of the magnetic levitated centrifugal pump. Courtesy of Levitronix.

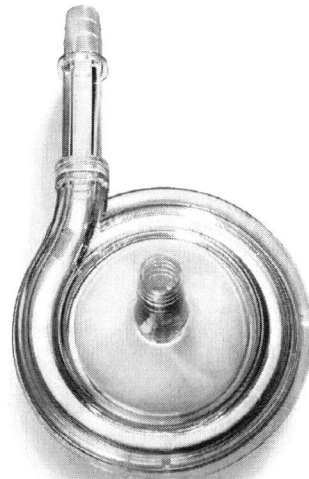

Figure 8-7. Rotaflow Pumphead, Pump rotor is balanced on a pivot bearing. The pumphead couples via magnets in the pump motor. When the pump is engaged the impeller spins as a function of rpm. Courtesy of Maquet Cardiopulmonary.

power switch (Figure 8-8). The unit is not servo regulated to inlet negative pressure.

Sorin Revolution (cleared for up to 6 hours of use by the US FDA for CPB, CE Mark)

The Sorin Revolution centrifugal pump features a seal-less, low friction bearing which improves pump head reliability and reduces heat buildup and resultant hemolysis (Figure 8-9). The Revolution pumphead is operated by the Sorin Centrifugal Pump (SCP) System, including the S3, S5, or C5 pump base modules. The system also incorporates an Electrical Remote-Controlled Tubing Clamp (ERC®) that is designed to improve the safety of operation. The ERC adds a safeguard against inadvertent air delivery during operation. When certain conditions are detected (low level, bubble, or retrograde flow), the ERC occludes the reinfusion line to minimize the danger of air delivery. The clamp can be opened and closed at any time by pressing the respective key on the control panel or by manually opening or closing the clamp head. This feature provides some servo regulatory controls that are unique to centrifugal pump technology.

Medtronic BPX-80+ and BPX-50 (cleared for up to 6 hours of continuous use by US FDA, CE Mark)

The Medtronic BPX pump design features a patented vertical cutwater outlet and a smooth vortex cone design that provides superior micro air retention. The disposable is controlled by a Bio-console 560 system (Figure 8-5). This pump has been used widely during clinical open heart surgery, but has been associated with a higher level of hemolysis with extended use.[29]

Levitronix Centrimag Pump (cleared for up to 6 hours of continuous use by US FDA for CPB, 30 days as a RVAD. CE Mark)

The Levitronix centrifugal pump is a magnetically levitated pump with no contact bearings as diagramed in Figure 8-6. The pumphead is disposable. The impeller is suspended and supported by a rotating magnetic field that provides no direct contact points with the pump housing during operation. Two sizes exist, one for adult use, the second for pediatric use. Both pumpheads are operated by the same hardware and both require flow probes to enable the system. The pumphead cannot be manually handcranked, so a backup system must be present if required. The complete system is shown in Figures 8-10, 8-11 and 8-12.

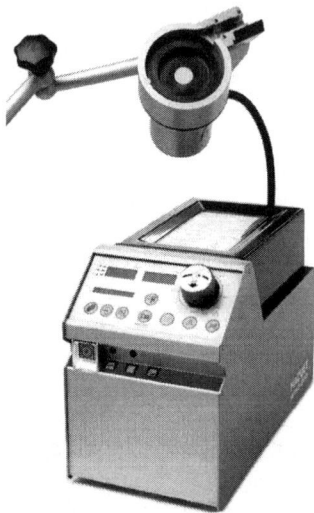

Figure 8-8. Rotaflow ICU Pump Console and System. Courtesy of Maquet Cardiopulmonary.

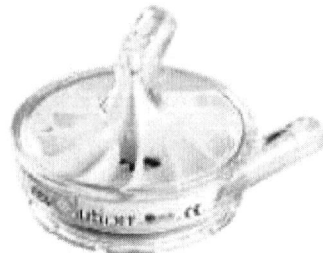

Figure 8-9. Sorin Revolution Pumphead. Courtesy of the Sorin Group.

Figures 8-10, 8-11 and 8-12. Levitronix Centrimag Drive Motor, Pumphead and Console. Courtesy of Levitronix.

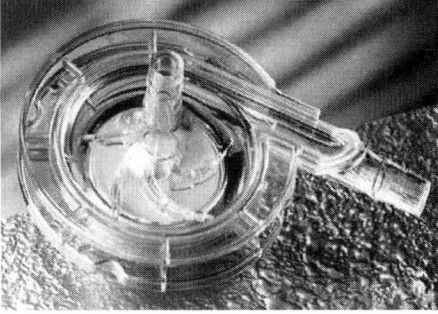

Figure 8-10. Levitronix PediMage Pumphead.

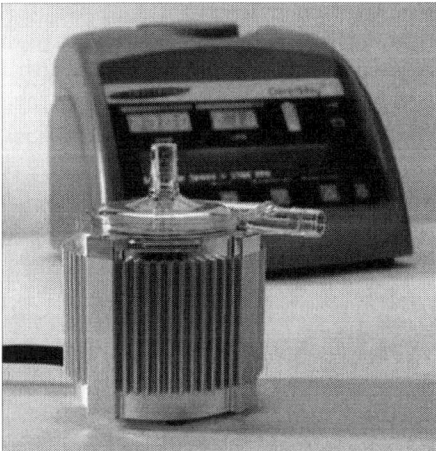

Figure 8-11. Levitronix System.

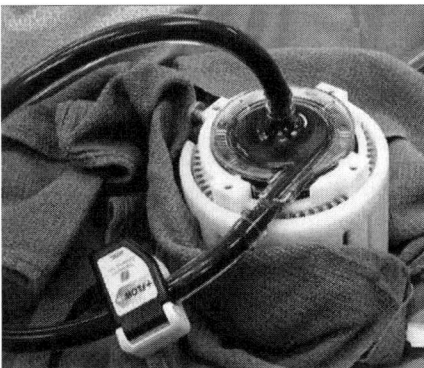

Figure 8-12. Pumphead in Operation.

Medos Delta Stream (Not available in the USA, 6 hours CPB-CE Mark)

The Medos DP2 and DP3 systems include a small disposable pumphead characterized by diagonally streamed impellers. High hydraulic performance is achieved through an optimal flow guide. A pivot bearing concept combined with magnetic coupling is CE approved for up to 6 hours. The pump works in conjunction with the Medos Delta Stream console offering flow and pressure control, touch screen monitoring, battery operation, and portability (Figure 8-13).

Gas exchange devices

The gas exchange device is designed to add oxygen and remove CO_2. The device must be of adequate size to provide for the anticipated metabolic requirements of the patient. The gas exchanger may contain several biomaterials including: silicone rubber, polypropylene (microporous hollow fiber), compressed surface polymethylpentene (PMP), polyvinylchloride (PVC), polyurethane as well as stainless steel.

The surface area and blood path mixing determine the maximum oxygenation capacity of any gas exchanger. The "rated flow" or "maximal oxygen delivery" is defined by the amount of desaturated (75%) blood that can be nearly fully saturated (95%) per minute. When used for total support the gas exchange device should

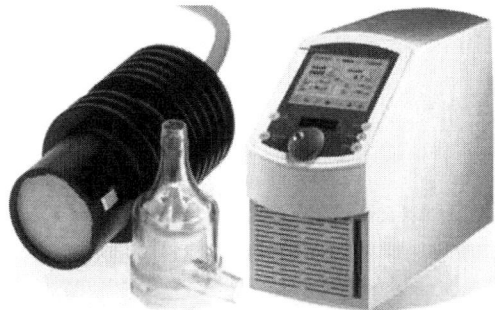

Figure 8-13. Medos Pump.

provide full oxygen and CO_2 exchange. The following features and characteristics uniquely describe each gas exchange device.

Rated Flow

A standard, called Rated Flow, has been established so that membrane gas exchangers can be compared. Rated Flow is the flow rate at which venous blood, with a saturation of 75% and hemoglobin of 12 gm/dL will exit the gas exchange device with a saturation of 95%.

Maximal Oxygen Delivery

The Maximal Oxygen Delivery of a gas exchange device is the amount of oxygen delivered per minute when running at rated flow. This is determined by calculating the difference in oxygen content between the outlet blood and the inlet blood to the gas exchanger. This difference is typically 4-5cc O_2/dL. Multiplying this by blood flow rate through the gas exchanger will yield the oxygen delivered by the gas exchanger in cc O_2/min. A gas exchange device with a rated flow of 2.0 L/min will offer a maximal oxygen delivery of 100 cc O_2/min. A device with a rated flow of 4.0 L/min will offer a maximal oxygen delivery of 200 cc O_2/min. The physiologic needs of the patient will determine the oxygen delivery required. Once the oxygen delivery requirements are appreciated, the associated rated flow can be determined and an appropriate gas exchange device can be chosen. A gas exchange device should be chosen that is capable of total support or greater.

Sweep gas

The gas blown through the gas exchange device and across the membrane is called the sweep gas. For most applications, sweep gas will be 100% oxygen. There are occasions during cardiac support or by institutional preference when the sweep gas will be a mixture of oxygen and compressed room air, thus requiring an oxygen-nitrogen blender. In some instances when the pCO_2 must be maintained, carbogen gas (5% CO_2, 95% O_2) or 100% CO_2 gas (in very small amounts) may be added into the sweep gas. Often a gas flow rate equal to the blood flow rate (1:1) is used to begin support. The gas to blood flow ratio is then adjusted to maintain the systemic pCO_2 at a desired range (i.e., 36-44 mmHg). Increasing the sweep gas flow rate will increase CO_2 clearance but will not effect oxygenation. Decreasing the sweep gas flow rate will increase the pCO_2, but will usually not effect oxygenation. Water vapor can condense within the gas compartment of the membrane lung and may be cleared by intermittently increasing sweep gas flow to a higher flow. If there is excessive water that has not been purged, the pCO_2 may rise.

ECLS can be used for CO_2 removal instead of oxygen delivery. Since membrane gas exchangers are more efficient at clearing CO_2 than delivering oxygen, the metabolic production of CO_2 can be removed with blood flows as low as 0.75L/min/m². In this situation, the gas exchange device size can be smaller than that required for full support with the gas: blood flow rate of 10:1 or greater.

Pressure gradients

Early generation membrane lungs were characterized by a long blood path and a high pressure gradient. These early designs included flat sheet silicone rubber membranes and the "blood inside" hollow fiber bundle configurations. Design modifications led to a hollow fiber concept with "gas inside" and blood circulating outside the fibers. This configuration resulted in significantly lower pressure gradients in the blood path.[35] This design principle ("gas inside" fiber bundle) has been applied to all subsequent device designs regardless of hollow fiber material. The first widely used biomaterial was microporous polypropylene. Although this material could be manufactured as a flat sheet, fibers provided more effective surface area and were relatively inexpensive to manufacture. These changes allowed for engineering designs to maximize secondary flows and mixing in the blood path. Thus optimizing gas exchange and allowing for smaller devices to be built. In addition, resistance to blood flow was lower, as was the associated pressure gradient. The lower resistance made these newer generation gas exchange devices more practical for long duration use.

Microporous polypropylene hollow fiber gas exchange devices are limited in longevity because over time, plasma will leak across the fiber eventually causing the device to fail.[36,37] Gas transfer normally occurs across a protein layer covering the micropores. Over time, exposure to phospholipids in the blood causes the surface tension at the blood/gas interface in the micropores to decrease. As the surface tension decreases, plasma begins to weep through the micropores into the gas side of the membrane. As a result, gas exchange efficiency falls and the membrane begins to fail.[38] This phenomenon limited the widespread application of polypropylene devices for long-term use.

A chemical cousin to polypropylene became available in early 2000 that showed promise as a plasma-leakage resistant hollow fiber. Polymethylpentene (PMP) fibers were fashioned into a gas exchange membrane efficient for extended use. PMP is a microporous material, however, compressing the fibers results in an outer surface with properties similar to that of a solid membrane. The material's compressed outer surface provides a more leak resistant property than the microporous polypropylene. Even though the PMP membranes are "solid-like," gas can still be entrained across the PMP material into the blood path if a large negative pressure is applied. Therefore, it is important to maintain positive pressure on the blood path side.

Polymethylpentene devices were first described in two pilot clinical studies. Peek, et al. showed the feasibility of PMP fibers in long-term ECLS support. The Medos HiLite was used in six patients in whose transfusion rates were significantly lower and plasma leakage was not observed.[39] Similarly, Horton et al. described an experience in 23 patients in which a single Quadrox-D device was used for up to 46 days in conjunction with a centrifugal pump.[40] No plasma leakage was observed in either series. Both of these devices soon became staples of this new generation of gas exchangers. The initial experience with the PMP devices demonstrated promise in durability, inflammatory response attenuation, and decreased transfusion requirements making these gas exchange devices well suited for long-term ECLS use.

Polymethylpentene fibers are produced by Membrana GmbH (Wuppertal, Germany) and have similar gas exchange characteristics as polypropylene. The material is more challenging to handle, so it is typically matted and either wound or stacked in relatively short blood path configurations. Current PMP hollow fiber devices have low pressure gradients and the fibers mimic more of a "solid hollow fiber" technology with minimal plasma leakage.[41]

Gas exchanger induced air embolism

Air or oxygen bubbles can pass through the gas exchange device into the blood path if the sweep gas pressure exceeds the pressure in the blood path. This can occur when the device blood path pressure is subatmospheric (which is often the case with a centrifugal pump). Air can also be pulled across microporous and PMP membranes when there is no blood flow and the device is above the level of the patient's heart. In this circumstance, the gas exchange device can drain by gravity into the dependent blood tubing, "de-priming" the device, pulling air into the blood path. While this is more likely with microporous membrane technologies, it is a possibility with silicone membranes if the membrane has been damaged.

The best way to minimize the risk of air embolization through the gas exchanger is by maintaining blood path pressures that are higher than the gas side pressure.[42] Pressure popoff valves can be placed in the gas supply line, sweep gas pressures can be servo regulated and the gas exchange device can be kept below the level of the patient's heart as strategies to minimize air embolism risk. The newer generation gas exchange devices and centrifugal pumps have improved patient safety making it more practical to move patients within and between hospitals. These moves often require repositioning the gas exchange device and manipulating blood flow. It is probable that at times, the gas exchange device will be above the level of the patient's heart while venous drainage pressures are subatmospheric. If blood flow were to suddenly stop (line kink, patient cough, clot in gas exchange device) the possibility of catastrophic air embolism exists.

Commercial gas exchange devices

A synopsis of many gas exchange devices including a description of their US regulatory status is in Table 8-2.

Maquet QUADROX- iD (CE Mark, cleared for up to 6 hours of continuous use by US FDA)

The Maquet QUADROX- iD (innovative diffusion membrane) device comes in an adult and pediatric size (Figures 8-14 and 8-15). Both devices are constructed of plasma resistant hydrophobic PMP hollow fibers and have a low device pressure gradient. The compressed surface of the PMP fiber reduces the risks of failure related to plasma leakage. It effectively prevents the formation of micro bubbles and

Table 8-2. Gas Exchanger Specifications.

Model	Quadrox ID Pediatric	Quadrox ID Adult	Medos Hilite 800LT	Medos Hilite 2400LT	Medos Hilite 7000LT
Material	PMP Fiber	PMP Fiber	PMP Fiber	PMP Fiber	PMP Fiber
Blood flow range	0.2-2.8 LPM	0.5-7.0 LPM	0.8 LPM	2.4 LPM	7.0 LPM
Priming volume	81 ml	250 ml	55 mL	95mL	275mL
Effective surface area	$0.8\ m^2$	$1.8\ m^2$	$0.32\ m^2$	$0.65\ m^2$	$1.9\ m^2$
Heat exchanger material	Polyurethane	Polyurethane	Polyester	Polyester	Polyester
Effective heat exchange surface area	$0.15\ m^2$	$0.6\ m^2$	$0.074\ m^2$	$0.074\ m^2$	$0.45\ m^2$
Blood inlet and outlet connection size	1/4 inch	3/8 inch	3/16-1/4 inch	1/4 inch	3/8 inch

Model	Novalung ILA	Novalung sLA	Medtronic Kolobow ECMO	Medtronic Kolobow Surgical	Sorin Lilliput 2 ECMO
Material	PMP Fiber	PMP Fiber	Silicone rubber	Silicone rubber	PMP Fiber
Blood flow range	0.5-4.5 LPM	0.5-4.5 LPM	1.0,1.2,1.8 LPM	4.5,5.5,6.5 LPM	2.3 LPM
Priming volume	225 ml	225 ml	90,100,175 mL	455,575,665 mL	90mL
Effective surface area	$1.3\ m^2$	$1.3\ m^2$	$0.6,0.8, 1.5\ m^2$	$2.5,3.5,4.5\ m^2$	$0.60\ m^2$
Heat exchanger material	None	None	None	Stainless Steel	Stainless Steel
Effective heat exchange surface area	Not applicable	Not applicable	Not applicable	unknown	$0.02\ m^2$
Blood inlet and outlet connection size	3/9 inch safety connector	3/8 inch	1/4 inch	3/8 inch	1/4 inch

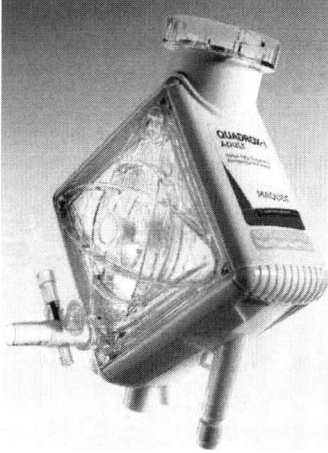

Figure 8-14. Quadrox iD-Adult.

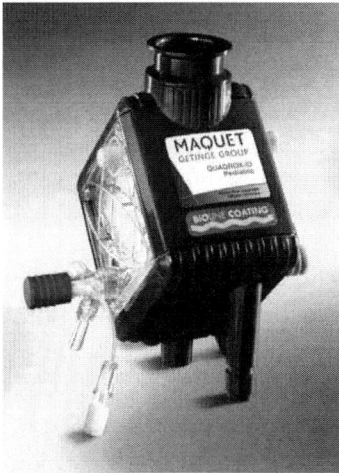

Figure 8-15. Quadrox iD-Pediatric.

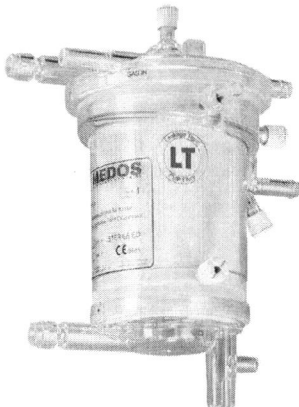

Figure 8-16. Medos HiLite Gas Exchanger: Exterior View.

protects against bacterial contamination from the gas side. The smaller QUADROX-iD Pediatric provides a smaller device for infant and pediatric patients. Combined with a lower static volume and surface area, high performance is similar to the larger adult version. High gas transfer rates of up to 180 ml/min for O_2 and up to 140 mmHg for CO_2 provides an optimal unit for smaller patients.

Medos Hilite LT (not available in the USA, CE Mark)

Medos Medizintechnik AG (Stolberg, Germany) produces three sizes of plasma tight PMP hollow fiber membrane devices for long-term support. The design incorporates the requirements inherent to several weeks of circulatory support. Each device has shown efficacy in providing effective gas exchange characteristics over a wide range of flow rates. The heat exchanger is integrated into the unit and results in a low priming volume with small foreign surface. The device is characterized by a low pressure differential between blood inlet and outlet. The Medos devices are suitable for use with roller or centrifugal pumps. The Medos LT device is illustrated in Figure 8-16. The figure shows the external and internal components in an exterior and cross section view. Three devices are manufactured based on surface area to meet the metabolic needs of all patient populations while attempting to limit surface area and reduce stagnant zones that could produce unwanted coagulation disorders related to low blood velocity states.

Medtronic ECMO and Medtronic Surgical Membrane Oxygenators (ECMO units cleared for > 6 hours of continuous use by US FDA, CE Mark. Surgical units cleared for 6 hours of use by US FDA, CE Mark)

The Kolobow silicone rubber device was state-of-the-art in gas exchangers during the

1970s, '80s, and '90s. The device's design resulted in a high blood path pressure and flow resistance. This was a result of the winding tension of the silicone rubber material and the relatively long blood path. The Kolobow membrane lung consists of a flat, reinforced silicone membrane envelope that is wound in a spiral coil. The silicone membrane acts as a highly gas-permeable barrier separating blood and gas compartments. Gas transfer occurs by simple molecular diffusion across the membrane. The device is manufactured in several sizes based on effective surface area. The smaller ECMO sized devices (0.6, 0.8, 1.5m²) require the use of a separate heat exchanger to maintain normothermia. The larger surgical membrane oxygenators (2.5, 3.5, 4.5m²) have an integrated stainless steel heat exchanger positioned proximal to the gas exchange compartment. This device has been used for extended support for decades and has been described in detail in the first three editions of the "Redbook."[1-3]

Novalung Lung Assist Devices (CE Mark. iLA devices not available in USA, sLA devices cleared for 6 hours of continuous use by US FDA for CPB, not available outside the USA)

Novalung GmbH (Heilbronn, Germany) manufactures two versions of a gas exchange device for support of respiratory failure. The Novalung Membrane Ventilator® (Figure 8-17) acts as a low resistance temporary artificial lung to allow oxygen and CO_2 transfer across its membrane fibers with or without the use of a blood pump. The largest experience with the device is for pumpless extracorporeal lung assist (PECLA) or arteriovenous CO_2 removal (AV-COR). In these applications of partial support, the native heart pumps arterial blood across the device and back into the venous circulation. Clearance of CO_2 via the device makes it possible to implement protective lung management strategies with the mechanical ventilator. The device is heparin coated and has a very low resistance to blood flow allowing perfusion to occur with or without a blood pump. The Novalung system simplifies the complexity of an extracorporeal circuit and clinical use has shown benefits and good feasibility in a wide number of etiologies including ARDS and COPD diagnoses.[43-46] The device has also been

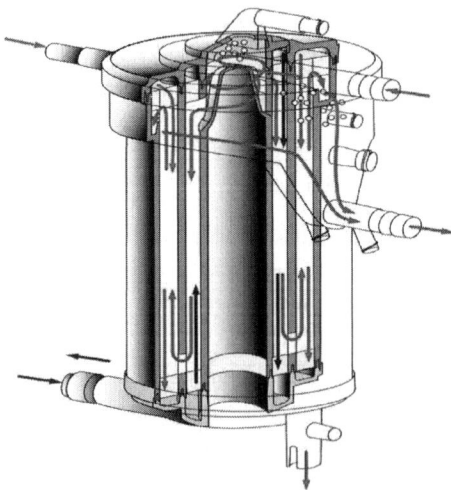

Figure 8-17. Cross Sectional view of Medos Gas Exchange Device.

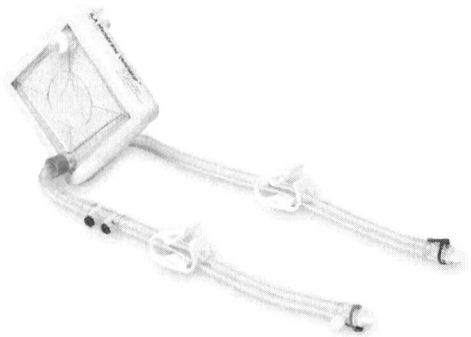

Figure 8-18. Novalung Membrane Ventilator.

used as an artificial lung to bridge a series of patients to lung transplant with or without a blood pump.[47-49]

Sorin Lilliput 2 ECMO (CE Mark. Not available in the USA or Japan)

The Sorin Lilliput 2 ECMO gas exchanger is a small to midrange blood outside the fibers unit made from PMP.[35] Validated for up to 5 days of extended support, the device has a phosphorylcholine surface coating, but operation requires the use of a blood pump. The device is produced in two sizes (Figures 8-18 and 8-19).

Nipro Biocube (available in Japan and Brazil)

Nipro Corporation, (Osaka, Japan) produces three sizes of plasma tight PMP hollow fiber membrane gas exchange devices. The Cube design allows for low priming volumes while maintaining gas exchange efficiency necessary for long-term support. The two smallest models are produced with or without an integral heat exchanger. The devices utilize a biocompatible coating which is heparin based with an ionic coupling promoting durability and anti-thrombogenic properties (see Table 8-3). The adult and infant sizes of the Nipro Biocube are shown in Figure 8-20a and 8-20b.

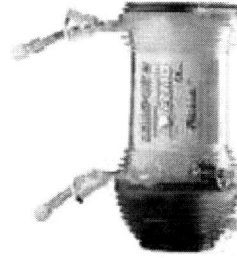

Figure 8-19. Sorin Lilliput 2 ECMO Device.

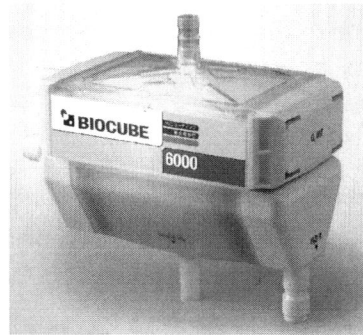

Figure 8-20a. Adult unit with integrated heat exchanger.

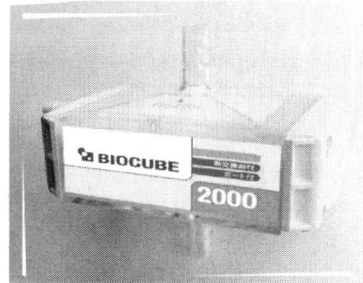

Figure 8-20b. Infant unit without heat exchanger.

Table 8-3. Nipro Biocube Sizes and Specification.

Model	BC2000P	BC4000P	BC6000P	BC6000	BC2000EL	BC4000EL
Blood flow range (L/min)	0.3-1.5	1.0-3.0	2.0-5.0	2.0-5.0	0.3-1.5	1.0-3.0
Priming volume (mL)	75	145	250	250	45	95
Fiber surface area (m^2)	0.4	0.8	1.3	1.3	0.4	0.8
Blood inlet port (in)	3/8	3/8	3/8	3/8	1/4	3/8
Blood outlet port (in)	3/8	3/8	3/8	3/8	1/4	3/8
Gas inlet port (in)	1/4	1/4	1/4	1/4	1/4	1/4
Heat exch surface area (m^2)	0.05	0.08	0.12	0.12	-	-
Sampling port	Female luer	Female luer	Female luer	-	-	-
Temp probe port	YS1400	YS1400	YS1400	-	-	-
Water connection	Hansen	Hansen	Hansen	Hansen	None	None

Circuit management

Circuit priming

The ECLS circuit is primed under sterile conditions with an isotonic balanced electrolyte solution resembling normal extracellular fluid including 4-5 mEq/L potassium. The prime is circulated through a reservoir bag until all bubbles are removed. Priming can be expedited by saturating the blood path with 100% CO_2 gas before adding the priming solution.

Microporous gas exchange devices prime quickly because gas in the circuit is purged through the micropores (even PMP surfaces) when delivered with positive pressure. The circuit can be primed at the time of use, or several days before use. Although there is variation amongst institutions, common practice is to maintain a circuit for up to 30 days once it has been primed.[50]

Before connecting to the patient, the circuit prime is warmed to 37°C by a water bath that circulates warm water across the heat exchanger. Support can be instituted with a crystalloid prime, but many centers add human albumin (12.5 gm) to "coat" the plastic surfaces and add an oncotic component. For adults, a crystalloid prime is practical and safe. This is also the case for larger children but infants require a blood-primed circuit. For infants, packed red cells are added to bring the hematocrit of the prime to 35-40%. When blood is added to the prime, heparin is also added as anticoagulation (1 unit per cc prime). Calcium is added to replace the calcium bound by the citrate in the bank blood. If time permits, it is helpful to verify the circuit's electrolyte composition and ionized calcium before starting support. For emergency use or ECPR, the prime can be crystalloid with the hemodilutional effects treated after the onset of support with diuretics, hemoconcentration, and/or transfusion.

Temperature management

During ECLS, the patient's blood volume is constantly being exposed to the ambient temperature of the environment as it circulates through the system. The sweep gas being blown over the membrane is cold and the evaporative losses across the membrane dissipate heat. It is common that patients on ECLS require active warming to maintain normal body temperature. This is almost always the case for the neonatal patient. Warming the gas source or employing topical warming methods in small patients can be effective. For larger patients, direct warming of the blood with the ECLS circuit is required.

A circuit heat exchanger is needed if it is necessary to control the blood and the patient temperature. While this typically means warming, circuit heat exchangers can also be used to offer cooling. Hypothermia is sometimes employed for neuroprotection[52] or to decrease the metabolic demand of a patient. Heat exchangers require an external recirculating water bath which circulates water through a coil or network of fibers in the blood path. The coil, or fiber network, is often integrated within the shell of the gas exchange device. The temperature of the circulating water bath is regulated to control the patient or blood path temperature. In general, the temperature of the water bath is maintained < 38.5° C to achieve normothermia. Although direct contact between the water path and the circulating blood is very rare, if blood or protein are present in the circulating water, or if unexplained hemolysis occurs, a breach in the heat exchanger should be suspected. Considering the water in the water bath is not sterile, the circuit will be contaminated. When not in use, the water bath should be cleaned and treated with a liquid antiseptic.[51]

Circuit Monitoring

The circuit may be outfitted with monitors that are designed to provide levels of safety, measure circuit function, and alert the health care personnel of abnormal conditions. The circuit can be equipped to measure the following:

Blood flowmeter

The extracorporeal blood flow is monitored most commonly with an ultrasonic flow detector. The flow meter may be a separate monitor or integrated into the blood pump. Integrated flow monitors are common with modern centrifugal pumps. Flow can also be calculated based on pump capacity and revolutions per minute, commonly done when using a roller pump. Standardized tubing sizes have been described for the various ranges of blood flow.[53]

Circuit pressures

Circuit pressures are commonly measured to determine the gradient across the gas exchange device or to measure the siphon effect (negative pressure) in the venous drainage line. An increase in the device's pressure gradient may be an indication of a kink in the circuit tubing or device thrombosis. Measuring post gas exchanger pressure would be necessary to determine the gradient across the device and to measure the return pressures to the patient. There could be associated alarms (lowest acceptable inlet pressure, highest acceptable outlet pressure) or control points for circuit servo regulation based on these pressure measurements.

Inlet and outlet pressures, relative to the gas exchange device and the pump, are common points for pressure measurement. A centrifugal pump is capable of generating extremes in negative pressure and monitoring the pump inlet pressure can be valuable when trying to minimize cavitation associated hemolysis. Cavitation causes local negative pressure fields. The red cells in these cavitation fields can be exposed to extreme negative pressure in excess of -750 mmHg. Gas will come out of solution causing the red cell membrane to lyse. The gas

will return to solution, but the free hemoglobin remains. A negative pressure <-600 mmHg typically does not induce cavitation or cause hemolysis unless the red cells are preconditioned by an air interface such as that observed with cardiotomy suction during CPB.[55]

Prior to the modern centrifugal pumps, the roller pump was the most common ECLS pump. The venous drainage inlet to the roller pump required gravity drainage. Gravity drainage resulted in a siphon, pulling the patient's blood to the roller pump. To create this siphon effect, it was necessary to have the pump in a dependent position, relative to the patient. The distance of separation was typically 100 – 150 cm. Most centers used servo regulated roller pumps so that the gravity siphon did not result in a suction pressure negative enough to cause cavitation. Under most circumstances, centrifugal pumps generate similar suction pressures and there is no cavitation or resulting hemolysis. When centrifugal pumps are used at high speeds (typically greater than 3000 RPM), the negative pressure generated within the pump head can exceed -700 mmHg when the venous line chatters or is momentarily occluded. The result of this momentary interruption of flow causes cavitation and hemolysis can occur within the pump head. If the venous line is occluded while the rotor is spinning at high speed, blood in the pump head is ejected but no blood fills the space. This results in an instant vacuum in the pump head, cavitation occurs, and the blood in the pump head is hemolyzed. When flow is reestablished the hemolyzed blood is perfused into the patient.

When "chattering" occurs in the venous line (due to hypovolemia, changes in patient position, changes in cannula position, changes in intra-thoracic pressure by coughing, etc.) the blood flow usually decreases. The common response would be to turn up the pump speed to try to increase the blood flow rate, but that simply adds to the problem. Each interruption in drainage can cause cavitation at high RPMs.

The correct response is to turn down the RPM, determine the cause of the intermittent occlusion, and implement a solution. In the absence of venous line occlusion, support may proceed at a high RPM for hours with no hemolysis until the venous line is occluded, so episodes of hemolysis seem to occur at mysterious and random intervals. The ideal centrifugal pump would be servo controlled by venous pressure as well as mixed venous oxygen saturation. Until that technology becomes available, the use of a venous inlet pressure monitoring, combined with a venous compliance chamber, will minimize the risk of negative pressure associated cavitation.[25] Both venous line compliance and pump inlet pressure must be factored in and clearly understood to avoid the potential hemolytic effects of a centrifugal pump when flow is intermittently interrupted. In settings such as this, the venous drainage pressure may be measured or monitored to establish a threshold of excessive negative pressure.[56]

Oxyhemoglobin saturation

The oxyhemoglobin saturation of the circuit blood can be measured by inserting an indwelling catheter through a specialized optical connector or by applying a wraparound fitting and sensor that encompasses the tubing. Oxyhemoglobin saturation is most useful on the venous side of the gas exchange device. If the ECLS mode is venoarterial, the oxyhemoglobin saturation of the venous drainage blood will be similar to the mixed venous saturation, which is commonly used to reflect overall metabolism and adequacy of support. If the mode of ECLS is venovenous, recirculation of arterialized blood will falsely elevate the oxyhemoglobin saturation for the venous blood making it less representative of metabolism and support. Measuring the oxyhemoglobin saturation of the arterialized blood that exits, the gas exchange device can offer helpful information about the performance of the gas exchange device. Blood gases can also

be measured from pre and post gas exchanger sites either by continuous monitoring or batch sampling. The value in measuring blood gasses is for information about acid-base status, CO_2 metabolism and membrane performance.

Circuit access sites

Most circuits have blood access sites in the circuit. The number of access sites should be minimized, but at least two are usually included: pre and post gas exchanger. Blood access sites should be avoided between the patient and the pump inlet because of the risk of entraining air. Although it is acceptable to use the circuit for all blood sampling and infusions, the patient may be accessed directly to give infusions, transfusions, or blood samples.

Alarms

Audible alarms should identify pressures or parameters that have exceeded preset safety settings. Alarms can reflect transmembrane device pressure gradients, negative or positive pressure in the blood path, excessive gas inlet pressure, and central power failure. Thrombosis or clotting within the device is suggested by increasing membrane lung pressure gradient and/or a drop in the flow rate. Pump speed can be controlled by defining limits of maximum and minimum flow with alarms to alert care providers. Measuring and controlling the centrifugal pump inlet pressure may prevent extremes in negative pressure, minimizing the risk of cavitation and hemolysis. Bubble detectors may also be used on the blood return line to protect patients from microemboli or catastrophic air embolus. Both pressure and bubble detector alarms can be used to clamp lines and regulate the blood pump, although any detected air must be removed from the circuit manually.

Emergency circuits

Emergency circuits should be available within minutes of need, should be fully primed with crystalloid, and ready to attach as soon as the patient is cannulated for emergency support. These circuits should also include safety features to prevent excessive negative pressure on the inlet side and high positive pressure on the outlet side to avoid errors during emergent cannulation and attachment. The emergency circuit may include a simple short term microporous gas exchange device and a centrifugal pump.

Refining circuit design: Simplicity and integrated systems

The question may be raised to as to whether future ECLS circuits can be simplified to fit on a smaller cart or IV pole. Can the circuit be adapted so that a single caregiver model is safe and practical? As ECLS expands into more patient subpopulations with wider indications for use, the circuit's design will require simplicity and automation. Ideally, the circuit should be designed to require less hands-on maintenance. Medical industry has taken a renewed interest in this area by adapting more sophisticated technologies for longer-term use.[57]

This is evident in the evolution of left ventricular assist devices which require minimal bedside maintenance and offer durable support for years outside of the hospital setting. The ECLS circuit will likely follow this trend.

It is realistic to contemplate a simple and relatively smaller footprint for the ECLS system of the future. Components will be smaller. The system will have integrated feedback control, allowing sophisticated servo regulation with inherent safety. The compact system will be contained in a small wheeled cart or IV pole, which will lend itself to easy portability. Commercial systems are now available with many of these features. These systems will continue to evolve as a function of technology and patient care needs.

The Maquet Sprinter cart is a simple, portable cart that contains space for a centrifugal pump, gas exchange device, and normothermia heater unit (Figure 8-21). Such a system can be positioned on either side of the bed and may be used for routine care or intrahospital transport. Levitronix also produces a ventricular assist cart which can easily be adapted to accommodate a gas exchange device and supportive equipment (Figure 8-12).

ECLS systems can be made more compact by integrating multiple components. An example of this design concept exists in cardio-

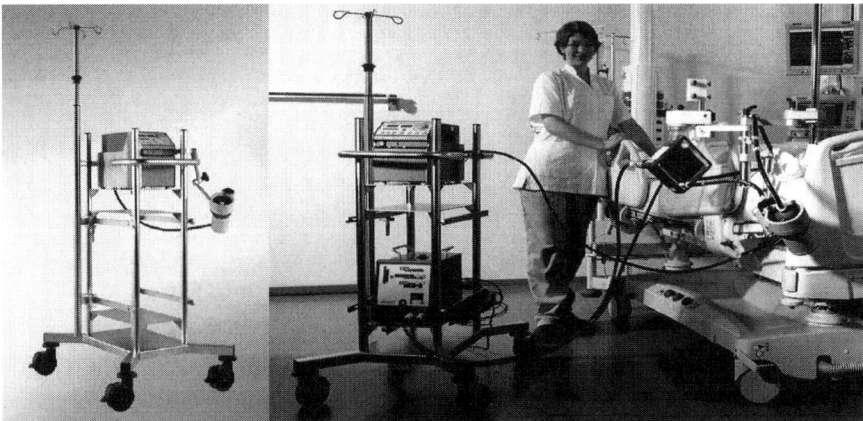

Figure 8-21. Maquet Sprinter Cart System.

pulmonary bypass with the Sorin Synergy. In this device, the arterial filter, heat exchanger, centrifugal pump, and venous and arterial bubble traps are integrated into a single housing. The Maquet CardioHelp system integrates three major components (gas exchanger, pump, heat exchanger) into a single product (Figures 8-22, 8-23 and 8-24). In theory, such a system can be positioned on or under the bed and would operate with a minimal number of controls. Such a system would potentially be easier to set up and initiate, as well as allow for easier patient transports. Such systems would simplify the use of ECPR, but may also be of significant value in the support of all patients. Again, training and mastery of such a system is essential for bedside personnel to correctly troubleshoot the system. Failure of one component would require replacing the entire system, which is certainly a drawback, yet such a system also lends itself well for feedback servo regulation of essential parameters (i.e., venous inlet pressure).

Summary: The circuit

The circuit is designed to provide complete mechanical support of the patient for an expected duration of days, weeks, or even months at a time. Each circuit can vary according to the patient, size, diagnosis, and expected length of use. The circuit is outfitted with various artificial organs that mechanically provide all cardiac and respiratory support that may be required. Similarly, the circuit must be adaptable to all vascular access pathways. Ideally the circuit should be simple, with only essential access sites, so that minimal manipulations of the circuitry are required to support the patient. Certain patients will be good candidates for extubation and ambulatory care while on ECMO. Therefore streamlining the system will continue and patient rehabilitation may become similar to that of patients with implantable ventricular assist devices. However, it is noted that due to the mechanical nature of the circuit, trained personnel must be available to the patient at all times to troubleshoot, diagnose, and implement

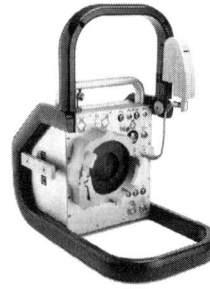

Figure 8-22. Maquet Cardiohelp System (rear view). Integrated component secures into back side of the module.

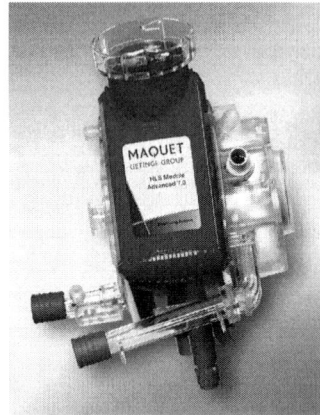

Figure 8-23. Maquet CardioHelp disposable component.

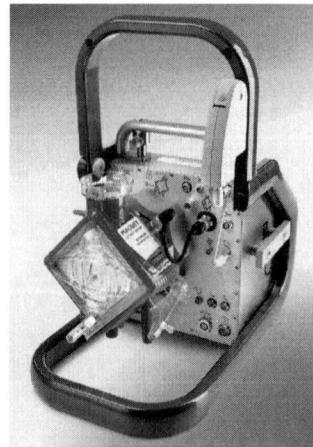

Figure 8-24. Assembled Maquet Cardio-Help System.

128

any changes the circuit may require from moment to moment. New, more durable components may be integrated together to provide a smaller, more portable system. Continued use and modifications of such circuits will define the optimal treatment parameters.

References

1. Hirschl RB. Devices, Chapter 10. In, Zwischenberger JB and Bartlett RH, eds. ECMO Extracorporeal Cardiopulmonary Support in Critical Care. Ann Arbor, Extracorporeal life Support Organization 1995; 159-184.
2. Hirschl RB. Devices, Chapter 12. In, Zwischenberger JB, Steinhorn RH, Bartlett RH, eds. ECMO Extracorporeal Cardiopulmonary Support in Critical Care 2nd ed. Ann Arbor, Extracorporeal life Support Organization 2000; 199-224.
3. Hansell DR. ECLS Equipment and Devices, Chapter 6. In, Van Meurs K, Lally KP, Peek G, Zwischenberger JB, eds. ECMO Extracorporeal Cardiopulmonary Support in Critical Care 3rd ed. Ann Arbor, Extracorporeal life Support Organization 2005; 107-119.
4. Kolobow T, Bowman RL. Construction and evaluation of an alveolar membrane heart lung. Trans Am Soc Artif Intern Organs 1963; 9:238-245.
5. Kern F, Schulman SR, Lawson DS, Darling EM. Extracorporeal Circulation and Circulatory Assist Devices in the Pediatric Patient. In: Pediatric Cardiac Anesthesia, 3rd ed., Ed. Lake C, Appleton and Lange, Stamford, CT 1998; 219-257.
6. Toomasian JM, Kerby KA, Chapman RA, Heiss KF, Hirschl RB, Bartlett RH. Performance of a rupture- resistant polyvinylchloride tubing. Proc Amer Acad Cardiovasc Perf 1987; 8:56-59.
7. Snyder E, McElwee D, Harb H, et al. Investigation of Fatigue Failure of S-65-HL "Super Tygon" Roller Pump Tubing. J Extracorp Tech 1996; 28:79-87.
8. Peek GJ, Wong K, Morrison C, Killer HM and Firmin RK. Tubing failure during prolonged roller pump use: a laboratory study. Perfusion 1999; 14:443-452.
9. McDonald JV, Green TP, Steinhorn RH. The role of the centrifugal pump in hemolysis during neonatal extracorporeal support. ASAIO J 1997; 43(1):35-8.
10. Kawahito K. and Nose Y., Hemolysis in different centrifugal pumps. Artificial Organs 1997; 21(4):323-6.
11. Augustin S, Horton A, Butt W, Bennett and Horton S. Centrifugal pump inlet pressure site affects measurement. Perfusion 2010; 25(5):313-320.
12. Peek GJ, Firmin RK. The inflammatory and coagulative response to prolonged extracorporeal membrane oxygenation. ASAIO J 1999; 45(4): 250-63.
13. Ranucci M, Pazzaglia A, Isgro G, Gazzaniga A, et al. Closed, phosphorylcholine-coated circuit and reduction of systemic heparinization for cardiopulmonary bypass: the intraoperative ECMO concept. Int J Artif Org 2002; 25(9):875-81.
14. Bahaaldin B, Shen I, Karamlou T, et al. Extracorporeal Life Support in Neonates, Infants, and Children after repair of Congenital Heart Disease: Modern Era Results in a Single Institution. Ann Thorac Surg 2005; 80:15-20.
15. ELSO Guidelines Version 1.1 April 2009; Page 5.
16. Reed CC and Stafford TB. Circuits. In: Reed and Stafford, ed. Texas Medical Press, 2nd ed; Cardiopulmonary Bypass 1985; 263—271.
17. Public Health Notification: PVC Devices Containing the Plasticizer DEHP. www.fda.gov/cdrh/ost/dehp-pvc.pdf 2002.
18. Center for Devices and Radiological Health. US Food and Drug Administration: safety assessment of di(2-ethylhexyl)phthalate released from PVC medical devices. http://www.fda.gov/cdrh/ost/dehp-pvc.pdf 2001.
19. Burkhart HM, Joyner, N, Niles S, Ploessl J, et al. Presence of Plasticizer Di-2(ethylhexyl) phthalate in Primed Extracorporeal Circulation Circuits. ASAIO J 2007; 53(3):365-367.
20. De Mol AC, Van Heijst AF, Van der Staak FH, Liem KD. Disturbed cerebral circulation during opening of the venoarterial bypass bridge

in extracorporeal membrane oxygenation. Int J Artif Organs 2008; 31(3):266-71.

21. Van Heijst A, Liem D, Van Der Staak F, Klaessens J, Festen C, De Haan T, Geven W, Van De Bor M. Hemodynamic changes during opening of the bridge in venoarterial extracorporeal membrane oxygenation. Pediatr Crit Care Med 2001; 2(3):265-270.

22. Liem KD, Kollée LA, Klaessens JH, Geven WB, Festen C, De Haan AF, Oeseburg B. Disturbance of cerebral oxygenation and hemodynamics related to the opening of the bypass bridge during veno-arterial extracorporeal membrane oxygenation. Pediatr Res 1995; 38(1):124-9.

23. Chambers SD, Ceccio SL, Annich GA, Bartlett RH. Extreme negative pressure does not cause erythrocyte damage in flowing blood. ASAIO J 1999; 45:431-5

24. Pedersen TH, Videm V, Svennevig JL et al. Extracorporeal membrane oxygenation using a centrifugal pump and a servo regulator to prevent negative inlet pressure. Ann Thorac Surg 1997; 63(5): 1333–39.

25. Tamari Y, Lee-Sensiba K, King S, and Hall MH: An Improved Bladder for Pump Control during ECMO. J Extracorpor Technol 1999; 31: 84-90.

26. ELSO Guidelines Version 1.1 April 2009 Page 6.

27. Leaf J.D., Dyson C., and Emerson R. Comparison Study of Connector and Tubing Blow-Off Line Pressures. J Extracorp Tech. 1982; 14(3):385-390.

28. Steinhorn RH, Isham-Schopf B, Smith C, et al. Hemolysis during long-term extracorporeal membrane oxygenation. J Pediatr 1989; 115:625-630.

29. McDonald JV, Green TP, Steinhorn RH. The role of the centrifugal pump in hemolysis during neonatal extracorporeal support. ASAIO J 1997; 43(1):35-8.

30. Tamari Y, Lee-Sensiba K, Leonard EF, Parnell V, and Torolani AJ. The Effects of pressure and flow on hemolysis caused by

Bio-Medicus centrifugal pumps and roller pumps: Guidelines for choosing a blood pump. J Thorac Cardiovasc Surg 1993; 106(6): 997-1007.

31. Lawson DS, Lawson AF, Walczak R, et al. North American Neonatal Extracorporeal Membrane Oxygenation (ECMO) Devices and Team Roles: 2008 Survey Results of Extracorporeal Life Support Organization (ELSO) Centers. J Extracorp Technol 2008; 40:166-174.

32. Khan NU, Al-Aloul M, Shah R, Yonan N. Early experience with the Levitronix Centrimag® device for extra-corporeal membrane oxygenation following lung transplantation. Eur J Cardiothorac Surg 2008; 34:1262-1264.

33. Mendler N, Podechtl F, Feil G, Hiltmann P and Sebening F. Seal-less Centrifugal Blood Pump with Magnetically Suspended Rotor: Rot-a-Flow. Artificial Organs 1995; 19(7):620-624.

34. Lawson DS, Ing R, Cheifetz IM, et al. Hemolytic characteristics of three commercially available centrifugal blood pumps. Pediatr Crit Care Med 2005; 6:573-577.

35. Schaadt J. Fiber Manufacturing, Membrane Classification, and Winding Technologies Associated with Membrane Oxygenators. J Extracorp Technol 1998; 30:30-34.

36. Thiara APS, Hoel TN, Kristiansen F, et al. Evaluation of oxygenators and centrifugal pumps for long-term pediatric extracorporeal membrane oxygenation. Perfusion 2007; 22:323–326.

37. Eash HJ, Jones HM, Hattler BG, Federspiel WJ. Evaluation of plasma resistant hollow fiber membranes for artificial lungs. ASAIO J 2004; 50:491–97.

38. Montoya JP, Shanley CJ, Merz SI, et al: Plasma leakage through microporous membranes. Role of phospholipids. ASAIO J 1992; 38: M399–405.

39. Peek GJ, Killer HM, Reeves R, Sosnowski AW, Firmin RK. Early experience with a

polymethyl pentene oxygenator for adult extracorporeal life support. ASAIO J 2002; September; 48(5):480-2.

40. Horton S, Thuys C, Bennett M, Augustin S, Rosenberg M, Brizard C. Experience with the Jostra Rotaflow and QuadroxD oxygenator for ECMO. Perfusion 2004; January; 19(1):17-23.

41. Eash HJ, Jones HM, Hattler BG, Federspiel WJ. Evaluation of plasma resistant hollow fiber membranes for artificial lungs. ASAIO J 2004; 50:491–97.

42. ELSO Guidelines Version 1.1 April 2009 Page 7

43. Elliot SC, Paramasivam K, Oram J, Bodenham AR, Howell SJ, Mallick A. Pumpless extracorporeal carbon dioxide removal for life-threatening asthma. Crit Care Med 2007; 35: 945-8.

44. Zimmermann M, Bein T, Arlt M, Philipp A, Rupprecht L, Mueller T, Lubnow M, Graf BM, Schlitt HJ. Pumpless extracorporeal interventional lung assist in patients with acute respiratory distress syndrome: a prospective pilot study. Critical Care 2009; 13: R10.

45. Weber-Carstens S, Bercker S, Hommel M, Deja M, MacGuill M, Dreykluft C, Kaisers U. Hypercapnia in late-phase ALI/ARDS: providing spontaneous breathing using pumpless extracorporeal lung assist. Intensive Care Med. DOI 10.1007/s00134-009-1426-3, 2009.

46. Taylor K, Holtby H. Emergency Interventional Lung Assist for Pulmonary Hypertension. Anesth Analg 2009; 109:382–5.

47. Fischer S, Hoeper MM, Tomaszek S, Simon A, Gottlieb J, Welte T, Haverich A, Strueber M. Bridge to lung transplantation with the extracorporeal membrane ventilator Novalung in the veno-venous mode: the initial Hannover experience. ASAIO J 2007; Mar-Apr;53(2):168-70

48. Fischer S, Simon AR, Welte T, et al., Bridge to lung transplantation with the novel pumpless interventional lung assist device

NovaLung. J Thorac Cardiovasc Surg 2006; 131(3):719-23.

49. Strueber M, HoeperMM, Fischer S, Cypel M, Warnecke G, Gottlieb J, Pierre C, Welte T, Haverich A, Simon AR, Keshavjee S. Bridge to thoracic organ transplantation in patients with pulmonary arterial hypertension using a pumpless lung assist device. Am J Transplant 2009; 9: 853–857.

50. Walczak R, Lawson DS, Kaemmer D, et al. Evaluation of a pre-primed microporous hollow fiber membrane for rapid response neonatal ECMO. Perfusion 2005; 20:269-275.

51. Stovall SH, Wisdom C, McKamie W, Ware W, Dedman H, Fiser RT. Nosocomial transmission of Cupriavidus pauculus during extracorporeal membrane oxygenation. ASAIO J 2010; 56(5):486-7.

52. Amberman K and Shen I. Minimizing reperfusion injuries: successful resuscitation using eCPR after cardiac arrest on a post-operative Norwood patient. J Extra Corpor Technol 2010; 42(3):238-41.

53. ELSO Guidelines Version 1.1 April 2009 Page 8.

54. Pohlmann JR, Toomasian JM, Hampton CE, Cook KE, Annich GM, Bartlett RH. The synergistic effect of subatmospheric pressure and the air-blood interface on hemolysis. ASAIO J 2009; 55: 469-73.

55. Chambers SD, Ceccio SL, Annich GA, Bartlett RH. Extreme negative pressure does not cause erythrocyte damage in flowing blood. ASAIO J 1999; 45:431-5.

56. Tamari Y, Lee-Sensiba K, Ganju R, Chan R, Hall MH: A new bladder allows kinetic venous augmentation with a roller pump. Perfusion 1999; 14:453-459.

57. Palanzo D, Qiu F, Baer L, Clark JB, Myers JL and Undar A. Evolution of the Extracorporeal Life Support Circuitry. Artif Org 2010; 34(11):869-873.

9

Vascular Access for Extracorporeal Support

Thomas Pranikoff MD FACS , Michael H. Hines MD FACS

Introduction

The establishment and maintenance of adequate vascular access is essential for extracorporeal life support (ECLS). Cannulation techniques vary depending on the type of support needed, patient age and size, and clinical situation. This chapter will review general principles and elaborate on some specific situations commonly encountered while providing adequate vascular access.

Principles

Patient Management Pre-ECLS

Management of critically ill patients prior to the initiation of extracorporeal life support can be challenging. The decision regarding where to cannulate the patient (e.g., in the ICU, operating room (OR), emergency department, etc.) needs to be well thought out. Adequate monitoring and nursing care are essential. The ability to transport the patient safely with adequate ventilation and hemodynamic support should be considered. Required equipment (cannulae, surgical instruments, circuit, and components) and personnel (OR and ECLS) must be available.

The procedure should be explained to the family and informed consent obtained. Mean-while, blood products including packed cells and platelets should be ordered from the blood bank. Cannulation may be performed either in the ICU or operating room, or other suitable locations. The patient should be adequately sedated or anesthetized to facilitate safe cannulation, reduce anxiety and discomfort, and minimize the likelihood of air embolism, while also considering the hemodynamic effects of these medications. We commonly use a combination of fentanyl and rocuronium in children, with additional benzodiazepine sedation in adults as indicated. After the vessels have been surgically exposed or a guidewire placed during percutaneous access, the patient is systemically heparinized (100 units/kg) and a period of at least 30 seconds and up to three minutes allowed for adequate anticoagulation before placing the cannulae into the vascular system, depending on the urgency of cannulation.

Type of Support

Extracorporeal support may be provided in two principle ways: 1) venovenous (VV) ECMO which provides excellent respiratory support, and 2) venoarterial (VA) ECMO which provides both cardiac and respiratory support. Because of several advantages discussed below, VV ECMO is preferred for respiratory support.

A comparison between VV and VA ECMO is shown in Table 9-1.

VA ECMO removes blood from the systemic venous circulation, usually from the right atrium via the right internal jugular or femoral vein, and returns the blood to the systemic arterial circulation in the aortic arch via the right common carotid artery or distal aorta via the femoral artery. In VV ECMO, blood is drained from the venous circulation and returned back to the venous circulation either through a single double lumen cannula in the right atrium via the jugular vein or by using two cannulae in the femoral (drainage) and jugular (inflow) veins. VV ECMO offers several advantages over VA ECMO including: 1) the avoidance of arterial cannulation, potential arterial embolization, and distal limb ischemia or stroke; 2) the elimination of arterial ligation or repair at the completion of the ECMO run; 3) the preservation of pulmonary blood flow with well oxygenated blood with its beneficial vasodilatory effect; 4) the preservation of native pulsatile arterial flow, and; 5) the absence of any negative hemodynamic effects, such as the increase in afterload observed with VA ECMO.

Selection of the mode of support depends on the clinical situation (Figure 9-1). In patients considered for ECLS for severe hypoxemia, some degree of cardiac dysfunction is commonly present. Often patients are on significant inotropic and vasopressor support, and have hypotension or hypoperfusion. While there may be true cardiac dysfunction related to sepsis and the inflammatory response, often patients have significant hypotension because of diseased lungs, increased pulmonary vascular resistance and extremely high ventilator pressures. This usually results in poor left ventricular preload, despite very high right sided pressures, and can even result in right ventricular dysfunction and failure. When cardiac function is normal, VV ECMO is clearly indicated. However when cardiac dysfunction is present, a judgment should be made as to the degree of dysfunction and whether it is from a primary cardiac etiology or secondary to high levels of respiratory support (high airway pressure, PEEP). If on echocardiographic evaluation there is no clear evidence of true RV failure, or if the LV is contracting but poorly filled, VV ECMO should be strongly considered, and will usually provide excellent gas exchange, along with dramatic improvement in LV filling, and RV afterload reduction as the ventilator settings are reduced to "rest" levels. The vast majority of patients with ARDS

Table 9-1. Comparison of VV and VA bypass.

	Venoarterial (VA)	Venovenous (VV)
Cannulation Site	V: IJ, FV, RA A: RCCA, Ax, Fem, Ao	IJ, FV, saphenous v., RA
PaO_2	60-150 mmHg	45-80 mmHg
Indicator of O_2 adequacy	SvO_2, PvO_2	PaO_2, cerebral SvO_2, transmembrane $DavO_2$
Cardiac Effects	↓preload, ↑afterload, ↓pulse pressure, LV blood → coronary O_2	negligible
O_2 delivery capacity	High	moderate
Circulatory support	Partial to complete	No <u>direct</u> effect
Pulmonary circulation		
R→L shunt	↓SaO_2 in aorta	↑SaO_2 in aorta
L→R shunt	May cause pulmonary congestion and systemic hypoperfusion	May cause pulmonary congestion and systemic hypoperfusion

and other forms of respiratory failure will be well supported with VV ECMO and usually tolerate relatively rapid weaning of inotropes and vasopressors. Those patients who do not improve once on VV ECMO, require relatively urgent reevaluation of cardiac function with echocardiography.

With primary cardiac dysfunction, VA ECMO is required. The preferred method in infants and children is by cutdown exposure of the right jugular vein and common carotid artery. VA support in adults can be achieved using several different cannulation configurations. Jugular venous drainage and carotid artery inflow, as used in infants, can provide excellent hemodynamic support, especially for combined cardiac and pulmonary dysfunction. It provides excellent perfusion to all branches of the aortic arch and distal aorta, but increases LV afterload. However, importantly, up to 15% of adults will develop ischemic brain injury after carotid artery ligation, particularly in the setting of hypoxemia and hypotension. Jugular (or femoral) venous drainage with femoral artery inflow provides adequate distal perfusion, but can fail to perfuse the aortic arch if some native cardiac function is preserved and the LV is still able to eject. If the patient has concomitant pulmonary dysfunction, the coronary arteries and aortic arch (i.e., brain) will be perfused with poorly oxygenated blood from the LV, and not see the well-oxygenated pump blood. This problem can be solved with the placement of an additional cannula from the infusion limb of the ECMO circuit into the right internal jugular vein, to create venoarterial-venous (VA-V) ECMO.[1] This increases oxygenation of the right ventricular blood much like VV ECMO while still providing the hemodynamic support of VA ECMO. Increased afterload from VA ECMO may prevent the failing left ventricle from ejecting blood and result in high left atrial pressure that causes pulmonary edema. This can be managed by venting the left atrium, either by draining blood from the left atrium into the venous side of the circuit from direct cannulation of the left atrium or LV apex through a left thoracotomy or by catheter based balloon atrial septostomy.

Cannulation of the femoral artery may be performed either percutaneously or by direct cutdown on the vessel. With either method, depending on the size of the cannula, distal ischemia may result. Several methods of managing this situation have been described. Placement of a distal perfusion catheter directly into the femoral artery can be performed by an open technique, feeding it off the arterial limb of the circuit. An alternative approach is to place an end-to-side PTFE vascular graft to the common femoral artery and cannulate the graft directly, which allows bidirectional flow.[2] This technique may be used primarily in children and smaller women to prevent likely distal ischemia when the artery is found to be small, or as a treatment for distal ischemia. In this case the graft is usually placed on the contralateral femoral artery, and once flow established, the original cannula is removed and the artery repaired. When the leg appears ischemic following percutaneous placement of the arterial catheter, a retrograde arterial line can be placed into either the dorsalis pedis or posterior tibial artery by cutdown and the distal pressure measured. If this is less than 50 mmHg, the catheter can be perfused by a line from the perfusion limb of the circuit.[3]

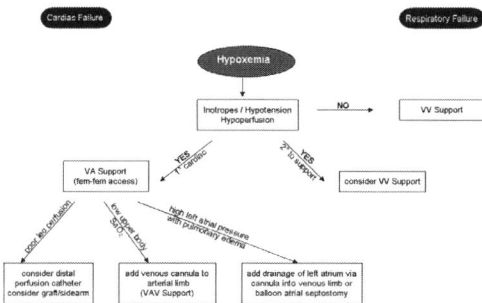

Figure 9-1. Algorithm for cannulation.

Cannula considerations

During ECLS it is important to use a drainage (venous) cannula with the largest lumen and shortest length possible, particularly when using a roller pump since venous drainage is achieved by gravity siphon. In this system, if preload is adequate, the limiting factor determining maximum flow is cannula resistance which is directly proportional to the length and inversely proportional to the fourth power of the luminal radius. This simple relationship becomes more complicated for non-uniformly shaped devices. Cannula size is standardly reported according to the outer diameter. Identically-sized cannulae may vary in inner diameter according to the wall thickness of the material used. A simple method to describe the pressure/flow characteristics of vascular cannulae has been developed. Catheters are tested for their pressure/flow relationship and an "M-number" determined which represents a resistive factor that can then be used to approximate the expected flow at a specific pressure difference.[4,5] These values for a typical ECLS situation using a typical pressure gradient of 100 cmH$_2$O siphon are demonstrated in Table 9-2.

Venous cannulae generally have both end and side holes to allow flow even if the end of the cannula is occluded. Arterial cannulae generally have only end holes to minimize turbulence in the high velocity system, though some arterial inflow cannulas with multiple holes are available. The cannula should resist kinking while remaining flexible and thin-walled to offer the least resistance possible. Wire wound cannulae (e.g., Biomedicus, Avalon) are very resilient to kinking while the thin-walled double lumen cannulae are more prone to kink.

Vascular access for ECLS in the neonate is particularly challenging due to the small vessel size. The route of access depends on the method used. VA ECMO is indicated for cardiac support but may be necessary for respiratory support in neonates where the access vein is too small to accept the smallest available double lumen cannula (12F).

For VA access, the preferred site for venous drainage is the right atrium via the right internal jugular vein and the aortic arch via the right common carotid artery for arterial infusion. The internal jugular vein and carotid artery are relatively large in the neonate and usually simple to cannulate. For VV access, a double lumen cannula is placed into the right atrium via the right internal jugular vein and is carefully positioned so that the "arterial" inflow is directed toward the tricuspid valve to minimize recirculation back into the ECMO circuit.

Selection of technique

Access for VA ECMO by cutdown over the carotid artery requires arterial ligation to prevent leakage around the cannula and possible distal embolization from flow past the cannula.

Table 9-2. Commonly used ECLS cannulae.

Manufacturer	Size (F)	Length (cm)	M#	Flow@100cmH$_2$O
Venous Cannulae (Single Lumen)				
Biomedicus	8	25	4.35	0.5
	10	25	3.9	0.9
	12	25	3.55	1.5
	14	25	3.35	2
	15	50	3.65	1.3
	17	50	3.4	1.9
	19	50	3.15	2.6
21	21	50	2.9	3.2
	23	50	2.65	5
	25	50	2.55	6
	27	50	2.4	6.5
	29	50	2.3	8
DLP	17	53	3.3	2.2
	21	53	3.05	3
	28	65	2.5	5.5
RMI	18	52	3.2	2.5
	20	52	3	3
	28	52	2.3	8
Venous Cannulae (Double Lumen)				
Origen	12	6	3.9V 4.7A	0.9
	15	8	3.5V 4.3A	1.6
	18	15	3.4V 3.8A	1.9
Jostra	12		4.1V 4.6A	0.8
	15		3.6V 4.6A	1.4
Covidien	14	10	3.5V 5.1A	1.6
Avalon	16	13	3.6V 4.2A	1.7
	19	20	3.3V 3.8A	2
	20	29	3.4V 3.7A	1.8
	23	29	3.1V 3.4A	2.6
	27	29	2.7V 3.1A	4.4
	31	29	2.5V 2.8A	6
Arterial Cannulae				
Biomedicus	8	25	4.4	0.5
	10	25	4	0.9
	12	25	3.55	1.5
	14	25	3.25	2.4
	15	37	3.3	2.2
	17	37	3.05	3
	19	37	2.8	3.8
	21	37	2.6	5
	23	38	2.4	6.5
DLP	8	23	4.5	0.4
	14	23	3.3	2.2
	16	23	3	3
	17	17	2.95	3.2
	21	17	2.65	5
RMI	18	15	3	3
	20	25	3	3
	20	15	2.8	3.8
	22	25	3.1	2.9

In infants and small children the carotid artery is usually safe to ligate without major sequelae.[6] The incidence of neurologic impairment after carotid ligation was similar for ECMO survivors and conventionally managed babies in the UK Collaborative ECMO Trial.[7] Schumacher et al. showed that the right side is more commonly involved when brain lesions are seen after carotid ligation,[8] although this lateralization was not found in another study of 74 infants after carotid artery ligation.[9] Cannulation for VV ECMO can be performed either using a similar technique or without vessel ligation via a percutaneous or semi-open technique. While jugular vein ligation is usually tolerated, there is evidence that this may produce high venous pressure which can exacerbate cerebral ischemia.[10] Percutaneous access utilizes the Seldinger technique to place the cannula. Because the size of the vessel in relation to the cannula is unknown, vessel disruption is a risk. For this reason, our preferred method in infants is the semi-open technique.[11] This technique requires a small incision to visualize the size of the vein as an aid to select the correct cannula size (usually 12F or 15F in a newborn). Cannula insertion is then made percutaneously well above the incision, including the entrance into the vein, but the cannula can be visualized passing down the vein through this incision if desired. With this technique, vessel ligation is not utilized. This has several advantages: cephalad flow into the cannula increases the amount of deoxygenated blood available to enter the bypass circuit, the vessel may remain patent after decannulation (and can be recannulated if needed), and kinking of the cannula at the vessel is reduced because the vessel is not fixed to the cannula with a ligature which can act as a fulcrum around which the cannula kinks. This also makes adjustment of cannula depth much simpler.

Cannula Insertion for Neonatal ECLS

VV/VA cannulation - open technique[12]

Preoperative

Vascular cannulation and decannulation are usually performed in the neonatal or pediatric intensive care unit under adequate sedation and neuromuscular blockade. Neuromuscular blockade is especially important in preventing the potentially lethal complication of an air embolus during introduction of the venous cannula. The instruments and sterile procedures used are identical to those used in the operating room. Heparin sodium (100 units/kg) is drawn up for subsequent administration.

Anesthesia. Local anesthesia is administered by infiltration of 1% lidocaine.

Operation

Position of patient. The patient is placed supine with the head turned to the left. A roll is placed transversely beneath the shoulders. Special attention is paid to assuring that the endotracheal tube is positioned to prevent kinking under the drapes during the procedure. This can be accomplished by using a piece of suction tubing split lengthwise and placed over the tube at the connector to prevent kinking. Unlike in the operating room, access to the patient by anesthesia or ICU physicians is limited, and so end-tidal CO_2 monitoring is also useful to assure the tube does not become kinked during the procedure. The chest, neck, and right side of the face are aseptically prepared and draped.

Incision (Figure 9-2). A transverse cervical incision approximately 2-3 cm in length is made one finger's breadth above the clavicle over the lower aspect of the right sternocleidomastoid muscle were the two heads of the muscle divide.

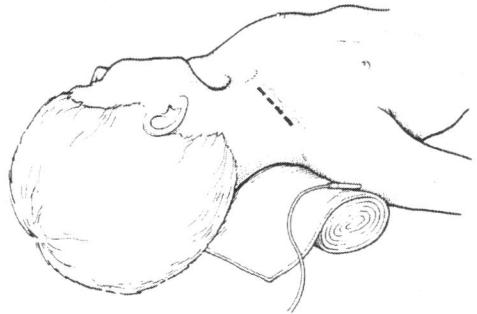

Figure 9.2. Patient positioning.

Exposure of the carotid sheath (Figure 9-3). The platysma muscle and subcutaneous tissues are divided with electrocautery and the sternocleidomastoid muscle exposed. Dissection is continued bluntly between the sternal and clavicular heads of the muscle. The omohyoid muscle will be seen superiorly. It may be necessary to divide the omohyoid muscle tendon to expose the carotid sheath. Two alternating self-retaining retractors are placed.

Dissection of the vessels (Figure 9-4). The carotid sheath is opened and the internal jugular vein, common carotid artery, and vagus nerve are identified and isolated. Dissection is progressed proximally and distally along the vessels, dissecting the vein first. Special care should be taken while dissecting the vein to avoid induction of spasm, which makes subsequent introduction of a large venous cannula difficult. Manipulation of the vein therefore should be minimized. There is often a branch on the medial aspect of the internal jugular vein which must be ligated. Ligatures of 2/0 silk

are placed proximally and distally around the internal jugular vein. The common carotid artery lies medial and posterior and has no branches, which facilitates dissection. Ligatures of 2/0 silk are also placed around the carotid artery. The vagus nerve should be identified.

Once vessel dissection is completed, heparin (100 units/kg) is administered intravenously. During the waiting period, papaverine or lidocaine may be instilled into the wound to overcome any vasospasm present.

Arteriotomy/venotomy (Figure 9-5). For venoarterial ECMO the arterial cannula is chosen (usually 8 or 10Fr) and marked with a 2/0 silk ligature, left uncut, at a point that will allow the tip of the cannula to lie at the ostium of the brachiocephalic artery (about 2.5 cm). The venous cannula (usually 10-14 Fr.) is similarly marked at a point equal to the distance from the venotomy to the right atrium (roughly 6 cm). A smooth round-tipped obturator is placed into the venous cannula to allow smooth guidance of the cannula into the vein, and to prevent blood

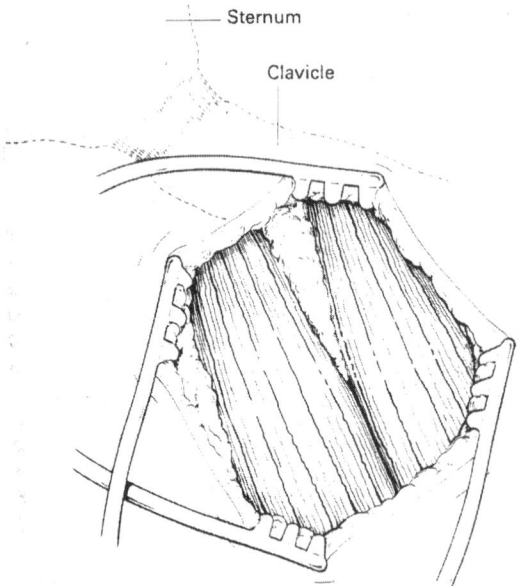

Figure 9-3. Superficial dissection.

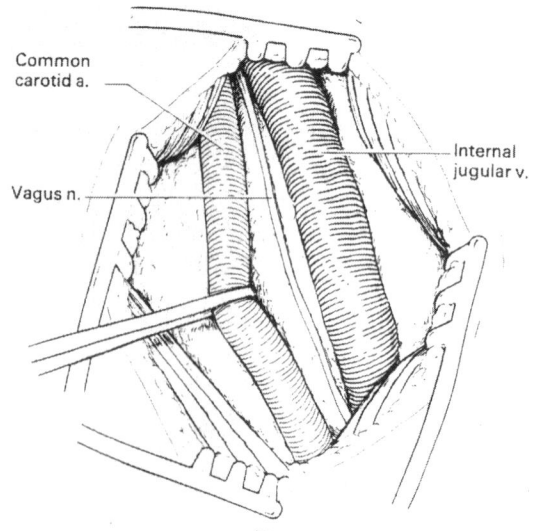

Figure 9-4. Deep dissection with exposed internal jugular vein, common carotid artery, and vagus nerve.

from flowing out through the side holes during introduction into the vessel. The common carotid artery is ligated distally. Proximal control is obtained with the use of an angled vascular clamp. A transverse arteriotomy is made near the distal ligature. Full thickness stay sutures of 6/0 polypropylene may be placed on the proximal edge of the artery to prevent subintimal dissection during cannula insertion. Following arterial cannulation, a venotomy is performed in similar fashion. Gentle retraction of the caudal ligature around the vein can preclude the need for a vascular clamp during venotomy and venous cannulation. Stay sutures are also not routinely necessary for venous cannulation.

Cannula placement (Figure 9-6). The cannulae are carefully placed into the artery and vein and secured using two circumferential 2/0 silk ligatures. A small piece of silastic vessel loop can be left inside the ligatures to protect the vessels from injury during decannulation when the ligatures are sharply divided. The ends of the marking ligatures are tied to the most distal cir-

cumferential ligature for extra security. Careful placement of the securing ligatures close to the arteriotomy to minimize the length of damaged vessel may accommodate primary repair of the carotid during decannulation after short ECMO runs. Immediately after each cannula is secured, it is carefully de-aired via back-bleeding and filling with heparinized saline. For venovenous ECMO, the double lumen cannula is placed into the venotomy and advanced to place the tip in the mid-right atrium. It is crucial to maintain the arterial reinfusion (red) port anteriorly while securing for proper orientation to minimize recirculation of reinfused blood.

Wound closure (Figure 9-7). The wound is irrigated with saline and hemostasis obtained. The skin is closed with continuous monofilament suture around the cannulas after open cannulation. The wound is dressed with gauze. The cannulae are sutured to the skin with several 2/0 silk sutures. Special attention should be directed to affixing the cannulae securely to the bed.

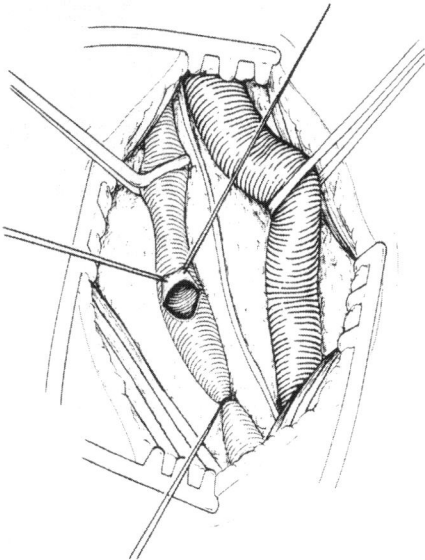

Figure 9-5. Carotid artery ligated distally and proximal arteriotomy.

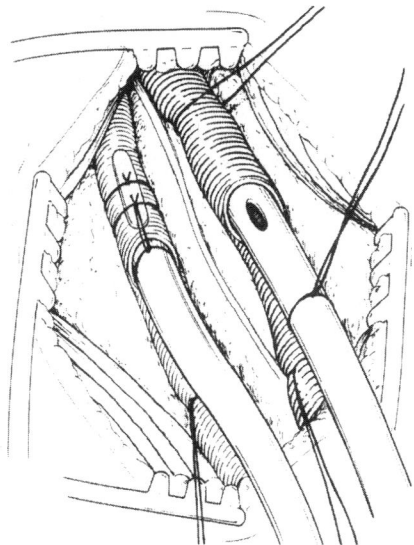

Figure 9-6. Arterial cannula secured. Venous cannula being inserted.

Decannulation. After the patient has successfully weaned from ECMO support following recovery of cardiac and pulmonary function, decannulation can take place. Depending on surgeon preference and potential for carotid reconstruction after short ECMO runs, this may be done at beside in the ICU, or may be done in the operating room. The wound in prepped and draped in a sterile fashion including significant length of the cannulae and tubing to allow manipulation. The wound is opened and the vessels and ligatures exposed. An additional ligature is placed around the cannula and the vein proximal to the insertion site, and then the cannula clamped, removed, and the ligature secured. A vascular clamp can be used as well but is usually not necessary. Attempts have been made to repair the vein, but are probably not necessary and often do not remain patent. If the ECMO run has been relatively short (less than 5–7 days or so), reconstruction of the artery may be considered. While the benefit of this is theoretical and as of yet unproven, many surgeons believe it is beneficial as long as the artery appears healthy and the intima is not damaged above and below the level of the repair. After obtaining vascular control proximally and distally with silk loops and clamps in place, the arterial cannula is clamped and removed, and the vascular clamps closed. The area of the arteriotomy is excised and the proximal and distal artery carefully inspected. If the intima is intact, the artery can be reconstructed in end to end fashion using standard vascular techniques, often with slight spatulation of the ends of the vessels. If there is any intimal damage, laminated clot, intimal contusion, etc., then the risk of clot and embolization may make reconstruction contraindicated. In that case the vessel is ligated on both ends, and the wound irrigated and closed. After longer ECMO runs, carotid reconstruction is not usually recommended, and the artery is ligated as the cannula is removed. Keeping the ligatures relatively close together may be beneficial for those few cases that require re-cannulation for a second run of ECMO.

VV Cannulation - semi-open technique[13]

Incision and vein exposure (Figure 9-8). A transverse cervical incision approximately 1.5-2 cm in length is made 2 cm above the right clavicle between the heads of the sternocleidomastoid muscle. The platysma is divided with electrocautery and the anterior surface of the internal jugular vein is exposed with minimal dissection. The vessel is observed and the appropriate size venovenous ECMO cannula is

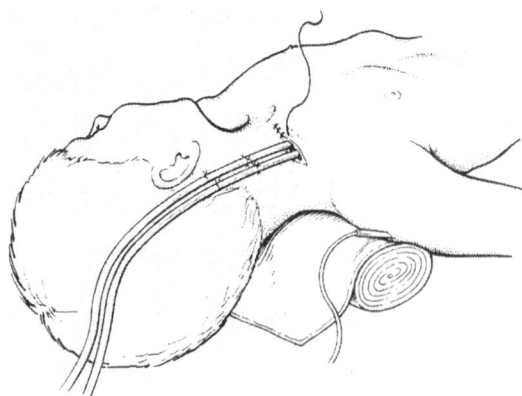

Figure 9-7. Cannulas secured to skin. Wound closed.

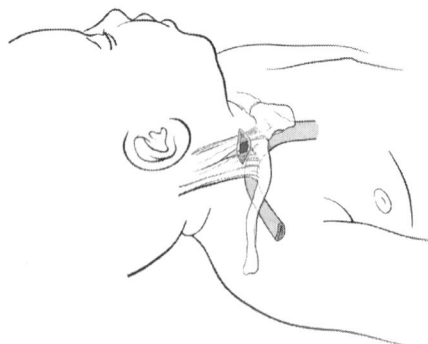

Figure 9-8. Superficial dissection exposing anterior surface of internal jugular vein.

selected (12 and 15 F available from Origen Biomedical Inc, Austin, Texas USA, and 14 F available from Covidien [formerly Kendall, Mansfield MA, USA]).

Guidewire placement (Figure 9-9). The cannula skin exit position is selected so that the cannula will lie behind the right ear when the head is returned to the midline. The needle or angiocath is placed through the skin about 2 cm superior to the incision and into the internal jugular vein, preferentially entering above the level of the incision to allow complete tissue coverage around the venous insertion site. A 0.035 inch diameter guidewire is advanced and the needle or catheter withdrawn. A Teflon guiding obturator is placed over the guidewire into the vessel and right atrium. The skin exit is slightly enlarged with a scalpel. The skin should not be over dilated or problems with bleeding around the cannula may be encountered.

Cannula placement (Figure 9-10). Following adequate heparinization the selected cannula is advanced over the Teflon obturator into the vein under direct vision to confirm entrance into the vein. The arterial (red) port of the cannula must be directed anteriorly to allow the arterial blood to cross the tricuspid valve and minimize recirculation of circuit blood. The tip of the cannula is placed at 6-9 cm from the skin.

Wound closure and cannula fixation (Figure 9-11). The relatively low venous pressure allows adequate hemostasis around the venotomy site without any ligature. This prevents kinking of the thin-walled cannula which often occurs at the area of a ligature if used around the vessel. Repositioning of the cannula only requires removing the skin sutures, repositioning the cannula, and replacing skin sutures. The cannula is fixed to the skin with several 2-0 silk sutures. The incision is closed with a monofilament suture, or may be closed with absorbable sutures.

Decannulation. After respiratory failure has resolved to allow ventilation without extracorporeal support, cannulation can be performed by removing the skin sutures, pulling the cannula, and holding pressure on the catheter exit site for five minutes or until bleeding stops. Care must be taken to rapidly remove the entire cannula to prevent air from entering the side holes while the end of the cannula remains in the vessel.

Cannula Insertion for Pediatric ECLS

Children older than infants have different access needs which are more similar to adults. Vessels are larger and make more options for access available. Venovenous ECMO is still used preferentially for respiratory support.

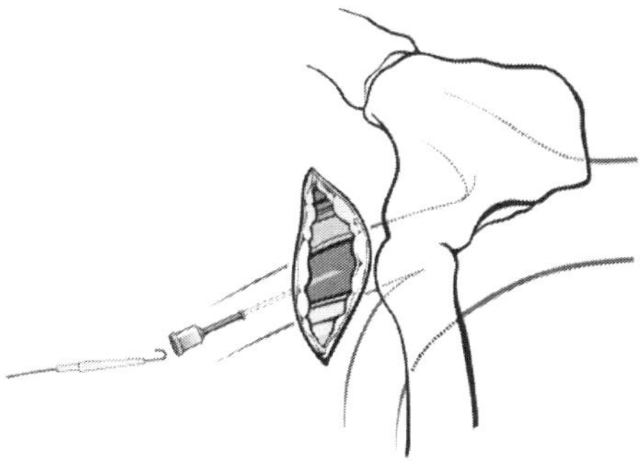

Figure 9-9. Introducer needle inserted through superior skin flap into vein.

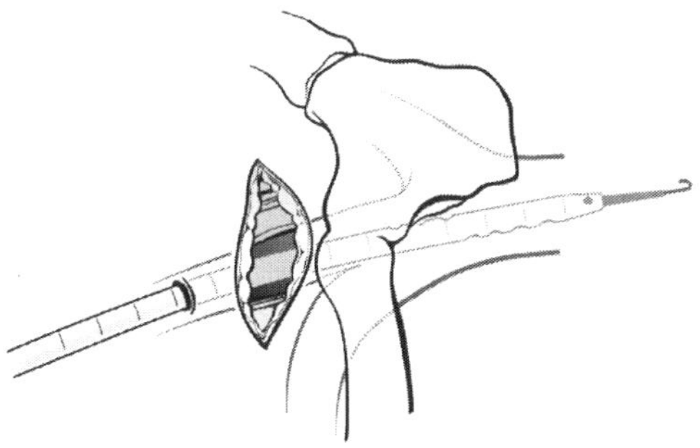

Figure 9-10. Cannula, dilator, and guidewire inserted into vein under direct vision.

Venoarterial ECMO is reserved for cardiac support, including postoperative patients who fail to wean from cardiopulmonary bypass after heart surgery. Children who are not yet old enough to walk have smaller femoral vessels which may be unsuitable to use for ECMO access. For this reason, in this group (<10 kg) a double lumen cannula in the jugular vein for venovenous bypass, or single lumen cannulae in the jugular vein and carotid artery can be used for VA ECMO. Rarely a small child with respiratory failure has a jugular vein which is too small to allow a large enough double lumen cannula for adequate flow on VV bypass, and must be placed on VA ECMO.

Venovenous ECMO

As described above, VV bypass in small children can be achieved using a double lumen cannula either placed by a modified Seldinger technique as described above or entirely percutaneously if the vein is judged to be of adequate size to receive the cannula. Children >10 kg usually have large enough veins to allow a two-cannula technique by placing cannulae in both the femoral and jugular veins.[14] The selection of cannulae is again based on two criteria: 1) the largest cannula that the vein will accept based on surgical judgment, and; 2) a large enough

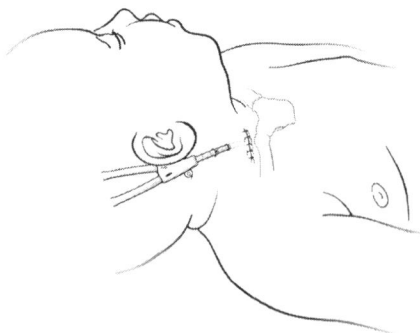

Figure 9-11. Cannula secured to skin. Wound closed.

drainage cannula to allow for enough flow (100 cc/kg/min) which can be estimated by the M-number. The issue of which cannula to use for drainage and reinfusion has two potential solutions. The jugular vein cannula will often allow more drainage. If the end of this cannula is in the atrium and preload is adequate, it can drain until the atrium collapses around the cannula and the pump flow is interrupted by servo regulation. Flow is thought to be higher in this situation because the atrium is spherical in shape compared to the cylindrical shape of the femoral or iliac vein. However, if pump blood is directed toward and reinfused into the femoral vein cannula, recirculation is often significant. This may be due to the blood draining into the right atrium from the inferior vena cava, directed preferentially into the jugular cannula before mixing occurs. Rich et al. showed that draining blood from the femoral cannula and reinfusing into the jugular cannula results in higher arterial saturation (i.e., oxygen delivery), even though the total flow achievable is less, because recirculation is decreased.[15] We prefer this method of bypass and try to use a femoral cannula that reaches the intrahepatic vena cava which is large and does not collapse.

Venoarterial ECMO

For cardiac failure, most pediatric patients are cannulated through the neck using the jugular vein and carotid artery by cutdown. Patients placed on bypass after cardiac surgery may utilize their cannulation sites in the chest used for cardiopulmonary bypass.

Cannula Insertion for Adult ECLS

Venovenous ECMO

Cannulation for adult VV ECMO may be achieved by one of two techniques. The first uses two cannulae placed in the jugular and femoral veins. These cannulae can be placed safely by a percutaneous method.[16] A large cannula (23-29F) should be placed for drainage and a somewhat smaller cannula (21-23F) for venous reinfusion. It is especially important for the venous cannula to have side holes in addition to an end hole to maximize drainage and allow flow to continue if the end becomes obstructed. While early adult ECMO experience used internal jugular cannulae to drain from the right atrium, and returned blood was infused into the femoral vein and inferior vena cava, this was sometimes accompanied by significant recirculation issues. The development of longer and larger, thinner walled, wire reinforced cannulae led to a preferred method of IVC drainage via the femoral approach, and right internal jugular infusion. This technique allowed for high flow rates with minimal recirculation. It is important to place the IVC cannula within the intrahepatic portion of the cava to essentially eliminate the issue of venous collapse around the cannula, frequently seen in the soft intraabdominal IVC. This often leads to the insertion of a second cannula in the other femoral vessel, but this is rarely if ever needed if an adequate size cannula is properly placed in the high IVC (intrahepatic). Patients with IVC filters or umbrellas in place who require VV ECMO support can still be supported with the older technique of right atrial drainage and reinfusion into the femoral venous system below the device. Subclavian vein cannulation for infusion has also been used successfully in patients with occluded or unavailable internal jugular access. A new double lumen cannula has recently become available which allows for venovenous bypass using a single cannula in larger patients. This cannula, Avalon Elite™ (Avalon Laboratories, LLC., Rancho Dominguez, CA, USA), has a novel design which incorporates drainage from both the inferior and superior vena cava and the infusion port has a deflectable inner membrane that directs blood across the tricuspid valve. These features help limit recirculation. Recirculation is a problem which can

be solved as described in the above section on pediatric cannulation. In addition, the cannula is wire-reinforced to resist kinking. The Avalon Elite™ cannulae come in varied sizes ranging from 13-31F making them sized for children and adults. Preliminary results from a number of centers demonstrate good performance.[17] Because the cannula is designed to drain both the superior and inferior vena cava, it requires placement through the right atrium with the tip in the IVC. Placement of the cannula is aided by fluoroscopy and echocardiography. Viewing the course of the entire cannula during placement with fluoroscopy assures that placement is accurate. It is particularly helpful to aid in assuring that the guidewire crosses the atrium and is well into the inferior vena cava. Then as the cannula is advanced over the guidewire, fluoroscopy allows direct confirmation that the guidewire continues to remain straight and that the tip follows the course into the inferior vena cava. On occasion during cannula advancement, the guidewire will "kick up" into the right atrium and needs to be repositioned well into the IVC before the cannula is further advanced. Unlike fluoroscopy, echocardiography is particularly helpful to confirm optimal placement of the tip into the IVC and evaluate whether flow from the infusion port is directed through the tricuspid valve to minimize recirculation. However echocardiography alone does not allow visualization of the entire cannula and guidewire as it is inserted. While experience is still limited, it appears that the two techniques may be complimentary in safely inserting this very large cannula into position.

Venoarterial ECMO

Techniques for cannulation to provide venoarterial extracorporeal support in adults parallel those used in pediatric patients with a few exceptions, primarily related to the arterial access. Unlike children, adult patients are less likely to have extensive collateral circulation and in fact, may have significantly compromised arterial circulation so that cannulation with even small arterial cannulae can lead to distal ischemia. In addition to tolerating carotid cannulation much less well than children, leg ischemia is a significant issue in adults, particularly with increased age, and must be identified and dealt with early in its course. Some centers routinely insert additional distal perfusion catheters in place as previously described to prevent leg ischemia during femoral cannulation and perfusion.

In general, adult femoral vessels are usually large enough to accommodate percutaneous insertion of perfusion cannulas unless there is a suspicion or history of significant peripheral vascular disease. If the urgency of the support will allow it, the use of fluoroscopy and potential use of contrast injection can be invaluable in these cases. In more urgent cases, open exposure of the artery and palpation for an appropriate insertion site may facilitate insertion and prevent complications such as leaking and local femoral or retrograde aortic dissection. At other times, particularly in obese patients, open cannulation may be required if the artery cannot be located percutaneously. While the presence of a bounding pulse is usually a fair indication that percutaneous cannulation can proceed, the vast majority of patients that require VA ECMO for cardiovascular reasons are obviously unlikely to have a bounding pulse. Exceptions may occur during resuscitations, particularly with the use of catecholamines, where transient hypertension may occur, providing an adequate target for cannulation as well as some reassurance as to the lack of severe peripheral vascular disease. In addition, the palpation of a pulse during external cardiac massage is also a relatively good indicator that the artery is sufficiently patent to be cannulated percutaneously.

Other options for arterial access are also available and have been used successfully in more complicated cases where adults have either significant peripheral vascular disease or some other contraindication to femoral can-

nulation (e.g., burns, open wound, Dacron grafts in place, etc.). While a few have supported the use of the carotid artery, primarily in Europe, the most common alternative site utilized in the United States is the axillary artery. Use of this artery can be accomplished on either side and does require an open incision. While the artery can be cannulated directly, the issues of arm ischemia and bleeding essentially prohibit its safe use for long term support. Instead, most surgeons employ the use of a Dacron or PTFE side graft sewn to the axillary artery, which can then be tunneled out through a separate incision, and the primary cutdown incision closed. As with all these techniques, extra care should be taken both for wound care, and for securing and stabilizing the cannulas to the patient.

While the open technique may make cannulation easier and reduce the risk of arterial injury, the additional time and equipment required, as well as the added risk of leaking around the cannula and later wound infection, must all be weighed by the surgeon in deciding how to proceed.

Once the patient no longer requires VA ECMO support, venous decannulation can be performed as previously described for the vein (i.e., direct pressure for percutaneously placed line, ligation of the jugular vein for cutdown placement). Arterial decannulation is more complicated. Some surgeons prefer direct visualization of the artery with direct suture repair after cannula removal. Others, however, find that direct pressure may be all that is needed for percutaneously placed arterial cannulae. The larger the cannula is in relation to the artery, the more likely a pseudoaneurysm or arterial stenosis will result. An alternative to this method is venous patch angioplasty, a technique used for removing arterial cannulae placed by cutdown. In this technique, the vessel is controlled by a clamp and the cannula is removed. A diamond shaped patch of vein is then sutured into the defect which both closes the hole and prevents stricture at the repair.

Transthoracic Cannulation

There are circumstances when cervical or femoral access for venoarterial extracorporeal support is either not possible or practical, particularly when treating patients who have failed to wean from cardiopulmonary bypass or who have undergone post-sternotomy resuscitation. In these circumstances, direct cannulation of the arterial and venous system is performed using techniques and cannulas commonly used with cardiopulmonary bypass. Pursestring sutures of some sort are placed in the ascending aorta and (usually) directly in the right atrium, and brought through snares that allow the suture to be tightened around the cannula and secured, preventing leaking of blood around the cannula and, in the case of the venous side, preventing entraining of air into the system. While in the operating room the cannulas are usually lightly secured to the drapes or left lying on the field. It is critical to secure the cannulas in a more "permanent" fashion when providing more prolonged extracorporeal support, and particularly for safety during transport. In general this involves suturing the cannula to the chest wall at some point, and then closing the wound with an artificial dressing, usually made of some sort of plastic or elastic, with the cannulas exiting between the suture line between the material and the skin. If the patient becomes more lightly sedated and moves, or attempts to breathe or cough, the sternal edges can separate and put tension on the cannulas, risking dislodgement. This is best prevented by using one or two heavy sutures or sternal wires to stabilize the sternal edges. The authors find this provides more than adequate stabilization of the support apparatus, and prefer it over continuous muscle relaxation with its significant potential sequelae.

Cannulation Complications

Cannulation of patients for ECMO can be quite challenging and problems are frequently encountered. By adequately preparing the patient, serious complications can usually be avoided. Proper training and support of the surgeon performing these procedures will allow most of these problems to be managed without poor outcomes.

Difficult venous cannulation

This may occur because the vein is too small, the catheter is too big, or there is a left-sided SVC without an innominate vein. The clavicle or first rib can sometimes obstruct if the patient's head is hyperextended or hyper-rotated. Try to reposition the head. There may also be severe mediastinal shift which may be present with diaphragmatic hernia or pneumothorax or effusion.

Complete division of the jugular vein

Especially in small newborns, it may be difficult to introduce the venous cannula and during attempts to do this, the vein may become divided. This makes further attempts to introduce the cannula more difficult. Vascular control is the primary goal. This is best done with a vascular clamp. Once this has been done, placing a guidewire may be helpful to introduce the cannula. Placing stay sutures to provide traction during cannula placement will help. A ligature should be placed around the vein to tie in the cannula. At decannulation, a pursestring suture may be used to control bleeding.

Proximal vein lost in mediastinum

During a difficult venous cannulation when the cannula does not thread easily, sudden loss of resistance may be due to division of the vein which may retract into the mediastinum. Bleeding may be controlled by direct pressure with a finger. If the vein end can be retrieved with a forceps, cannulation may be performed as above with vein division. Otherwise, if no other suitable vein is available for access, median sternotomy and access via a thoracic approach may be needed. If other access is available, control can almost always be achieved by suturing fascia to cover the hole where the vein was lost and applying direct pressure.

No flow after catheter placement

If there is no flow after placement of the cannula, the cannula and circuit tubing should be examined for kinking. Chest radiography or fluoroscopy should be used to assess the position of the venous cannula and reposition or replace as needed.

Intrathoracic perforation

Sudden cessation of flow with hemodynamic instability may be due to intrathoracic vessel or right atrial perforation. This situation requires immediate median sternotomy and vascular repair, with subsequent direct transthoracic cannulation.

References

1. Miskulin J, Annich G, Grams R, Boules T, McGillicuddy J, Hirschl R, Bartlett R. Venous-arteriovenous cannulation for adult ECMO patients with cardiogenic shock. 14th Annual ELSO Conference, September 10-12, 2004, Chicago, IL

2. Vaders Salm TJ. Prevention of lower extremity ischemia during cardiopulmonary bypass via femoral cannulation. Ann Thorac Surg 1997; 63:251-2.

3. Bartlett RH, personal communication.

4. Montoya JP, Merz SI, Bartlett RH. A standardized system for describing flow/pressure relationships in vascular access devices. Trans Am Soc Artif Intern Organs 1991; 37:4-8.

5. Sinard JM, Merz SI, Hatcher MD, et al. Evaluation of extracorporeal perfusion catheters using a standardized measurement technique-- The M-number. Trans Am Soc Artif Intern Organs 1991; 37:60-4.

6. Streltz LJ, Bej MD, Graziani LJ, et al. Utility of serial EEGs in neonates during extracorporeal membrane oxygenation. Pediatric Neurology 1992; 8:190-6.

7. UK collaborative randomized trial of neonatal extracorporeal membrane oxygenation. UK Collaborative ECMO Trial Group. Lancet 1996; 348:75-82.

8. Schumacher RE, Barks JD, Johnston MV, et al. Right-sided brain lesions in infants following extracorporeal membrane oxygenation. Pediatrics 1988; 82:155-61.

9. Lazar EL, Abramson SJ, Weinstein S, et al. Neuroimaging of brain injury in neonates treated with extracorporeal membrane oxygenation: Lessons learned from serial examinations. J Pediatr Surgery 1994; 29:186-91.

10. Walker LK, Short BL, Traystman RJ. Impairment of cerebral autoregulation during venovenous extracorporeal membrane oxygenation in the newborn lamb. Critical Care Med 1996; 24:2001-6.

11. Peek GJ, Firmin RK, Moore HM, et al. Cannulation of neonates for venovenous extracorporeal life support. Annals of Thoracic Surgery 1996; 61:1291-2.

12. Pranikoff T, Hirschl RB. Neonatal extracorporeal membrane oxygenation. In: Carter DC, Russell RCG, eds. Rob and Smith's Operative Surgery, 5th edition, London: Butterworth-Heinemann. 1995. Reprinted with permission of the authors and Edward Arnold.

13. Pranikoff T, Hirschl RB. Neonatal extracorporeal membrane oxygenation. In: Carter DC, Russell RCG, eds. Rob and Smith's Operative Surgery, 6th edition, London: Butterworth-Heinemann. 2005. Reprinted with permission of the authors and Edward Arnold.

14. Foley DS, Swaniker F, Pranikoff T, Bartlett RH, Hirschl RB. Percutaneous cannulation for venovenous extracorporeal life support (ECLS). J Pediatr Surg 2000; 35:943-7.

15. Rich PB, Awad SS, Crotti S, Hirschl RB, Bartlett RH, Schreiner RJ. A prospective comparison of atrio-femoral and femoro-atrial flow in adult venovenous extracorporeal life support. J Thorac Cardiovasc Surg 1998; 116:628-32.

16. Pranikoff T, Hirschl RB, Remenapp R, Swaniker F, Bartlett RH. Venovenous extracorporeal life support via percutaneous cannulation in 94 patients. Chest 1999; 115:818-22.

17. Bermudez CA, Rocha RV Sappington PL, Toyoda Y, Murray HN, Boujoukos AJ. Initial experience with single cannulation for venovenous extracorporeal oxygenation in adults. Ann Thorac Surg 2010; 90:991-5.

10

Management of Blood Flow and Gas Exchange during ECLS

Robert H Bartlett MD, Joseph B Zwischenberger MD

The Guidelines for managing blood flow and gas exchange during ECLS are:

A. Criteria for selecting circuit components

The circuit is planned to be capable of total support for the patient involved, unless the intent is specifically partial support (i.e., CO_2 removal for asthma)

1. Blood flow for cardiac support

Access is always venoarterial. The circuit components are selected to support blood flow 3 L/m²/min (neonates 100 cc/kg/min; pediatrics 80 cc/kg/min; adults 60 cc/kg/min.) The best measure of adequate systemic perfusion is venous saturation greater than 70%. Achieving a desired flow is determined by vascular access, drainage tubing resistance, and pump properties.

2. Blood flow and gas exchange for respiratory failure (VA or VV)

The oxygenator and blood flow should be capable of oxygen delivery and CO_2 removal at least equal to the normal metabolism of the patient (i.e., an oxygen delivery of 6 cc/kg/min for neonates; children 4-5 cc/kg/min; adults 3 cc/kg/min), This will usually equate to VV blood flows of 120 ml/kg/min for neonates down to

60-80 ml/kg/min for adults. Oxygen delivery capability is determined by blood flow, hemoglobin concentration, inlet hemoglobin saturation, and oxygenator properties. Carbon dioxide removal always exceeds oxygen delivery when the circuit is planned for full support.

3. Selective CO_2 removal

Using extracorporeal circulation primarily for CO_2 removal was first described by Kolobow and Gattinoni in animal models in the 1970s.[1] Gattinoni reported a large series in 1980 with 50% survival.[2] The circuit flow and membrane were large enough to support oxygenation if needed. In 1999 Conrad, Zwischenberger, and others demonstrated selective CO_2 removal with low blood flow achieved with a femoral arteriovenous shunt (AVCO2R).[3-6] Intervention Lung Assist (ILA) or pumpless extracorporeal assist (PECLA) are other terms for AVCO2R using the Novalung device.[7] The incidence of occasional femoral artery complications has led to venovenous access as the preferred access for AVCO2R. If the circuit is planned for CO_2 removal only, access can be venoarterial, venovenous or arteriovenous. Typical blood flow is approximately 25% of cardiac output, which is sufficient to remove the CO_2 produced by metabolism (3-6 cc/kg/min). AVCO2R at low flow does not supply enough oxygenation

149

for major support. CO_2 removal is determined by the blood flow and the sweep gas rate, the inlet PCO_2 and the membrane lung properties.

B. Management during ECLS

1. Blood flow

After cannulation blood flow is gradually increased to mix the circulating blood with the prime, then, blood flow is increased until maximum flow is achieved. This is done to determine the maximum flow possible based on the patient and the cannula resistance. After determining maximum possible flow, the blood flow is decreased to the lowest level that will provide adequate support at rest settings. For VA access, the pump flow is decreased until the arterial pulse pressure is at least 10 mmHg (to assure continuous flow through the heart and lungs during ECLS). This is often not possible when the heart function is very poor, so total extracorporeal flow is required. The physiologic goals (mean arterial pressure, arterial and venous saturation) are set and blood flow is regulated to meet the goals.

For VV access, adequate support is defined as arterial saturation greater than 85% and actual venous saturation greater than 60% at rest settings. For VV access, flow is decreased from maximal until the arterial saturation is at the desired level (greater than 85%). The physiologic goals (mean arterial pressure, arterial and venous saturation) are set and blood flow is regulated to meet the goals.

2. Oxygenation

As long as the blood flow is below rated flow for that oxygenator (and the inlet saturation is 70% or higher) the oxyhemoglobin saturation at the outlet of the oxygenator should be greater than 95%. Usually the outlet saturation

will be 100% and the PO_2 will be over 300. If the outlet saturation at or below the rated flow is less than 95%, the oxygenator is not working at full efficiency (due to irregular flow, clotting, water in the gas phase). It may be necessary to change the oxygenator.

Oxygen added from the circuit should be adequate for full support (3 to 6 cc/kg/min). This will result in systemic saturation greater than 95% (VA) or over 85% (VV) at low ventilator settings and FiO_2. If O_2 added is less than adequate the cause is low flow (limited by resistance in the drainage cannula), anemia, or oxygenator malfunction. If the oxygen added by the circuit is inadequate it is necessary to increase the venous drainage, increase the hematocrit, or change the oxygenator

3. CO_2 clearance

CO_2 transfer across the oxygenator will exceed oxygen transfer. CO_2 clearance is controlled by the sweep gas. Initially the gas to blood flow ratio is set at 1:1 and titrated to maintain the pCO_2 in the desired range. An alternative is to use carbogen (5% CO_2/95% O_2) as the sweep gas. If CO_2 clearance is decreased but oxygenation is adequate the cause is usually water accumulation in the gas phase. If the initial $PaCO_2$ is greater than 70, the $PaCO_2$ should be normalized over several hours rather than immediately in order to avoid swings of cerebral perfusion related to CO_2 and pH.

4. Hemodynamics

During **VV support** the patient is dependent on his own hemodynamic physiology. Appropriate medications and infusions are used to control cardiac output, blood pressure, and resistance.

During **VA support** hemodynamics are controlled by the blood flow (pump flow plus native cardiac output) and vascular resistance. Because the pulse pressure is low the mean systemic arterial pressure will be somewhat lower than normal pressure (40 to 50 mmHg for a newborn, 50 to 70 mmHg for a child or adult). In addition, patients placed on ECLS for cardiac support are on high doses of pressors when ECLS is begun. As these drugs are titrated down, resistance falls and systemic pressure falls proportionately. If the systemic perfusion pressure is inadequate (low urine output, poor perfusion) pressure can be increased by adding blood or low doses of pressor drugs. Systemic vasodilatation requiring pressor drugs is common in patients in septic shock. Although the mean arterial pressure may be low, systemic perfusion may be completely adequate. Systemic perfusion is best measured by mixed venous blood saturation. If venous saturation is greater than 75% systemic oxygen delivery is adequate even though the pressure may be low. If systemic oxygen delivery is not adequate (venous saturation less than 70%) the pump flow is increase until perfusion is adequate. If extra blood volume is required to gain extra flow, transfused blood is used, rather than adding more crystalloid solution.

C. Ventilator management

Whether the patient is on either VV or VA mode, the ventilator should be managed at low settings to allow lung rest. For patients with respiratory failure, a common mistake is to try to recruit lung volume during the acute inflammatory stage early in ECLS. Typical rest settings include low rate (<10) with long inspiratory time (2:1 I:E ratio, low FiO_2 [under 40%] and low plateau inspiratory pressure [under 25 cm H_2O]). PEEP is usually set between 5-15 cmH_2O, balancing mean airway pressure against venous return. The resultant tidal volume will range from 1 to 5 cc/kg.

Spontaneous breathing is encouraged by maintaining the patient awake as tolerated. In an awake patient, continuous positive airway P (CPAP) at 10-20 cm H_2O is a good method of airway and ventilator management. If the patient is on VA ECLS for cardiac support, and lung function is adequate, the patient can be extubated and managed awake with spontaneous breathing. If the patient is on VV for respiratory support, one approach is to extubate the patient and allow spontaneous breathing with the patient awake. This is the preferred approach for patients bridging to elective lung transplant.

If the systemic gas exchange is not adequate at these rest settings (arterial sat < 95%VA or 85%VV, or $PaCO_2$ > 40) the solution is to improve extracorporeal gas exchange, not return the ventilator to higher settings.

If there is a **major pulmonary air leak** or interstitial emphysema the ventilator pressure can be reduced or turned off altogether for hours or days until the leak seals. This will lead to significant atelectasis in addition to the primary lung disease, and lung recruitment will be necessary when returning to mechanical ventilation. If the patient develops a pneumothorax, placement of a chest tube is not an automatic response. Even placing a small tube may result in significant bleeding ultimately requiring thoracotomy. A small pneumothorax (less than 20%) with no hemodynamic compromise is best treated by waiting for absorption. An enlarging pneumothorax or a pneumothorax causing hemodynamic compromise requires external drainage. This is best done using the technique most familiar to the operator. This could be a small catheter placed by Seldinger technique, or a surgical thoracostomy with placement of a chest tube. (see procedures, section 9)

Lung recruitment maneuvers (prolonged inflation at 25 to 30 cm of H_2O for one to two minutes) can be used when acute inflammation has subsided. When lung recovery begins, spontaneous breathing will enhance recovery. Adjusting the sedation drugs to allow spontaneous breathing, adjusting the sweep gas to maintain the infusion blood PCO_2 over 40 mmHg, and putting the ventilator in assist mode may speed lung recovery.

Patient arterial blood gases are the result of infusion blood mixing with the blood in the aorta (VA) or right atrium (VV). The infusion blood is typically PCO_2 40 mmHg, PO_2 500 mmHg, saturation 100%, oxygen content 22 ccO_2/dL.

In **VV mode** infusion blood mixes with systemic venous return blood. At typical blood flow, the ratio of infusion blood to deoxygenated right atrial blood is usually around 3:1. This results in PCO_2 41, PO_2 40-50, sat 80-90%, content 17-18 ccO_2/dL in the pulmonary artery. If there is no native lung function, this will be the composition of gases in the arterial blood (see chapter 2). It is important to realize that systemic arterial saturation around 80% is typical during VV support. As long as the hematocrit is over 40% and cardiac function is good, systemic oxygen delivery will be adequate at this level of hypoxemia. Any native lung function will increase systemic oxygenation over 85% sat, but do not increase ventilator settings or FiO_2 above rest settings to increase SaO_2. Increase blood flow or hemoglobin instead.

In **VA mode** infusion blood mixes with blood in the aorta. The ratio of infusion to native aortic blood flow is typically 8:1. If native lung function is normal (i.e., in cardiac support) and the FiO_2 is 0.2, this results in PCO_2 40, PO_2 200, sat 100%, content 21 ccO_2/dL. If there is no native lung function this mixing results in PCO_2 40.5, PO_2 100, sat 98%, content 20 ccO/dL. NOTE: The forgoing is true if infusion blood goes to the aortic root (as in carotid or direct arch perfusion). If the infusion blood is going into the femoral artery and flow is retrograde, the mixing will occur somewhere in the mid aorta, the higher the flow rate, the higher the level of mixing. During severe respiratory failure, at typical VA flow rate (80% of full cardiac output) this can result in desaturated blood from the left ventricle perfusing the aortic arch and coronaries and fully saturated infusion blood perfusing the lower 2/3 of the body. This can occur in large children and adults. This can be managed by including SVC blood in the venous drainage, or by infusing some infusion blood into the right atrium (VVA). See patient specific protocols for further discussion.

Comment on the Guidelines: These guidelines are complete for managing flow and gas exchange for all types of patients. Application of the guidelines for physiologic management is described in Chapter 2. Some points deserving emphasis are:

1. Oxygenation and hemodynamic support are determined by blood flow. The limiting factor to blood flow is the resistance in the drainage cannula. If drainage is not adequate to allow the required flow, some improvement can be achieved by: 1) adding blood volume (blood, not crystalloid; the volume must stay in the vascular space) and / or 2) increasing suction by increasing gravity siphon or allowing more suction with a centrifugal pump. If these maneuvers do not achieve the desired flow another drainage cannula should be added.

2. Oxygenation is limited first by flow, then by oxygenation capacity of the blood going into the oxygenator. For optimal function of the oxygenator the hematocrit should be normal (45-48%), at least over 40%. Any risk of transfusion is trivial compared to the risk of poor oxygen delivery, or steps taken to try to increase flow in anemia. The other limitation of oxygenation is high saturation of blood entering the oxygenator. This occurs only during recirculation with VV access. If the inlet saturation is over 80% recirculation is occurring, and is addressed by repositioning the access cannulas.

3. Management of flow and oxygenation is based on the oxygen kinetic physiology described in Chapter 2. Any problem in perfusion or oxygenation can be solved by applying these principles.

4. CO_2 clearance is limited by sweep gas flow rate, (as $PaCO_2$ is regulated by minute ventilation in the normal lung). Most oxygenators are designed to operate at a ratio of 1:1, sweep gas to blood flow. If that is not sufficient to maintain the desired $PaCO_2$, the sweep gas is simply increased. This problem is usually caused by water in the gas phase of the oxygenator, and is solved by intermittent high flow (10 L/min).

5. Maintaining a normal hemoglobin is essential for normal oxygenator function, but is not common practice in patient care because of the risks of transfusion (primarily hepatitis). There is also an increased rate of infection when old blood is infused (older than 3 weeks), Both these risks are very small compared to the risk of dying from heart or lung failure exacerbated by anemia. You may have to read Chapter 2 to your blood bank director to explain the unique requirements of an ECLS system.

6. In VA support it is important to keep some blood flowing through the heart and lungs to avoid clotting. In severe cardiac failure the heart may not eject, even when the ECMO flow is turned down. If that happens, there are two risks. 1) The left atrium will gradually fill with bronchial venous blood creating high pulmonary capillary pressure and pulmonary edema. The left atrium must be decompressed by inserting a drainage cannula into the LA or PA, or by creating an atrial septostomy. Ideally every ECLS patient should have a PA catheter to monitor PCW pressure, and to manage the patient when weaning, or if pulmonary arterial hypertension occurs. 2) Blood clotting will occur in the heart and pulmonary vessels, even with systemic anticoagulation.

7. The best single monitor is continuous venous saturation in the drainage blood. This is usually the only monitor required for management.

Figures 10-1 and 10-2

Blood Flow Algorithm: VA Access

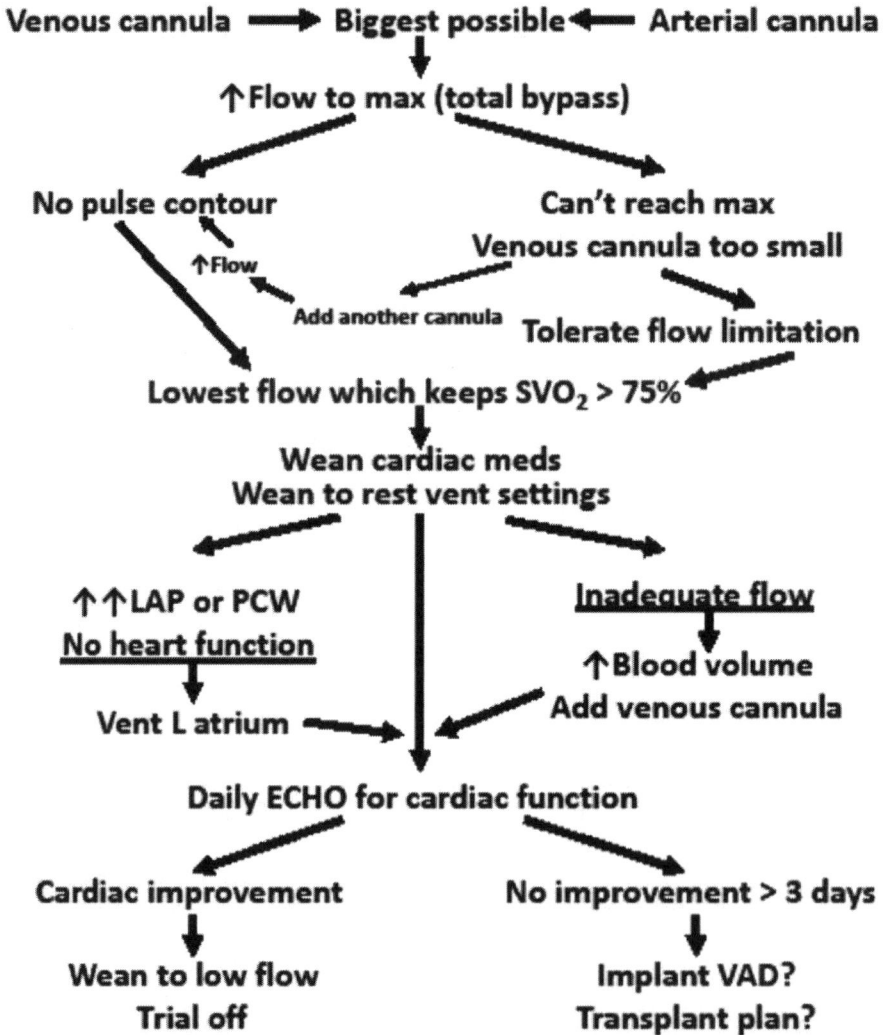

Venous cannula ➡ Biggest possible ⬅ Arterial cannula

↑Flow to max (total bypass)

No pulse contour   Can't reach max
                        Venous cannula too small

↑Flow

Add another cannula   Tolerate flow limitation

Lowest flow which keeps SVO$_2$ > 75%

Wean cardiac meds
Wean to rest vent settings

↑↑LAP or PCW   Inadequate flow
No heart function
                        ↑Blood volume
Vent L atrium   Add venous cannula

Daily ECHO for cardiac function

Cardiac improvement   No improvement > 3 days

Wean to low flow   Implant VAD?
Trial off   Transplant plan?

Figure 10-1. Algorithm for blood flow and gas exchange in VA ECLS

Blood Flow Algorithm: VV Access

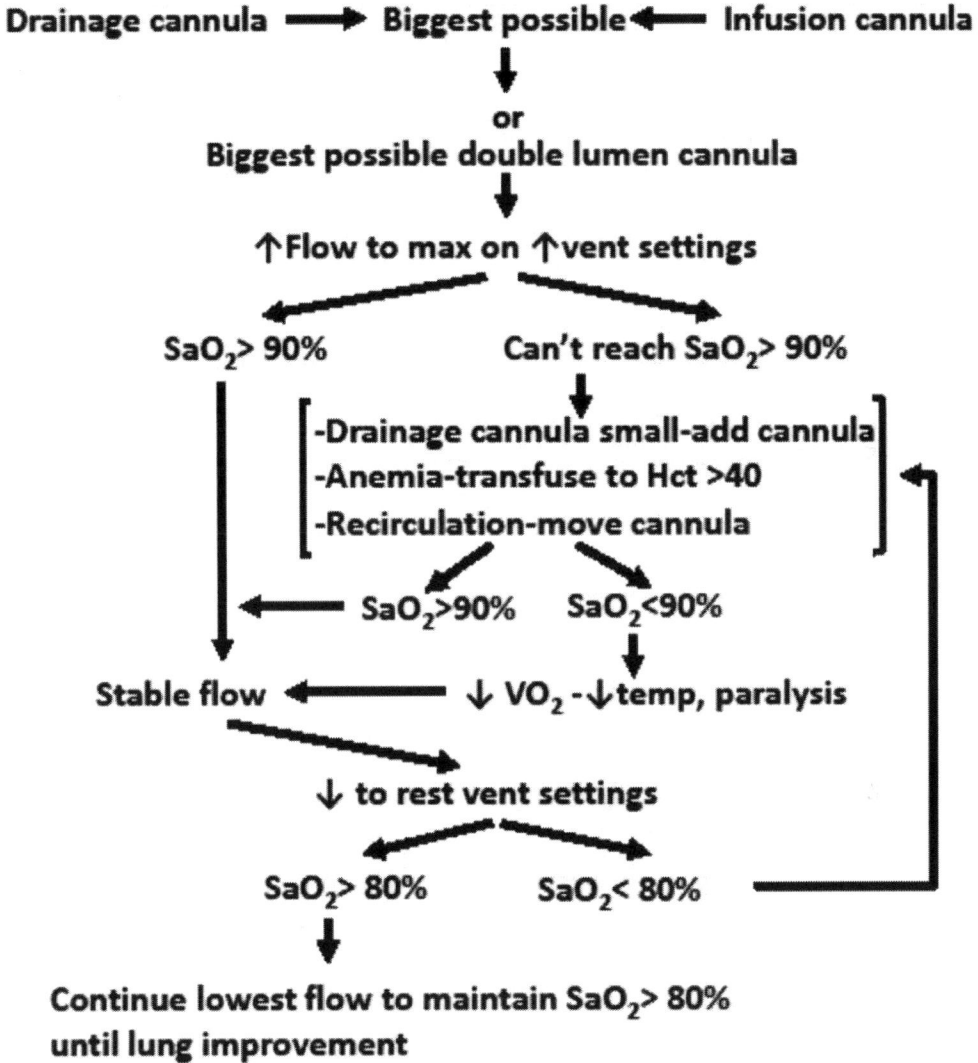

Drainage cannula ➡ Biggest possible ⬅ Infusion cannula

↓

or

Biggest possible double lumen cannula

↓

↑Flow to max on ↑vent settings

SaO_2> 90%   Can't reach SaO_2> 90%

↓

-Drainage cannula small-add cannula
-Anemia-transfuse to Hct >40
-Recirculation-move cannula

SaO_2>90% SaO_2<90%

Stable flow ⬅ ↓ VO_2 -↓temp, paralysis

↓ to rest vent settings

SaO_2> 80% SaO_2< 80%

Continue lowest flow to maintain SaO_2> 80%
until lung improvement

Figure 10- 2. Algorithm for blood flow and gas exchange in VV ECLS

References

1. Gattinoni L, Kolobow T, Tomlinson T, et al. Low-frequency positive pressure ventilation with extracorporeal CO_2 removal (LFPPV-ECCO2R): an experimental study. Anesth Analg 1978;57(4):470-477.
2. Gattinoni L, Agostoni A, Pesenti A, et al. Treatment of acute respiratory failure with low-frequency positive-pressure ventilation and extracorporeal removal of CO_2. Lancet 1980;2(8189):292-294.
3. Conrad SA, Brown EG. Heming TA, Bidani A: Mathematical analysis of extracorporeal arteriovenous CO2 exchange. Proceedings 13th Annual Houston Conference on Biomedical Engineering Research. Presented at the 13th Annual Conference, Houston, TX, Feb 16, 1995.
4. Conrad SA, Brown EG, Grier LR, Baier J, Heming T, Zwischenberger JB, Bidani A: Arteriovenous extracorporeal carbon dioxide removal (AVCO2R): a mathematical model and experimental evaluation. ASAIO Journal 1998; 44(4): 267-277.
5. Conrad SA, Zwischenberger JB, Grier LR, Alpard SK, Bidani A: Total arteriovenous carbon dioxide removal (AVCO2R) in acute respiratory failure: A phase I clinical study. Intensive Care Med. 2001; 27(8):1340-1351.
6. Zwischenberger JB, Conrad SA, Alpard SK, et al. Percutaneous extracorporeal arteriovenous CO_2 removal for severe respiratory failure. Ann Thorac Surg 1999;68(1):181-187.
7. Florchinger B, Philipp A, Klose A, et al. Pumpless extracorporeal lung assist: a 10-year institutional experience. Ann Thorac Surg 1008;86(2)410-417.

11

Anticoagulation and Bleeding During ECLS

Laurance L. Lequier MD, Gail M. Annich MD MS FRCP(C), M. Patricia Massicotte MD

Anticoagulation

An ideal anticoagulant for ECLS should inhibit platelet and coagulation system activation within the extracorporeal circuit, be easily titrated to clinical effect, yet still allow enough endogenous coagulation activity to prevent bleeding in the patient. Such an ideal anticoagulant is not currently available and therefore unfractionated heparin (UNFH) remains the default anticoagulant for ECLS.

The anticoagulant effect of UNFH is mediated by its interaction with two endogenous anticoagulants: antithrombin (AT) and tissue factor pathway inhibitor (TFPI). AT is produced in the liver and is a natural inhibitor of all serine proteases (except for fVIIa and protein C) and the majority of its anticoagulant effect results from inhibition of thrombin and fXa.[1] AT also inactivates kallikrein and plasmin, also involved in blood coagulation. Since AT inhibits most of the coagulation enzymes to varying degree, it is an important endogenous anticoagulant protein. UNFH is a complex glycosaminoglycan that binds to AT via a pentasaccharide sequence that is only present in approximately one third of UNFH molecules.[2] Once bound together, the UNFH-AT complex has a 1000 times inhibitory effect on coagulation protein activity as compared to antithrombin alone.[1] The UNFH-AT complex potentiates the inhibition of activated proteins, fXa, fIXa, fXIa, fXIIa and, to a lesser extent, fIIa (thrombin). The inhibition of thrombin requires that both AT and thrombin bind to UNFH, while the inhibition of fXa requires only the binding of AT to UNFH.[3] UNFH inhibits thrombin after it is formed, but it does not inhibit thrombin formation nor does it inhibit thrombin already bound to fibrin. UNFH increases the antithrombotic effect of TFPI by 2 - 4 times by increasing its affinity for fXa.[4]

Unfractionated heparin management

Every ECLS program has developed their own policies and procedures for anticoagulation and monitoring of UNFH anticoagulation based on the published literature, the protocols of other ECLS centers, the Extracorporeal Life Support Organization (ELSO) guidelines, and their own historical experience. Despite all the information available, every ECLS patient is unique resulting in many challenges with effectively anticoagulating the extracorporeal circuit, while avoiding any patient related bleeding or thrombosis complications. Evidence based guidelines state that anticoagulation is necessary during ECLS, however there have been no safety and efficacy studies to determine how much anticoagulation is necessary.[5] The effect of UNFH can be measured using a number of tests including activated clotting time (ACT), activated partial thromboplastin time (APTT), antifactor Xa level and thromboelastography (TEG). As will be discussed later, studies have demonstrated poor correlation between these tests. Proper studies using these tests during ECLS have not been carried out to determine the best test to monitor UNFH effect and patient outcomes. As a result, protocols for anticoagulation vary between clinical centers.

In most centers, patients usually receive an initial bolus of UNFH of between 50-100 units per kg body weight at the time of cannulation for ECLS. The bolus dose can be adjusted based on clinical factors such as evidence of preexisting bleeding, if for instance the patient has had recent surgery or CPB, and whether or not the UNFH given during CPB has been reversed to any degree with protamine. An UNFH infusion will be connected to the ECLS circuit immediately following initiation of ECLS. When the measured ACT drops to 300 seconds or lower, the UNFH infusion is usually initiated at 10-20 units/kg/hr, unless there is excessive bleeding. Patients who are experiencing significant bleeding or who have just had cardiac surgery may not be started on UNFH immediately. UNFH infusion rates will be titrated by the ECLS specialist to maintain the ACT within the ordered daily parameters.

The standard goal ACT parameter range is 180-220 seconds, but will vary from center to center depending on local experience and the type of monitoring equipment being used.[6] This is a starting guideline, and will be adjusted based on specific patient condition and response to anticoagulation therapy. Generally, a lower range of ACTs are desired for patients at increased risk for bleeding or who are having clinical bleeding, while higher ACTs are accepted when there appears to be clot developing anywhere in the ECLS circuit. Adequate goal ACTs are typically achieved with infusion rates of 20-50 units/kg/hour of UNFH. There is constant activation of coagulation as described earlier and significant UNFH consumption, thus

the UNFH infusion needs to maintained, and often increased, during the course of ECLS. This is especially true in neonates who have historically been described as having an increased UNFH requirement to achieve the same effect as older children.[7] An early study of 5 consecutive neonates on ECLS showed that more than 50% of administered UNFH was eliminated by the extracorporeal circuit and components alone.[8] The administration of platelets, increased urine output or the use of renal replacement therapy, result in an increased UNFH requirement to maintain goal ACTs.

Since UNFH is dependent on circulating AT for most of its anticoagulant activity, it may be helpful to measure AT levels, particularly in the patient who has a high UNFH requirement.[9] This is especially true for infants where it has been identified that they not only require a higher dose of UNFH to reach therapeutic target levels, but that they also demonstrate greater variation in UNFH dosing.[10,11] As well, one study revealed that neonates undergoing initiation of ECLS support had AT levels < 30% (<0.3 u/ml) of normal adult values.[12] Pooled plasma and recombinant AT concentrate are now available and can be administered to patients with low levels (< 30-50% of normal activity) and results in a significant decrease in markers of prothrombin activation.[13] Some centers will use AT administration (50 u/kg) if the AT levels are below 0.7 to 0.5 u/ml. The UNFH infusion is decreased by 25% prior to AT replacement because of the potential for significant augmentation of UNFH's anticoagulant effect. In one program, continuous infusion of AT to achieve levels of 100% was shown to decrease bleeding complications in a small number of neonates on ECLS.[14] The use of AT concentrate is preferred over the administration of fresh frozen plasma (FFP) for this purpose; as giving standard bolus infusions of FFP does not easily achieve adequate AT levels in patients on ECLS due to the AT concentration in FFP, 1 u/ml.[15] As a result, frequent boluses of FFP or continuous FFP infusions may be needed to ultimately achieve an increased AT level using FFP alone.

Unfractionated Heparin Monitoring

A number of different blood tests are currently used during ECLS to monitor hemostasis and the effect of UNFH including the ACT, APTT, antifactor Xa, and the TEG.

The ACT has been used for decades, and still is, to monitor heparin therapy in extracorporeal applications. Whole blood is mixed with one of two 'activators' (celite or kaolin) to provide a global functional test of hemostasis. A landmark study by Green et al. of target UNFH concentration (by thrombin time dilution method) of 0.1-0.25 u/ml correlated to an ACT range of 120-205 seconds (r = 0.55 for individual values, r = 0.95 for mean values) in a series of nine infants on ECLS.[16] The ACT required multiple serial determinations to improve accuracy, but because it was a low cost, bedside test, available around the clock, it was felt that the precision of the ACT was reliable enough to achieve target UNFH concentrations. The optimal UNFH concentration to provide adequate anticoagulation, but avoid bleeding complications, has not been determined in proper studies. Measuring ex vivo UNFH concentrations (by protamine titration) is both reliable and reproducible, but it is not as readily available or easy to automate.[17] Outside of ECLS applications, many institutions use the antifactor Xa assay as the gold standard test to monitor and manipulate the management of UNFH and low molecular weight heparin (LMWH) therapy.[18]

The antifactor Xa assay is not a measure of UNFH concentration, but rather a measure of UNFH effect, based on the ability of UNFH to catalyze AT's inhibition of factor Xa. Patient plasma is added to a test reagent that contains excess factor Xa. UNFH from the patient's plasma will bind AT and inhibit Xa. The amount of UNFH in the test plasma is inversely proportional to the amount of residual Xa, which is used to calculate the antifactor Xa level.[19] The ACT has been shown to have poor correlation to antifactor Xa in both children and adults undergoing CPB for cardiac surgery.[20,21,22] The reasons for this poor correlation, particularly when considering children on CPB, include platelet dysfunction and coagulopathy, hypothermia and hemodilution, and an immature coagulation system including lower AT levels.[23] Interestingly, Urlesberger et al. demonstrated that UNFH levels as measured by antifactor Xa assay of 0.2-0.5 u/ml not only correlated poorly to ACT values, but also remained much more stable throughout the course of neonatal ECLS than did ACTs.[24] A more recent, prospective study of 12 neonates on ECLS by Nankervis et al. not only confirmed poor correlation of ACT to anti factor Xa levels and heparin dose, but revealed a positive correlation between heparin dose and antifactor Xa (r = 0.75).[25]

Use of the APTT during ECLS suggests that infants and young children demonstrate an increased sensitivity to UNFH as indicated by a prolonged APTT with less than age appropriate UNFH doses.[26] The APTT is a plasma test activated by phospholipids which provides a measure of hemostasis in the absence of cellular components. In adults, an APTT of 1.5-2.5 times baseline provides safety, efficacy, and correlates to an UNFH concentration of 0.2-0.4 u/ml.[27] In a study of critically ill, non-ECLS adult patients, the APTT was better able to distinguish between low and moderate levels of anticoagulation than did the ACT.[28] Baseline APTT levels change significantly with age as part of developmental hemostasis, and similar studies in non-ECLS infants and children demonstrated that the APTT had poor correlation to antifactor Xa levels.[29,30] However, a recent retrospective review comparing TEG to standard anticoagulation results in pediatric patients on ECLS showed poor correlation of TEG to APTT, but moderate correlation of APTT to ACT (r = 0.56).[31] Although not formally studied, the APTT may be a useful test in adults where moderate doses of UNFH are used, including ECLS, but likely less reliable in pediatric populations. Many adult ECLS programs use the APTT instead of the ACT to monitor and adjust UNFH therapy and there are point-of-care devices that provide bedside APTT results.

There is significant variability in response to UNFH therapy in adults, and this is even more problematic in the pediatric population. Infants have decreased levels of the coagulation inhibitor AT (as low as 30% adult levels) compared to older children and adults (100%), which alters their response to UNFH and may result in inadequate anticoagulation when using ACT alone to guide heparin dosing. As well, infants have physiologically low concentrations of vitamin K dependent factors (II, VII, IX, and X), and contact factors (XI, XII, prekallikrein, and HMWK) which gradually rise to near adult levels by 6 - 12 months of age.[32] Despite these lower levels of coagulation factors, healthy infants do not seem to have bleeding tendencies and can form clot effectively. In fact, TEG studies of healthy infants revealed normal coagulation function in neonates and older infants and that infants 1 - 3 months of age may be more coagulable.[33]

The thromboelastogram (TEG) was introduced into clinical practice more than 50 years ago, and is classically used to analyze the different phases of anticoagulation of patients during CPB. The TEG is a whole blood point-of-care test of the viscoelastic properties of blood clot formation that provides information regarding the integrity of the coagulation cascade,

platelet function, platelet-fibrin interactions, and fibrinolysis.[14] Clotting of a whole blood sample is followed from initial fibrin clot formation (R = reaction time), which is prolonged in factor deficiencies or the use of exogenous anticoagulant or deficiencies of fibrinogen and platelets (K = coagulation time), through clot acceleration (alpha angle), and maximum clot strength (MA = maximum amplitude), which is dependent on platelet interaction with fibrin, and ultimately to fibrinolysis (LY 30) (Figure 11-1).[34] Some typical pathophysiologic TEG tracings are shown in Figure 11-2. Paired TEG samples, one with kaolin (kTEG) and one with kaolin-heparinase (hTEG), allows for assessment of coagulation in the presence of UNFH and corrected for UNFH. TEG provides information relating to multiple phases of coagulation in whole blood, relevant to ECLS

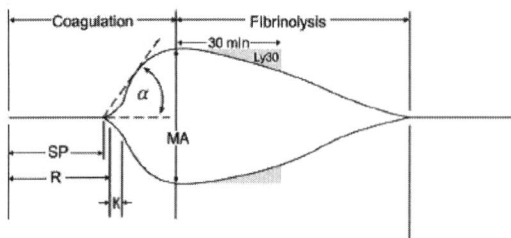

Normal
R;K;MA;Angle=Normal

Anticoagulants/Hemophilia
Factor Deficiency
R;K=Prolonged
MA;Angle=Decreased

Platelet Blockers
Thrombocytopenia/Thrombocytopathy
R-Normal;K=Prolonged
Angle=Normal
MA=Very Decreased

Fibrinolysis (UK,SK or t-PA)
Presence of t-PA
R=Normal
MA=Continuous Decrease
LY30>7.5%
LY60>15%

Hypercoagulability
R;K=Decreased
MA;Angle=Increased

D.I.C.
Stage 1
Hypercoagulable state with
secondary fibrinolysis

Stage 2
Hypercoagulable state

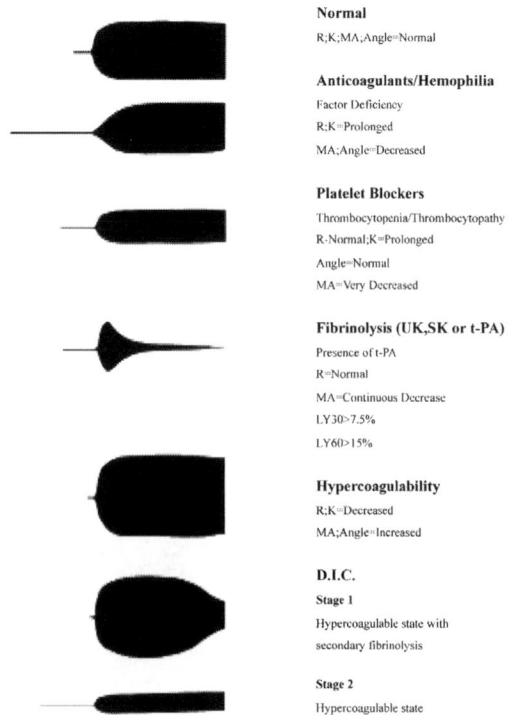

Figure 11-1. Components of a thromboelastogram tracing.

Figure 11-2. Typical pathophysiologic TEG tracings.

patients since more than one reason for coagulation abnormalities may be present.[31] Studies are needed to clarify the role for TEG monitoring in ECLS applications, especially in children.

The majority of ECLS centers use the ACT to dictate UNFH dosage.[35] Unfortunately, the ACT is not only affected by UNFH but also platelets and other coagulation factors. A prolonged ACT, for example, may be due to a true high UNFH level and therefore indicate that the amount of UNFH being given should be reduced. However, it may also be due to decreased fibrinogen, platelets, or other coagulation factors in which case the true plasma UNFH level and therefore UNFH dose may be appropriate. Because of the potential shortcomings of UNFH and the ACT, it may be useful to complement regular whole blood ACT measurements, intermittently, with more elaborate tests like an antifactor Xa assay.

A recent retrospective review of over six hundred consecutive pediatric venoarterial ECLS patients from a single center, over a twenty year time period, was conducted to determine anticoagulation associated factors that may affect patient outcome.[36] The UNFH protocol consisted of maintaining a standard ACT range of 180-220 seconds (mean ACT 227 +/- 50 seconds). The mean UNFH dose was 45 +/- 21 u/kg/hr. Multiple logistic regressions were used to assess the impact of ACT, UNFH dose, and other factors on survival. Increased hourly dose per kg of UNFH was the only significant correlate for improved survival (Figure 11-3). There was no difference in ACT range between survivors and non-survivors. There was moderate correlation of ACT to UNFH dose of survivors (r = 0.48). Cardiac patients received less UNFH than noncardiac ECLS patients and any previous surgery was associated with increased likelihood of death.

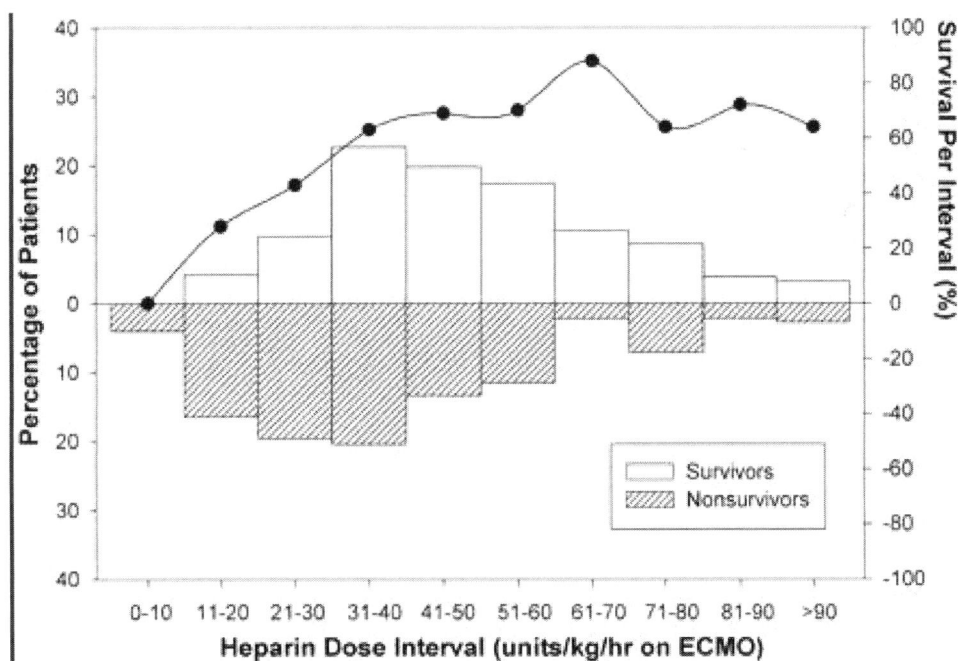

Figure 11-3. Empirical histograms show the percentage of patients in each of 10 intervals of heparin dose for survivors (open bars) and nonsurvivors (patterned bars). (From Baird CW, Zurakowski D, Robinson B et al. Anticoagulation and Pediatric Extracorporeal Membrane Oxygenation: Impact of ACT and Heparin Dose on Survival. Ann Thorac Surg. 2007;83:912-920.)

The authors conclude that ACT measurements alone may be too insensitive to maintain adequate long-term anticoagulation for patients on ECLS and other methods, such as UNFH serum concentrations or antifactor Xa levels, should be used. AT levels were not measured in this study, but it may be that many patients had low AT and therefore required much higher doses of UNFH to get effective anticoagulation, and this in turn was associated with improved survival.

A protocol described in two separate publications by Urlesberger and Muntean supports daily establishment of ACT ranges based on UNFH effect as measured by the antifactor Xa levels and AT levels.[37,38] These levels can be measured more frequently if there is clinical bleeding or thrombosis issues. As well, given that the ACT is more likely to overestimate UNFH effect in children and this may lead to inadequate anticoagulation and possible thrombosis, some ECLS programs have adopted a minimum heparin dose of 10-20 u/kg/hour despite the ACT value. Experts in anticoagulation can be helpful to help tailor your individual anticoagulation protocols.

Extracorporeal Circuit Modifications

UNFH anticoagulation allows for many different extracorporeal circuit applications, but its efficacy is compromised by its relative ineffectiveness toward platelets. An ideal anticoagulation strategy for ECLS would be to modify the extracorporeal circuit to make it as nonthrombogenic as vascular endothelium. Among other things, endothelial cells produce prostacyclin and nitric oxide (NO) which inhibit thrombin induced platelet adhesion and activation as a way to maintain the fluidity of blood.[67] Both prostacyclin and NO, exogenously added to extracorporeal circuits along with UNFH in an effort to inhibit the interaction between platelets and extracorporeal surfaces, have been shown to reduce platelet activation and consumption.[40,41] In one of these studies, ex-

perimental circuits were used and nafamostat mesylate (a serine protease inhibitor) was also administered.[40]

In the presence of NO, platelets become reversibly anesthetized, and, therefore, do not become activated during contact with the extracorporeal circuit. The half-life of NO is extremely short in plasma, as hemoglobin very quickly eliminates it (<1 second). This allows for rapid reversal of its inhibitory effects on platelets and allows them to quickly function at the sites where hemostasis is necessary. NO and the creation of NO releasing polymers have been successfully demonstrated in a rabbit model of VV ECLS.[42] MAHAMA/NO was the first compound to be incorporated into a polymer matrix applied to an extracorporeal circuit that, upon exposure to blood, locally released NO at its surface and without systemic heparinization. The MAHAMA/NO-doped circuits showed significantly decreased platelet consumption when compared to both the heparinized and non-heparinized control groups. Since this success further development of more lipophilic NO donor compounds that remain within the polymer or are covalently attached to the structural backbone of the polymer have been developed to prevent the leaching of the NO donor systemically.[43] Most recently a discrete, lipophilic analogue of MAHAMA/NO, DBHD/NO was synthesized and tested in an AV rabbit model of extracorporeal circulation (ECC).[44] The results exceeded expectations with the compound remaining within the organic phase, no leaching of the donor and allowing for precise NO release/control at the surface allowing determination of the exact NO flux required at the surface to prevent platelet activation and adhesion during ECC without systemic anticoagulation.

Many centers are using heparin bonded or surface treated circuits (there are a number of different formulations available) in an effort to make their circuits more biocompatible and limit or eliminate the need for anticoagulation during cardiopulmonary bypass and ECLS.

Some have shown that the use of these circuits reduces platelet activation, fibrinolysis, and the inflammatory response.[45] Others have demonstrated decreased blood loss and need for blood product replacement when heparin-bonded circuits were used.[46,47] However, the useful effects of the coated circuits may be measured in hours and be too short-lived to be of benefit in longer runs of ECLS that can last for days to weeks. Although, the benefit of a heparin-bonded or otherwise surface-treated circuit may be that it allows for delayed initiation of anticoagulation at the start of ECLS particularly when there are bleeding concerns as for instance immediately postoperatively or post extracorporeal cardiopulmonary resuscitation (ECPR).

One program described a "multi-system therapy protocol" to not only achieve both frequent and accurate UNFH dosing, but also by using dipyridamole to stabilize platelet function, aspirin to inhibit platelet aggregation, aprotinin to prevent excessive fibrinolysis, and pentoxifylline to reduce blood viscosity.[48] This protocol resulted in reduced bleeding and was associated with improved survival in a group of ECLS patients compared to a group of historical control patients in which UNFH therapy and ACT monitoring alone were used for anticoagulation.

The challenges with UNFH including poor bioavailability, how to accurately measure anticoagulation effect, reliance on AT levels, and development of heparin induced thrombocytopenia (HIT) have resulted in the development of novel anticoagulants. HIT is an immune mediated disorder in which IgG antibodies bind to a complex of UNFH and platelet factor-4 before binding to platelet Fc receptors causing platelet activation and destruction.[49] The diagnosis of HIT can be confirmed by testing for heparin-induced platelet aggregation using the gold standard test, C14 serotonin assay. The measurement of platelet factor-4 antibodies using the Elisa test is less sensitive with a high false positivity, but more easily carried out by laboratories. Warkentin et al. have reported on

the probability of a positive C14 serotonin assay based on the results of the Elisa test.[50]

Novel Anticoagulation

The novel anticoagulants, direct thrombin inhibitors (DTIs) have several theoretical advantages over UNFH, especially in children.[51] First, they bind thrombin directly, independent of AT, making them more reliable in patients with low or fluctuating AT levels. Second, they do not bind to other plasma proteins or cells and therefore are not prone to day to day changes in serum chemistry or blood cell counts. Third, DTIs inhibit clot-bound and circulating thrombin which may lead to improved efficacy. Finally, they do not cause HIT. As a result, novel anticoagulants including DTIs may be required during ECLS. DTIs are a relatively new class of short-acting anticoagulants that bind to active sites on thrombin directly, and demonstrate more predictable pharmacokinetics and reduce thrombin generation to a greater degree when compared to UNFH.[52] Dosing is adjusted by maintaining APTT ratios of 1.5-2.5 times normal values. One potential problem, which probably limits the use of DTIs, more so in CPB than ECLS, is the lack of an antidote in the way that UNFH has in the form of protamine. However, unlike in CPB, the need to reverse anticoagulant effect on ECLS would rarely occur. If needed, in cases of severe bleeding, given their relatively short half lives, DTI anticoagulation can be decreased or discontinued and its effect allowed to wear off. As well, studies have demonstrated that the anticoagulant effect of DTIs can be reversed with recombinant activated factor VIIa (rFVIIa).[53]

Three synthetic DTIs, argatroban, bivalirudin, and lepirudin, have been used in CPB, ECLS, and VAD supports, mainly in the context of preexisting or suspected HIT.[54-57] There are multiple case reports using argatroban in both adults and children. Effective argatroban dose ranged from 0.2-10 ug/kg/min based on therapeutic ACTs and/or APTTs. A study of sham ECLS circuits demonstrated significantly less thrombin generation in circuits anticoagulated with argatroban compared to those anticoagulated with UNFH.[58] Interestingly, one DTI case report with lepirudin demonstrated good linear correlation between ACT and APTT during lepirudin anticoagulation (r = 0.88).[57] DTIs could provide a more predictable dosing regimen that allows for consistent anticoagulant effect with less bleeding compared to UNFH making them useful in ECLS, not just in cases of HIT.[59] The advantage of acting independent of AT, renders these novel anticoagulants especially appealing for use in ECLS for infants and children. However, there are few studies studying the pharmacokinetics and pharmacodynamics of these agents and none definitively establishing safety and efficacy in cohorts which may require their usage.

Ventricular Assist Devices

Thrombin is generated in a similar manner during the use of ventricular assist devices (VADs). Activation of coagulation occurs via a similar mechanism as with traditional ECMO. There are no proper clinical studies establishing safety and efficacy of antithrombotic therapy in VADs however, anticoagulation and antiplatelet therapy is recommended.[60]

Clinical Consequences

Bleeding

Bleeding complications are frequently encountered during the provision of ECLS and are the principal cause of morbidity and mortality. ECLS produces a consumptive coagulopathy that continues as long as blood circulates over non-endothelial cell surfaces. Interventions to reduce nonsurgical bleeding necessarily increase the likelihood that more thrombin will be generated and more fibrin formed. Similarly, therapy that suppresses coagulation increases the possibility of bleeding. In addition to the need for anticoagulation to maintain patency of the extracorporeal circuit, patients who require ECLS may be predisposed to bleeding in a number of ways. Infants are the most likely population to receive extracorporeal support and are known to have, at baseline, lower levels of coagulation factors than do older children and adults.[61] Patients with cardiorespiratory compromise severe enough to require ECLS can demonstrate various degrees of disseminated intravascular coagulation (DIC). In one study, more than two thirds of infants and children demonstrated significant coagulation factor deficiencies prior to being placed on ECLS.[62] Over half of these patients continued to have coagulation factor deficiency despite factor replacement at the time of cannulation for ECLS. Ongoing consumption of platelets and coagulation factors, in the extracorporeal circuit during ECLS, further increases the chance of bleeding complications.

Bleeding may occur in a number of anatomic sites. Surgical site bleeding, the most common source of bleeding, is reported in 6-32% of ECLS patients with the highest incidence occurring in patients who have had recent cardiac surgery.[63] Intracranial hemorrhage, the most potentially devastating bleeding complication occurs in 3-6% of patients who have received ECLS with neonates having the highest incidence. Hypoxemia, acidosis, and cardiovascular instability prior to initiation of ECLS, prematurity, coagulopathy, and jugular vein and carotid artery ligation all increase the risk for intracranial hemorrhage.[64] The development of any significant bleeding may require alteration in the degree of anticoagulation being used, and intracranial hemorrhage may ultimately require discontinuation of ECLS.

During ECLS, in an effort to reduce the risk of bleeding complications and/or to treat clinical bleeding as a result of consumption of platelets and coagulation factors, regular blood product replacement will be required. The replacement of blood products is currently not evidence based but by protocol in most centers and based on clinical experience, historical literature, and guideline recommendations than as a result of well conducted research studies. Transfusions of packed red blood cells are given as needed to replace any blood loss and maintain a near normal hematocrit (> 35%). The INR (PT) is a good test of the status of the hemostatic pathway and not affected by UNFH. Fresh frozen plasma (FFP) is administered in aliquots of 5-10 ml/kg as needed if the INR is > 1.5-2.0 and/or if there is significant bleeding. FFP may also be used, as previously described, in an effort to increase the AT level when UNFH dosing has been escalated without achieving target ACT, but pooled or recombinant AT administration is preferred. Cryoprecipitate can be given if the fibrinogen level is < 100 mg/dL.

There is a significant relationship between platelet count and hemorrhagic complications on ECLS and platelet administration decreases the incidence of bleeding complications.[38,65] Frequent platelet transfusions of 10 ml/kg, or 1 unit per 5 kg, are given to maintain a platelet count >100,000 cells/mm³ in most patients, particularly neonates. The threshold for platelet transfusion may be reduced in older patients with an inherent lower risk of intracranial hemorrhage and who are stable on ECLS. There may be significant platelet dysfunction despite regular platelet transfusions. Determination of platelet function by standard platelet aggregation tests requires large blood volumes thus is challenging during ECLS. The TEG can measure the integrity of platelet activity.[66] Performance of platelet mapping using the arachidonic acid and adenosine diphosphate agonists, as an extension of the TEG may assist in the evaluation of platelet function, although not formally validated.

Often the level of anticoagulation accepted may be reduced if there is clinically significant bleeding. Newer ECLS circuitry and components that are heparin-bonded or surface-treated may allow for a number of hours of minimal to no UNFH therapy in an effort to reduce or control completely patient bleeding, particularly following CPB-facilitated cardiac surgery, or other surgical manipulations. Surgical exploration with careful hemostasis may be required in some cases. Topical agents such as oxidized cellulose (Surgicel), gelatin sponge (Gelfoam) thrombin and fibrinogen sealant (Tisseel) can be used at the surgical sites to help control oozing.[34]

Additional agents, such as aminocaproic acid (Amicar), tranexamic acid (TEA), and aprotinin, all inhibitors of fibrinolysis, have been used successfully to manage significant surgical site bleeding.[67-69] Amicar was shown to reduce the incidence of surgical bleeding in ECLS patients, particularly cardiac surgery patients while TEA reduced postoperative blood loss associated with congenital diaphragmatic hernia (CDH) repair while on ECLS. Subsequently, both Amicar and TEA are used in many centers to prevent hemorrhage in ECLS patients having surgical procedures. Aprotinin, however, has been shown to be associated with renal dysfunction following cardiac surgery making its use controversial.[70]

There are several reports of using activated recombinant factor VII (rVIIa) for refractory bleeding during ECLS despite platelet transfusion and correction of all other coagulation factor deficiencies.[71,72] rVIIa enhances the rate of thrombin formation and is given in a dose range of 40-90 ug/kg. In multiple series, following treatment with rVIIa, patients had significant reduction in chest tube drainage and reduced need for packed red blood cell transfusions. The rate of patient thromboembolic complications (25-30%) seen in the series reviewed, was not significantly higher than the rate of the same complications in ECLS patients that did not receive rVIIa. However, increased circuit clot and pre/post-membrane pressures was seen occasionally and led to a need to change out the circuit in a small number of patients. As well, there have been a few case reports of fatal thrombosis after administration of rVIIa on ECLS, so one must be extremely careful.[73-75] Thus, some centers will administer lower doses of rVIIa (25-50 ug/kg) and if more than one dose is required they do not repeat the dose more than every two to four hours.

Thrombosis

Thrombosis in the patient may occur due to an inability to modulate the activation of coagulation initiated in the extracorporeal circuit despite using anticoagulant therapy. Although some thromboses may be large and readily clinically apparent, many thrombotic events are likely not reported because they are subclinical or occult. In a single center adult series of postcardiotomy ECLS patients, 50% of patients who died underwent autopsy, and ¾ had clinically unrecognized, postoperative, thromboembolic complications.[76] These included venous thromboses, systemic thromboemboli, cerebral infarction, and bowel ischemia. As well, the longer a patient received ECLS, the more likely there was to be a thromboembolic complication. A similar autopsy series of 29 ECLS children published recently demonstrated that 69% of autopsies revealed evidence for systemic thromboses, with thrombosis being significantly more common in children who had congenital cardiac disease.[77] There was no correlation of this prevalence of thrombosis to results of coagulation testing or duration of ECLS. Therefore, it is very likely that the true incidence of thromboembolic complications is underestimated in ECLS patients as a whole, especially in the absence of objective testing. When color Doppler sonography was used in a prospective series of pediatric ECLS patients, significant venous thrombosis was identified in 20% of subjects.[78]

Thrombosis in the ECLS circuit is more likely to occur during periods of low flow or inadequate circuit anticoagulation, for a variety of reasons. The ELSO registry reports significant circuit or component clots occur in 20% of patients.[63] Clots can be found anywhere in the circuit, especially at sites of stasis or turbulent flow and are more common on the venous (pre-oxygenator) side of the circuit than on the arterial (post-oxygenator) side. The membrane oxygenator and bridge tubing are the most commonly reported sites for clot formation, although it is hoped that this decreases significantly with the newer ECLS equipment (oxygenator, pumps, circuits) that are now available. Extensive clot formation, particularly if it is associated with significant hemolysis, may require that the entire circuit be replaced.

Conclusions

During the last 50 years, we have learned to circulate, oxygenate, and ventilate blood outside of the body, but to this day, we still do not command the blood-surface interface. This limitation severely restricts the use of ECLS patients, particularly those who have consumptive coagulopathy or preexisting coagulation and/or organ dysfunction prior to the initiation of ECLS. Control of the blood-surface interface promises huge benefits to critical care medicine by allowing ECLS to give time for organ recovery. Many unanswered questions exist concerning therapies to maintain the hemostatic balance during ECLS exist including the optimal combination, duration and dosage of antithrombotic agents needed to limit bleeding and thrombotic complications. Properly designed clinical studies determining the pharmacokinetics and pharmacodynamics, as well as safety and efficacy of therapies are urgently required. The ELSO participants are in a unique position to design and complete these studies.

References

1. Pratt C, Church F. Antithrombin: structure and function. Semin Hematol. 1991;28:3-9.
2. Wu Y, Sheffield W, Blajchman M. Defining the heparin binding domain of antithrombin. Blood Coagul Fibrinolysis. 1994;5:83-95.
3. Danielsson A, Raub E, Lindahl U, et al. Role of ternary complexes, in which heparin binds bothantithrombin and proteinase, in the acceleration of the reactions between antithrombin and thrombin or factor Xa. J Biol Chem. 1986;261:15467-15473
4. Huang ZF, Wun TC, Broze GJ Jr. Kinetics of factor Xa inhibition by tissue factor pathway inhibitor. J Biol Chem. 1993;268:26950-26955.
5. Monagle P, Chalmers E, Chan A, et al. Antithrombotic therapy in neonates and children: American College of Chest Physicians Evidenced-Based Clinical Practice Guidelines (8th edition). Chest. 2008133:887S-968S.
6. Fleming GM, Gupta M, Cooley E, et al. Maintaining the standard:a quality assurance study for new equipment in the Michigan ECMO program. ASAIO J. 2007;53:556-560.
7. Schmidt B, Ofosu FA, Mitchell, et al. Anticoagulation effects of heparin in neonatal plasma. Pediatr Res. 1989;25:405-408.
8. Green TP, Isham-Schopf B, Irmiter RJ et al. Inactivation of heparin during extracorporeal circulation in infants. Clin Pharmacol Ther. 1990;48:148-154.
9. Shapiro A. Antithrombin deficiency in special clinical syndromes - Part I: Extracorporeal Membrane Oxygenation. Seminars in Hematology. 1995;32:33-36.
10. Andrew M, Marzinotto V, Massicotte P, et al. Heparin therapy in pediatric patients: a prospective cohort study. Pediatr Res. 1994;35:78-83.
11. Schmidt B, Andrew M. Neonatal thrombosis: report of a prospective Canadian and international registry. Pediatrics. 1995;96:939-943.
12. Arnold P, Jackson S, Wallis J, et al. Coagulation factor activity during neonatal extracorporeal membrane oxygenation. Intensive Care Med. 2001;27:1395-1400.
13. Pollock ME, Owings JT, Gosselin RC. ATIII replacement during infant extracorporeal support. Thromb Haemost. 1995;73:936.
14. Agati S, Ciccarello, Salvo D, et al. Use of a Novel Anticoagulation strategy During ECMO in a Pediatric Population. ASAIO J. 2006;52:513-516.
15. Thureen PJ, Loomis M. Manco-Johnson M, et al. Randomized trial of albumin versus plasma for correction of ATIII deficiency in neonatal ECMO. Second annual meeting of ELSO 1990 (Abstract 50).
16. Green TP, Isham-Schopf B, Steinhorn RH, et al. Whole blood activated clotting time in infants during extracorporeal membrane oxygenation. Crit Care Med. 1990;18:494-498.
17. Olson J, Arkin C, Brandt J, et al. Laboratory monitoring of unfractionated heparin therapy. Arch Pathol Lab Med. 1998;122:782-798.
18. Hirsh J, Raschke R. Heparin and low-molecular-weight heparin. Chest. 2004;126:188S-203S.
19. Newall F, Johnston L, Ignjatovic, et al. Unfractionated heparin therapy in Infants and Children. Pediatrics. 2009;123:e510-e518.
20. Gruenwald C, deSouza V, Chan AK, Andrew M. Whole blood heparin concentrations do not correlate with plasma antifactor Xa heparin concentrations in pediatric patients undergoing cardiopulmonary bypass. Perfusion. 2000;15:203-209.
21. Guzetta NA, Monitz HG, Fernandez JD, et al. Correlations Between Activated Clotting Time Values and Heparin Concentration Measurements in Young Infants Undergoing Cardiopulmonary Bypass. Anesthesia-Analgesia. 2010;111:173-179.

22. Raymond PD, Ray MJ, Callen SN, Marsh NA. Heparin monitoring during cardiac surgery. Part 2: Calculating the overestimation of heparin by the activated clotting time. Perfusion. 2003;18:277-281.

23. Martindale SJ, Shayevitz AL, Joist JH, et al. The activated coagulation time: suitability for monitoring heparin effect and neutralization during pediatric cardiac surgery. J Cardiovasc Vasc Anesth. 1996;10:458-463.

24. Urlesberger B, Zobel G, Zenz W, et al. Activation of the clotting system during extracorporeal membrane oxygenation in term newborn infants. J Pediatr. 1996;129:264-268.

25. Nankervis CA, Preston TJ, Dysart KC, et al. Assessing Heparin Dosing in Neonates on Venoarterial Extracorporeal Membrane Oxygenation. ASAIO J. 2007; 53:111-114.

26. Chan AK, Berry L, Monagle P, et al. Decreased concentrations of heparinoids are required to inhibit thrombin generation in plasma from newborns and children compared to plasma from adults. Thromb Hemostat. 2002;87:606-613.

27. Brill-Edwards P, Ginsberg J, Johnston M, Hirsh J. Establishing a therapeutic range for heparin therapy. Ann Intern Med. 1993;119:104-109.

28. De Waele JJ, Van Cauwenberghe S, Hoste E, et al. The use of activated clotting time for monitoring heparin therapy in critically ill patients. Intensive Care Med. 2003;29:325-328.

29. Chan AK, Black L, Ing C, et al. Utility of aPTT in monitoring unfractionated heparin in children. Thromb Res. 2006;122:135-136.

30. Kuhle S, Eulmesekian P, Kavanagh B, et al. Lack of correlation between heparin dose and standard clinical monitoring tests in treatment with unfractionated heparin in critically ill children. Haematologica. 2007;92:554-557.

31. Alexander DC, Butt WW, Best JD, et al. Correlation of thromboelastography with standard tests of anticoagulation in paediatric patients receiving extracorporeal life support. Thrombosis Research. 2010;125:387-392.

32. Monagle P. Anticoagulation in the young. Heart. 2004;90:808-812.

33. Miller BE, Bailey JM, Mancuso TJ, et al. Functional maturity of the coagulation system in children: an evaluation using thromboelastography. Anesth Analog. 1997;84;745-748.

34. Yeh T Jr., Kavarana MN. Cardiopulmonary bypass and the coagulation system. Progress Ped Cardiol. 2005;21:87-115.

35. Graves DF, Chernin JM, Kurusz M, Zwischenberger JB. Anticoagulation practices during neonatal extracorporeal membrane oxygenation: survey results. Perfusion. 1996;11:461-466.

36. Baird CW, Zurakowski D, Robinson B et al. Anticoagulation and Pediatric Extracorporeal Membrane Oxygenation: Impact of ACT and Heparin Dose on Survival. Ann Thorac Surg. 2007;83:912-920.

37. Urlesberger B, Zobel G, Zenz W, et al. Activation of the clotting system during extracorporeal membrane oxygenation in term newborn infants. J Pediatr. 1996;129:264-268.

38. Muntean W. Coagulation and anticoagulation in extracorporeal membrane oxygenation. Artificial Organs. 1999;23:979-983.

39. Radomski MW, Palmer RMJ, Moncada S. The anti-aggregating properties of vascular endothelium: interactions between prostacycline and nitric oxide. Br J Pharmacol. 1987;92:639-646.

40. Skogby M, Friberg G, Adrian K, Mellgren K. Pharmacological inhibition of plasma coagulation and platelet activation during experimental long-term perfusion. Scand Cardiovasc J; 37:222-227.

41. Jacobson J. Nitric oxide: platelet protectant properties during cardiopulmonary bypass/ECMO. J Extra Corpor Technol. 2002;34:144-147.

42. Annich GM, Meinhardt JP, Mowery KA et al. Reduced platelet activation and thrombosis in extracorporeal circuits coated with nitric oxide release polymers. Crit Care Med. 2000;28:915-920.

43. Batchelor MM, Reoma SL, Fleser PS, Nuthakki VK, Callahan RE, Shanley CJ, Politis JK, Elmore J, Merz SI, Meyerhoff ME. More lipophilic dialkyldiamine-based diazeniumdiolates: synthesis, characterization, and application in preparing thromboresistant nitric oxide release polymeric coatings. J Med Chem 2003;46:5153-5161.

44. Skrzypchak AM, Lafayette NG, Bartlett RH, Zhou Z, Frost MC, Meyerhoff ME, Annich GM. Effect of varying nitric oxide release to prevent platelet consumption and preserve platelet function in an in vivo model of extracorporeal circulation. Perfusion 2007;22:193-200.

45. Palatianos GM, Foroulis CN, Vassili, MI et al. A prospective, double-blind study of the efficacy of the bioline surface-heparinized extracorporeal perfusion circuit. Ann Thorac Surg. 2003;76:129-135.

46. Marcolin R, Bonbino M, Pesenti A, et al. Venovenous ELS with heparin bonded circuits. Int J Artif Organs. 1995;18:624-626.

47. Tayama E, Hayashida N. Akasu K, et al. Biocompatibility of heparin-coated extracorporeal bypass circuits: New heparin bonded bioline system. Artif Organs. 2000;24:618-623.

48. Glauber M, Szefner J, Senni M, Gamba, A et al. Reduction of hemorrhagic complications during mechanically assisted circulation with the use of a multi-system anticoagulation protocol. Artificial Organs. 1995;18:649-655.

49. Kelton JC. The pathophysiology of heparin-induced thrombocytopenia: Biological basis for treatment. Chest. 2005;127:9S-20S.

50. Warkentin TE, Sheppard JA, Moore JC, et al. Laboratory testing for antibodies that cause heparin-induced thrombocytopenia: how much class do we need? J Lab Clin Med. 2005;146:341-346

51. Young G. New Anticoagulants in Children. Hematology. 2008:245-250.

52. Bates SM, Weitz JI. The mechanism of action of thrombin inhibitors. J. Invasive Cardiol. 2000;12:1-12.

53. Young G, Yonekawa KE, Nakagawa PA, et al. Recombinant activated factor VII effectively reverses the anticoagulant effects of heparin, enoxaparin, fondaparinux, argatroban and bivalirudin. Blood Coag Fibrin. 2007;18:547-553.

54. Beiderlinden M, Treschan T, Gorlinger K, Peters J. Argatroban in Extracorporeal Membrane Oxygenation. Artificial Organs. 2007;31:461-465

55. Scott KL, Grier LR, Conrad SA. Heparin-induced thrombocytopenia in a pediatric patient receiving extracorporeal membrane oxygenation managed with argatroban. Pediatr Crit Care Med. 2006;7:473-475.

56. Koster a, Weng U, Bottcher W, Gromann T, et al. Successful use of Bivalirudin as anticoagulant for ECMO in a patient with HIT. Ann Thorac Surg. 2007;83:1865-1867.

57. Balasubramanian SK, Tiruvoipati R, Chatterjee S, et al. Extracorporeal Membrane Oxygenation with Lepirudin Anticoagulation for Heparin Induced Thrombocytopenia. ASAIO J. 2005;5:477-479.

58. Young G, Yonekawa KE, Nakagawa P, Nugent DJ. Argatroban as an alternative to heparin in extracorporeal membrane oxygenation circuits. Perfusion. 2004;19:283-288.

59. Chan VHT, Monagle P, Massicotte P, Chan AKC. Novel pediatric anticoagulants: a

review of the current literature. Coagul Fibrinolysis. 2010;21:144-151.

60. Monagle P, Chalmers E, Chan A, et al. Antithrombotic therapy in neonates and children: American College of Chest Physicians Evidenced-Based Clinical Practice Guidelines (8th edition). Chest. 2008133:887S-968S.

61. Andrew M, Paes B, Johnston M. Development of the hemostatic system in the neonate and young infant. Am J Pediatr Hematol Oncol. 1990;12:95-104.

62. McManus ML, Kevy SV, Bower LK, et al. Coagulation factor deficiencies during initiation of extracorporeal membrane oxygenation. J Pediatr. 1995;126:900-904.

63. Extracorporeal Life Support Organization. Registry Report. Ann Arbor: University of Michigan; January 2010.

64. Bulas D, Glass P. Neonatal ECMO: neuroimaging and neurodevelopmental outcome. Seminars in Perinatology. 2005;29:58-65.

65. Stallion A, Cofer BR, Rafferty JA, et al. The significant relationship between platelet count and haemorrhagic complications on ECMO. Perfusion. 1994; 9:265-269.

66. Oliver WC. Anticoagulation and coagulation Management for ECMO. Seminars in Cardiothoracic and Vascular Anesthesia. 2009; 13:154-175.

67. Downard CD, Betit P, Chang RW, Garza JJ, Arnold JH, Wilson JM. Impact of Amicar on hemorrhagic complications of ECMO: A ten year review. J Pediatr Surg. 2003; 38:1212-1216.

68. van der Staak FH, de Haan AF, Geven WB, Festen C. Surgical repair of congenital diaphragmatic hernia during extracorporeal membrane oxygenation: hemorrhagic complications and the effect of tranexamic acid. J Pediatr Surg. 1997; 32:594-599.

69. Biswas AK, Lewis L, Sommerauer JF. Aprotinin in the management of life-threatening bleeding during extracorporeal life support. Perfusion. 2000;15:211-216.

70. Mangano DT, Tudor IC, Dietzel C, et al. The Risk Associated with Aprotinin in Cardiac Surgery. NEJM. 2006 354;: 353-365.

71. Dominguez TE, Mitchell M, Friess SH, et al. Use of recombinant factor VIIa for refractory hemorrhage during extracorporeal membrane oxygenation. Pediatr Crit Care Med. 2005;6:348-351.

72. Niebler, RA, Punzalan, RC, Marchan M, et al. Activated recombinant factor VII for refractory bleeding during extracorporeal membrane oxygenation. Pediatr Crit Care Med. 2009; 10; 1-5.

73. Bui JD, Despotis GD, Trulock EP, et al. Fatal thrombosis after administration of activated prothrombin complex concentrates and recombinant Factor VII. Jn Thorac Cardiovasc Surg. 2002; 124:852-854.

74. Syburra T, Lachat M, Genoni M, Wilhelm MJ. Fatal Outcome of Recombinant Factor VIIa in Heart Transplantation With Extracorporeal Membrane Oxygenation. Ann Thorac Surg. 2010;89:1643-1645.

75. Velik-Sachner C, Sergi C, Fries D, et al. Use of recombinant factor VIIa led to thrombotic occlusion of the truncus brachiocephalicus in a neonate supported on ECMO. Anesth Analog. 2005; 101:924.

76. Rastan AJ, Lachmann N, Walther tT, et al. Autopsy findings in patients on postcardiotomy extracorporeal membrane oxygenation (ECMO). Int J Artif Organs. 2006; 29:1121-1131.

77. Reed RC, Rutledge JC. Laboratory and clinical predictors of thrombosis and hemorrhage in 29 pediatric ECMO nonsurvivors. Pediatr Dev Pathol. 2001;

78. Riccabona M, Kuttnig-Haim M, Dacar D, et al. Venous thrombosis in and after extracorporeal membrane oxygenation: detection and follow-up by color Doppler sonography. Eur Radiol 1997; 7:1383-1386.

12

Analgesia, Sedation, Neuromuscular Blockade, and Temperature Control During ECLS

William Lynch MD, Gail Annich MD MS FRCP(C)

Analgesia and Sedation

Analgesics and sedation are ubiquitous in modern intensive care units. This pharmacologic approach is intended to relieve pain, minimize anxiety, offer amnesia, and minimize oxygen consumption and carbon dioxide production. The sedated patient is less apt to remove lines, endotracheal tubes, and vascular cannulae. The sedated patient is one more likely to breath synchronously with the mechanical ventilator. A chemically "calmed" patient is an easily "controlled" patient. While the "calmed" and "controlled" intensive careunit (ICU) patient was considered the compassionate standard two decades ago, this paradigm has shifted dramatically to promote "animation" and "liberation." We now recognize that the endotracheal tube violates the airway rather than protecting it. Clinical trials demonstrate noninvasive ventilation reduces infections and complications seen with endotracheal intubation while improving survival.[1,2] We realize that mechanical ventilation can injure the lung, stimulate systemic inflammation, and cause death.[3,4] Sedative infusions, once thought essential for humane care, can be stopped daily in the sickest ICU patient. The result being decreased time on the ventilator, fewer days in the ICU, and improved survival while decreasing ICU related posttraumatic stress disorder.[5,6,7] Finally, we have learned it is both practical and beneficial to mobilize the critically ill patient; again achieving improved survival and functional outcomes for these patients.[8]

ECLS technology has matured sufficiently such that there is a new "safety profile." ECLS is being used earlier in the time course of the patient's illness instead of being reserved as a "rescue" or "salvage" strategy with little opportunity for benefit. ECLS is also being used in the awake and active patient. All the benefits of "animation" and "liberation" can be realized even in the patient supported with ECLS.[9]

This chapter will review common strategies for analgesia, sedation, and chemical paralysis in the ECLS patient. Delirium in the ICU will also be reviewed. And lastly, hypothermia in the setting of ECLS will be discussed.

Pharmacology and ECLS

Accurate dosing of drugs in the ICU, such as sedation and analgesia, contribute to reduction in morbidity and mortality by reducing side effects, duration of use, and adverse reactions.[10] Critical illness changes the pharmacodynamics and pharmacokinetics of most drugs. The pharmacology of patients supported with ECLS is not as well understood. ECLS patients have an increased blood volume and volume of distribution as a consequence of the extracorporeal circuit. These patients often have impaired hepatic and renal function. There are also effects from the polyvinyl chloride (PVC) tubing and membrane oxygenators that cause these patients to be unique in comparison to the typical ICU patient.

The ECLS circuit as described in detail in Chapter 8 and 10 consists of PVC tubing, connectors, pump, and a membrane oxygenator (MO). Membrane materials are made from different polymers. The most commonly used membranes in ECLS are polypropylene, silicone, and polymethyl pentene (PMP). The pharmacokinetics of sedative, analgesic, and antibiotic medications has been studied in relationship to the ECLS circuit. Clinical observations commonly show the dosing of these medications to be far greater than when used in non-ECLS patients.[11,12,13] The PVC tubing and MO add a large volume of distribution, increased blood volume and offer a large surface area for adsorption of drugs onto a polymer surface.[11,14,15] This drug adsorption reduces the bioavailability of the first drug dose while affecting the overall drug clearance. Mulla et al. evaluated sedative drug losses in an in vitro model. This two-phase model looked at loss of lorazepam, midazolam, diazepam, and propofol while on ECLS. There was uptake of drugs with losses of 40-98% in the order of propofol>diazepam>midazolam>lorazepam. In addition to the circuit materials, the circuit prime with albumin, blood, electrolyte solutions, buffers, and temperature manipulations all impact drug availability while on ECLS. Further, the investigations suggested ECLS circuits extracted significant amounts of sedative drugs and the effect decreased with increased use of the circuit. More drug adsorption was due to the PVC tubing than to the silicone membrane.

Tibboel et al. looked at drug absorption of commonly used drugs (midazolam, morphine, cefazolin, meropenem, vancomycin) in ECMO circuits with silicone and polypropylene hollow fiber membranes. Significant drug absorption occurred with both membranes correlating with increased lipophilicity of the drugs. The polypropylene membrane demonstrated significantly less drug absorption when compared with the silicone membrane.[16]

It is necessary therefore to recognize the potential impact of the ECLS circuitry and its priming solutions with respect to drug distribution and effect. Drug elimination and clearance is reduced, volume of distribution is increased, and drugs are sequestered by the polymeric components of the ECLS circuitry. This constellation of events leads to low bioavailability of many commonly used ICU medications.

Indications for Sedation and Analgesia

The ECLS patient should be considered as any other patient in an intensive care unit. The ICU patient typically needs sedation and analgesia. This is the case with the ECLS patient. These patients will have widely varying sedation and analgesia needs and therefore this management must be individualized on a case to case basis. While the use of analgesic, sedative, and antipsychotic medications is commonplace in the ICU, achieving the optimal effect is challenging. Unpredictable pharmacokinetics can result in inappropriate dosing and effect. Under treatment can perpetuate pain, agitation, ventilator dyssynchrony, self-extubation, removal of central lines, and ICU related posttraumatic stress disorder (PTSD). Over treatment is associated with prolonged mechanical ventilation, hospital acquired infections, delirium, increased length of stay, and also is associated with PTSD.[5,17,18]

ECLS is offered for respiratory failure when conventional respiratory support fails. Even though physiologic requirements of oxygen and carbon dioxide can be effectively managed, these patients commonly have dyspnea, which remains a source of distress. Excessive coughing also remains a cause for distress and opiates may alleviate both of these consequences of respiratory failure. Sedation can reduce oxygen consumption by 15% in the mechanically ventilated patient. Sedation will also offer amnesia but the evidence does not support improved outcomes when measured by survival or length of stay. It does however seem appropriate to offer amnesia for painful or distressing procedures of short duration.

Delirium is quite common in the ICU resulting in increased length of stay and increased healthcare costs. Delirium is most noticeable when patients are unruly and aggressive, however, hypoactive delirium is much more common. Antipsychotics such as haloperidol can be effective with aggressive delirium but can exacerbate hypoactive delirium. Delirium can be the result of disturbed sleep-wake cycles, medications, infection, and withdrawal or encephalopathy.[20]

Analgesia

Pain is a common experience for almost all ICU patients. The need for analgesia is due to numerous factors including surgery, trauma, chronic pain, endotracheal tube irritation, procedures, and ICU related immobility. Failure to recognize pain can lead to agitation and inappropriate administration of sedatives. Consensus opinion recommends an aggressive strategy to managing pain[21] however; discerning pain is difficult in this critically ill patient population.

The physiologic response to pain can be increased endogenous catecholamines, increased metabolism, myocardial ischemia, anxiety, sleep deprivation, and delirium. Adequate analgesia can ameliorate these consequences. The assessment of pain can be challenging in patients supported with ECLS. It is typical that these patients will be heavily sedated during the early stage of their ECLS course. In addition these patients have commonly been in an ICU setting on mechanical ventilators and sedation for days to weeks prior to ECLS support. Neurologic assessment is difficult because commu-

nication with the patient is hindered. Modifying sedation strategies can be complicated by withdrawal. Pain scales and scoring systems can be useful tools when trying to quantify pain as an objective strategy to offer analgesics and sedatives; however, these scales are more practical and reliable when the patient is aware and can communicate. This is not always the case with the ECLS patient.

The ECLS patient is anticoagulated, most commonly with heparin. Anticoagulation limits the avenues of analgesia to enteral, intravenous, or transdermal delivery. Most commonly, intravenous analgesia is the option of choice because of the variable absorption of the enteral and transdermal routes. Regional techniques of analgesia are hindered by the unacceptable risk related to the anticoagulated patient. This is also the case for subcutaneous and intramuscular injections of analgesics and sedation.

Continuous infusions are most typical, however; recent critical care literature questions the validity of this approach. Continuous opioid infusions have been associated with significant bioaccumulation and subsequent delayed awakening and prolonged ICU length of stay. The theoretical benefit of continuous intravenous infusions is that there are fewer fluctuations in serum drug concentrations, thus limiting under- or overdosing.[22] Remembering the altered pharmacokinetics and pharmacodynamics related to ECLS, analgesic dosing and management is challenging.

Opiate withdrawal needs to be appreciated. The signs and symptoms are vague and nonspecific, often suggesting other causes for physiologic stress: pupillary dilation, sweating, tachycardia, hypertension, fever, tachypnea, nausea, vomiting, muscle aches, insomnia, and restlessness.[20]

Sedation

Sedation Strategies in ECLS

Sedation strategies for ECLS practices are local and program specific. Programs have been surveyed to understand practice patterns.[23,24] One survey asked the respondents to provide reasons for sedation. Most common responses were: decrease anxiety, decrease pain, induce amnesia, facilitate synchronous breathing with the ventilator, prevent patients from removing lines, to decreased oxygen consumption and CO_2 production, manage withdrawal, staff wishes, parent wishes, and other. The medications most commonly delivered were: morphine, midazolam, propofol, and fentanyl.

These surveys suggest that analgesia and sedation is offered to critically ill patients on ECLS in a similar fashion and with a similar rationale as for other critically ill patients.[20,22]

Assessing Level of Sedation

Adequacy of sedation is difficult to assess in critically ill patients supported with or without ECLS. Several assessment scales are in use and these are appropriate for any ICU patient including ECLS patients. Scales are helpful guides but adequacy of sedation remains a subjective bedside skill. It is important to recognize that the ECLS patient should be treated in a similar fashion to the ICU patient. Adequacy of sedation assessment should be part of the daily evaluation. Daily sedation "holidays" and spontaneous breathing trials need to remain part of the critical care strategy for ECLS patients.[20,22]

Drugs used for Sedation

1. Opiates

Opioid agonists exert activity against central and peripheral receptors. The clinically important receptors are the mu and kappa receptors. There are two mu receptor subtypes. The mu-1 subtype is responsible for analgesia. Mu-2 subtype receptors mediate nausea, vomiting, constipation, euphoria, and respiratory depression. The kappa receptors are responsible for the sedation effects and miosis.[20,22]

a. Pharmacodynamics:

i. Central Nervous System

Primary effect is analgesia as mediated via the mu and kappa receptors. There is mild to moderate anxiolysis.[20,22]

ii. Cardiovascular System

Opiates will have little effect on the euvolemic patient. However, in patients sustaining blood pressure via the hyperactive sympathetics, hypotension can result with opioids. This hypotensive response can be exaggerated when benzodiazepines are also being given. This synergy is not understood. Meperidine, with a structure similar to atropine, can cause tachycardia. The other opioids will typically decrease heart rate as a consequence of decreasing sympathetic activity. Morphine and Meperidine may cause histamine release. Remifentanil can cause bradycardia and hypotension.[20,22]

iii. Respiratory System

Opiates cause a dose related centrally mediated respiratory depression. Respiratory depression is mu-2 receptor mediated in the medulla.

Typically there is decreased respiratory rate with preserved tidal volumes. The response to increased CO_2 is ameliorated and the ventilatory response to hypoxia is obliterated.[20]

iv. Other

Meperidine can blunt postoperative shivering. Nausea, vomiting, and decreased gastrointestinal motility are side effects of the opiates. Other effects can be itching and urinary retention.[20,22]

b. Drugs

i. Fentanyl

Fentanyl is a highly lipophilic synthetic opioid. It has a rapid onset of action (1-3 minutes) and short duration of activity. Fentanyl can be given as bolus or continuous infusion. Fentanyl redistributes into peripheral tissues and will accumulate if used for extended periods. Fentanyl has little effect on the cardiovascular system. Fentanyl will be absorbed by silicone membrane oxygenators.[16,20,22]

ii. Morphine

Morphine is a naturally occurring opioid. Intravenous morphine has a slow onset of action (5-10 minutes) as a consequence of its low lipid solubility. Morphine will also have a long duration of action (up to 7 hours) and is effective in bolus administration. The majority of morphine is metabolized in the liver to morpine-6-glucuronide and morphine-3-glucuronide. Morphine-6-glucuronide has analgesic activity and will accumulate in the setting of renal impairment. Morphine can cause pronounced histamine release, which can cause vasodilation and hypotension.[20,22]

iii. Meperidine

Meperidine is a weak mu agonist. Meperidine undergoes hepatic metabolism and renal elimination. The metabolite normeperidine is a CNS stimulant and can precipitate seizures in the setting of renal failure and/or prolonged use. It is contraindicated in patients receiving monoamine oxidase inhibitors. It has little advantage over other opioids and is not commonly used in the ICU.[20,22]

iv. Hydromorphone

Hydromorphone is a semisynthetic mu-agonist with a similar pharmacokinetic profile as morphine but is approximately ten times more potent. Hydromorphone can be used in hemodynamically unstable patients. It does not cause a histamine release. Hydromorphone undergoes glucuronidation into inactive metabolites and is considered the drug of choice in renal insufficiency.[22]

2. *Benzodiazepines*

a. Pharmacodynamics

Benzodiazepines are the most commonly used sedatives in the ICU and with ECLS patients. They exert their effect by binding the gamma-aminobutyric acid (GABA) receptor complex. Benzodiazepines induce amnesia, respiratory depression and can be opioid sparing.[20,22] Three drugs in this class are commonly used in the ICU: diazepam, midazolam, and lorazepam. Midazolam is most commonly used in ECLS patients.[16,22] Benzodiazepines are absorbed by PVC tubing and membranes used in ECLS circuits.

i. Central Nervous System

Benzodiazepines cause dose dependent suppression of awareness. They induce amnesia. A paradoxical state of agitation can occur, most commonly in the geriatric patient. Benzodiazepines have anticonvulsive effects.

ii. Cardiovascular System

Benzodiazepines have little effect on the hemodynamics of a euvolemic patient.

iii. Respiratory System

Benzodiazepines cause a dose dependent centrally mediated respiratory depression that is not as pronounced as that caused by opioids. Benzodiazepines can obliterate the ventilatory response to hypoxia. Benzodiazepines will cause decreased tidal volume with increased respiratory rate.[20]

b. Drugs

i. Midazolam

Midazolam has a rapid onset of action (0.5-5 minutes) with short duration of effect. Elimination is via hepatic metabolism to hydroxylated metabolites, which are conjugated and excreted in the urine. The active metabolite, alpha-hydroxymidazolam accumulates in renal failure. Midazolam will accumulate in peripheral tissues during continuous intravenous infusions. Obese patients and elderly patients with impaired hepatic and renal function may be prone to prolonged effects.[20,22] Midazolam is the most commonly used benzodiazepine in ECLS patients.[16]

ii. Lorazepam

Lorazepam has slower onset of action than midazolam (~5 minutes). It has lower lipid solubility and increased time to cross the blood brain barrier. Duration of action is longer. There is less accumulation in the periphery.[20]

iii. Diazepam

Diazepam has an onset of action and duration between that of midazolam and lorazepam. Diazepam is rarely given as continuous infusion. Elimination is via hepatic metabolism and is prolonged in liver disease and in the elderly.

3. Propofol

Propofol is a rapid acting anesthetic with quick onset (1-5 minutes) and short duration. It is highly lipid soluble and quickly crosses the blood brain barrier. Propofol is commonly used in the ICU as a continuous infusion. The drug is metabolized mainly in the liver to inactive metabolites, which are excreted by the kidneys. The side effect profile is limited.

Propofol infusion syndrome (PRIS) is rare but manifests as fever, myocardial failure, acidosis, and rhabdomyolysis in the presence of lipemic plasma.[25] Many of these symptoms will be masked while on ECLS, so care should be taken to look for this complex. Following triglycerides and looking for evidence of rhabdomyolysis is prudent. Pancreatitis can also be a consequence of prolonged, high dose propofol infusions[22,25].

a. Pharmacodynamics

i. Central Nervous System

Propofol is a dose dependent hypnotic. It is a potent amnestic and anxiolytic. Propofol does not offer analgesia.

ii. Cardiovascular System

Propofol can cause significant hypotension in the hypovolemic patient. This is mainly due to decreased preload as a consequence of vasodilation of venous capacitance vessels. Propofol is a mild myocardial depressant. Care must be taken when using this drug in patients with marginal cardiac function. The myocardial oxygen consumption is decreased and the myocardial oxygen supply-demand ratio is conserved. This allows propofol to be used in the setting of ischemic heart disease with depressed function.

iii. Respiratory System

The response to CO_2 accumulation is blunted and apnea may occur. There is typically increased respiratory rate with decreased tidal volumes.

iv. Other

Propofol is delivered in via intralipid carrier. Hypertriglyceridemia can result and is an indication to discontinue use. It is necessary to adjust caloric intake, considering the lipid calories related to propofol use.

4. *Haloperidol*

Haloperidol is antipsychotic butyrophenone commonly used as sedation. It appears to antagonize dopamine, especially in the basal ganglia. Haloperidol induces a state of tranquility. Haloperidol can be given orally, intramuscularly and as intravenous bolus and infusions. In the ICU setting, and for patients on ECLS, it is usually given intravenously. Intramuscular is not appropriate in an anticoagulated patient on ECLS.

a. Pharmacodynamics

i. Central Nervous System

Haloperidol produces CNS depression resulting in a calm and detached patient. Haloperidol is often used to help control agitated and hyperactive patients in the ICU. There is no analgesic effect; however, it does appear to potentiate opioids. Haloperidol is often the drug of choice for patients with agitation refractory to other medications.[20,22]

ii. Cardiovascular System

Haloperidol will cause mild hypotension secondary to alpha-1-blocking effects. Haloperidol can prolong the QT interval and has been reported to result in torsade de pointes.

iii. Respiratory System

Haloperidol does not appear to cause direct respiratory depression.

iv. Other

Extrapyramidal effects can occasionally be a consequence of haloperidol use. This is more common with oral haloperidol than with the intravenous form. Diphenhydramine is the treatment. More concerning is neuroleptic malignant syndrome, which can be life threatening. Symptoms are fever, muscle rigidity and mental status changes. Bromocriptine, dantrolene and pancuronium have all been used successfully to reverse this syndrome.[20]

5. *Dexmedetomidine*

Dexmedetomidine is a centrally acting alpha-2-agonist. It promotes anxiolysis and sedation without respiratory depression. Patients will remain sedated if undisturbed but will arouse easily when disturbed. This facilitates frequent neurologic exams. Dexmedetomidine can be safely used in extubated patients.[22,25,26] A recent randomized control trial looked at dexmedetomidine and midazolam in an adult ICU. There was no difference between dexmedetomidine and midazolam in time at targeted sedation level in mechanically ventilated ICU patients. At comparable sedation levels, dexmedetomidine-treated patients spent less time on the ventilator, experienced less delirium, and developed less tachycardia and hypertension. The most notable adverse effect of dexmedetomidine was bradycardia.[26,27]

a. Pharmacodynamics

i. Central Nervous System

Centrally acting alpha-2-agonist acting in the locus ceruleus and the spinal cord. The result is anxiolysis, analgesia, and attenuation of the stress response.

ii. Cardiovascular System

Bradycardia and hypotension can result. It has been reported to lead to complete heart block.[25]

iii. Respiratory System

No significant respiratory depression.

Neuromuscular Blockade

The most common reason to use neuromuscular blockade in the ICU is for respiratory failure refractory to mechanical ventilation. Use has diminished over that last 20 years because of related complications. When neuromuscular blockade is used, it is mandatory to offer adequate sedation. In the setting of ECLS, neuromuscular blockade is commonly used during cannulation, however; it is usually not necessary once ECLS support has been initiated.

Nondepolarizing agents are used in the ICU when necessary. These mediations competitively inhibit the acetylcholine receptors without activating it. Succinylcholine is the only depolarizing neuromuscular blocking agent. It is used to facilitate endotracheal intubation but is not used as a continuous infusion in the ICU.

1. Drugs

a. Pancuronium

Pancuronium has a long half-life with duration of action for 60-90 minutes after a single dose. It increases the heart rate, has active metabolites, and is renally cleared. These characteristics limit its use in the ICU.

b. Vecuronium

Vecuronium has a shorter half-life than Pancuronium, lasting for about 30 minutes after a single dose. Half the drug is cleared via the liver and a third by the kidneys. There are active metabolites, which can lead to prolonged effect.

c. Rocuronium

Rocuronium has a rapid onset of action. It is practical for endotracheal intubation when Succinylcholine is contraindicated (burns, renal failure, upper motor neuron lesions). The metabolites have minimal neuromuscular blocking effects.

d. Cisatracurium

Cisatricurium is an isomer of atracurium. It has a rapid onset of action and lasts for 25-30 minutes. The drug is inactivated in the plasma by ester hydrolysis and Hofmann elimination. Because of its short half-life, it must be administered as a continuous infusion. This is the most frequently used neuromuscular blocking agent in the ICU.

2. *Monitoring Level of Neuromuscular Blockade*

The depth of neuromuscular blockade is monitored with peripheral nerve stimulators. The stimulator delivers four sequential stimuli and adequate neuromuscular blockade is achieved if 2-3 pulses result in muscular twitch.[25]

3. *Complications of Neuromuscular Blockade*

Prolonged weakness after neuromuscular blockade is the most concerning complication. Prolonged recovery is defined by an increase in time to recovery that is 50% to 100% longer than the blockade was used. There can also be a rare syndrome with acute paresis and myonecrosis. Concerns over complications of neuromuscular blockade have led to a dramatic decrease in their use in the ICU. These complications can be more prevalent in the setting of concomitant corticosteroid use.[28]

Delirium

Delirium is an independent risk factor for mortality in ICU patients.[29] The hyperactive, agitated form is more easily recognized; however, the hypoactive and quiet form is more common. The hallmark characteristic of delirium, which differentiates it from chronic states like dementia, is the acuteness of onset in a period of days to weeks.[25] Delirium can be defined by the presence of four clinical features: 1) acuteness of onset; 2) fluctuating course; 3) inattention; 4) disorganized cognition.[31,32]

Delirium is thought to be an imbalance in neurotransmitters that modulate cognitive function, behavior and mood.[22] Causal factors might be reduction in cerebral metabolism, in-

fection, hypoxia, withdrawal, benzodiazepines, and narcotics.

The ECLS patient is at risk for delirium as are all ICU patients. Delirium assessment tools, like the Confusion Assessment Method for the ICU (CAM-ICU) should be employed. Daily sedation liberation and spontaneous breathing trials should also be used for the ECLS patient. The ECLS circuitry and technology can be a distraction from offering expected and proven ICU care that should be directed at liberating patients from sedation with efforts to mobilize.

Temperature Control

Introduction and Clinical Criteria for Therapeutic Hypothermia

Therapeutic hypothermia for the prevention of ischemic brain injury was first introduced in the 1950s with its use during cardiac surgery.[33,34] Since that time, mild hypothermia (32-34^0 C) has been used for many neurologic conditions, which include traumatic brain injury, stroke, and anoxic brain injury after cardiac arrest.[35,36] In 2003, the International Liaison Committee on Resuscitation published recommendations for therapeutic hypothermia after two large randomized controlled trials (performed in Europe and Australia) for therapeutic hypothermia demonstrated efficacy in unconscious adults who suffered out-of-hospital cardiac arrest from shockable arrhythmias. Recommendations extended to consideration for other patients as well[37,38] and in 2005 this led to the American Heart Association and European Resuscitation Council including therapeutic hypothermia in their advanced life support guidelines. Neonatal trials have also demonstrated improved outcome using therapeutic hypothermia for the neonate who has suffered perinatal hypoxic ischemic neurologic injury; the hypothermia is achieved with either whole body cooling or cool cap cooling techniques and is now a recommended therapy in neonatal clinical care.[39,40] In response to these results, the pediatric community is presently undergoing a National Institutes of Health funded, multicenter randomized controlled trial in North America; Therapeutic Hypothermia After Pediatric Cardiac Arrest (THAPCA).[41] The results are anticipated to be similar to those found in both the adult and neonatal populations.

The precise mechanisms of how induced hypothermia is neuroprotective is not entirely understood, and it is likely that several different properties of hypothermia act both alone and in concert with other physiological mechanisms to affect this neuroprotection. What is known is that there is a cascade of destructive processes that unfold in the injured brain within minutes to hours post injury leading to post resuscitation cerebral disease as well as reperfusion injury.[33] It is also well understood that the development of fever independently results in adverse outcomes in patients with neurologic injury. This has therefore led to the understanding that temperature control and manipulation are important aspects of neuro intensive care and as such utilization of hypothermia aids in the reduction of metabolic rate and cerebral oxygen demand, which in turn can decrease intracranial pressure and cerebral edema.[42,43] The relevance of this therapy to the ECLS patient is para-

mount, as the majority of ECLS patients have the potential for suffering a neurologic injury, or have already suffered a neurologic injury prior to the initiation of ECLS. Therefore this therapeutic modality must be understood and potentially implemented in those patients who may benefit from it.

Definitions

It is important to understand the various definitions and terminology used in the field of therapeutic temperature manipulation.[33] Table 12-1 shows all of the definitions to be aware of with the most important ones for the purposes of this chapter being *controlled normothermia*, *induced hypothermia*, and *therapeutic hypothermia*.

1. *Controlled Normothermia* is a regular practice in neuro intensive care and is part of regular ECLS patient care and management. It means reducing or increasing body temperature within a normal range (36.0-37.5 ^{0}C) while controlling the side-effects that may result, such as shivering.

2. *Induced Normothermia* is the intentional reduction of the core body temperature to below 36.0 ^{0}C.

Table 12-1. Definitions for Temperature Control, Manipulation and Range.

Temperature Control and Manipulation	Definition
Hypothermia	Core Body Temperature of <36 ^{0}C
Induced Hypothermia	Deliberate reduction of core body temperature to <36 ^{0}C
Therapeutic Hypothermia	Maintenance of induced hypothermia
Controlled Normothermia	Reducing fever/temperature to maintain normal core body temperature of 36 ^{0}C-37.5 ^{0}C
Accidental Hypothermia	Reduction of core body temperature to <36 ^{0}C from accidental cold exposure, i.e. drowning, mountaineering, etc.

Temperature Range	Definition
Mild Therapeutic Hypothermia	Maintenance of hypothermia between 34 ^{0}C-35.9 ^{0}C
Moderate Therapeutic Hypothermia	Maintenance of hypothermia between 32 ^{0}C-33.9 ^{0}C
Moderate/Deep Therapeutic Hypothermia	Maintenance of hypothermia between 30.0 ^{0}C-31.9 ^{0}C
Deep Therapeutic Hypothermia	Maintenance of hypothermia <30 ^{0}C

3. *Therapeutic Hypothermia* is the maintenance of induced hypothermia while controlling any deleterious effects including shivering, electrolyte imbalance, and hemodynamic instability.

In addition to understanding the above definitions, it must also be understood that accidental hypothermia and its effects are not the same as therapeutic hypothermia management and care since the physiologic responses between the two are quite different as is their management.

Induction of Hypothermia

Induction of hypothermia results in the body's counter-regulatory responses attempting to decrease the heat loss and prevent the hypothermia. As core temperature drops to below 36.5 ^{0}C, vasoconstriction of cutaneous vasculature occurs. In addition shivering begins once the temperature drops to 1^{0}C below the vasoconstriction threshold to around 35.5 ^{0}C. Shivering results in an increased rate of metabolism and oxygen consumption along with an increased work of breathing, increased heart rate, and stress-like response.[44-47] In the awake patient these responses increase O$_2$ consumption by 40-100%, which is of course undesirable in the neurologically injured patient. With the intentional induction of hypothermia, these counter regulatory physiologic responses must be controlled. Effective management is via aggressive sedation of the patient to counteract shivering and the associated hemodynamic responses (see Table 12-2 for list of frequently used medications for the control of shivering).[33,34] With control of the counter-regulatory responses, induced hypothermia actually results in a slowing of the heart rate.

There are a variety of devices and methods for induction of hypothermia, but for the purpose of this chapter, temperature manipulation during ECLS is achieved by adjustment of the heat exchanger, the mechanics, and details of which are well described in Chapter 8. What is important to note is that temperature manipulation is an important vital sign in ECLS management one that requires hourly recording and at times frequent manipulation. The surface area of the ECLS circuit results in significant heat loss from the patient and therefore all ECLS patients require continuous heating of the circuit to maintain normal body temperature.

Table 12-2. Medications Frequently Used for Control of Shivering

Drug	Effect on Shivering
Magnesium	Muscle relaxation; Prevention of rewarming Mg depletion
Propofol	Brief-acting anesthetic, quick on and off. Concern for hypotension
Benzodiazepines	Amnestic, muscle relaxation. Some sedative qualities. Less hypotension
Opiates	Short acting: Fentanyl, effective but can develop tolerance quickly. Long acting: Morphine both analgesia and sedation
Dexmedetomidine	Moderately effective in conjunction with other therapies. Bradycardia and hypotension can occur
Clonidine	Moderately effective, similar effects to Dexmedetomidine
Meperidine	Rapidly effective with rigor abating effect. Good sedative qualities
Muscle Relaxants	Complete abating of shivering with no sedative qualities

Physiologic Responses to Hypothermia and Their Management

1. Hemodynamic Effects

The cardiovascular effects of frequent occurrence are: a mild increase in blood pressure and central venous pressure due to peripheral vasoconstriction; a slight increase in mixed venous saturation due to a decrease in metabolic rate; and an associated decrease in heart rate (bradycardia) with a cardiac output that is less or equal to the decrease in metabolic rate. Hypotension can also occur although this is less frequent. It must be anticipated however, and is related to an associated cold diuresis, which occurs with induced hypothermia and can be even more prevalent in the traumatic brain injured patient as they may have also received osmotic diuretics to control ICP. Bradycardia has already been mentioned but in addition to this common arrhythmia the PR interval and QT interval can both lengthen during hypothermia and once the temperature drops below 30 °C between 28-30 °C, other arrhythmias can occur and usually start with atrial type but can progress to ventricular fibrillation.[48-50]

2. Electrolyte Disorders

Electrolyte abnormalities are frequent during induced therapeutic hypothermia. It is important to maintain K, Mg, P, and Ca at high normal levels as their loss can be significant. It is also important to closely monitor them upon rewarming, as they can then rise above normal levels and most specifically this has been seen with K.[50-51]

3. Coagulation Deregulation

It is well known that platelet functionality is compromised during hypothermia and in conjunction with a decrease in platelet number.

This could present a risk for hemorrhage in patients undergoing therapeutic hypothermia. In addition the transformation of the zymogens of the coagulation cascade to active factors is slowed and thus this can further affect normal hemostasis. During therapeutic hypothermia, bleeding is not frequently seen but the risks for bleeding must be acknowledged. In the ECLS patient undergoing therapeutic hypothermia, the risk is enhanced and more concerning, thus meticulous monitoring is necessary to prevent any catastrophic events. With this deregulation of normal hemostasis, catheter associated thrombosis can increase, occurring within both the venous and arterial systems.[52-55] Daily surveillance of line insertion sites and the surrounding area must be carried out to detect early thrombus formation. Most often removal of the line results in spontaneous resolution of the thrombus. In the ECLS patient undergoing therapeutic hypothermia the risk is less, as they are systemically anticoagulated but should a thrombus occur, line removal would not occur until the patient has weaned from ECLS.

4. Suppression of Inflammatory Response

There is an intermediate frequency of infection, including catheter associated blood stream infections during therapeutic hypothermia. The normal inflammatory response is suppressed with cooling, particularly in the airways and in wounds. This is also a risk of ECLS itself such that the two therapies do place the patient at increased risk for infection and therefore acute awareness for infection and judicious use of antibiotics is recommended.[33]

5. Insulin Resistance

Hyperglycemia is frequently seen during induction and maintenance of therapeutic hypothermia. There is an induced insulin resistance such that often patients >3 years of age may not require glucose containing intravenous fluids.

Higher doses of insulin are required to control the hyperglycemia, but again upon rewarming this must be watched very closely so as to prevent hypoglycemia.[56-61]

6. Laboratory Value Derangements

There are frequent laboratory derangements seen during therapeutic hypothermia, but for most of these no interventions are needed. In addition some of the lab values can be influenced by temperature itself (such as pH, blood gas values, and coagulation parameters) so these must be temperature corrected to obtain the accurate value. Lab values that frequently become abnormal are: lactate, amylase, and liver enzymes which all go up; white blood cell count and platelets which are mildly decreased; hematocrit which may show a mild increase; and pH which usually shows a mild decrease.[33,62-64] For patients on ECLS these derangements can also be seen and close monitoring is all that is usually required.

7. Decreased Drug Clearance

Drug clearance and metabolism is usually slowed during therapeutic hypothermia and this is a frequent occurrence. It is most likely due to a slowing of liver enzymatic activity. Often infusion rates and bolus doses of drugs need to be increased to achieve the same effect. In combination with ECLS, which in itself is well known for decreasing drug effect due to increased volume of distribution, can result in a significant challenge most specifically with sedative/analgesia management.[34]

8. Skin Injury

The organ most vulnerable to adverse consequences from therapeutic hypothermia is the skin. The cooling process results in peripheral vasoconstriction and therefore compromise to the skin of the immobilized patient. These patients need to be placed on specialty beds that can continuously alter pressure points and in addition they will need frequent body position shifts to prevent pressure sores and skin breakdown. If shivering is profound and cannot be controlled by effective sedation management, the patient will need to undergo neuromuscular blockade and automatically will need to be placed on long term EEG monitoring.[33,34] The monitoring electrodes themselves cause prolonged pressure in one spot and this can result in skin breakdown as well. When these patients are on ECLS, moving their positions becomes more challenging, risky, and difficult, and the use of specialty beds is not common but may need to be considered for certain patients with a large body habitus.

9. Shivering

Shivering is the most frequent and common side effect to therapeutic hypothermia. As discussed above, it is the body's physiologic response/attempts to rewarm after vasoconstriction is ineffectual and the core body temperature drops below 35.5 °C.[44-47] Every attempt should be made to try and control the shivering with sedatives and muscle relaxant medications with the goal to avoid long term neuromuscular blockade if at all possible. The following medications are frequently used: magnesium sulfate infusion for muscle relaxation, quick acting opiates or meperidine for analgesia, benzodiazepines for anxiolysis, propofol for sedation in the adult population, and brief-acting neuromuscular block to gain control of the shivering.[33,34] It must be noted that animal studies have demonstrated that poorly sedated animals with neuromuscular blockade during therapeutic hypothermia had no beneficial effect from the therapy; whereas, those animals that were adequately sedated and neuromuscular blocked showed recovery and possible benefit from the therapeutic hypothermia.[65,66] Other medications that can be used to reduce shivering are clonidine and dexmedetomidine. Shivering will increase metabolic rate and increase ICP, therefore a clear strategy of how to control this response is imperative to the success of this therapy.

The benefits of neurologic recovery with induced and therapeutic hypothermia warrant its use in a select group of patients, which include traumatic brain injury and witnessed cardiorespiratory arrest as well as perinatal hypoxic ischemic injury at birth. In addition the results of the pediatric trial will likely add to the selection of patients who may benefit from this therapy. As with all aspects of care for ECLS patients, critical therapies and management must be incorporated into their care and therefore a clear understanding of induced and therapeutic hypothermia must also be known and utilized in the appropriate patient population.

Accidental Hypothermia and ECLS

A brief discussion must also be had regarding accidental hypothermia and the rewarming of these patients using ECLS. Early case reports in which cardiopulmonary bypass was used to resuscitate patients who had suffered severe hypothermia and cardiac arrest demonstrated success and as the use of ECLS began to expand, ECLS became a more manageable and desirable method by which to provide this resuscitation. This use of ECLS has been explored and studied in geographic areas that have a high incidence of accidental hypothermia.[67-69] The basics of this resuscitation are early implementation of ECLS with rapid warming. The shortest time from discovery of the victim to femoral arterial and venous cannulation will improve chances for survival with minimal sequelae. The initiation of VA ECLS allows for cardiovascular support while a stepwise, swift, controlled increase in the patient's body temperature can be carried out utilizing the circuit heat exchanger. Because the patient is on VA ECLS they can be fully supported as myocardial function returns

and ventricular arrhythmias requiring defibrillation +/- medicinal intervention occur which can jeopardize adequate perfusion in the patient not on ECLS.[67-69]

Successful outcomes/survival in accidental hypothermia are related to the rapidity with which these patients can be rescued, transported, and placed on ECLS for rewarming. In addition, studies showing successful outcome were in centers with organized rescue teams, a young patient population with minimal comorbidities, minimal to no preceding asphyxia, and deep hypothermia, <28 ^{0}C.[68] Aside from case reports, survival after deep hypothermia and prolonged cardiac arrest is rare without ECLS intervention.[70-72] The early implementation of ECLS and rewarming in select populations appears to be a valid therapeutic intervention that could result in a good outcome. It is therefore important, as a center that performs ECLS, to be aware of these protocols and when they should be implemented.

References

1. Brochard L, Mancebo J, Wysocki M, et al. Noninvasive ventilation for acute exacerbations of chronic obstructive pulmonary disease. N Engl J Med 1995; 333:817-22.
2. Kramer N, Meyer TJ, Meharg J, et al. Randomized, prospective trial of noninvasive positive pressure ventilation in acute respiratory failure. Am J Respir Crit Care Med 1995; 151:1799-806.
3. Ranieri VM, Suter PM, Tortorella C, et al. Effect of mechanical ventilation on inflammatory mediators in patients with acute respiratory distress syndrome: a randomized controlled trial. JAMA 1999; 282:54-61.
4. Brower RG, Matthay MA, Morris A, et al. N Engl J Med 2000; 342:1301-8.
5. Kress JP, Pohlman AS, O'Connor MF, et al. Daily interruption of sedative infusions in critically ill patients undergoing mechanical ventilation. N Engl J Med 2000; 342:1471-7.
6. Girard TD, Kress JP, Fuchs BD, et al. Efficacy and safety of a paired sedation and ventilator weaning protocol for mechanically ventilated patients in intensive care (Awakening and Breathing Controlled trial): a randomized controlled trial. Lancet 2008; 371:126-34.
7. Kress JP, Gehlbach B, Lacy M, et al. The long-term psychological effects of daily sedative interruption on critically ill patients. Am J Respir Crit Care Med 2003; 168:1457-61.
8. Schweickert WD, Pohlman MC, Pohlman AS, et al. Early physical and occupational therapy in mechanically ventilated, critically ill patients: a randomized controlled trial. Lancet 2009; 373:1874-82.
9. Herridge MS, Tansey CM, Matté A, et al. Functional disability 5 years after acute respiratory distress syndrome. N Engl J Med 2011; 364:1293-304.
10. Bhatt-Mehta V, Annich G. Sedative clearance during extracorporeal membrane oxygenation. Perfusion 2005; 20: 309-15.
11. H Mulla, G Lawson, C von Anrep, et al. In vitro evaluation of sedative drug losses during extracorporeal membrane oxygenation. Perfusion 2000 15: 21.
12. Burda G, Trittenwein G. Issues of Pharmacology in Pediatric Cardiac Extracorporeal Membrane Oxygenation with Special Reference to Analgesia and Sedation. Artificial Organs 1999;23:1015-19.
13. Ahsman MJ, Hanekamp M,Wildschut ED, et al. Population Pharmacokinetics of Midazolam and Its Metabolites during Venoarterial Extracorporeal Membrane Oxygenation in Neaonates. Clin Pharmacokinet 2010; 49(6): 407-19.
14. Mulla H, Lawson G, von Anrep C, et al . In vitro evaluation of sedative drug losses during extracorporeal membrane oxygenation. Perfusion 2000; 15: 21_/26.
15. Mulla H, Lawson G, Woodland ED, et al. Effects of extracorporeal membrane oxygenation circuits on drug disposition. Curr Ther Res 2000; 61: 838_/48.
16. Wildschut ED, Ahsman MJ, Allegaet K, et al. Determinants of drug absorption in different ECMO circuits. Intensive Care Med 2010; 36:2109-16.
17. Buck ML. Pharmacokinetic changes during extracorporeal membrane oxygenation. Clin Pharmacokinet 2003; 42: 403_/17.
18. Sessler CN, Varney K. Patient-focused sedation and analgesia in the ICU. Chest. 2008;133(2):552-565.
19. Kollef MH, Levy NT, Ahrens TS, et al. The use of continuous iv sedation is associated with prolongation of mechanical ventilation. Chest. 1998;114(2):541-548.
20. Gelbach B, Kress JP. Pain control, sedation, and the use of muscle relaxants. In: Principles of Critical Care; 3rd Edition. Editors Hall JB, Schmidt GA, Wood LDH. McGraw-Hill. 2005

21. Jacobi J, Fraser GL, Coursin DB, et al. Clinical practice guidelines for the sustained use of sedatives and analgesics in the critically ill adult. Crit Care Med 2002; 30:119.

22. McMillian WD, Taylor S, Lat I. Sedation, analgesia, and delirium in the critically ill patient. J Pharm Prac 2011; 24(1):27-34.

23. Frenckner B, Tibboel D. Sedation and management of pain on ECLS. In: ECMO Extracorporeal Cardiopulmonary support in critical care. 3rd edition. Editors Van Meurs K, Lally KP, Peek G, Zwischenberger JB. 2005. ELSO, Ann Arbor, Michigan

24. DeBerry BB, Lynch JE, Chernin JM, et al. A survey for pain and sedation medications in pediatric patients during extracorporeal membrane oxygenation. Perfusion 2005; 20:139-43.

25. Diedrich DA, Brown DR. Propofol infusion syndrome in the ICU. J Intensive Care Med 2011; 26:59-72.

26. Riker RR, Shehabi Y, Bokesch PM, et al. Dexmedetomidine vs midazolam for sedation of critically ill patients: a randomized trial. JAMA. 2009;301(5):489-499.

27. Pandharipande PP, Pun BT,Herr DL, et al. Effect of sedation with dexmedetomidine vs lorazepam on acute brain dysfunction in mechanically ventilated patients: the MENDS randomized controlled trial. JAMA. 2007;298(22):2644-2653.

28. Hansen-Flaschen JH, Brazinsky S, Basile C, Lanken PN. Use of sedating drugs and neuromuscular blocking agents in patients requiring mechanical ventilation for respiratory failure: A national survey. JAMA 1991; 66: 2870-

29. Ely EW, Shintani A, Truman B, et al. Delirium as a predictor of mortality in mechanically ventilated patients in the intensive care unit. JAMA. 2004;291(14):1753-1762.

30. Ely EW, Gautam S, Margolin R, et al. The impact of delirium in the intensive care unit on hospital length of stay. Intensive Care Med. 2001;27(12):1892-1900.

31. Bergeron N, Dubois MJ, Dumont M, et al. Intensive Care Delirium Screening Checklist: evaluation of a new screening tool. Intensive Care Med. 2001;27(5):859-864.

32. Ely EW, Inouye SK, Bernard GR, et al. Delirium in mechanically ventilated patients: validity and reliability of the confusion assessment method for the intensive care unit (CAM-ICU). JAMA. 2001;286(21):2703-2710.

33. Polderman KH. Induced hypothermia and fever control for prevention and treatment of neurological injuries. Lancet 2008; 371: 1955–1969.

34. Arpino PA, Greer DM. Practical Pharmacologic aspects of therapeutic hypothermia after cardiac arrest. Pharmacotherapy Volume 28, Number 1, 2008.

35. Vandam DV, Butnap TK. Hypothermia. N Engl J Med 1959;261:546–53.

36. Benson DW, Williams GR, Spencer FC, Yates AJ. The use of hypothermia after cardiac arrest. Anesth Analg 1958;38:423–8.

37. Nolan JP, Deakin CD, Soar J, et al: European Resuscitation Council Guidelines for Resuscitation 2005. Section 4. Adult Advanced Life Support. Resuscitation 2005; 67(Suppl 1):S39 –S86.

38. Kees H. Polderman KH, Ingeborg H. Therapeutic Hypothermia and Controlled normothermia in the intensive care unit: practical considerations, side effects, and cooling methods Crit Care Med 2009 Vol. 37, No. 3

39. Jacobs SE, Morley CJ, Inder TE, et al. For the infant cooling evaluation collaboration: whole-body hypothermia for term And near-term newborns with hypoxic-ischemic encephalopathy. Arch Pediatr Adolesc Med/ Vol 165 (No. 8), Aug 2011.

40. Tagin MA, Woolcott CG, Vincer MJ, et al. Hypothermia for neonatal hypoxic ischemic encephalopathy: An updated systematic review and meta-analysis. Arch Pediatr

Adolesc Med Published Online February 6, 2012

41. Http://www.thapca.org

42. Zeiner A, Holzer M, Sterz F, et al. Hyperthermia after cardiac arrest is associated with an unfavorable neurologic outcome. Arch Intern Med 2001; 161:2007–2012.

43. Diringer MN, Reaven NL, Funk SE, et al. Elevated body temperature independently contributes to increased length of stay in neurologic intensive care unit patients. Crit Care Med 2004; 32:1489 –1495.

44. Frank SM, Fleisher LA, Breslow MJ, et a.: Perioperative maintenance of normothermia reduces the incidence of morbid cardiac events. A randomized clinical trial. *JAMA* 1997; 277:1127–1134.

45. Frank SM, Beattie C, Christopherson R, et al. Unintentional hypothermia is associated with postoperative myocardial ischemia. The Perioperative Ischemia Randomized Anesthesia Trial Study Group. Anesthesiology 1993; 78:468 – 476.

46. Leslie K, Sessler DI. Perioperative hypothermia in the high-risk surgical patient. Best Pract Res Clin Anaesthesiol 2003; 17: 485– 498.

47. De Witte J, Sessler DI. Perioperative Shivering: Physiology and Pharmacology. Anesthesiology 2002; 96:467– 484.

48. Leduc J. Catecholamine production and release in exposure and acclimation to cold. Acta Physiol Scand 1961;183(Suppl): 1–101.

49. Frank SM, Higgins MS, Breslow MJ, et al. The catecholamine, cortisol, and hemodynamic responses to mild perioperative hypothermia: A Randomized Clinical Trial. Anesthesiology 1995;82:83–93.

50. Zeiner A, Sunder-Plassmann G, Sterz F, et al. The effect of mild therapeutic hypothermia on renal function after cardiopulmonary resuscitation in men. Resuscitation 2004;60:253–61.

51. Polderman KH, Peerdeman SM, Girbes AR. Hypophosphatemia and hypomagnesemia induced by cooling in patients with severe head injury. J Neurosurg 2001;94: 697–705.

52. Patt A, Mccroskey B, Moore E. Hypothermia-induced coagulopathies in trauma. Surg Clin North Am 1988;68:775–85.

53. Valeri CR, Macgregor H, Cassidy G, et al. Effects of temperature on bleeding time and clotting time in normal male and female volunteers. Crit Care Med 1995;23:698–704.

54. Michelson AD, Macgregor H, Barnard MR, at al. Hypothermia-induced reversible platelet dysfunction. Thromb Haemost 1994; 71:633– 640

55. Watts DD, Trask A, Soeken K, et al. Hypothermic Coagulopathy in Trauma: Effect of varying levels of hypothermia on enzyme speed, platelet function, and fibrinolytic activity. J Trauma 1998; 44:846 – 854.

56. Van Den Berghe G, Wouters P, Weekers F, et al. Intensive insulin therapy in the critically ill patients. N Engl J Med 2001; 345: 1359 –1367.

57. Van Den Berghe G, Wilmera,Hermans G, et al. Intensive insulin therapy in the medical ICU. N Engl J Med 2006; 354:449–461.

58. Lundgren J, Smith ML, Siesjo BK. Influence of moderate hypothermia on ischemic brain damage incurred under hyperglycemic conditions. Exp Brain Res 1991; 84: 91–101.

59. De Courten-Myeres GM, Kleinholz M, Wagner KR, et al. Normoglycemia (not hypoglycemia) optimizes outcome from middle cerebral artery occlusion. J Cereb Blood Flow Metab 1994; 14:227–236.

60. Capesse, Huntd, Malmbergk, etal. Stress hyperglycemia and prognosis of stroke in non-diabetic and diabetic patients: A Systematic Overview. Stroke 2001; 32: 2426 –2432

61. Polderman KH, Girbes ARJ. Intensive insulin therapy: Of harm and health, of hypes

and hypoglycemia. Crit Care Med 2006; 34: 246 –248.

62. Kern FH, Greeley WJ: Pro. pH-stat management of blood gases is not preferable to alpha-stat in patients undergoing brain cooling for cardiac surgery. J Cardiothorac Vasc Anesth 1995; 9:215–218.

63. Burrows FA: Con. pH-stat management of blood gases is preferable to alpha-stat in patients undergoing brain cooling for cardiac surgery. J Cardiothorac Vasc Anesth 1995; 9:219 –221.

64. Laussen PC. Optimal blood gas management during deep hypothermic paediatric cardiac surgery: Alpha-stat is easy, but pH-stat may be preferable. Paediatr Anaesth 2002; 12:199 –204.

65. Thoresen M, Satas S, Loberg EM, et al. Twenty-four hours of mild hypothermia in unsedated newborn pigs starting after a severe global hypoxic-ischemic insult is not neuroprotective. Pediatr Res 2001; 50: 405– 411.

66. Tooley JR, Satas S, Porter H, et al. Head cooling with mild systemic hypothermia in anesthetized piglets is neuroprotective. Ann Neurol 2003; 53:65–72.

67. Saxena P, Shehatha J, Boyt A, et al. Role of extracorporeal management of accidental deep hypothermia. Department of Cardiothoracic Surgery, University of Western Australia, Sir Charles Gairdner Hospital, Nedlands, WA 6009, Australia Heart, Lung and Circulation 2009;18:410–418

68. Walpoth BH, Walpoth-Aslan BN, Mattle HP, et al. Outcome Of Survivors Of Accidental Deep Hypothermia And Circulatory Arrest Treated With Extracorporeal Blood Warming. N Engl J Med 1997;337:1500-5

69. Farstada M, Andersenb KS, Kollera ME, et al. Rewarming from accidental hypothermia by extracorporeal circulation. A retrospective study. European Journal of Cardio-thoracic Surgery 20 (2001) 58-64.

70. Herity B, Daly L, Bourke GJ, Horgan JM. Hypothermia and mortality and morbidity: an epidemiological analysis. J Epidemiol Community Health 1991;45:19-23.

71. Hauty MG, Esrig BC, Hill JG, Long WB. Prognostic factors in severe accidental hypothermia: experience from the Mt. Hood tragedy. J Trauma 1987;27:1107-12.

72. Kornberger E, Mair P. Important aspects in the treatment of severe accidental hypothermia: the Innsbruck experience. J Neurosurg Anesthesiol 1996;8:83-7.

13

Renal Function and Renal Supportive Therapy during ECMO

Geoffrey M. Fleming MD, Patrick D. Brophy MD

Renal Function

One of the primary roles of the kidney when functioning normally is to provide fluid and electrolyte homeostasis in addition to toxin clearance. The kidney is also a vital metabolic and endocrine organ, producing antioxidants such as glutathione and hormones such as erythropoietin. Determining inadequate function of an organ requires identifying lapses in normal performance metrics, and currently renal dysfunction is based solely upon alterations of the detoxifying component of function with elevated serum creatinine. Emerging data support fluid regulation disorders in defining renal insufficiency, however most artificial renal support is currently provided by classical indications for dialytic therapy that include electrolyte disturbances, severe acidosis, and acute kidney injury.

Defining Kidney Dysfunction

As many as 30 definitions of renal failure exist in the literature, yet recent consensus definitions and guidelines are becoming more widespread. Traditionally, these definitions have been determined by an increase in serum creatinine or decline in urine output below absolute threshold values. For many studies in the literature these thresholds were determined by local expert opinion. The variety in definitions makes it difficult to compare incidence, therapeutics, and outcomes across multiple studies. The Acute Dialysis Quality Initiative (ADQI) group published consensus definition of acute kidney injury for adults[1] with a graded severity **R**isk **I**njury **F**ailure **L**oss and **E**nd stage kidney disease (RIFLE), which were modified for use in pediatric patients (pRIFLE).[2] Further refinement of these criteria were undertaken by the Acute Kidney Injury Network (AKIN) with an emphasis on the spectrum of renal disease and a preferential nomenclature of Acute Kidney Injury (AKI) encompassing the 'at risk' to 'overt failure' spectrum.[3] The AKIN definition of AKI is staged 1-3 similarly to the **R I F** stages of RIFLE criteria, based on absolute *changes* in serum creatinine. In both models, classification is based on a *change* in glomerular filtration rate (GFR) or urine output in the previous hours rather than absolute threshold values, thereby individualizing it to the patient.

Yet, despite newer staged consensus definitions of AKI using the AKIN, pRIFLE, and RIFLE criteria, definitions of renal failure rely upon serum creatinine measurements. Although this biomarker is readily available in most medical facilities, it is flawed in that it is known to overestimate GFR.[4-7] Additionally, in acute kidney injury the rise in serum creatinine used to define organ failure is delayed approximately

24-48 hours from the insult. Furthermore, neonatal definitions of AKI are hampered by the normally depressed GFR (~50ml/min/1.73m^2) in term newborns[8] who have maternal serum creatinine levels and thus the pRIFLE criteria have not been validated in this group. Although not an issue in chronic kidney disease and failure, these difficulties affect timing of definition and organ support in the acute setting. Consequently, current research is focused on appropriate biomarkers that would aid in the diagnosis of acute kidney injury, especially in the critically ill patient. Multiple markers are under study, some of which have performed well in select patient populations to date, and the reader is directed to comprehensive reviews of the subject.[9-11] In the future, the definition of acute kidney injury will likely be driven by a combination of markers of organ function, including biomarkers, as is the case for myocardial infarction and current troponin use.

To date, the Extracorporeal Life Support Organization (ELSO) Registry has indicated "renal complications" on the registry data collection form using serum creatinine and the need for dialytic therapies. Serum creatinine levels indicative of renal complications during ECMO have been defined as levels 1.5– 3 mg/dL or > 3 mg/dL, which clearly are inadequate thresholds for the smallest patients in whom normal creatinine levels are in the 0.3-1 mg/dl range. These factors become important when understanding the incidence and effect of AKI during ECMO in a variety of populations.

Acute Kidney Injury

In the intensive care units (ICUs) of countries where ECMO is available, secondary etiologies of AKI predominate in both adults and children. AKI in the pediatric ICU occurs commonly, with an incidence of 4.5-8.5% depending on the definition used.[12-17] A recent multicenter, multinational study of adult ICUs found an incidence of 5.7% among critically ill adults.[18] The leading cause of AKI in high-income countries is ischemia associated with natural disease and advanced therapies: cardiopulmonary bypass, acute tubular necrosis, and the systemic inflammatory response syndrome (SIRS) of severe sepsis. These data represent a shift in epidemiology away from primary renal disease presenting to the ICU, likely due to improved outpatient surveillance and an increase in the number of patients requiring advanced therapies, such as open heart surgery with chronic multisystem illness. The association of cardiopulmonary bypass (CPB) with AKI is important as some elements are similar to the ECMO environment, as well as the growing number of both adult and neonatal/pediatric patients that are supported with ECMO following CPB. Multiple mechanisms have been proposed for CPB-induced AKI, including ischemia/reperfusion, inflammation, oxidative stress, and altered nitric oxide biology.[19-21] As yet no therapeutic intervention has substantially reduced the development of AKI after CPB.

The current incidence of AKI during ECMO is discernable from two sources. First, there are a variety of single center studies of various patient groups on ECMO that offer the advantages of describing and controlling for variables which contribute to the development of AKI. Second, data published from the ELSO Registry have the advantages of reflecting international multicenter experience but are hampered by the registry's restrictive definition of AKI. For neonates supported with ECMO, the single center incidence of AKI has ranged from 22-71% depending on the indication for support, with a higher incidence of AKI in the post-CPB group.[22,23] Published data from the ELSO Registry for neonatal AKI ranged from 10-22% using creatinine data only, with no ELSO registry-based publications of pediatric and adult AKI incidence.[24-28] For non-neonatal pediatric patients, the incidence of AKI approximates 12-30% in single center studies[29-31] and 50% among adult patients.[32,33] With the inclusion of the need for renal supportive therapy (RST) in the definition of AKI, the incidence in these groups among single centers increases substantially.[22,29-32,34,35] The most recent ELSO International Summary[36] renal complication data are summarized in Table 13-1. It is evident that the incidence of AKI as reported by single center experiences is quite different from the cumulative ELSO data for some patient groups, likely reflecting varying definitions of AKI.

Fluid Overload

The critically ill pediatric population has been the most recent target of studies evaluating the effect of fluid overload (FO). This concept has been previously alluded to in studies of critically ill adult patients in whom a mortality benefit was noted with reversal of fluid overload in the first days of illness.[37,38] To date, numerous observational studies of pediatric patients have demonstrated that fluid overload is associated with higher mortality.[39-42] In these retrospective studies, FO > 10% is associated with higher mortality when controlling for severity of illness. Data from the Prospective Pediatric Continuous Renal Replacement Therapy (ppCRRT)

Registry Group[43] demonstrated that % fluid overload is associated with mortality and survival is improved if dry weight was attained during continuous renal replacement therapy (CRRT), as compared to those who did not attain dry weight (76% vs. 36% respectively).[44,45] This issue of fluid overload as a biomarker of critical illness associated with worse outcomes is now being followed in the adult literature with newfound attention.[46-48] To date, causality has not been established between FO and mortality, however the association is clear.

Data regarding FO during ECMO originated in the 1990s in the neonatal population. Roy et al. noted that neonatal respiratory failure patients supported with venovenous (VV) ECMO had more fluid accumulation and lower urine output when compared to the control group receiving conventional support.[49] Other investigators have reported an association of fluid overload during ECMO as well as with the duration and the need for ECMO support. Utilizing sodium bromide to measure extracellular fluid space (ECF) and deuterium oxide to measure total body water (TBW), neonates with respiratory failure on ECMO demonstrate an elevation in both TBW and ECF during the

Table 13-1. Cumulative Renal Complications data from the ELSO Registry defined as AKI and the need for renal supportive therapy (RST) divided by age group, support indication and category of complication.[36] SCr = Serum Creatinine

Age Group	Support Indication	AKI Category	Number	Incidence
Neonatal	Respiratory	SCr 1.5-3 mg/dL	1735	7.1%
		SCr > 3 mg/dL	334	1.4%
		RST	4700	19.3%
	Cardiac	SCr 1.5-3 mg/dL	584	13.4%
		SCr > 3 mg/dL	74	1.7%
		RST	1827	41.8%
Pediatric	Respiratory	SCr 1.5-3 mg/dL	464	9.8%
		SCr > 3 mg/dL	219	4.6%
		RST	1999	42.4%
	Cardiac	SCr 1.5-3 mg/dL	636	12.4%
		SCr > 3 mg/dL	248	4.8%
		RST	1963	38.3%
Adult	Respiratory	SCr 1.5-3 mg/dL	442	20.3%
		SCr > 3 mg/dL	288	13.2%
		RST	1119	51.3%
	Cardiac	SCr 1.5-3 mg/dL	449	31.8%
		SCr > 3 mg/dL	313	22.2%
		RST	693	49%

run. Return of these values to baseline correlates with improved lung function and separation from ECLS.[50] Additional data demonstrate the peak weight gain of infants on ECMO for respiratory support is 7% above birth weight and occurs in the first 25% of total ECMO duration. A gradual decline in weight back to 2% above birth weight occurs during the ECMO run through increased urinary flow and insensible losses through the artificial lung, ventilator circuit, and skin.[51] Finally, others reported that FO is common during neonatal ECMO with a mean increase of 20% in body weight above birth weight.[52]

There are no systematic data regarding fluid overload during ECMO in non-neonatal patients. Swaniker et al. report experience with pediatric patients in whom body weight increased during ECMO support with gains as much as 35% above dry weight for some.[53] Hoover et al. compared pediatric patients on ECMO without RST with a group on ECMO with RST. The group receiving continuous venovenous hemofiltration (CVVH) during the ECMO course demonstrated a significantly lower fluid balance among survivors when compared to those surviving with ECMO support alone, 25 ml/kg/day vs. 40 ml/kg/day respectively.[30] More recent retrospective data comparing survivors of either ECMO alone or ECMO+CVVH report the indication for RST was FO in 52% of the cases.[31] No such data are reported for adults on ECMO.

ECMO and Serum Electrolytes

Electrolyte disturbances are common in the critically ill population secondary to multiple factors.[54] Resuscitation with large volumes of fluids may alter electrolytes secondary to the fluid's composition, e.g., hyperchloremic metabolic acidosis (with or without hypernatremia) with vigorous saline resuscitation, or hyperkalemia with massive transfusion of packed red blood cells, particularly in small infants.[55-58] Hormonal milieu changes during critical illness may also occur, e.g., hyponatremia secondary to relative excess of antidiuretic hormone during illness in pediatric patients.[59,60] For those patients who require ECMO support, the circuit priming practices of an institution may affect serum electrolytes. Circuit priming without blood is performed with isotonic fluids and causes little to no electrolyte disturbances unless the prime is calcium free. Blood priming is done with packed red blood cells from the blood bank that are "reconstituted" to resemble whole blood. The combination of fluids and additives used varies from center to center, with the majority utilizing isotonic crystalloid, calcium, fresh frozen plasma, and a buffering agent in the form of tromethamine or sodium bicarbonate. Little published data exist regarding the usual electrolyte ranges seen in patients on ECMO, but the goal would be the same as for other critically ill patients. Single center neonatal data demonstrate that the mean sodium rises over the course of ECMO as compared to controls but remains in the normal range < 145 mEq/L.[49] Potassium levels remain fairly stable within the normal range, but total carbon dioxide rises over the course of ECMO as compared to controls, from 21 mg/dL to 31 mg/dL. This may be due to bicarbonate supplementation and generation of bicarbonate from acetate or citrate in TPN and blood products. Data from the ELSO registry published in 1994 describe the prevalence of electrolyte abnormalities from 1%-4%, with hypokalemia ($K^+ < 2.5$ mEq/L) occurring the most frequently, and hyponatremia (< 125 mEq/L) and hypercalcemia (>12 mg/dL) occurring the least frequently.[24]

Supporting Renal Function

Indications for RST

As presented in the introduction of the chapter, renal supportive therapy is meant to supplement the function of the kidney to maintain homeostasis. Among classical indications for RST, the detoxification function most often drives therapy; however, fluid management and nutritional support are gaining popularity as indications for RST. Recent survey results indicate that treating or preventing fluid overload accounted for 59% of the RST indications on ECMO, whereas AKI accounted only for 35%.[61] Of note, electrolyte disturbances and "other" accounted for only 6% of the total indications for RST on ECMO. Although these data are limited by the study design including the scope of inquiry, they do reflect current center-specific practices as reported by Program Directors or Program Coordinators of ECMO.

RST Basics: Nomenclature

Since the initial description of "vivi-diffusion" in 1913 by Dr. Abel[62] a flurry of nomenclature has appeared in the literature to describe renal supportive therapy. The list is long and includes peritoneal dialysis (PD), intermittent hemodialysis (IHD), sustained low- efficiency dialysis (SLED), extended daily dialysis (EDD), and continuous renal replacement therapy (CRRT). The continuous extracorporeal therapies (CRRT) are comprised of slow continuous ultrafiltration (SCUF), continuous venovenous hemofiltration (CVVH), continuous venovenous hemodialysis (CVVHD), or a combination of convective and diffusive therapies, continuous venovenous hemodiafiltration (CVVHDF). Early continuous therapies included continuous arteriovenous support and are all but abandoned today for the modern pump-driven venovenous systems. However, arteriovenous support may still be technically found on ECMO with a shunt from post-pump returning to the pre-pump circuit. The most important differences in the nomenclature of therapy exist in the physiology of the therapy reviewed below.

RST Basics: Physiology

RST employs two primary physiologies for solute and fluid movement with sequestration of blood on one side of a semipermeable membrane. Convective clearance is the most frequently used mode currently with RST during ECMO, with > 80% of centers reporting using SCUF or CVVH.[61] Convection (Hemofiltration or Ultrafiltration) utilizes a transmembrane pressure gradient that is increased as needed to "push" water through the membrane. This bulk flow of plasma water "drags" solute with it (convective mass transfer) in the formation of **ultrafiltrate**. In diffusive clearance (Dialysis), solute moves down its concentration gradient from areas of high concentration to low concentration. The solute must be of appropriate size and charge to pass through a semipermeable membrane. By passing fluid across the membrane countercurrent to blood flow, equilibration of plasma and **dialysate** solute concentrations occur. This process may remove or add solute to the plasma water space dependent upon the relative concentrations in dialysate and plasma. Water will also move along a gradient, in this case the osmolar or osmotic gradient, in effect "following" the solute.

Diffusive clearance is more effective at removal of small solutes, such as serum ions and urea, than for larger solutes. Both convection and diffusion provide nearly equivalent small solute removal, but larger molecular removal is superior with convective clearance. Convection demonstrates increased middle molecule (500 – 5000 Dalton) clearance, with vancomycin often quoted as the representative "middle molecule." Using convection to remove isotonic plasma water is considered slow continuous ultrafiltration (SCUF) and may lead to large volume shifts during therapy. SCUF has the potential to cause significant problems with electrolytes, particularly in neonatal or smaller pediatric patients. Since plasma water is removed during this process, attention must be paid to the intravenous fluids and nutrition administered to the patient. If these solutions are composed of hypotonic mixtures they can lead to significant and rapid electrolyte derangements (particularly hyponatremia) that can be fatal if not monitored closely. To offset the large fluid shifts of hemofiltration, convective therapies usually include a filter replacement fluid (FRF) that is administered into the patient to maintain near isovolemia. Fluid given is removed in equal quantities for isovolemic hemofiltration and over time the plasma composition will eventually resemble the FRF allowing for solute management. During hemofiltration the fluid out is often greater than the FRF in, so as to provide a slow, steady fluid removal for the patient. The provision of this therapy over SCUF affords a safer and controlled fluid removal.

Although these two models suggest very simple and predictable solute and fluid movement, the processes are in reality quite complex. Diffusion gradients change dependent upon blood flow rates, dialysate flow rates, and starting concentration gradients. Additionally, convection allows for larger solute to be pushed/pulled through the membrane with fluid transfer, conferring additional solute clearance properties. Finally, the combination of diffusion and convection across the membrane alter the properties of individual methods in a complex manner. The clearance delivered from either convection or diffusion can be calculated and is relative to blood flow rate and freedom of movement of the solute of interest across the membrane. Detailed discussion of these calculations is beyond the scope of this chapter and the reader is referred to a recent review for further reading.[63]

RST on ECMO

Connecting to the ECMO circuit

Regardless of the modality employed, blood must interface with the semipermeable membrane across which solute and fluid transfer will occur. Concerns for providing RST during critical illness often has centered on the hemodynamic stability of the patient with regards to blood flowing into the extracorporeal RST circuit. The addition of a RST circuit to the existing ECMO circuit should not affect hemodynamic instability with isovolemic therapy and the RST circuit may access blood flow through a variety of setups.

The simplest form of RST on ECMO is the inclusion of a modern hemodiafilter as a circuit in parallel off the main ECMO circuit. This often draws flow from the post-pump (arterial) limb of the ECMO circuit with return to the pre-pump (venous) limb (Figure 13-1). For most,

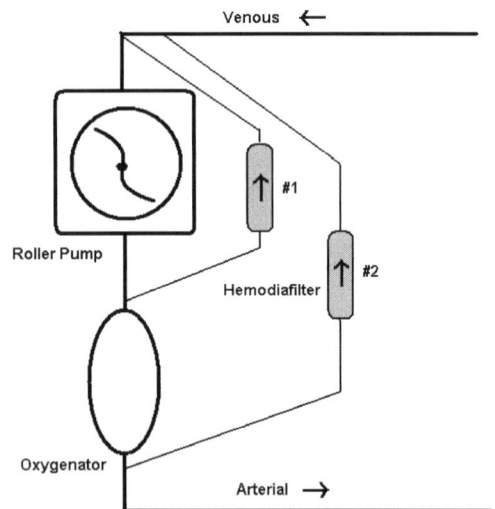

Figure 13-1. Schematic of parallel circuitry for RST on ECMO with a hemodiafilter as a shunt off the main circuit. Circuits # 1 and # 2 differ by pre-oxygenator vs. post-oxygenator source of blood. Arrows delineate direction of blood flow.

this hemodiafilter is used to provide convective clearance and generation of ultrafiltrate that can be quite large given the blood flow rates and circuit pressures on ECMO. Centers utilize two primary methods of regulating and measuring the flow of ultrafiltrate generated. A volume based approach utilizes standard intravenous infusion pumps connected to the effluent port of the hemodiafilter and fluid is removed from the system at the rate programmed into the IV pump. The "fluid source" for the IV pump is the ultrafiltrate portion of the hemodiafilter rather than the infusion bag for standard IV infusions.[30] Filter replacement fluids can be delivered into the ECMO circuit or into the patient directly to maintain euvolemia. If no specific FRF is utilized, the patient's TPN and other fluids become the FRF and can result in electrolyte disturbances if attention is not given to fluid tonicity (see SCUF above). Despite the seemingly ideal method for fluid control, IV infusion pumps have long been known to contain significant error. Jenkins et al. documented an error of up to 12.5% which was dependent upon inlet and outlet pressures with IV infusion pumps.[64] When used to control CVVH on ECMO, the error with IV infusion pumps were as great as 40%.[65] Weight-based control of ultrafiltration production utilizes scales for monitoring the total fluid produced, although "control" is a misnomer as the weight-based systems monitor rather than determine ultrafiltrate production. To reduce the flow of ultrafiltrate, hydrostatic pressure is increased within the ultrafiltrate compartment using clamps on the effluent port of the hemodiafilter or by placing the UF collection bag above the level of the hemodiafilter.[22,52] The next level of complexity of RST on ECMO utilizes a separate blood pump into the shunt circuitry to regulate blood flow through the hemodiafilter.[22,52] Although early descriptions of RST on ECMO utilize this method, it is rarely seen today. Instead, the nearly universal availability of pump regulated/driven RST machines for use in critically ill patients has

led to the substitution of these machines for the stand-alone pump in the hemodiafilter circuit. The benefits of the modern RST machine include accuracy and industry monitored precision in fluid management as well as additional alarm profiles to alert the bedside caregivers to changes within the circuit. Yet despite the feeling of security from using commercially available CRRT equipment, investigators are finding errors in hourly fluid control and measurement. (Personal communication of unpublished data, Matthew L Paden M.D., Children's Healthcare of Atlanta, Emory University, Atlanta, Georgia) The CRRT machine is connected primarily to the venous limb of the ECMO circuit in roller-pump setups (Figure 13-2) and post-pump in the case of centrifugal ECMO pumps where access pressures may affect CRRT machine function (depending on type used).[31,66] Any RST machine can theoretically be attached to an ECMO circuit and recent survey results report that a variety of manufacturers are represented.[61]

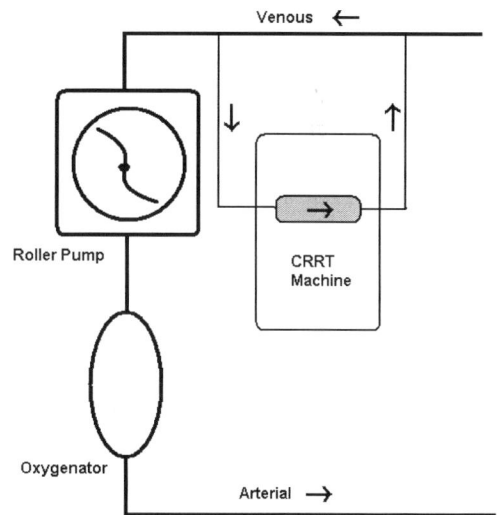

Figure 13-2. Schematic of connection of a separate pump driven machine for RST on ECMO with a roller pump. Connection sites may occur anywhere along the venous limb for roller pump ECMO circuits. Arrows delineate direction of blood flow.

No uniform method of providing RST on ECMO exists and many centers have local practices that are shaped by equipment and experience. For many centers the inclusion of a specific stopcock in the circuit or a smaller lumen resistance pigtail connection provides the necessary step for delivering RST on ECMO. Despite these differences, similar issues arise in the practical aspects of delivering RST on ECMO and are reviewed elsewhere.[67]

Effect of RST on Nutrition

Nutrition in the critically ill is likely as important or more important than many other therapies provided. Much work has been done, especially in the adult critically ill population, looking at the effects of nutrition on outcomes. Enteral nutrition has been shown to be protective in critically ill adults, likely due to reduced bacterial translocation and inflammatory responses.[68,69] The type of enteral nutrition has been studied, including immune modulating formulae that have been proposed as beneficial in the critically ill.[70,71] Enteral nutrition has been demonstrated to be safe in critically ill patients on ECMO in the neonatal and pediatric populations receiving either VV or VA ECMO.[72-74] Guidelines exist to guide enteral nutrition in adults with AKI on CRRT but have no pediatric counterpart.[75]

Guidelines for adult nutrition during AKI focus on the increased energy expenditure and caloric needs during this phase of illness. Specific attention is paid to nitrogen balance and adequate protein supplementation, especially enteral feeding with standard formulae during CRRT for AKI.[75] Although no study has looked specifically at enteral nutrition during CRRT for AKI in the pediatric population, researchers have looked at specific components of nutrition. The first important study made recommendations regarding protein supplementation during CRRT, suggesting > 2 g/kg/day be prescribed to compensate for losses through the hemodiafil-

ter.[76] Additionally, the authors examined specific amino acid losses and found glutamic acid, glutamine, cysteine, and arginine had sieving coefficients equal to urea, with the potential for substantial removal during therapy. Subsequent work through the ppCRRT registry found variable nutrition prescriptions despite the above data, with a substantial delay (5 days) to achieve > 2 g/kg/day protein prescription.[77] Despite this delay, no difference in protein prescription was seen relative to survival or the development of multiple organ dysfunction. The route of nutritional support was not documented in this study to gain insight in to enteral vs. parenteral nutrition. Additional single center data demonstrate a negative nitrogen balance in the first days of CRRT with nearly 20% of amino acid intake lost in the hemodiafilter.[78] In conjunction with amino acid losses, both selenium and folate losses were documented during CRRT. These losses have a potential but unknown effect on immune function and DNA synthesis during recovery from critical illness requiring CRRT. Although the authors comment that the predominant form of feeding was parenteral, they made no statements regarding the adequacy of either route and suggested it as an area for further study.

Outcomes

The presence of AKI and/or fluid overload is associated with reduced survival in the critically ill population in both children and adults, with numerous studies demonstrating this association.[12-14,16,18,79-83] Specific subgroups of patients are more affected than others as seen in postsurgical cardiac critical illness where the presence of AKI significantly increases the risk of mortality. This is true for both adult[80,81] and pediatric patients[84-86] after cardiopulmonary bypass and is important as these groups represent a growing population supported with ECMO. In studies of adult AKI the increased risk of mortality progresses stepwise with increased levels of AKI. Using the RIFLE criteria, the **R**isk,

Injury and Failure categories are associated with a continuous increasing risk of mortality in a variety of patient groups.[82,87] Although not as robustly demonstrated as in the adult population, the pRIFLE also has been associated with graded increasing risk of mortality in pediatric patients.[88] The association of fluid overload and mortality has been discussed in the previous section and its presence conveys increased risk of mortality in both children[39-42,44,45] and adults.[37,38,46-48]

The decreased survival associated with AKI in critical illness is also evident in the subgroup supported with ECMO. In the neonatal and pediatric population survival is reported to range 0-63% for those with AKI and/or RST during ECMO support, with a trend toward improved survival in the modern era.[22,24,29-31,35,89-93] The magnitude of this effect is dependent upon multiple variables including era of study, age group, subgroup of support indication, and single center vs. ELSO Registry derived data. Table 13-2 reports survival from the most recent ELSO Registry report and it is evident that survival with any form of AKI or RST is reduced as compared to the entire age group + support indication cohort. For most of the groups, the addition of RST to ECMO appeared to improve outcome as compared to AKI alone yet the ELSO registry does not adequately distinguish those on RST for FO vs. AKI to determine a causal relationship for the survival differences. In some single center studies those on ECMO with RST had a reduced survival as compared to those not requiring RST.[30,31,89] This phenomenon is seen in the wider critically ill population and is thought to be a marker of severity of illness rather than a sign that RST causes harm. Trials comparing RST in the critically ill have demonstrated an increased mortality risk with continuous therapies compared to intermittent therapies, although this is probably secondary to patient selection bias as sicker patients were supported with continuous therapies.[94-96] Although no trial has randomized critically ill patients to RST vs. no renal support, observational data from a recent pRIFLE study demonstrated that 66% patients with F level AKI who were not supported with RST died within 24 hours.[2] In fact, in more recent single center studies of patients receiving both RST, and ECMO support,[31] survival approximates critically ill

Table 13-2. Cumulative survival data from the ELSO Registry defined for renal complications during ECMO divided by age group, support indication and category of complication. Survival reflects data for the AKI category subgroup and total group survival reflects survival by support indication for the entire cohort.[36]

Age Group	Support Indication	AKI Category	AKI Survival	Cohort Survival
Neonatal	Respiratory	SCr 1.5-3 mg/dL	52%	75%
		SCr > 3 mg/dL	36%	
		RST	50%	
	Cardiac	SCr 1.5-3 mg/dL	22%	39%
		SCr > 3 mg/dL	22%	
		RST	22.6%	
Pediatric	Respiratory	SCr 1.5-3 mg/dL	31%	56%
		SCr > 3 mg/dL	27%	
		RST	38.8%	
	Cardiac	SCr 1.5-3 mg/dL	27.7%	47%
		SCr > 3 mg/dL	29%	
		RST	33.3%	
Adult	Respiratory	SCr 1.5-3 mg/dL	36%	53%
		SCr > 3 mg/dL	38%	
		RST	42.7%	
	Cardiac	SCr 1.5-3 mg/dL	31%	34%
		SCr > 3 mg/dL	25%	
		RST	23.5%	

patients requiring RST alone.[44] Significantly more study is required to determine the effect of AKI, FO and RST on ECMO outcomes for a variety of patient subgroups and will be driven by more detailed data collection of renal specific variables in this population.

The status of renal function after AKI during critical illness is another important outcome measure as it affects both cost and complexity of long-term medical care. In adults with AKI during critical illness, a large multicenter study of RST dose intensity demonstrated 15-18% of adults have complete recovery of renal function and 9% have partial recovery, with 15-16% discharged home free of dialysis.[97] A large European multicenter study found similar results with 12% requiring RST 6 months after AKI during critical illness.[98] To date, there are no similar results in pediatric patients reflecting multicenter renal outcomes after AKI. Single center experiences with RST during ECMO report near uniform recovery of renal function. Data from the University of Michigan from 1990-1999 report that 93% recovered renal function among survivors of ECMO with RST.[91] Paden et al. report 96% of ECMO+CVVH survivors at Children's Healthcare of Atlanta had renal recovery prior to discharge from 1997-2007, with non-recovery occurring in patients with primary (intrinsic) renal disease.[91] Outside of the United States, Cavagnaro et al. report their experience from Chile with an extraordinary survival rate of 83% overall and complete renal recovery in all six patients studied.[99] As yet, there are no renal recovery data recorded in the ELSO registry to address this question on a broader level.

Conclusions

AKI is common among critically ill patients, substantially affects mortality, and is a significant contributor to the multiple organ dysfunction syndrome in both children and adults. Newer consensus definitions of AKI will help future studies define the disease under study and allow for extrapolation of findings. However, current organ specific biomarkers for renal dysfunction lag substantially behind other disciplines such as troponin in cardiac dysfunction. Also emerging in the literature is the importance of fluid overload as a marker of renal dysfunction and is now a significant indication for RST during ECMO. Although the connection between fluid overload and outcomes is associative, there are emerging data that support resolving FO by extracorporeal means to improve outcomes.

These trends in the critically ill population are mirrored in the population on ECMO. To date we have insufficient data to answer some basic questions, such as the true incidence of AKI in the ECMO population. Yet both AKI and FO have been shown to affect outcomes in the cohort on ECMO, with the true effect likely underestimated due to the limited definition of AKI in the ELSO Registry at present. Using more renal specific data collection in the ELSO registry, investigators hope to answer basic questions such as incidence of AKI and FO during ECMO and their effect on outcomes. Subsequent work will then evaluate the impact of RST during ECMO on patient outcomes. Other important areas for further research include the best method of performing RST on ECMO, including site of connection and equipment to use, as well as the effect of mode (convection vs. diffusion) of RST on outcomes. Finally, the implementation of RST early in the course or ECMO may have a profound effect on prevention of FO, modulation of cytokines, and hence patient outcomes in both the short and long term.

References

1. Bellomo R, Ronco C, Kellum JA, Mehta RL, Palevsky P. Acute renal failure - definition, outcome measures, animal models, fluid therapy and information technology needs: the Second International Consensus Conference of the Acute Dialysis Quality Initiative (ADQI) Group. Crit Care. Aug 2004;8(4):R204-212.

2. Akcan-Arikan A, Zappitelli M, Loftis LL, Washburn KK, Jefferson LS, Goldstein SL. Modified RIFLE criteria in critically ill children with acute kidney injury. Kidney Int. May 2007;71(10):1028-1035.

3. Mehta RL, Kellum JA, Shah SV, et al. Acute Kidney Injury Network: report of an initiative to improve outcomes in acute kidney injury. Crit Care. 2007;11(2):R31.

4. Chantler C, Garnett ES, Parsons V, Veall N. Glomerular filtration rate measurement in man by the single injection methods using 51Cr-EDTA. Clin Sci. Aug 1969;37(1):169-180.

5. Moore AE, Park-Holohan SJ, Blake GM, Fogelman I. Conventional measurements of GFR using 51Cr-EDTA overestimate true renal clearance by 10 percent. Eur J Nucl Med Mol Imaging. Jan 2003;30(1):4-8.

6. Proulx NL, Akbari A, Garg AX, Rostom A, Jaffey J, Clark HD. Measured creatinine clearance from timed urine collections substantially overestimates glomerular filtration rate in patients with liver cirrhosis: a systematic review and individual patient meta-analysis. Nephrol Dial Transplant. Aug 2005;20(8):1617-1622.

7. Shemesh O, Golbetz H, Kriss JP, Myers BD. Limitations of creatinine as a filtration marker in glomerulopathic patients. Kidney Int. Nov 1985;28(5):830-838.

8. Arant BS, Jr. Postnatal development of renal function during the first year of life. Pediatr Nephrol. Jul 1987;1(3):308-313.

9. Devarajan P. The future of pediatric acute kidney injury management--biomarkers. Semin Nephrol. Sep 2008;28(5):493-498.

10. Edelstein CL. Biomarkers of acute kidney injury. Adv Chronic Kidney Dis. Jul 2008;15(3):222-234.

11. Trof RJ, Di Maggio F, Leemreis J, Groeneveld AB. Biomarkers of acute renal injury and renal failure. Shock. Sep 2006;26(3):245-253.

12. Bailey D, Phan V, Litalien C, et al. Risk factors of acute renal failure in critically ill children: A prospective descriptive epidemiological study. Pediatr Crit Care Med. Jan 2007;8(1):29-35.

13. Bunchman TE, McBryde KD, Mottes TE, Gardner JJ, Maxvold NJ, Brophy PD. Pediatric acute renal failure: outcome by modality and disease. Pediatr Nephrol. Dec 2001;16(12):1067-1071.

14. Chang JW, Tsai HL, Wang HH, Yang LY. Outcome and risk factors for mortality in children with acute renal failure. Clin Nephrol. Dec 2008;70(6):485-489.

15. Hui-Stickle S, Brewer ED, Goldstein SL. Pediatric ARF epidemiology at a tertiary care center from 1999 to 2001. Am J Kidney Dis. Jan 2005;45(1):96-101.

16. Moghal NE, Brocklebank JT, Meadow SR. A review of acute renal failure in children: incidence, etiology and outcome. Clin Nephrol. Feb 1998;49(2):91-95.

17. Williams DM, Sreedhar SS, Mickell JJ, Chan JC. Acute kidney failure: a pediatric experience over 20 years. Arch Pediatr Adolesc Med. Sep 2002;156(9):893-900.

18. Uchino S, Kellum JA, Bellomo R, et al. Acute renal failure in critically ill patients: a multinational, multicenter study. JAMA. Aug 17 2005;294(7):813-818.

19. Alonso de Vega JM, Diaz J, Serrano E, Carbonell LF. Oxidative stress in critically ill patients with systemic inflammatory response syndrome. Crit Care Med. Aug 2002;30(8):1782-1786.

20. Bellomo R, Auriemma S, Fabbri A, et al. The pathophysiology of cardiac surgery-associated acute kidney injury (CSA-AKI). Int J Artif Organs. Feb 2008;31(2):166-178.

21. Chatterjee PK. Novel pharmacological approaches to the treatment of renal ischemia-reperfusion injury: a comprehensive review. Naunyn Schmiedebergs Arch Pharmacol. Oct 2007;376(1-2):1-43.

22. Sell LL, Cullen ML, Whittlesey GC, Lerner GR, Klein MD. Experience with renal failure during extracorporeal membrane oxygenation: treatment with continuous hemofiltration. J Pediatr Surg. Jul 1987;22(7):600-602.

23. Smith AH, Hardison DC, Worden CR, Fleming GM, Taylor MB. Acute renal failure during extracorporeal support in the pediatric cardiac patient. ASAIO J. Jul-Aug 2009;55(4):412-416.

24. Zwischenberger JB, Nguyen TT, Upp JR, Jr., et al. Complications of neonatal extracorporeal membrane oxygenation. Collective experience from the Extracorporeal Life Support Organization. J Thorac Cardiovasc Surg. Mar 1994;107(3):838-848; discussion 848-839.

25. Haines NM, Rycus PT, Zwischenberger JB, Bartlett RH, Undar A. Extracorporeal Life Support Registry Report 2008: neonatal and pediatric cardiac cases. Asaio J. Jan-Feb 2009;55(1):111-116.

26. Meyer DM, Jessen ME. Results of extracorporeal membrane oxygenation in neonates with sepsis. The Extracorporeal Life Support Organization experience. J Thorac Cardiovasc Surg. Mar 1995;109(3):419-425; discussion 425-417.

27. Meyer DM, Jessen ME, Eberhart RC. Neonatal extracorporeal membrane oxygenation complicated by sepsis. Extracorporeal Life Support Organization. Ann Thorac Surg. Apr 1995;59(4):975-980.

28. Rajagopal SK, Almond CS, Laussen PC, Rycus PT, Wypij D, Thiagarajan RR. Extracorporeal membrane oxygenation for the support of infants, children, and young adults with acute myocarditis: a review of the Extracorporeal Life Support Organization registry. Crit Care Med. Feb 2010;38(2):382-387.

29. Zahraa JN, Moler FW, Annich GM, Maxvold NJ, Bartlett RH, Custer JR. Venovenous versus venoarterial extracorporeal life support for pediatric respiratory failure: are there differences in survival and acute complications? Crit Care Med. Feb 2000;28(2):521-525.

30. Hoover NG, Heard M, Reid C, et al. Enhanced fluid management with continuous venovenous hemofiltration in pediatric respiratory failure patients receiving extracorporeal membrane oxygenation support. Intensive Care Med. Dec 2008;34(12):2241-2247.

31. Paden ML, Warshaw BL, Heard ML, Fortenberry JD. Recovery of renal function and survival after continuous renal replacement therapy during extracorporeal membrane oxygenation. Pediatr Crit Care Med. May 6 2010.

32. Muehrcke DD, McCarthy PM, Stewart RW, et al. Extracorporeal membrane oxygenation for postcardiotomy cardiogenic shock. Ann Thorac Surg. Feb 1996;61(2):684-691.

33. Yap HJ, Chen YC, Fang JT, Huang CC. Combination of continuous renal replacement therapies (CRRT) and extracorporeal membrane oxygenation (ECMO) for advanced cardiac patients. Ren Fail. Mar 2003;25(2):183-193.

34. Maclaren G, Butt W, Best D, Donath S, Taylor A. Extracorporeal membrane oxygenation for refractory septic shock in children: one institution's experience. Pediatr Crit Care Med. Sep 2007;8(5):447-451.

35. Weber TR, Connors RH, Tracy TF, Jr., Bailey PV, Stephens C, Keenan W. Prognostic determinants in extracorporeal membrane oxygenation for respiratory

failure in newborns. Ann Thorac Surg. Nov 1990;50(5):720-723.

36. ELSO. ECLS Registry Report: International Summary. Extracorporeal Life Support Organization, Ann Arbor MI. July, 2010 2010.

37. Alsous F, Khamiees M, DeGirolamo A, Amoateng-Adjepong Y, Manthous CA. Negative fluid balance predicts survival in patients with septic shock: a retrospective pilot study. Chest. Jun 2000;117(6):1749-1754.

38. Schuller D, Mitchell JP, Calandrino FS, Schuster DP. Fluid balance during pulmonary edema. Is fluid gain a marker or a cause of poor outcome? Chest. Oct 1991;100(4):1068-1075.

39. Foland JA, Fortenberry JD, Warshaw BL, et al. Fluid overload before continuous hemofiltration and survival in critically ill children: a retrospective analysis. Crit Care Med. Aug 2004;32(8):1771-1776.

40. Gillespie RS, Seidel K, Symons JM. Effect of fluid overload and dose of replacement fluid on survival in hemofiltration. Pediatr Nephrol. Dec 2004;19(12):1394-1399.

41. Goldstein SL, Currier H, Graf C, Cosio CC, Brewer ED, Sachdeva R. Outcome in children receiving continuous venovenous hemofiltration. Pediatrics. Jun 2001;107(6):1309-1312.

42. Michael M, Kuehnle I, Goldstein SL. Fluid overload and acute renal failure in pediatric stem cell transplant patients. Pediatr Nephrol. Jan 2004;19(1):91-95.

43. Goldstein SL, Somers MJ, Brophy PD, et al. The Prospective Pediatric Continuous Renal Replacement Therapy (ppCRRT) Registry: design, development and data assessed. Int J Artif Organs. Jan 2004;27(1):9-14.

44. Goldstein SL, Somers MJ, Baum MA, et al. Pediatric patients with multi-organ dysfunction syndrome receiving continuous renal replacement therapy. Kidney Int. Feb 2005;67(2):653-658.

45. Sutherland SM, Zappitelli M, Alexander SR, et al. Fluid overload and mortality in children receiving continuous renal replacement therapy: the prospective pediatric continuous renal replacement therapy registry. Am J Kidney Dis. Feb 2010;55(2):316-325.

46. Bagshaw SM, Brophy PD, Cruz D, Ronco C. Fluid balance as a biomarker: impact of fluid overload on outcome in critically ill patients with acute kidney injury. Crit Care. 2008;12(4):169.

47. Bagshaw SM, Cruz DN. Fluid overload as a biomarker of heart failure and acute kidney injury. Contrib Nephrol. 2010;164:54-68.

48. Payen D, de Pont AC, Sakr Y, Spies C, Reinhart K, Vincent JL. A positive fluid balance is associated with a worse outcome in patients with acute renal failure. Crit Care. 2008;12(3):R74.

49. Roy BJ, Cornish JD, Clark RH. Venovenous extracorporeal membrane oxygenation affects renal function. Pediatrics. Apr 1995;95(4):573-578.

50. Anderson HL, 3rd, Coran AG, Drongowski RA, Ha HJ, Bartlett RH. Extracellular fluid and total body water changes in neonates undergoing extracorporeal membrane oxygenation. J Pediatr Surg. Aug 1992;27(8):1003-1007; discussion 1007-1008.

51. Kelly RE, Jr., Phillips JD, Foglia RP, et al. Pulmonary edema and fluid mobilization as determinants of the duration of ECMO support. J Pediatr Surg. Sep 1991;26(9):1016-1022.

52. Heiss KF, Pettit B, Hirschl RB, Cilley RE, Chapman R, Bartlett RH. Renal insufficiency and volume overload in neonatal ECMO managed by continuous ultrafiltration. ASAIO Trans. Jul-Sep 1987;33(3):557-560.

53. Swaniker F, Kolla S, Moler F, et al. Extracorporeal life support outcome for 128 pediatric patients with respiratory failure. J Pediatr Surg. Feb 2000;35(2):197-202.

54. Sedlacek M, Schoolwerth AC, Remillard BD. Electrolyte disturbances in the intensive care unit. Semin Dial. Nov-Dec 2006;19(6):496-501.

55. Brown KA, Bissonnette B, MacDonald M, Poon AO. Hyperkalaemia during massive blood transfusion in paediatric craniofacial surgery. Can J Anaesth. May 1990;37(4 Pt 1):401-408.

56. Hall TL, Barnes A, Miller JR, Bethencourt DM, Nestor L. Neonatal mortality following transfusion of red cells with high plasma potassium levels. Transfusion. Jul 1993;33(7):606-609.

57. Ratcliffe JM, Elliott MJ, Wyse RK, Hunter S, Alberti KG. The metabolic load of stored blood. Implications for major transfusions in infants. Arch Dis Child. Dec 1986;61(12):1208-1214.

58. Scanlon JW, Krakaur R. Hyperkalemia following exchange transfusion. J Pediatr. Jan 1980;96(1):108-110.

59. Bohn D. The problem of acute hyponatremia in hospitalized children: the solution is in the solution. Pediatr Crit Care Med. Nov 2008;9(6):658-659.

60. Halberthal M, Halperin ML, Bohn D. Lesson of the week: Acute hyponatraemia in children admitted to hospital: retrospective analysis of factors contributing to its development and resolution. BMJ. Mar 31 2001;322(7289):780-782.

61. Fleming G, Askenazi DJ, Zappitelli M, Paden ML. RRT on ECMO Study Group: Center Practice Survey Results. 21st Annual Extracorporeal Life Support Organization Conference. St Petersburg, Florida2010.

62. McCarthy LJ. Plasmapheresis--the Indiana connection. Transfus Sci. 1990;11(2):161-163.

63. Fleming G. Renal Replacement Therapy Review: Past, Present and Future. Organogenesis. 2011;7(1).

64. Jenkins R, Harrison H, Chen B, Arnold D, Funk J. Accuracy of intravenous infusion pumps in continuous renal replacement therapies. ASAIO J. Oct-Dec 1992;38(4):808-810.

65. Sanchez C, Lopez-Herce J, Garcia E, Moreno de Guerra M, Moral R, Carrillo A. Continuous venovenous renal replacement therapy using a conventional infusion pump. ASAIO J. Jul-Aug 2001;47(4):321-324.

66. Santiago MJ, Sanchez A, Lopez-Herce J, et al. The use of continuous renal replacement therapy in series with extracorporeal membrane oxygenation. Kidney Int. Dec 2009;76(12):1289-1292.

67. Hardison DC, Fleming GM. Hemofiltration and Hemodialysis on ECMO. In: Short B, Williams L., ed. ECMO Specialist Training Manual. Ann Arbor, Michigan: Extracorporeal Life Support Organization; 2010:189-196.

68. Artinian V, Krayem H, DiGiovine B. Effects of early enteral feeding on the outcome of critically ill mechanically ventilated medical patients. Chest. Apr 2006;129(4):960-967.

69. Khalid I, Doshi P, DiGiovine B. Early enteral nutrition and outcomes of critically ill patients treated with vasopressors and mechanical ventilation. Am J Crit Care. May 2010;19(3):261-268.

70. Atkinson S, Sieffert E, Bihari D. A prospective, randomized, double-blind, controlled clinical trial of enteral immunonutrition in the critically ill. Guy's Hospital Intensive Care Group. Crit Care Med. Jul 1998;26(7):1164-1172.

71. Galban C, Montejo JC, Mesejo A, et al. An immune-enhancing enteral diet reduces mortality rate and episodes of bacteremia in septic intensive care unit patients. Crit Care Med. Mar 2000;28(3):643-648.

72. Hanekamp MN, Spoel M, Sharman-Koendjbiharie I, Peters JW, Albers MJ, Tibboel D. Routine enteral nutrition in neonates on extracorporeal membrane oxygenation.

Pediatr Crit Care Med. May 2005;6(3):275-279.

73. Pettignano R, Heard M, Davis R, Labuz M, Hart M. Total enteral nutrition versus total parenteral nutrition during pediatric extracorporeal membrane oxygenation. Crit Care Med. Feb 1998;26(2):358-363.

74. Piena M, Albers MJ, Van Haard PM, Gischler S, Tibboel D. Introduction of enteral feeding in neonates on extracorporeal membrane oxygenation after evaluation of intestinal permeability changes. J Pediatr Surg. Jan 1998;33(1):30-34.

75. Cano NJ, Aparicio M, Brunori G, et al. ESPEN Guidelines on Parenteral Nutrition: adult renal failure. Clin Nutr. Aug 2009;28(4):401-414.

76. Maxvold NJ, Smoyer WE, Custer JR, Bunchman TE. Amino acid loss and nitrogen balance in critically ill children with acute renal failure: a prospective comparison between classic hemofiltration and hemofiltration with dialysis. Crit Care Med. Apr 2000;28(4):1161-1165.

77. Zappitelli M, Goldstein SL, Symons JM, et al. Protein and calorie prescription for children and young adults receiving continuous renal replacement therapy: a report from the Prospective Pediatric Continuous Renal Replacement Therapy Registry Group. Crit Care Med. Dec 2008;36(12):3239-3245.

78. Zappitelli M, Juarez M, Castillo L, Coss-Bu J, Goldstein SL. Continuous renal replacement therapy amino acid, trace metal and folate clearance in critically ill children. Intensive Care Med. Apr 2009;35(4):698-706.

79. Bagshaw SM, George C, Bellomo R. A comparison of the RIFLE and AKIN criteria for acute kidney injury in critically ill patients. Nephrol Dial Transplant. May 2008;23(5):1569-1574.

80. D'Onofrio A, Cruz D, Bolgan I, et al. RIFLE criteria for cardiac surgery-associated acute kidney injury: risk factors and outcomes. Congest Heart Fail. Jul 2010;16 Suppl 1:S32-36.

81. Lassnigg A, Schmid ER, Hiesmayr M, et al. Impact of minimal increases in serum creatinine on outcome in patients after cardiothoracic surgery: do we have to revise current definitions of acute renal failure? Crit Care Med. Apr 2008;36(4):1129-1137.

82. Uchino S, Bellomo R, Goldsmith D, Bates S, Ronco C. An assessment of the RIFLE criteria for acute renal failure in hospitalized patients. Crit Care Med. Jul 2006;34(7):1913-1917.

83. Symons JM, Chua AN, Somers MJ, et al. Demographic characteristics of pediatric continuous renal replacement therapy: a report of the prospective pediatric continuous renal replacement therapy registry. Clin J Am Soc Nephrol. Jul 2007;2(4):732-738.

84. Chesney RW, Kaplan BS, Freedom RM, Haller JA, Drummond KN. Acute renal failure: an important complication of cardiac surgery in infants. J Pediatr. Sep 1975;87(3):381-388.

85. Dimopoulos K, Diller GP, Koltsida E, et al. Prevalence, predictors, and prognostic value of renal dysfunction in adults with congenital heart disease. Circulation. May 6 2008;117(18):2320-2328.

86. Giuffre RM, Tam KH, Williams WW, Freedom RM. Acute renal failure complicating pediatric cardiac surgery: a comparison of survivors and nonsurvivors following acute peritoneal dialysis. Pediatr Cardiol. Oct 1992;13(4):208-213.

87. Lin CY, Chen YC, Tsai FC, et al. RIFLE classification is predictive of short-term prognosis in critically ill patients with acute renal failure supported by extracorporeal membrane oxygenation. Nephrol Dial Transplant. Oct 2006;21(10):2867-2873.

88. Schneider J, Khemani R, Grushkin C, Bart R. Serum creatinine as stratified in the RIFLE score for acute kidney injury is associated with mortality and length of stay

for children in the pediatric intensive care unit. Crit Care Med. Mar 2010;38(3):933-939.

89. Adolph V, Heaton J, Steiner R, Bonis S, Falterman K, Arensman R. Extracorporeal membrane oxygenation for nonneonatal respiratory failure. J Pediatr Surg. Mar 1991;26(3):326-330; discussion 330-322.

90. Duncan BW, Hraska V, Jonas RA, et al. Mechanical circulatory support in children with cardiac disease. J Thorac Cardiovasc Surg. Mar 1999;117(3):529-542.

91. Meyer RJ, Brophy PD, Bunchman TE, et al. Survival and renal function in pediatric patients following extracorporeal life support with hemofiltration. Pediatr Crit Care Med. Jul 2001;2(3):238-242.

92. Shaheen IS, Harvey B, Watson AR, Pandya HC, Mayer A, Thomas D. Continuous venovenous hemofiltration with or without extracorporeal membrane oxygenation in children. Pediatr Crit Care Med. Jul 2007;8(4):362-365.

93. Askenazi D. Acute Kidney Injurya nd Renal Replacement Therapy independently predict mortality in neonatal and pediatric noncardiac patients on extracorporeal membrane oxygenation. Pediatric Critical Care Medicine. 2010;11(5).

94. Kellum JA, Angus DC, Johnson JP, et al. Continuous versus intermittent renal replacement therapy: a meta-analysis. Intensive Care Med. Jan 2002;28(1):29-37.

95. Mehta RL, McDonald B, Gabbai FB, et al. A randomized clinical trial of continuous versus intermittent dialysis for acute renal failure. Kidney Int. Sep 2001;60(3):1154-1163.

96. Tonelli M, Manns B, Feller-Kopman D. Acute renal failure in the intensive care unit: a systematic review of the impact of dialytic modality on mortality and renal recovery. Am J Kidney Dis. Nov 2002;40(5):875-885.

97. Palevsky PM, Zhang JH, O'Connor TZ, et al. Intensity of renal support in critically ill patients with acute kidney injury. N Engl J Med. Jul 3 2008;359(1):7-20.

98. Delannoy B, Floccard B, Thiolliere F, et al. Six-month outcome in acute kidney injury requiring renal replacement therapy in the ICU: a multicentre prospective study. Intensive Care Med. Nov 2009;35(11):1907-1915.

99. Cavagnaro F, Kattan J, Godoy L, et al. Continuous renal replacement therapy in neonates and young infants during extracorporeal membrane oxygenation. Int J Artif Organs. Mar 2007;30(3):220-226.

14

Infections and ECMO

William Lynch, MD

ECMO patients are similar to all critically ill patients in that they are at risk for infections as a consequence of being in an intensive care unit (ICU). Ventilators, central lines, bladder catheters, surgical incisions, traumatic injuries, hospitals contaminated with resistant organisms, and the well-intended care provider are all sources of infection for ECMO patients.

Infections and ECMO have an associated epidemiology and microbiology, strategies for prophylaxis and treatment, and some important technology-related features that make diagnosing infections different than in other ICU patients. These aspects of infections in patients on ECMO will be the focus of this chapter.

The ELSO Task Force on Infection completed a review of this topic in 2010 and their findings and suggested Guidelines are available on the ELSO website, http://www.elso.med. umich.edu/.

Epidemiology

ECMO has been used in the ICU for almost 40 years. ELSO has collected data on many of these patients for over 20 years. Clearly there is an associated risk of infection in these patients and a recent review of the ELSO Registry has been published.[1] This report was a result of the ELSO Task Force on Infections, which was convened in 2009.

Bizzarro and colleagues[1] reviewed the ELSO Registry from 1998 through 2008. During this decade, there were 2,418 culture-proven infections reported in 20,741 ECMO patients. This was a prevalence of 11.7% with a rate of infection of 15.4% per 1000 ECMO days. The ELSO Registry reports as of 2011, 6.0% culture-proven infections were found in all neonatal respiratory cases, 18.3% in pediatric respiratory cases, and 21.3% in adult respiratory cases. While this represents accumulated data since 1986, it is representative of the yearly rate of infections in each patient group in the decade examined by Bizzarro. Culture-proven infections in adults have consistently had the highest prevalence and incidence whereas neonatal patients have had the lowest.

The Registry segregates patients into age groups (neonates, pediatric, and adult patients) and by ECMO indications (respiratory, cardiac, and ECPR). In addition, the Registry collects data by duration of ECMO run. Considering age groups and indication, the ECPR group has the highest rate of infection in all age groups, the highest rate being 42.8% in adults supported with ECPR. Considering age groups and modes of support, VA ECMO had the highest rates of infection in each age group. The trend shows an increased prevalence of infection as duration of ECMO persists. This trend is consistent in all age groups and again, older patients tend to have higher prevalence of culture-proven infections. Similar to other medical device-related infections,[2,3] the duration of ECMO support is associated with increased incidence of infection.

The relationship between risk of infection and duration of ECMO support has been studied and reported previously. These same reports demonstrate the association between increased mortality and presence of infection while on ECMO.[4-8] Until recently, the Registry has not recorded dates or sources of the positive cultures. Without this data, it is difficult to comment on whether infections lead to longer runs or longer runs lead to infections.

Microbiology

The Registry collects data on causal organisms for these infections. The source of the infection (sputum, blood, urine, wound) has recently been added as a data field. For the decade discussed above, the most commonly identified organism in the combined groups and the neonates was coagulase-negative staphylococcus. The most commonly identified organism in the pediatric and adult patient groups was candida,[1] followed by pseudomonas species.

The ELSO Registry data on infections in ECMO patients is supported by other studies. The infections of neonatal and pediatric ECMO are most typically coagulase-negative staphylococci. The incidence of fungal infections climbs with duration of support. Patients supported in the setting of cardiac failure in this patient group are more prone to infection, especially in the setting of open chest.[8-11] Adult ECMO patients seem most susceptible to fungal infections as duration of support continues, with some studies documenting bloodstream infections to be the most common in this patient group.[12,13]

The literature and ELSO Data Registry reviews are consistent in suggesting the offending microbes in ECMO are commonly those associated with medical device-related infections. Coagulase-negative staphylococci,

pseudomonas and candida species are also common hospital-acquired infections in the ICU setting. When there is suspicion of infection during ECMO, empiric antimicrobial therapy should target these organisms (e.g. glycopeptide + anti-pseudomonal beta-lactam +/- triazole).

Prophylaxis

It is clear that the mortality of the patient who develops nosocomial infection while on ECMO is higher than those without infections. Antibiotic prophylaxis to prevent infection to the patient or contamination of the circuit seems logical and justified. However, there are few data in the literature to support this practice. Polling the ECMO community, the disparity in practice habits reflects the uncertainty in this area. The ICU literature is replete in evidence supporting the concept of avoiding unnecessary antimicrobial therapy. Optimizing agent selection, dose, and duration of therapy is balanced against acceptable rate of complications and the consequence of resistance organisms.[14] ECMO patients are unique in some respects but are still critically ill patients with many of the same management considerations.

Cannulation can be considered similar to central line placement. Sterile technique should be used and skin flora controlled by prepping the cannulation site. Hair should be clipped off and use of a razor avoided. If there is a surgical cutdown used for cannulation, the wound should be considered clean and a single dose of a first generation cephalosporin (e.g. cephazolin) 30 minutes prior to incision is appropriate. There is no evidence supporting continuation of these antibiotics once support is established. There is evidence that prophylactic antibiotics may play a role in minimizing the risk of mediastinitis in the open chest ECMO patient, with coverage directed at gram-positive skin flora. ECMO patients supported for longer than two weeks, those supported for cardiac failure, and those with open chests are at risk for developing fungal infections. Some centers offer antifungal prophylaxis in these patient groups.[15]

Diagnosis of Infections while on ECMO

Infections can lead to the systemic inflammatory response syndrome (SIRS) and sepsis. Intervening early can be lifesaving while overreacting can result in life-threatening drug reactions and promote resistant organisms. Typical systemic responses to infection and SIRS can include temperature change (hypothermia or fever), tachypnea, leukocytosis, leukopenia, or thrombocytopenia (see Chapter 28). Sepsis can include all these features with the addition of hemodynamic collapse and malperfusion. ECMO controls the body temperature, gas exchange, and can be used to support hemodynamics. Upon initiation of ECMO (or with circuit changes) blood exposure to biomaterials (cannulas, tubing, oxygenator membranes) will often result in stimulation of the inflammatory cascade, resulting in a brief (up to 6 hours) and self-limited period of instability that can resemble SIRS. In addition, the blood/biomaterial interaction can result in leukocytosis, leukopenia, and thrombocytopenia. For these reasons, recognizing infection while on ECMO can be challenging.

Temperature control while on ECMO is necessary because the blood volume is constantly being exposed to ambient temperature as it passes though the extracorporeal circuit. Blood typically requires rewarming, especially in the neonate. Fever is not common on ECMO but can be detected by a fall in the amount of heat supplied by the heat exchanger. Fever typically is associated with increased metabolism. In mechanically ventilated patients not on ECMO, increased minute ventilation, as a consequence of climbing CO_2 production with increasing metabolic rate, can often be an early sign of SIRS/sepsis. The ECMO patient will also increase CO_2 production in this circumstance. Increasing the sweep rate would normalize pCO_2.

Recognizing the need to increase sweep can be a subtle sign of SIRS/sepsis while on ECMO.

Leukocytosis, leukopenia, and thrombocytopenia are difficult to interpret in the setting of ECMO as they lack specificity. It is not unusual for some of these conditions to set in shortly after initiating ECMO and then stabilizing to define a new baseline. As leukocytosis, leukopenia, and/or thrombocytopenia worsen relative to the new baseline, SIRS/sepsis should be considered as a cause. However, other circuit-related conditions such as thrombosis may cause similar changes.

Hemodynamic changes that set in once ECMO is established can be a manifestation of SIRS/sepsis. However, other conditions can also change hemodynamics. In VV ECMO, aggressive diuresis and/or CVVHDF (continuous venovenous hemodiafiltration) is used to return the patient to their dry weight. Tachycardia, hypotension, and inability to provide adequate drainage suggest hypovolemia. These can also be the hemodynamic changes associated with significant infection. VA ECMO support should be able to control hemodynamics but changes in support requirements (pump flow, associate pressors, sweep rate) will reflect changes in physiology.

Changes in hemostasis can also suggest infection, SIRS, and sepsis in the ECMO patient. Changes can suggest thrombosis or circuit contamination. Markers such as C-reactive protein, antithrombin-III, D-dimers, fibrinogen levels along with platelet count, white blood cell count, and differential will reflect changes suggestive of intravascular coagulopathy. This could be a consequence of circuit thrombosis and contamination. Some centers use changes in these markers to help guide elective circuit changes.[16]

These factors make the ECMO patient unique from others in the ICU in that the typical characteristics that suggest infection are not reliable. However, appreciating changes in the patient (and circuit) are necessary when trying to recognize infection. In critical care, it is common for our patients to change daily, sometimes hourly. It is necessary to look for changes and to be able to interpret them. Anticipating changes is even more important. The ECMO physician must appreciate the physiology of the patient and the physiology of the circuit to be able to best interpret the needs of the patient.

Surveillance

Infections on ECMO worsen outcomes and infections are difficult to recognize. A strategy of surveillance seems logical. Unfortunately, there is little in the literature to support this line of thinking. Daily blood cultures, routine tracheal aspirates or bronchoalveolar lavage, and surveillance cultures added 10-12 days into an ECMO run have all been studied without evidence of improved outcomes.[17-19] Given the lack of evidence and the significant cost of cultures, it is not recommended to perform surveillance cultures for patients on ECMO. Clinical suspicion should lead towards cultures as indicated.

Treatment

Treatment of documented infections should follow the same principles as for all patients in the intensive care units. Specific choice of antibiotics should be a function of the organisms being treated. Consideration for the altered volume of distribution as a consequence of the circuit might impact dosing of certain antibiotics. There is no evidence that the polymethyl pentene oxygenator has an affinity for antibiotics that might impact present recommended dosing guidelines. There is a body of literature on the silicone membrane oxygenator that demonstrates affinity for lipophilic medications affects bioavailability.[20,21]

Empiric therapy started prior to initiating ECMO should be continued and completed as indicated. Antibiotics used at the time of cannulation should be single-dose first generation cephalosporins for surgical cannulation. Patients with a picture of sepsis should be treated with broad spectrum antibiotics, considering the likely source of sepsis. ECMO patients that demonstrate sepsis after 1-2 weeks of ECMO should be covered for candida species, staphylococci, and pseudomonas species as part of the empiric strategy.

Circuit Management when Considering Infection.

Circuits are commonly built and prepared ahead of time. Many centers will have circuits placed on carts with pumps and necessary monitoring in place in order to minimize the setup time at initiation. Some centers will pre-prime the circuits with a glucose-free, crystalloid-based solution so that this is not necessary at initiation. The ELSO ID Task Force considered the infection-related consequences of this practice. The task force had three member centers prime several circuits of various sizes and cultures were drawn over a 30-day period. Sterile techniques were used to build the circuits. Crystalloid solutions without glucose were used. All cultures were without evidence of growth over this 30-day period. These results suggest it is safe to pre-prime circuits with glucose-free crystalloid solutions for up to 30 days prior to use.

Once support is established, circuit management with regards to infection is similar to care provided for any central line. Blood draws should not take place via the circuit unless absolutely necessary. Needleless hubs are recommended over Luer type connectors. Chlorhexidine should be used instead of alcohol or Betadine. If medications must be delivered via the circuit, preference should be for continuous infusions over bolus medications so that breaks in the circuit are minimized.

Circuit contamination is difficult to recognize. Surveillance cultures have not been demonstrated to reliably predict patient or circuit-related infection. Changes in hemostasis suggesting thrombosis of the circuit can be a subtle clue to circuit contamination indicating a new circuit is necessary.

Discussion

Standard ICU practices should apply to patients on ECMO. Hospital-acquired infections continue to be a risk for these patients. Guidelines to minimize ventilator-associated pneumonia should be adhered to. Unless contraindicated, the head of the bed should be elevated. Airway suctioning and pulmonary toilet should be performed as often as necessary. Tracheostomy, extubation, and elimination of the ventilator should also be considered. Along with this comes liberation from sedation. Central line associated bloodstream infections are a risk for the ECMO patient. Central lines can be removed if necessary and new ones placed if anticoagulation is appropriately adjusted around the time of the line change. Enteral nutrition should be offered when appropriate. Overfeeding should be avoided.

Physical therapy should not be denied to the ECMO patient. Special attention should be offered to cannula security when a patient is being moved. Special consideration should be offered to the anticoagulated patient. These factors make the ECMO patient different than most ICU patients but the ECMO patient is equally at risk for all ICU related complications.

The ECMO patient should be considered as all patients in a critical care unit and while unique, ECMO does not preclude well-accepted standards of ICU care.

References

1. Bizzaro MJ, Conrad SA, Kaufman DA, Rycus P. Infections acquired during extracorporeal membrane oxygenation in neonates, children and adults. Pediatr Crit Care Med 2011; 12:277-281.
2. Souweine B, Traore O, Aublet-Cuvelier B. Dialysis and central venous catheter infections in critically ill patients: Results of a prospective study. Crit Care Med 1999; 27:2394-2398.
3. Maki DG, Tambyah PA: Engineering out the risk for infection with urinary catheters. Emerg Infect Dis 2001; 7:342-347.
4. Meyer DM, Jessen ME, Eberhart RC. Neonatal extracorporeal membrane oxygenation complicated by sepsis. Ann Thorac Surg 1995; 59:975-980.
5. Brown KL, Ridout DA, Shaw M, Dodkins I, Smith LC, O'Callaghan MA, Goldman AP, Macqueen S, Hartley JC. Healthcare associated infection in pediatric patients on extracorporeal life support: The role of multidisciplinary surveillance. Pediatr Crit Care Med 2006; 7(6): 546-50.
6. Sun HY, Ko WJ, Tsia PR, Sun CC, Chang YY, Lee CW, Chen YC. Infections occurring during extracorporeal membrane oxygenation use in adult patients. J Thorac Cardiovasc Surg 2010;140:1125-1132.
7. Douglass BH, Keenan AL, Purohit DM. Bacterial and fungal infections in neonates undergoing venoarterial extracorporeal membrane oxygenation: an analysis of the registry data of the extracorporeal life support organization. Artif Organs 1996 Mar;20(3):202-8.
8. O'Neill JM, Schutze GE, Heulitt MJ, Simpson PM, Taylor BJ. Nosocomial infections during extracorporeal membrane oxygenation. Intensive Care Med 2001 Aug;27(8):1247-53.
9. Schultze GE, Heulitt MJ. Infections during extracorporeal life support. J Pediatr Surg 1995;30: 809-812.
10. Douglas BH, Keenan AL, Purohit DM. Bacterial and fungal infection in neonates undergoing venoarterial extracorporeal membrane oxygenation: an analysis of the registry data of the extracorporeal life support organization. Artif Organs 1996;20:202-208
11. Coffin SE, BelMann Polin R. Nosocomial infections in neonates receiving extracorporeal membrane oxygenation. Infect Control Hosp Epidemiol 1997;18:93-96.
12. Burket JS, Bartlett RH, Hyde KV, Chenoweth CE. Nosocomial infections in adult patients undergoing extracorporeal membrane oxygenation. Clin Infect Dis 1999; 28:828-833.
13. Sun H, Ko W, Tsai P, Sun C, Chang Y, Lee C, Chen Y. Infections occurring during extracorporeal membrane oxygenation use in adult patients. J Thorac Cardiovasc Surg 2010;140:1125-32.
14. Arnold HM, Micek ST, Skrupky LP, Kollef MH. Antibiotic stewardship in the intensive care unit. Semin Respir Crit Care Med 2011; 32:215-17.
15. Gardner AH, Prodhan P, Stovall SH, Gossett JM, Stern JE, Wilson CD, Fiser RT. Fungal infections and antifungal prophylaxis in pediatric cardiac extracorporeal life support. J Thorac Cardiovasc Surg 2012; 143:689-95.
16. Muller T, Lubnow M, Philipp A, Schneider-Brachert W, Camboni D, Schmid C, Lehle K. Risk of circuit infection in septic patients on extracorporeal membrane oxygenation: a preliminary study. Artif Organs 2011; 35:E84-90.
17. Kaczala GW, Paulus SC, Al-Dajani N, Jang W, Blondel-Hill E, Dobson S, Cogswell A, Singh AJ. Bloodstream infection in pediatric ECLS: usefulness of daily blood culture monitoring and predictive value of biologic

markers. The British Columbia experience. Pediatric Surg Int 2009; 25:169-73.

18. Steiner CK, Stewart DL, Bond SJ, Hornung CA, McKay VJ. Predictors of acquiring a nosocomial bloodstream infection on extracorporeal membrane oxygenation. J Pediatric Surg 2001; 36:387-92.

19. Elerian LF, Sparks JW, Meyer TA, Zwischenberger JB, Doski J, Goretsky MJ, Warner BW, Cheu HW, lally KP. Usefulness of surveillance cultures in neonatal extracorporeal membrane oxygenation. ASAIO Journal 2001; 47:220-23.

20. Ahsman MJ, Wildeschut ED, Tibboel D, Mathot RA. Pharmacokinetics of cefotaxime and desacetylcefotaxime in infants during extracorporeal membrane oxygenation. Antimicrob Agents Chemother 2010; 54:1734-41.

21. Wildeschut ED, Ahsman MJ, Allegaert K, Mathot RAA, Tibboel D. Determinants of drug absorption in different ECMO circuits. Intensive Care Med 2010; 36:2109-16.

15

Procedures on ECMO

William R. Lynch MD, Jay M. Wilson MD, Robert H. Bartlett MD

Procedures Guidelines

Procedures from venipuncture to liver transplantation can be done with success during ECLS. When an operation is necessary, coagulation should be optimized (anticoagulation minimized) as described in the section on anticoagulation. Even small operations like chest tube placement are done with extensive use of electrocautery. For the surgeon, the procedure is like operating on any coagulopathic patient. Note there are no references in this chapter, but rather guidelines of proper procedure to follow from ECMO clinicians who have been exposed to the majority of these procedural interventions on ECMO.

Comments on Procedures on ECMO

The paragraph in the ELSO Guidelines is short, but says it all in the last sentence. The surgeon or intensivist who is going to do an invasive procedure is expected to be experienced in operating on coagulopathic and anticoagulated patients.

Preoperative management begins with asking is the procedure really necessary? If so, how urgent is it? Placing a chest tube can usually wait until coagulation is normalized; repairing a puncture in the right atrium must be done immediately. When time allows systemic anticoagulation can be decreased or stopped altogether and platelet count increased to 100,000 before operation, if the operation is being done to stop bleeding (at a cannulation or trach site for example)

Adjuvant medications. Coagulation is normalized as much as possible as described above. Actively reversing heparin effect with protamine is possible but not recommended because it frequently results in clotting of the circuit. Aprotinin is an antifibrinolytic, diminishes the inflammatory response stimulated by ECLS systems, and can preserve platelet function. All of these characteristics are attractive for a medication to diminish bleeding in ECLS patients. However, because of complications related to this medication, it is no longer available in the US and many other countries. Procedures done on anticoagulated patients can usually be done with minimal blood loss, but normal fibrinolysis results in recurrent bleeding days later. This can be inhibited with antifibrinolytic drugs such as Amicar (epsilon aminocaproic acid) or tranexamic acid. Some centers advise giving Amicar routinely to all ECMO patients to minimize fibrinolysis at cannulation and other operative sites. It is reasonable to give Amicar following major procedures on ECMO, with the caution that clotting may be more prominent in the circuit. Amicar is usually given with a loading dose (100-150 mg/kg) followed by a maintenance infusion (10-25 mg/kg/hr), considering lower dosing for renal failure. Amicar can also be used in preparation for a procedure (e.g., tracheostomy, thoracotomy, laparotomy). Loading dose and continuous infusion is given. In this setting, heparin should be continued with typical ACT target of 1½ times normal (160-200 seconds) to minimize risk of catastrophic circuit thrombosis. Heparin could be discontinued prior to the procedure, recognizing there will be risk to the circuit. ECMO flows should be maximized, remaining at or above 100 cc/kg/hr.

Emergency Procedures. The only emergency procedures that must be done immediately, before normalizing coagulation status are conditions causing massive bleeding. In ECMO, this generally relates to cannulation site complications (intrathoracic puncture of major vessels or cardiac chambers or inadvertent decannulation).

Postoperative management is different than most procedures because of the ongoing need for major anticoagulation following the operation. Hemostasis is optimized with electrocautery before closing. Under most circumstances it is best to leave the tissues open and cover the wound with a plastic drape with drains under the drape, usually with active suction on the drains. This is discussed below with regard to specific procedures.

Specific procedures

Adding a cannulation site for a patient already on ECMO: additional cannulas are generally placed by percutaneous access using ultrasound guidance to identify the vessels. If open cannulation is required, a small incision with dissection to identify the vessel then puncture, placement of a wire, placement of the catheter is the best approach. This semi-Seldinger technique is favored over extensively dissecting the vessel and placing the cannula directly. Minimizing the tissue trauma of dissection will minimize associated bleeding. Surgical dissection is best done with electrocautery.

Tracheostomy: Tracheostomy is generally done using the Ciaglia technique with needle puncture into the trachea, passage of a wire into the trachea with bronchoscopic guidance, and progressive dilatation leading to placement of the tracheostomy tube. This procedure is often done with only a small skin incision. In ECMO patients the authors favor small dissection all the way to the trachea with hemostasis to avoid blind puncture through the thyroid or major vessels in the neck. Electrocautery is again recommended if incision is made.

Chest tube placement: When the chest tube is placed for pneumothorax it can be placed using the Seldinger technique over a wire using a small catheter. Bleeding can still occur with this approach but is less than if the chest tube is placed with incision and dissection. For pneumothorax, a chest tube or catheter should only be considered if there is suggestion of tamponade physiology (tension pneumothorax, tension hemothorax). For fluid in the chest, it is reasonable to try to pass a drainage catheter over a wire, but usually a large tube is required to drain blood or empyema fluid. In this case the dissection is carried out all the way from the skin to the pleural space with electrocautery and the catheter placed directly. In the anticoagulated ECLS patient, a hemothorax can evolve into a tension hemothorax and drainage will be required. Loss of venous drainage can be a consequence of tamponade physiology resulting from either air or blood.

Thoracotomy: Thoracotomy is usually carried out for bleeding following lung injury, cardiac puncture, or bleeding following chest tube placement. In this circumstance, a full anterolateral thoracotomy or clamshell bilateral thoracotomy is used to allow good exposure. Control of the local bleeding should be done directly along with electrocautery hemostasis of the raw surfaces. When the thoracotomy is done for bleeding, recurrent bleeding will almost invariably occur. It is wise to leave the chest wall open with drains on suction, covered with a plastic drape. If the patient has had a recent sternotomy leading to the bleeding site, the chest is re-explored through the sternotomy. This should be left open to evaluate the inevitable recurrent bleeding. If thoracotomy is done for ligation of patent ductus arteriosus, a small left forth interspace anterolateral thoracotomy is used and the chest is closed with a drain after this operation. If the thoracotomy is for lung biopsy, this can be done via thoracoscope with a low threshold for converting to an open procedure to control bleeding.

Repair of diaphragmatic hernia: The timing of hernia repair in congenital diaphragmatic hernia (CDH) patients on ECMO is controversial. Repair can be done from early in the course or waiting until the patient is off ECMO. When CDH repair is done on ECMO, coagulation is normalized as much as possible. An abdominal approach is used, hemostasis established thoroughly with cautery, and hernia repaired in the usual fashion with the exception that the posterior diaphragmatic leaf is not dissected out as this rarely results in the ability to achieve a primary repair and is frequently the source of postoperative bleeding on ECMO. Instead the patch, which is almost always needed for CDH patients sick enough to require ECMO, is cut slightly larger and sutured directly to the undissected posterior diaphragmatic rim. For the posterolateral sutures, which frequently need to be placed around a rib, the rib and neurovascular bundle is grasped with an Allis clamp and pulled forward allowing the suture to pass behind the rib without injuring the neurovascular finally topical thrombin can be sprayed onto all suture lines to contain small areas of hemorrhage. Some surgeons routinely use a chest tube to identify and treat postoperative intrathoracic bleeding if it occurs. Suction drains can also be placed in the abdomen to identify potential bleeding. Some of these cases may require a decompressive "silo" in the abdominal wall, but this is usually not necessary if the diaphragmatic patch is made large enough.

Soft tissue operations: For debridement of burns, management of lacerations, soft tissue injury, or necrotizing fasciitis, coagulation is normalized as much as possible and the operation is completed as needed. Re-bleeding will inevitably occur. It is best to leave the entire wound open, covered with a plastic drape placing vacuum drains underneath.

Amputation: Sometimes a distal limb is infarcted because of the vascular access cannula or because of injury prior to ECMO. In this circumstance amputation can be delayed until the patient is off ECMO by applying a completely occlusive tourniquet above the infarcted area and packing the dead limb in ice until the patient is off ECMO.

Uterine bleeding: Menstrual bleeding is rarely a significant issue during ECMO. Bleeding from the uterus following complication of pregnancy can be a significant problem. It is generally managed by packing the uterus combined with suction drains. Hysterectomy is rarely if ever required.

Skeletal procedures: Placement of pins, rods, and fixation devices can be done as in any anticoagulated patient.

Craniotomy: Craniotomy can be done for intracranial bleeding, either in the subdural space or in the brain parenchyma. If the patient is remaining on ECMO it is best to leave the bone flap off, close the scalp, and leave suction drains. It is rare for the bleed to be something that can undergo surgical correction, but when it can then this intervention must be considered.

Peripherally inserted central venous catheter (PICC Lines): With the increased use of these lines as an alternative to temporary central venous catheters, these lines are a safer alternative to place in a coagulopathic patient and therefore in a patient on ECMO as well. It is not infrequent that unstable patients who requirement emergent placement on ECMO often have preexisting central access used for the venous cannulation, especially if that line is in the right internal jugular. This then leaves the patient without any central access except through the circuit. In these instances placement of a PICC can be done and because of the peripheral approach for their placement, the site can have local control for bleeding.

16

Weaning, Trialing and Futility

William R. Lynch MD

Once ECLS is initiated, the goals of support are defined. The support goals will help establish the strategy of care and should be the fundamental first decision prior to offering ECLS. Are the goals achievable? Is meaningful survival possible? Does the risk/benefit equation favor ECLS when considered against other options? Can the system of care accommodate a patient on ECLS? If these questions are considered, ECLS can be an appropriate option for the patient. Once offered, the goals for ECLS will drive daily decision making for the ECLS team. ECLS should be discontinued once these goals have been achieved or when it becomes apparent that the goals are unobtainable.

Weaning ECLS is the process necessary to recognize whether or not a patient has improved enough to be sustained without ECLS. Trialing is the process of temporarily discontinuing ECLS in order to demonstrate that a patient can survive without ECLS. Futility is the realization that meaningful survival is no longer possible and obligates that ECLS, and perhaps all life support, be discontinued. Appreciating the pathophysiology of the specific patient is necessary when choosing patients, designing circuits, deciding the appropriate ECLS mode, and defining the strategy of support. Once these decisions are made (all functions of the patient's pathophysiology) goals of care can be established. These patient specific "goals

of care" allow the family and care providers to focus on what is achievable. If the goals are being met, continuing support is appropriate. If complications occur that change the goals of care or make it impossible to achieve them, this must be recognized.

When extracorporeal support has decreased to the point that it is contributing less than 30% of native organ function, it may be possible to separate from ECLS and a "trial off" is indicated. As long as ECLS support is more than 30 to 50%, there is no indication to trial off unless there are special circumstances, such as uncontrolled bleeding.

Weaning the Neonatal Patient

Weaning the neonate can be gradually achieved as native cardiopulmonary function returns. Decreasing pump flow over time by 10-20 cc/kg/min is typical. This can be done for venoarterial or venovenous ECMO as a strategy of weaning. Neonatal circuits are ¼ inch and care must be taken to protect the circuit from thrombosis as flows are decreased. Cannula flow should be maintained greater than 40-50 cc/min to protect the cannulas from thrombosing. Minimum circuit blood flow in a ¼" circuit should be approximately 100 cc/minute. Some centers refer to this minimum circuit flow as "idle" flow. Minimum oxygenator flows are device dependent and it is necessary to be aware of the specifications of the particular oxygenator being used. Some neonatal centers use an oxygenator that has a recommended minimum flow that is higher than the flow necessary to support a neonatal patient. In this circumstance, oxygenator blood flow can be greater than patient blood flow by employing a post oxygenator shunt, diverting blood flow back the circuit. During the weaning process, gas exchange is shifted from ECMO back to the native lung. Appropriate native lung support (mechanical ventilation, iNO, surfactant, high frequency ventilation) is typically offered. The patient hemodynamics and gas exchange are monitored as is the patient's overall appearance. Venoarterial (VA) and venovenous (VV) modes are common ECMO strategies in this patient category.[1] The process of trialing off of VV ECMO is different than trialing off of VA ECMO. The trialing process will be described later in this chapter.

Weaning the Pediatric Respiratory Patient

As native lung function returns, weaning from ECMO support can be considered. If VA support is used, venous drainage blood will represent mixed venous saturation (SvO_2). An $SvO_2 > 65$-70% typically indicates adequate oxygen delivery to support tissue level metabolism. ECMO flow can be slowly decreased over time to maintain $SvO_2 > 65$-70%. The weaning process begins by decreasing circuit flow 10-20 cc/kg/min and then reassessing the patient.[2,3] If hemodynamics, gas exchange and tissue level perfusion remain stable, the initial weaning step has been tolerated. VV support can also be weaned by decreasing ECMO pump flow as native lung function recovers. Sweep gas flow may also be decreased as a means of assessing native lung recovery. Sweep can be slowly decreased over time while monitoring the patient's minute volume, respiratory rate, and end tidal CO_2. As native lung function returns, more CO_2 will be eliminated by the native lungs. Sweep gas flow rate over the membrane oxygenator will need to be decreased in order to maintain normal pCO_2.[4]

Weaning the Pediatric Cardiac Patient

Inotropes, vasoconstrictors, and vasodilators are typically necessary and should be used as weaning from ECMO progresses. Echocardiography is used to guide ventricular and valvular performance during weaning. As flows are decreased, tissue level perfusion is assessed by monitoring mixed venous saturation, acid-base status, lactate levels, and urine output. Near infrared spectroscopy (NIRS) is commonly used in neonatal and pediatric ICUs and this technology can also be valuable in monitoring satisfactory tissue level perfusion. Left ventricular vents are often used in the setting of severe cardiac failure necessitating ECMO support. The LV vent keeps the ventricle empty optimizing cardiac rest. The LV vent must be removed or clamped in order for weaning to take place. Weaning LV vent flow would precede attempts of weaning from ECMO. Return of pulsatile flow is an encouraging sign of recovering cardiac function. Prior to trialing, fluid balance should be optimized and renal replacement therapy is often necessary. Pulmonary function is commonly compromised in the setting of severe cardiac dysfunction. As cardiac function recovers, attention should also be directed at lung function. Lung function must be optimized so that it does not impose an undue stress on a fragile heart. At times, continuing ECMO to support the recovering lungs is necessary as part of a successful wean of ECMO in the setting of cardiac failure. Weaning from ECMO can be considered successful if perfusion can be maintained with relatively low levels of inotropes and vasoactive infusions when ECMO flows are decreased to 25-40 cc/kg/min.[5-7] Trialing is described below for VA ECMO.

Weaning the Adult Respiratory Patient

Venovenous is the mode of choice in adults in respiratory failure. The dual lumen/bi-caval cannula is available in sizes appropriate for almost all adult patients. As native lung function begins to improve, ECLS flows can be decreased. Ventilator support continues at rest settings with minimal pressure and FiO_2. The typical strategy is to wean ECMO support as native lung function returns, transitioning back to a protective mode of mechanical ventilation. Some ECMO centers prefer to have patients undergo tracheostomy while on ECMO to minimize associated risks of endotracheal intubation. Other ECMO centers avoid tracheostomy while patients are anticoagulated on ECMO, preferring to continue with endotracheal intubation until off of ECMO. Bleeding and the associated aspiration of blood can hinder recovery of lung function.

During the initial days of ECMO, it is common that ventilating volume is lost as the mechanical ventilator is adjusted to "rest settings." In some cases, as euvolemia is approached and the pulmonary inflammatory process has resolved, ventilating volume will return as compliance improves. In other circumstances, ventilating volume will need to be actively recruited. Recruitment strategies can include bronchoscopy with lavage, prone positioning, sitting position, gentle hand bagging, and by reestablishing PEEP. It is important to resist the urge to recruit the lungs too early because this will only further damage the already injured lungs. If the patient is successfully weaned from ECMO and transitioned to mechanical ventilation, tracheostomy can accelerate weaning from the ventilator.[8]

The injury that sometimes occurs in the setting of ARDS can be a progressive and irreversible fibrosis.[9] This picture can be suggested when the mean pulmonary artery pressure is consistently greater than two-thirds that of the systemic blood pressure. The unprepared right ventricle is at risk of failing. Right ventricular failure is difficult to predict and can happen suddenly. Tachycardia can be a subtle sign that RV failure is pending. Arrhythmias leading to ventricular tachycardia and fibrillation may occur. The failing RV can be supported by converting to VA ECMO but it is difficult to decide if the lung dysfunction is recoverable or terminal. There is anecdotal experience that the lung may recover if the patient is supported long enough. The current generation of oxygenators, cannulas, and pumps have changed the safety profile in ways that makes prolonged support more practical. With single sight neck cannulation, patients can be liberated from sedation, mechanical ventilation, and even the beds. Avoiding deconditioning is possible which allows select centers to consider offering weeks to months of support in these types of patients.[10,11] While possible, the logistics and practicality of long term support rarely leads to success. Many centers will consider right ventricular failure in the setting of ARDS support with ECMO to be an irreversible and fatal disease. Conversely, if there is no evidence of RV dysfunction and with pulmonary pressures less than half that of systemic pressures, lung recover can be realized. Support should be continued.

The present generation of ECMO technology is allowing new strategies of patient management to emerge. Until recently, many intensivists would only consider ECMO after salvage strategies (oscillators, airway pressure release ventilation, nitric oxide) had been attempted and failed. In their view, ECMO was unproven, complicated, dangerous salvage strategy and should only be considered as futility was approached. ECMO employed in that fashion has little chance to offer benefit. The present ECMO technology has a safety profile that allows patients to be awake, off sedation, out of bed and active. Early mobility has been demonstrated to shorten ICU stay and diminish ICU associated complications.[12-15] When one considers the advantages of single sight neck cannulation, it is practical and safe to get patients out of bed while still supported with ECMO. Extracorporeal gas exchange allows work of breathing to be attenuated, diminishing the stress and distress of activity.

Trialing and weaning is as discussed in pediatric respiratory failure. In many adults the ventilator can be eliminated prior to ECMO. It is practical to use ECMO to eliminate the mechanical ventilator and the endotracheal tube. ECMO can be used to support gas exchange during the acute inflammatory phase of respiratory failure. Early in this course, the patient typically benefits from sedation and airway control with either the endotracheal tube or tracheostomy. Some patients continue to have increased work of breathing for the first few days. The patient typically benefits from sedation during this early phase. As the work of breathing diminishes, it becomes possible to liberate the patient from sedation completely. As the patient emerges from sedation, extubation can be achieved. It is necessary to decrease the PEEP prior to extubation. Disconnecting the ventilator from the endotracheal tube prior to committing to extubation is valuable in demonstrating whether the patient will tolerate losing the last bit of PEEP. Once extubated, it is possible to start nutrition by mouth and physical therapy.

In the extubated ECMO patient, weaning support can proceed by either decreasing flow, decreasing sweep, or a combination of the two. It is possible to slowly wean extracorporeal support without reverting back to mechanical ventilation. Alternatively, noninvasive ventilation can be included as part of the weaning process.

Weaning the Adult Cardiac Patient

VA ECMO will be the required mode for these patients and weaning is similar to that described for the Pediatric Cardiac Patient. Support goals are providing perfusion while the heart recovers. Echocardiography provides the best assessment of native cardiac function if the

chest is closed. In the setting of post-cardiotomy stun, it is not unusual for the chest to be left open. If there is minimal cardiac function, the left ventricle will require a decompressive vent or shunt. In the adult setting, cardiac function should recover in 3-5 days. During this time frame, alternative strategies of support such as a left ventricular assist device, artificial heart, and/or heart transplantation should be considered. Neurologic function should be assessed. Bleeding should be minimized. Markers of perfusion (mixed venous saturations, lactate production, neurologic function, renal function) are monitored as weaning takes place. Success is realized if perfusion can be maintained with modest pressor and inotropic infusions, protective ventilation strategies, and with ECLS providing less than 30% of overall support.[5,6] If the patient cannot be weaned in 4-5 days the alternative is to proceed to a VAD, or consider termination if the patient is not a VAD or transplant candidate.

Trialing off ECMO

The approach to "trialing off" depends on the mode of cannulation. Trialing off for veno-venous ECMO is quite simple. VV ECMO is essentially a venous shunt that does not support cardiac function. As native pulmonary function recovers, trialing off is accomplished by disconnecting the sweep gas from the oxygenator. Appropriate support of native lung function (protective ventilator strategies at minimal FiO_2 if mechanically ventilated; supplemental oxygen or non invasive ventilation if extubated) should be established prior to the trial. ECLS pump blood flow does not need to be adjusted nor does the strategy of anticoagulation. The gas inlet and outlet ports to the oxygenator can be capped off to eliminate gas transport across the membrane from "room air." The patient SaO_2, pCO_2, respiratory rate, minute volume (if available) should be followed along with hemodynamics and overall patient appearance.

If these parameters demonstrate acceptable native lung function over a couple of hours, it is appropriate to move towards decannulation.

Venoarterial ECMO trial off is more involved. VA ECMO should be considered an arterialized right to left shunt and oxygen must always be supplied to the oxygenator. In order to trial off when supported with VA ECMO, clamps must be applied to the drainage and return blood lines. By eliminating ECMO flow to and from the patient, native organ function (lung, heart, or both) can be evaluated. If VA ECMO was being used to support respiratory failure, preparations should be made to offer appropriate support with supplemental oxygen or gentle mechanical ventilation. The VA trial requires clamping of the drainage and infusion blood lines between the patient and the bridge. ECLS is effectively discontinued and the patient must be sustained by native organ function. In order to preserve the ECLS circuit, flow is continued through a "bridge" which connects the arterial and venous limbs of the circuit. Anticoagulation to the patient is maintained. If the anticoagulation was being delivered via the circuit, this needs to be moved to the patient. Clamps are released for brief periods every 10-20 minutes so that stagnant flow does not result in thrombosis. A trial can be safely offered for 2-3 hours and if the patient can be sustained with protective ventilation and modest inotrope and pressor support, the trial can be considered a success and ECLS support can be discontinued. It is best to remove the cannulas once ECLS is discontinued. It is possible to leave cannulas in place for up to 24 hours or more. If this is done, a low dose heparinized solution is infused to minimize thrombosis of the cannulas. The rationale for keeping cannulas in place for brief periods after discontinuing support could be that the decannulating surgeon is not immediately available. Another reason to keep cannulas in place after discontinuing support would be for the patient who remains tenuous.

Decannulation

Heparin should be discontinued 30-60 minutes prior to removing the cannulas to optimize hemostasis. Cannulas placed by direct cutdown will need to be removed by direct cutdown. Neonates and small children supported with VA ECMO are typically cannulated via the right neck. The carotid and internal jugular vein are usually ligated at the time of decannulation.

When removing a venous cannula from the neck there is risk that air can be entrained in this low-pressure system via the cannula side holes. This risk can be minimized by having the patient hold their breath, Valsalva, or by using short acting paralytics for mechanically ventilated patients. In larger patients, the femoral veins and arteries are possible cannulation vessels. If surgical cutdown was used for cannulation, this same approach is necessary or decannulation. The femoral vein can often be ligated but usually repair is done. The femoral artery typically needs to be reconstructed. A vein patch, prosthetic patch, or interposition graft is used. If cannulation of the femoral vessels was done percutaneously, these cannulas can often be removed simply by pulling and holding pressure. Percutaneous femoral venous cannulas can almost always be managed in this fashion. A percutaneous femoral artery cannula can be pulled with pressure, or removed in the operating room with direct repair.

Futility

ECLS should be discontinued if there is no longer hope for healthy survival. This could be a consequence of severe brain injury, unrecoverable heart and/or lung injury, worsening multi-organ failure and for patients without hope of organ replacement by ventricular assist devices or transplantation. The definition of "unrecoverable" is patient and organ specific. In each case, a reasonable expectation for organ recovery can be estimated based on the pathophysiology of the organ affected. It is important to establish the expectation for recovery early during the ECLS support. As an example, in the setting of cardiac failure, if native function has not recovered in 3-5 days in a patient who is not a VAD or transplant candidate, this would be considered futility in most centers. In lung failure, two weeks without return of any native function in a patient not considered a transplant candidate can be considered futile although lung recovery has been reported after 1-2 months of support. Futility remains a challenge to define in ECMO and throughout modern critical care medicine. There is ample conversation on the ethics of this topic in the literature.[16-17]

References

1. Shelley CL, Rees NJ. Management of the Neonate on ECMO. In: Short BL, Williams L, eds. ECMO specialist training manual. Third Edition. Ann Arbor, MI: Extracorporeal Life Support Organization; 2010: 129.

2. Van Meurs KP, Hintz SR, Sheehan AM. ECMO for neonatal respiratory failure. In: Van Meurs K, Lally KP, Peek G, Zwischenberger JB, eds. Extracorporeal cardiopulmonary support in critical care. Third edition. Ann Arbor, MI: Extracorporeal Life Support Organization; 2005: 281.

3. Sussman J. Management of the pediatric ECMO patient. In: Short BL, Williams L, eds. ECMO specialist training manual. Third Edition. Ann Arbor, MI: Extracorporeal Life Support Organization; 2010: 135-141.

4. Frenckner B, Palmer P. Management of the pediatric respiratory failure patient on ECLS. In: Van Meurs K, Lally KP, Peek G, Zwischenberger JB, eds. Extracorporeal cardiopulmonary support in critical care. Third edition. Ann Arbor, MI: Extracorporeal Life Support Organization; 2005: 363-81.

5. Ferroni R, Berger J, Schuette JJ. Management of the cardiac ECMO patient. In: Short BL, Williams L, eds. ECMO specialist training manual. Third Edition. Ann Arbor, MI: Extracorporeal Life Support Organization; 2010: 145-56.

6. Steinhorn DM. Termination of extracorporeal membrane oxygenation for cardiac support. Artificial Organs 1999. 23(11):1026-30.

7. Sarani B, Kormos RL. Adult cardiac failure: Management and use of ECMO. In: Van Meurs K, Lally KP, Peek G, Zwischenberger JB, eds. Extracorporeal cardiopulmonary support in critical care. Third edition. Ann Arbor, MI: Extracorporeal Life Support Organization; 2005: 467-75.

8. Bartlett RH. Management of ECLS in adult respiratory failure. In: Van Meurs K, Lally KP, Peek G, Zwischenberger JB, eds. Extracorporeal cardiopulmonary support in critical care. Third edition. Ann Arbor, MI: Extracorporeal Life Support Organization; 2005: 403-16.

9. Kress JP, Pohlman AS, O'Connor MF, Hall JB. Daily interruption of sedative infusions in critically ill patients undergoing mechanical ventilation. N Engl J Med 2000; 342:1471-7.

10. Girard TD, Kress JP, Fuchs BD, Thomason JWW, Schweickert WD, Pun BT, Taichman DB, Dunn JG, Pohlman AS, Kinniry PA, Jackson JC, Canonico AE, Light RW, Shintani AK, Thompson JL, Gordon SM, Hall JB, Dittus RS, Bernard GR, Ely EW. Efficacy and safety of a paired sedation and ventilator weaning protocol for mechanically ventilated patients in intensive care (Awakening and Breathing Controlled trial): a randomized controlled trial. Lancet 2008; 371:126-34.

11. Kress JP, Gehlbach B, Lacy M, Pliskin N, Pohlman AS, Hall JB. The long-term psychological effects of daily sedative interruption on critically ill patients. Am J Respir Crit Care Med 2003; 168:1457-61.

12. Schweickert WD, Pohlman MC, Pohlman AS, Nigos C, Pawlik AJ, Esbrook CL, Spears L, Miller M, Franczyk M, Deprizio D, Schmidt GA, Bowman A, Barr R, McCallister KE, Hall JB, Kress JP. Early physical and occupational therapy in mechanically ventilated, critically ill patients: a randomized controlled trial. Lancet 2009; 373:1874-82.

13. Herridge MS, Tansey CM, Matté A, Tomlinson G, Diaz-Granados N, Cooper A, Guest CB, Mazer CD, Mehta S, Stewart TE, Kudlow P, Cook D, Slutsky AS, Cheung AM, Canadian Critical Care Trials Group. Functional disability 5 years after acute

respiratory distress syndrome. N Engl J Med 2011; 364:1293-304.

14. Roberts RJ, de Wit M, Epstein SK, Didomenico D, Devlin JW. Predictors for daily interruption of sedation therapy by nurses: a prospective, multicenter study. J Crit Care 2010; 25:660.e1-7.

15. Wilkinson DJC, Savulescu J. Knowing when to stop: futility in the ICU. Current Opinions in Anesthesiology 2011, 24:160-165.

16. Luce JM. A history of resolving conflicts over end of life care in the intensive care units in the United States. Crit Care Med 2010, 38:1623-9.

17. Grossman E, Angelos P. Futility: What Cool Hand Luke can teach the surgical community. World J Surg 2009, 33:1338-40.

17

Neonatal Respiratory ECLS

Denise M. Suttner MD, Billie L. Short MD

Introduction

Extracorporeal membrane oxygenation (ECMO) also referred to as extracorporeal life support (ECLS) has saved thousands of lives in neonates with respiratory failure. According to the Extracorporeal Life Support Organization (ELSO) registry, neonates continue to have the best survival across all patient diagnoses. Since Dr. Robert Bartlett's first reports of survival of the sickest neonates after ECMO support, several clinical studies have shown its efficacy[1-3] and it is now considered the standard of care for the newborn with respiratory failure.

Diseases Treated

The most common neonatal diseases treated with ECMO include meconium aspiration syndrome (MAS), congenital diaphragmatic hernia (CDH), idiopathic pulmonary hypertension (PPHN/PFC), sepsis, and respiratory distress syndrome (RDS). ECMO has also been used with success in less common diseases including persistent air leak syndrome, hydrops fetalis, viral pneumonia, and cardiomyopathy; these are grouped together in the "other" category.[4] The ex-utero intrapartum treatment (EXIT) to ECMO procedure has also been successfully described for complex airway anomalies.[5] Until 2002, MAS as the primary cause of hypoxic respiratory failure (HRF) was the foremost reason neonates were placed on ECMO. Treatment strategies for HRF have changed significantly over the years and so too has the ECMO data.[6] Surfactant, high frequency ventilation (HFV), and inhaled nitric oxide (iNO) have dramatically decreased the need for ECMO in many newborns. To that end, recent data shows CDH and the "other" category, which used to be the least represented, surpassing MAS as leading indications for ECMO (Figure 17-1).[4]

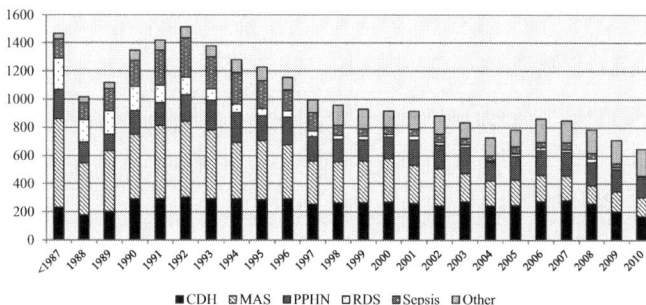

Figure 17-1. Neonatal ECLS diagnosis by year.[4]

225

Patient Selection Criteria

Indications

ECMO is considered a standard of care for infants meeting criteria as outlined in this section. ECMO therapy should be considered in term and late pre-term infants with hypoxic respiratory failure who have failed to improve with other medical therapies. Currently, the more complicated decision is the optimal time to initiate bypass: What defines "failure to improve on other medical therapies?" Three decades ago, when the ECMO pioneers developed entry criteria for the clinical trials that proved the efficacy of ECMO, the goal was to prevent patients from dying. In that era criteria for ECMO included Oxygenation Index (OI), Alveolar-arterial oxygen difference (A-aDO$_2$), and refractory hypoxia (Table 17-1).[7,8,9]

These measures were used to select the sickest neonates - those with a projected mortality of 80%. Standard medical therapy at that time included hyperventilation, hyperoxia, medically induced alkalosis, routine paralysis, and intravenous vasodilators. Over the years our knowledge and understanding of optimal medical management in newborns with respiratory failure have changed tremendously. Inhaled nitric oxide, surfactant, and HFV are used routinely, while hyperventilation, hyperoxia, and many others are now obsolete. As a result the degree-of-illness measures are difficult to translate from one epoch to another. Comparing an OI obtained on conventional ventilation to that calculated on high frequency ventilation is not necessarily accurate. Furthermore, as providers know all too well, predictors of mortality and morbidity can be institution dependent. Universal acceptance of any specific criterion for ECMO initiation is limited. One objective in instituting ECMO continues to be increased survival; however, ECMO is no longer considered merely a "last ditch effort." With improved technology and a better understanding of the risk and benefits of ECMO therapy, our rationale to cannulate is based just as much on decreasing morbidity as it is based on preventing death. Tools that predict morbidity are lacking and therefore many simply use "failure to respond to other therapies" as their indication for ECMO.

Table 17-1. Respiratory entry criteria.

AaDO$_2$[*]	>605-620mmHg[+] for 4-12hr.
Oxygenation index (OI)[□]	>35-60 for 0.5-6hr.
PaO$_2$	<60mmHg for 2-12hr.
Metabolic acidosis and shock	pH <7.25 for 2hr or with hypotension
Acute deterioration	PaO$_2$ <40mmHg

* At sea level
± Patm-47-PaCO$_2$-PaO$_2$/FiO$_2$
[□] Calculation is shown below

Beyond this, the most commonly used quantifier of disease severity for HRF remains the OI. Oxygenation Index Calculation:

$$OI = \frac{MAP \times FiO_2 \times 100}{Post\ ductal\ PaO_2}$$

MAP = (Mean Airway Pressure)

The initial trials used an OI ≥ 40 as enrollment criteria. Presently most centers still use an OI range of 40-45 as an indication for ECMO therapy. Schumacher et al. documented that patients who received ECMO when the OI was >25 but <40 had shorter and less costly hospital stays with a trend toward improved outcome. This study contained small numbers of patients and will eventually need repeating in a larger trial, but the results do indicate that earlier cannulation may reduce morbidity.[10] Radhakrishnan et al. compared the morbidity of patients with MAS with that in patients with all other respiratory conditions treated with ECMO (no-MAS). Data from the ELSO registry from 1989 to 2004 was utilized. Overall, MAS patients had a significantly higher survival rate and a significantly lower number of complications per patient in each category compared to the no-MAS patient. This information supports the consideration of relaxed ECMO entry criteria for the MAS patient. Grist et al. reviewed neonatal patients to determine if later cannulation correlated with increased mortality. Elevated CO_2 gradient, anion gap, and Viability Index [AGc + p(v-a)CO_2] correlated with a significantly higher risk of mortality (P < .05). The authors concluded that starting ECMO too late may cause reperfusion injury that reduces survival.[11] Because there is data to suggest improved outcome with earlier initiation of ECMO, it is recommended that any neonate requiring standard medical therapy with an OI of 25 should be cared for in an ECMO center, where timely initiation of ECMO can occur if the patient's condition deteriorates. Therapeutic options such as surfactant and iNO have certainly decreased the need for ECMO support in neonates with respiratory failure as witnessed by the sharp decline in neonatal respiratory numbers (Figure 17-2).[4,6,12] There is no question that in this patient population the need for ECMO is less; however, in 2010 almost 600 infants required ECLS because they failed other

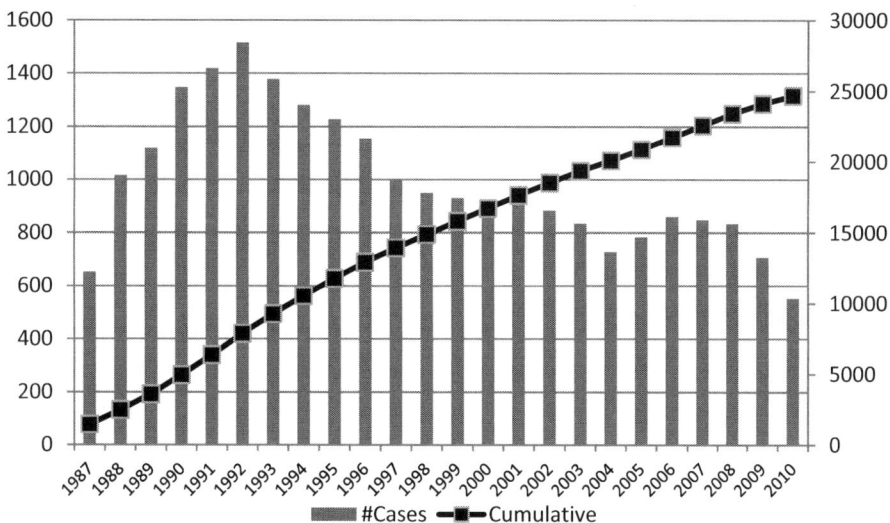

Figure 17-2. Annual and cumulative neonatal respiratory ECLS cases.[4]

therapeutic strategies.[4] While patients should be given the opportunity to respond to less invasive therapies, delaying ECMO cannulation is unacceptable. Regional ECMO centers should work with the non-ECMO centers in their area to establish a standard protocol regarding transfer criteria in order to prevent untimely delays.

The Pre-ECMO Evaluation

There are some patients with additional pathology who should not be considered for ECLS regardless of the degree of respiratory failure. Examples of patients in this category include those with lethal chromosomal disorders (such as Trisomy 13 or Trisomy 18), severe pre-existing brain damage, or with significant intracranial hemorrhage (Grade III or IV). Patients who were born with or who have developed other irreversible organ injury are ineligible for ECMO unless they are being considered for transplant. Even with progress, ECMO remains a high risk and resource intense intervention; it should only be utilized in those patients with a high likelihood of a meaningful survival. Pre-ECMO review of the history and physical and appropriate testing and consultation (if feasible) should be done prior to cannulation when major contraindications are of concern.

The Pre-ECMO Evaluation for Neonatal Respiratory Failure:

- Review of prenatal and delivery history
- Complete physical examination
- Chest and abdominal radiographs
- CBC, differential, platelet count
- Basic serum electrolytes with BUN and creatinine
- Renal ultrasound (if labs or prenatal history suggest renal disease)
- Coagulation factors (PT, PTT, Fibrinogen)
- Cranial ultrasound
- Cardiac ECHO
- Neurologic evaluation

Contraindications

Absolute
- Lethal malformations or lethal congenital anomalies
- Severe irreversible brain damage
- Grade III or greater intracranial hemorrhage (ICH)

Relative
- Birth weight < 1.6 kg
- Gestational age < 34 weeks
- Irreversible organ damage (unless considered for organ transplant)
- Disease states with a high probability of a poor prognosis
- Ventilation with 100% oxygen for ≥14 days

When there is concern about the appropriateness of ECLS, the specific issues should be discussed with the relevant medical subspecialists prior to cannulation. This allows an in-depth discussion about the risks of the procedure (including the risk of using valuable resources) versus the potential benefits. As ECMO therapy has become refined, with less risk and more data on outcome, it is less clear which neonates should be not be considered candidates for ECMO. Historically published absolute contraindications are now considered relative contraindications. Chapman et al. performed a cross-sectional study using a data collection survey to evaluate differences in practice related to ECMO criteria.[13] The lowest birth weight and gestational age at which respondents would consider placing a neonate on ECMO were frequently below recommended thresholds. There was wide variability in respondents' willingness to place neonates on ECMO in the presence of conditions such as intraventricular hemorrhage and hypoxic ischemic encephalopathy. The number of respondents who would never seek to override parental refusal of ECMO was equal to the number who would always do so.[13] This apparent confusion is more likely the product of more experience in ECLS, advancement in capabilities, and an increasingly complex patient population. Ultimately each patient should be evaluated individually, by a team of caregivers whose decision is solely based on what is in the patient's best interest.

Weight < 2 kg

For the past three decades, weight < 2kg has been at least a relative contraindication to ECMO. Despite years of experience, there remains debate regarding the lowest weight acceptable for cannulation. In other words, "How low really is too low for ECMO?" In 1999 Hardart found that weight was not an independent factor for developing ICH as was previously believed.[14] In 2004 Rozmierek et al. hypothesized that ECMO was effective and safe in babies under 2 kg and sought to examine outcome. All patients less than 30 days old in the ELSO registry (n = 14,305) were divided into those less than 2 kg (n = 663) and those more than 2 kg (n = 13,642). Multiple regression analysis determined factors that predicted survival rate and the lowest safe weight for ECMO. Overall survival rate lower in infants < 2 kg compared to infants ≥ 2 kg (53% versus 77%, P <.0001). Survival was significantly lower for patients with diaphragmatic hernia (CDH), bleeding, and ICH. In contrast to the findings by Hardart, the incidence of ICH was increased in babies < 2 kg (6% versus 4%, P <.05). Regression analysis determined that the lowest weight at which a survival rate of 40% could be achieved was 1.6 kg.[15] Forty percent survival is similar to that seen in patients with congenital heart disease that require ECMO. Cardiac surgery using cardiopulmonary bypass is now being done in patients less than 2 kg with encouraging results.[16]

For neck cannulations, cannula size may be a limiting factor, although 8Fr catheters may be sufficient for this population. The use of the smallest commercially available venous cannula (6Fr) and a small IV catheter have been reported. Venovenous ECLS support in patients < 2 kg is currently not an option since the smallest dual-lumen VV cannula available is only 12Fr. One must weigh the hazards of VA ECMO especially in what would surely be considered a high risk patient. Although technically feasible, with limited long-term follow up on patients < 2 kg, the question remains when it is the right thing to do. What we currently know is that in patients <1.6 kg traditional ECMO is not an option and that in patients > 2 kg it can be lifesaving. More investigation, particularly with regard to long-term developmental followup, is needed in the 1.6 to 2 kg population before it will become widely used in these patients.

Gestational age < 34 wks

Because of limited data and several testimonials, some centers feel comfortable providing ECMO to infants < 34 weeks if they are deemed "good candidates." At the time of this publication, a relative contraindication of <34 weeks is still universally recognized. The reason for refusing ECMO support to a premature infant is based on previous studies that have established a strong correlation between gestational age (GA) and intracranial hemorrhage (ICH). The idea of artificial cardiorespiratory support for the premature infant has been around for a half century. In the mid 1960s, ECMO was used as an "artificial placenta" in a group of premature infants.[17] Sufficient cardiorespiratory support was achieved; however, all infants died secondary to ICH. The same results occurred in the initial trials of ECMO. During the early years of clinical research on neonatal ECMO, 16 premature infants of less than 35 weeks gestational age were treated by Bartlett et al. and only four (25%) survived.[18] Intracranial hemorrhage occurred in 100% of the premature infants, prompting the authors to recommend that ECMO not be used in premature infants with respiratory failure.

The primary reason for refusing ECMO to a premature infant today is still based on the increased incidence of ICH identified in these initial trials. However, ECMO management has changed dramatically over time. To help understand the incidence of ICH in premature infants on ECMO, the records of those early cases were reviewed in detail. The findings were quite revealing: of the 16 patients, four had pre-ECMO conditions that would now be considered contraindications and five of the remaining patients had major technical complications that have become rare. Optimal anticoagulation was undefined and several of these premature infants had activated clotting times >700 seconds. The authors suggested that due to changes in practice, a survival of 50% or greater would likely be achieved using newer strategies.[19] As further proof of progress, a review of the ELSO data base from 1988 to 1991 showed a dramatic decrease in the rate of ICH and death compared to a decade earlier. During this period there was a 37% incidence of ICH in patients 32-35 weeks gestation compared to 100% as first reported.[20] Hardart also reviewed the ELSO registry for ICH rates in patients ≤ 37 weeks from 1992 to 2000. In this study, GA did not predict ICH unless combined with post-natal age (PNA) to calculate postconceptional age (PCA). Twenty-six percent of patients ≤32 weeks PCA developed ICH as compared with 6% of patients with PCA of 38 weeks (P .004).[21] More recently, a review of 21,218 neonatal ECMO runs in the ELSO registry from 1986 to 2006 evaluated the association between GA and outcome. Infants were divided into three groups: Late Preterm (LPT = 34 0/7 to 36 6/7 weeks), Early Term (ET = 37 0/7 to 38 6/7 weeks), and Full Term (FT = 39 0/7 to 42 6/7 weeks). Neonates with CDH, other major congenital defects or syndromes, or missing data were excluded, leaving 14,528 neonatal ECMO patients which met inclusion criteria. Late preterm infants experienced the highest mortality on ECMO (LP 26.2%, ET 18%, FT 11.2; P <0.001) and had longer ECMO runs. They also had higher rates of ICH (LP 12.3%, ET 7.6%, FT 3.6; P <0.0001) and other neurological complications on ECMO. Furthermore, they experienced increased mechanical, metabolic, and infectious complications on ECMO. The authors conclude that late preterm infants had poorer outcomes on ECMO than their more mature counterparts, underscoring their developmental immaturity and vulnerability.[22] Effective treatment of respiratory failure in premature infants remains an unsolved problem. Despite significant advances, given the complication rate in the more premature population, alterations in traditional ECMO may still be necessary before acceptance in patients <34 weeks gestation is universal. The development of an artificial placenta that maintains fetal circulation without systemic anticoagulation is the most appealing alternative.[23]

Intracranial hemorrhage

Grade III or IV ICH can be detected by head ultrasound. Patients with this degree of hemorrhage should not be offered ECMO because of the associated poor long-term prognosis.[24] This degree of hemorrhage is also likely to expand with exposure to the anticoagulated ECMO blood, further compromising the neurologic prognosis. Patients with pre-ECMO grade I or II ICH have been successfully managed on ECMO without extension of hemorrhage. Even in this less severe situation, diligent monitoring of clotting factors, platelets, bleeding times, anticoagulation, and imaging is required.

Irreversible organ damage

Although patients with irreversible organ damage should not be offered ECMO unless they are eligible for transplantation, determination of irreversibility of organ function can be difficult. If time permits, appropriate testing should be done to document underlying irreversible conditions prior to instituting ECMO. An example is a patient with respiratory failure and severe renal dysfunction evidenced by oliguria and elevated creatinine. A renal ultrasound prior to cannulation can help determine if the patient has renal agenesis leading to severely hypoplastic lungs, who therefore should not be offered ECMO.

One of the more difficult evaluations to perform prior to ECMO is a thorough neurologic evaluation, making it difficult to determine irreversible brain injury. Initial head ultrasounds can usually be obtained quickly, but may appear normal even in the face of significant ischemic injury. When time allows, imaging with MRI or CT combined with an EEG may prove more definitive.[25] Exclusive of grade III or IV ICH, there are no clear measurements that define how severe the damage must be in order to exclude an infant from receiving ECMO. Therefore, pre-ECMO evaluations to determine irreversibility of the organ damage, whether it be the brain or another organ, are not always available or precise enough to determine criteria for ECMO, i.e., denial of ECMO therapy. It is quite common and acceptable to proceed with ECLS support in cases where preexisting contraindications may exist, but cannot be confirmed. In these circumstances reevaluation and discussions on options with the parents should occur shortly after cannulation. If ECLS support is not in the patient's best interest, it should be discontinued.

Chromosomal abnormalities

Patients with physical findings suggestive of Trisomy 13, Trisomy 18, or other lethal syndrome should have a pre-ECMO dysmorphology evaluation if time allows. In those situations where time does not allow for a definitive diagnosis, the decision to initiate ECLS may be valid. However, once the diagnosis is confirmed most proceed with a discussion with the family about withdrawal of support.

Modes of neonatal ECMO

Neonates with respiratory failure that are candidates for ECMO can be supported with venovenous (VV) ECMO or venoarterial (VA) ECMO. In both, vascular access is achieved by cannulation of the neck. VA ECMO support requires one cannula in the internal carotid artery and one in the internal jugular vein. Newborns on VV ECMO are usually supported with one dual-lumen cannula placed in the internal jugular vein (IJ). VV ECMO is the preferred choice for most patients for several reasons; the biggest motivation is avoidance of carotid artery ligation. In pediatric and adult patients, more providers are using the less invasive percutaneous or semi-Seldinger techniques for cannula placement.[26] Because of the small vessel size in neonates, an open surgical technique is used to place the arterial cannula. In many institutions, the single venous or dual-lumen cannulae is also placed by this method. However, the semi-Seldinger procedure is preferred by some for venous insertion.[27] This involves exposure of the internal jugular vein, but does not require ligation of the vessel. The modified Seldinger method allows for a less complex cannulation, but with the potential for more risk given the small vessel size and location. Percutaneous access for VV ECMO in the neonatal population has also been described[28] but is not routinely performed.

Morbidity and mortality related to intracranial injury is significant for neonates on ECMO. Ligation of the internal jugular has been identified as a potential contributor to this injury through a mechanism of cerebral congestion and hypertension.[29] A cephalad cannula can be placed in the proximal IJ to decrease venous congestion. This cannula has the added benefits of improving venous drainage and decreasing the recirculation that occurs on VV ECMO. Cannulas placed in this position should be the largest possible to maximize drainage and decrease stasis. Although beneficial in theory, there is no clear evidence that neurologic outcomes differ because of cephalad drainage. A review of the ELSO registry data did not demonstrate significant differences in neonatal outcome or complication rates in those infants on VV ECMO with or without a cephalad catheter.[30]

VV ECMO

For neonatal VV ECMO a single double lumen venovenous cannula (DLVV) is inserted into the internal jugular vein.[31] There are several advantages to VV ECMO compared to VA ECMO and therefore it is the preferred mode of ECLS support in newborns with respiratory failure. The most critical are the potential benefits to the brain. As mentioned above, in VV ECMO ligation of the carotid artery is not required. VV ECMO, unlike VA ECMO, does not decrease cerebral blood flow velocities[32,33] or decrease cerebral oxygenation as noted during right carotid cannulation.[34,35,36]

Pre-ECMO patients are hypoxic and often poorly perfused making them particularly susceptible for reperfusion injury on initiation of VA ECMO. Hyperoxic reperfusion can promote inflammation and neuronal cell death[37] and hypocarbia decreases cerebral perfusion.[38] Hyperoxic and hypocarbic reperfusion are greater risks with VA ECMO compared to VV. On VA ECMO blood entering the cerebral circulation is under higher pressure, increasing the risk for reperfusion injury. For this reason extra attention must be paid to the post membrane arterial blood which will return directly into the systemic circulation. Prior to initiating ECMO, circuit blood should be ventilated and oxygenated. However, the membrane is very efficient; the blood can easily be over-oxygenated and hyperventilated. In an attempt to limit reperfusion injury and optimize perfusion to the brain, careful monitoring of sweep flow and FiO_2 is necessary. On initiation of ECMO, the flow rate in VA ECMO is gradually increased to avoid

immediate high pressure cerebral circulation. These problems are less of a threat on VV ECMO because the pump-arterial blood returns to the venous circulation, is mixed with venous blood, and only then is distributed to the lungs and body by the patient's own cardiac output. Short et al. has shown increased cerebral autoregulation impairment in an animal model after exposure to VA compared to VV ECMO[39,40] suggesting increased cerebral vulnerability using this mode. Further studies have shown that the altered cerebrovascular responses in vessels exposed to VA ECMO seem to be mediated through the nitric oxide pathway.[41] Perfusing highly oxygenated blood under high pressure into the cerebral circulation of a patient with impaired cerebral autoregulation increases the risk of reperfusion injury. The central nervous system is also better protected against possible blood clots or air emboli arising from the ECMO circuit on VV ECMO, because they are initially directed through the pulmonary rather than the systemic and cerebral circulations. These differences make VV ECMO a better choice for ECLS support in this critically ill patient population. Yet it is important to state that despite concerns about VA ECMO, there is no profound evidence that survival or neurologic outcome is improved by using VV.[42]

There are several additional advantages to VV ECMO: return of pump-arterial blood to the right side of the heart, elimination of increased afterload, maintenance of normal pulsatile blood flow, and safer weaning of circuit blood flow.

1. Return of pump-arterial blood to the right side of the heart is optimal for two main reasons. As described previously, if a blood clot or air embolus escapes the pump safety guards and is infused into the patient, the result could be catastrophic if it lodges directly in the coronary or cerebral circulation. With the patient on VV ECMO, the embolus would be injected into the right atrium

and filtered out by the pulmonary circulation. If right to left shunt physiology exists, of course, the embolus could still flow directly into the systemic circulation on VV ECMO with an equally devastating outcome as would occur on VA ECMO. Returning pump-arterial blood to the right side of the heart is additionally beneficial because the oxygenated blood mixes with the venous, improving the oxygen content of the blood returning to the pulmonary circulation and to the left heart. This could help decrease pulmonary vascular resistance and right ventricular afterload and also improves coronary artery oxygenation delivery which comes from the left ventricle. In a piglet model, Golej et al. found increased pro-inflammatory and decreased anti-inflammatory interleukins in the bronchoalveolar lavage fluid of VA ECMO animals compared to VV ECMO suggesting that the VA modality of ECMO leads to a more pronounced inflammatory reaction of the lung.

2. Decreased cardiac afterload is another example of how VV ECMO is advantageous. In VA ECMO the return of pump blood directly into the aorta increases afterload, which can hinder the recovery of cardiac function. By the nature of its circulation, VA ECMO support decreases preload and increases afterload. This physiology can contribute to the impaired cardiac function, sometimes referred to as "cardiac stun." This dilemma is eliminated by supporting the patient with VV ECMO.

3. Normal pulsatile flow is maintained on VV ECMO because cardiac output is completely dependent on the patient's intrinsic heart function. When compared to non-pulsatile flow, pulsatile flow decreases vascular resistance, decreases afterload, and improves organ perfusion. Renal blood flow is reported to be improved with pulsatile flow as well. However, experimental animal studies show comparable effects of VV and VA support on blood pressure, renal blood flow, and plasma renin activity.[43]

4. Lastly, weaning on VV ECMO is safer, requires less monitoring, and needs less interventions than VA (see below).

There are disadvantages to VV ECMO, but these are usually manageable. As there is no cardiac support with VV ECMO, there was initially a concern that a pre-ECMO requirement for high inotropic support mandated VA ECMO. It is now known that there is no specific level of inotropic medication that precludes VV ECMO for respiratory failure.[44] In fact, after initiation of VV ECMO, cardiac function has been shown to improve; inotropic support can typically be weaned to low dose and often is successfully discontinued.[45] A legitimate disadvantage to VV ECMO is the technical difficulty placing the dual-lumen cannula in small patients (< 2.5 kg) or in those with very small jugular veins. Finally, the neonate on VV ECMO will have a lower arterial oxygen saturation compared to a patient on VA ECMO. Since the arterial blood returns to the right atrium, there will be obligatory mixing of the oxygenated blood with the desaturated venous blood even with perfect cannula position. Adequate arterial oxygen saturations (SaO_2) in neonates on VV ECMO are $\geq 80\%$. In situations where the SaO_2 is < 92%, oxygen content is maintained by optimizing the hemoglobin. Resolution of metabolic acidosis, normal hemodynamics, and normal lactate are data measures reassuring the caregiver that adequate tissue oxygen delivery is being achieved.

Comparing mode of respiratory support over time, it is clear that VV ECMO is becoming more widely used. However, despite data and years of experience to support VV ECMO as the first mode to consider in all neonates with hypoxic respiratory failure, the ELSO registry data shows that many centers still primarily use VA (Figure 17-3).[4]

VA ECMO

Although VV ECMO is preferred for neonatal respiratory failure, there are some circumstances where VA ECMO is the only possibility. In neonates with primary cardiac failure as the indication for ECMO, VA ECMO is used because the arterial circulation is directly augmented by the pump. Secondary cardiac failure from profound respiratory failure can occur and some elect VA ECMO in these situations. However as previously discussed, there is no amount of pre-ECMO inotropic support that mandates VA ECMO. Other candidates for VA ECMO would include those who are too small for the smallest double lumen cannula (currently 12Fr). Finally, the issue of recirculation, which occurs on VV ECMO because of the single cannula flow dynamics, is eliminated when VA ECLS is utilized. Proper cannula positioning will diminish recirculation, so this benefit alone should not be used as a primary justification for choosing VA.

Unique to VA ECMO is the placement of a cannula into the internal carotid artery. After the patient is weaned off ECMO and ready for decannulation, both cannulas are surgically removed. Carotid reconstruction is performed in some centers.[49] Given the concern for long-term complications and the lack of conclusive evidence, most institutions do not routinely reconstruct the carotid artery.[48]

ECMO details

The neonatal ECMO team

All ECMO teams require a multidisciplinary group. In the case of neonates, this group is highly specialized and experienced in the care of critically ill newborns.

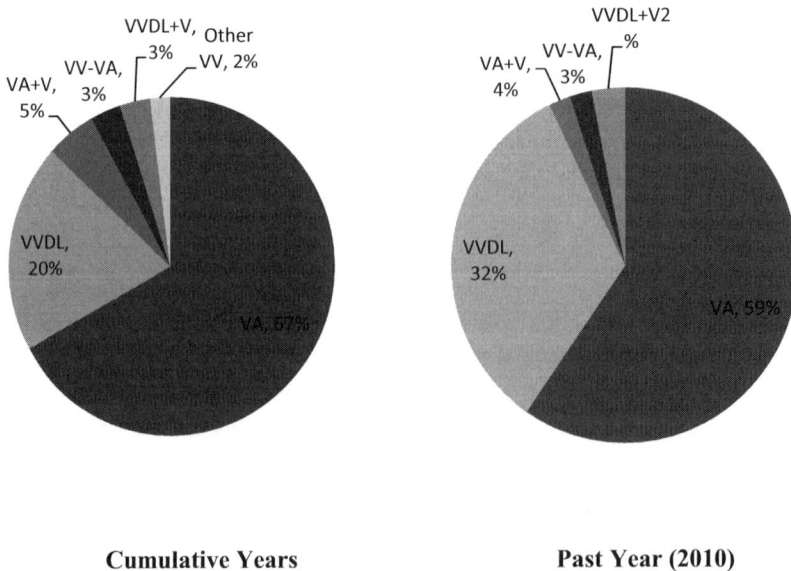

Cumulative Years   **Past Year (2010)**

Figure 17-3. Mode of ECMO support. VA= venoarterial; VVDL = venovenous dual lumen; VA+V=venoarterial + cephalad;VV-VA = venovenous converted to venoarterial.

Instituting pump flow

Even with careful technique, primed blood is often hypocarbic and hyperoxic as previously stated. Once the cannulas are placed and connected, the pump flow should be initiated at around 20 ml/kg/min and increased gradually over 5 to 10 minutes in order to achieve adequate oxygen delivery, while minimizing the risk of reperfusion injury. A monitoring device is placed on the venous tubing in order to determine adequate pump flow. On VA ECMO, pump flow is increased to achieve a venous saturation of 70 to 80%. On VV ECMO, pump flow is increased to the desirable patient oxygen saturation, usually $\geq$ 85%. In neonates with respiratory failure, adequate oxygen delivery is usually obtained with pump flows of 100 to 150 ml/kg/min.

Volume replacement

Volume replacement may be necessary when the patient initially goes on ECMO. Platelets are transfused just after initiation of flow to replace the loss due to dilution by the primed circuit. In some centers, plasma is transfused as part of the prime volume. In others, plasma is given only for documented coagulation derangements. After the initial stabilization period, volume replacement should be minimal and primarily given only to correct ECMO related anemia and thrombocytopenia. The obvious exception is septic shock, where capillary leak makes it impossible to maintain intravascular volume without fluid replacement. If volume transfusion is necessary to maintain pump flow, other causes of poor venous drainage must be excluded. A malpositioned, kinked, or inappropriately sized venous cannula needs to be repaired or replaced.

Management during ECLS

Fluids

Typical fluid management for the newborn infant can be used, starting with 80 ml/kg/day, increasing to 120 to 130 ml/kg/day over the first 4-5 days of the run. It is common to see lower sodium (0-2 meq/kg/day) and higher potassium (3-5 meq/kg/day) requirements than usual. During ECMO it is common to see a decrease in urine output that may be associated with acute renal failure. In most cases, urine output improves 12 to 24 hours after initiation of ECMO. Some centers routinely use diuretics to enhance diuresis, whereas others use diuretics only in cases where fluid overload is a problem. In patients who have had significant pre-ECMO hypoxia and hypoperfusion, renal insufficiency may persist for several days. Continuous renal replacement therapy (CRRT) should be considered if progressive fluid overload and electrolyte imbalance occur. The details of fluid management are fully presented in Chapter 13.

Nutrition

Neonates are born with very limited reserves and require close attention to nutritional support to enhance their growth and recovery. When neonates are sick enough to require ECMO, optimal weight gain is difficult to achieve due to their underlying illness and relative fluid intolerance. Critically ill neonates have relatively higher nutritional requirements, which makes early institution of nutritional support especially important.[47, 48] In patients on ECMO, this is generally provided via total parental nutrition (TPN) to allow for the rapid attainment of metabolic stabilization and adequate nutrition in the context of severe cardiorespiratory failure. Advancing TPN per normal newborn protocols is the routine. Enteral feeds are usually avoided because of concerns of splanchnic hypoperfusion and the risk of increasing intestinal ischemia or bacterial translocation. Large-scale studies have not been performed on the preferred route of nutrition in this specific patient population. When gastrointestinal function is normal and the patient is clinically stable, enteral nutrition (EN) is preferable to TPN in critically ill patients for a variety of reasons.[49] Enteral nutrition plays an important role in the maintenance of gut mucosal integrity and has been associated with improved gastrointestinal immunologic function and reduced septic morbidity, in both adults and children.[50,51,52] Hanekamp et al. retrospectively reviewed the feasibility and tolerance of routine enteral nutrition in neonates on VA ECMO over a five year period (January 1997 to January 2002). Feasibility was evaluated by recording the time needed for enteral nutrition to reach 40% of total fluid intake; tolerance was evaluated by reviewing data on enteral nutrition related morbidity. Sixty-seven of the 77 eligible patients received enteral feeding during ECMO. Thirty-six of these patients (54%) received 40% of total fluid intake as enteral nutrition within a median of three (range 2 - 4) days. Over the years there was a trend toward an increasing usage of enteral nutrition from 71% to 94% (P=.07). Enteral nutrition was temporarily discontinued in 16 patients, with 14 showing gastric retentions, one showing discomfort, and one showing aspiration. Symptoms of bilious vomiting, bloodstained stool, or abdominal distention were not present.[53] Despite some evidence for tolerance and benefit, there are animal studies that indicated decreased gut perfusion while on ECMO. If enteral feeds are done, close monitoring of feeding tolerance should be done to pick up any early signs of necrotizing enterocolitis.[54]

Ventilator management

Whether the patient is on VV or VA ECMO, the ventilator should be managed at low settings to allow lung rest and minimize ongoing lung injury. A common mistake is to try to recruit lung volume early in ECLS run during the acute inflammatory stage. Typical rest settings for a neonate on ECLS are PIP (15-22), PEEP (5-12), rate (12-20), and inspiratory time (0.5sec). Using low PEEP may lead to alveolar collapse and increased edema.[55] If the PEEP is set too high, venous return and hemodynamics may be impaired, which may be even more significant in patients with primary cardiac failure as the indication for ECMO.

Air Leak

Neonates with respiratory failure often have persistent air leak prior to ECMO and some patients will develop air leak while on ECMO. In both situations, it will usually resolve with decreasing ventilation. Ventilator settings should be decreased until no active air leak is visualized. This often means low CPAP settings or even "capping-off" the ETT for some period of time. Reexpanding the collapsed lung should be done gently over 24 to 48 hours depending on the severity of the air leak and may be best accomplished with HFV.

Cardiac Support

Critically ill newborns placed on ECLS are often on high doses of inotropic medications when ECLS is begun. As these drugs are titrated down, resistance falls and systemic pressure may also decrease. Although the mean arterial pressure may seem low, systemic perfusion may be completely adequate. In cases where the perfusion pressure is inadequate (low urine output, poor perfusion, elevated lactate, metabolic acidosis, low SvO_2) it can be improved by increasing pump flow, administrating blood transfusions, or adding inotropic medications. Patients on VV ECMO, who are completely dependent on their intrinsic cardiac function, may benefit from continued low dose inotropic medication. According to the ELSO registry, 19.7% of all patients receive some form of inotropic medication while on ECMO.[4] If a cephalad catheter is used in VV ECMO, saturation monitoring can be helpful to determine if cerebral perfusion (cerebral saturations $\geq 60\%$) is being maintained. Some centers use a cerebral saturation value of less than 55% as an indication to convert to VA ECMO. If extra blood volume is required to provide the extra flow and therefore oxygen delivery, it is preferable to transfuse blood or blood products rather than adding more crystalloid solution if the hematocrit is less than 40.

Hematology

Neonates are unique in their coagulation deficits, making an increased risk for bleeding a particular concern. Pre-ECMO coagulation studies should include platelet count, PT/PTT, and fibrinogen level, along with a baseline activated clotting time (ACT). Any abnormal levels should be investigated for cause, and attempts to correct prior to ECMO should be done with platelet, fresh frozen plasma, or cryoprecipitate transfusions. After initiation of ECMO it is common to require platelet transfusions within the first few hours and then once or twice per day. Some centers use thrombelastography (TEG) measurement to determine coagulation replacement needs. TEG as a method of assessing global hemostatic and fibrinolytic function has existed for some time and improved technology has led to increased usage. This is a relatively new technology for ECMO and its full use in this arena has not been determined.[47] The patient must remain systemically heparinized during the ECMO course. The activated clotting time (ACT) is the most commonly used and easiest bedside measure of whole blood clotting (see Chapter 11).

Infection control

Most centers use prophylactic antibiotics in their ECMO patients with the assumption that these will prevent nosocomial infections. This approach remains controversial and would require a multicenter trial to determine efficacy or risk associated with not using prophylactic antibiotics (see Chapter 14).

Neurology

Seizures, CNS infarction, and CNS hemorrhage are major complications reported in ECMO–treated neonates. There are multiple factors that have been implicated in the increased risk of intracranial injury in this patient population. The challenge is that the cause is almost certainly multifactorial and both pre-ECMO and on-ECMO events may contribute. The blood brain barrier in this age group is altered by ischemia, decreased perfusion, and acidosis, all common pre-ECMO events.[57] In a series by Hardart, gestational age, sepsis, acidosis, and coagulopathy were all associated with a higher incidence of ICH.[14,21] Using near infrared spectrophotometry, Liem et al. demonstrated changes on ECMO including increased cerebral blood volume, loss of autoregulation, reactive hyperperfusion, and hemodilution[58] all of which could increase the risk of ICH. Unstable ACTs, low platelet count, elevated pre-ECMO lactate are other factors that have been statistically associated with an increase in the development of ICH.[59,60,61] Diligent monitoring and treatment of clotting abnormalities and thrombocytopenia may decrease the risk associated with on-ECMO events.

Management: Even without ICH, the neonate on ECMO is at risk for neurologic injury and impaired neurodevelopmental outcome. The pre-ECMO patient is hypoxemic and often acidemic and hypotensive; these conditions can lead to encephalopathy and potentially permanent brain injury. Hypoxic ischemic encephalopathy (HIE) is a persistent challenge in the care of neonates. Hypothermia is the only therapy that has been shown to significantly impact neurodevelopmental outcome in this patient population.[62] Hypothermia is associated with a wide range of physiologic changes affecting every organ system, including an increased tendency for bleeding. Fortunately, lack of serious adverse effects of moderate hypothermia therapy in term and near-term newborns with moderate to severe hypoxic ischemic encephalopathy has been shown in several trials.[63] Therefore, it seems logical to apply the same treatment to newborns with respiratory failure that require ECMO. A small number of infants with HIE who were being cooled developed severe PPHN and subsequently required ECMO.[64] The NEST trial is an ongoing multicenter randomized controlled study in the United Kingdom designed to test whether cooling to 34°C for the first 48 to 72 hours on ECMO leads to subsequent improvement in health status.

Monitoring: On-ECMO neurologic complications are a particular concern in this patient population. Detecting intracranial hemorrhage and seizures as soon as they occur is critical, as interventions may be possible and may improve outcome. This is often difficult given levels of sedation and the limited capability of current monitoring devices. Bleeding into the head or brain parenchyma, which can be extensive and fatal, is the most serious ECLS complication. Head ultrasounds (HUS) are easily performed at the bedside and can usually detect intracranial bleeding. They should be performed every 24 hours for at least the first three days in stable neonates[65] on ECLS and then per institution protocol. If the patient is unstable from a hemodynamic or coagulation standpoint, daily HUS should be considered. If bleeding is detected, the degree of bleeding will guide therapy. For a small bleed, coagulation status should be optimized and repeat HUS should be performed twice per day to detect any extension. For

extending bleeds, or bleeds that are moderate to large, the patient should be weaned from ECMO as quickly as possible. For severe ICH withdrawal of ECLS is indicated because of the poor neurologic prognosis.

Apart from easily detected ICH, identifying cerebral injury and interpreting the importance of the injury in these critically ill newborns is difficult. However, compared to years past, better devices do exist. Noninvasive cerebral oximetry has moved from the research laboratory into clinical settings. Cerebral oximetry saturations have been shown to correlate with actual cerebral venous saturation in patients on VV ECMO, suggesting cerebral oximetry as a means to monitor brain oxygenation.[66] Fenik demonstrated utility using this modality compared to arterial oxygen saturation (SpO_2) to detect low cerebral oxygenation events in pre-ECMO and ECMO patients.[67] The technique is safe, but there is a wide range of values considered to be normal and developmental outcome data in this population is lacking. Significant abnormalities obtained by electroencephalogram (EEG) can be helpful in diagnosing neurologic injury.[68] Continuous bedside EEGs are more commonly used in neonatal ICUs and in combination with other measures are often useful. CT has been shown to be superior to HUS in detecting ICH and should be considered in situations where HUS is likely to have underestimated the degree of hemorrhage. Until recently, obtaining a CT scan meant moving the patient and ECMO circuit to the radiology suite. This is resource intensive and has some inherent danger to the patient, although it has frequently been done. Portable CT scanners are now available and eliminate many of the problems associated with moving the ECMO patient to the CT suite. In most cases, prognosticating neurologic injury requires several data points. Repeated measures that suggest a poor neurologic outcome are grounds for discontinuing ECMO, sparing the family and medical providers a prolonged intensive care course leading to a tragic outcome.

Sedation

Neonates on ECLS can usually be successfully managed with light sedation, typically a prn narcotic +/- a benzodiazepine. Paralysis and high dose continuous narcotic infusions should be reserved for the rare ECLS patient such as a newborn with CDH that has significant intestinal distension from swallowed air. Neuroprotective agents in neonates with hypoxic-ischemic encephalopathy have failed to prove beneficial. However, encouraging data has been shown with the use of hypothermia in this patient population as previously described.

Weaning

Newborns with respiratory failure are ready for a weaning trial once there is adequate pulmonary recovery. Beyond this vague description, no absolute weaning criteria exist. The ECMO clinician considers several factors in reaching this conclusion, including at least moderate resolution of the underlying disease process. Evidence of recovery includes: improved chest radiograph and lung compliance, stable hemodynamics on minimal inotropes, and resolution of capillary leak. Further reassurance that the disease process is resolving is improved patient SaO_2 on VV ECMO and SvO_2 on VA ECMO.

On VA ECMO weaning involves the gradual decrease in ECMO flow over a period of time until idle flow is reached ($\sim$10-20 ml/kg/min). As the flow is decreased there is an increased chance of clot formation; measures of anticoagulation should be performed more frequently and ACT levels should be increased. The ventilator must also be adjusted as more blood is circulated through the patient's lungs. During the period of weaning, vital signs, pulse oximetry, and blood gases need to be carefully monitored. Idle flow can be maintained for several hours if necessary to ensure the infant is tolerating minimal support. At this point some institutions advocate a "trial-off" ECMO with-

out actually removing the cannulas. The cannulas are clamped and blood gases are checked to ensure the infant is ready to decannulate. This "trial off" usually lasts no more than two hours and frequently the necessary information is obtained within an hour. During this time, there are several important considerations. Pump flow, which is now isolated from the patient, is increased to 150-200 ml/min to diminish clot formation. Sweep gas must be removed from the circuit to prevent air extravasation. For trials lasting more than 15 minutes, the heparin drip is moved from the circuit to the patient. The cannulas must be unclamped briefly (flashed) every 10 to 15 minutes. Vital signs, ACTs, and blood gases are obtained every 15 minutes. Other centers have had success avoiding this "trial-off" step in neonates with respiratory failure whose ECMO course has been straight forward. A 4 to 6 hour idling period with good blood gases usually indicates that the patient will successfully come off ECMO. Risks associated with a "trial-off" are related to the cannula being clamped off with no flow. Stagnant blood has a high likelihood of forming clots, which could be dislodged into the circulation while flashing the cannulas. As a result it is advantageous to avoid the trial off period on VA ECMO if at all possible.

In VV ECMO weaning is more straightforward. Pump flow is gradually weaned over several hours to a minimum of $\sim$200 ml/min. Oxygen to the membrane is weaned to room air and then the sweep gas is gradually weaned off completely. A "trial-off" is then completed by "capping off" the membrane. Because the membrane is very efficient, the inlet and outlet gas ports both need to be covered or capped to prevent any air entry. Because no direct circulatory support is provided by VV ECMO, this maneuver is equivalent to a complete "trial-off" ECMO. Once the membrane is completely capped, it is no longer helping with oxygenation or ventilation; venous blood is simply circulating on the right side of the heart. During this period, vital signs, pulse oximetry, and serial blood gases are obtained; similar to measures taken during a "trial-off" in VA ECMO. If the data is reassuring, the patient is considered ready for decannulation. Since it is not necessary to wean the pump flow below 200 ml/min on VV ECMO, there is no need to increase the ACTs or clamp off the cannulas at any point. This minimizes the risk of bleeding and clot formation and allows for an extended evaluation "off ECMO" prior to actual decannulation.

Procedures

Procedures on ECMO-treated newborns are sometimes necessary, making consideration of benefit versus risk critical. Refer to Chapter 15 for on-ECMO procedure details. The EXIT to ECMO procedure is unique to neonates and therefore is discussed briefly.

EXIT procedure

Due to anticipated respiratory or cardiac failure, some in-utero diagnosis predict an almost certain need for ECMO. In these situations the ex-utero intrapartum treatment (EXIT) procedure has been used to transition the fetus to extracorporeal support while still receiving placental support. In utero diagnosis of severe airway anomaly, obstructive neck mass, complicated CDH, pulmonary sequestration, and cystic adenomatoid malformation are conditions where this has been done successfully.[69,70,71] A multidisciplinary team and extensive planning are essential in order to optimally manage the mother and the fetus. The goal of the EXIT to ECMO procedure is a stepwise treatment approach and a smooth hemodynamic transition to the ex-utero environment while avoiding hypoxemia, acidosis, lung injury, and hemodynamic instability.

Surgery on ECMO

Repair of congenital diaphragmatic hernia (CDH) is the one surgery that is unique to neonates on ECMO. CDH is among the most complex pathophysiologic states in neonates. Because of the technical difficulty and physiologic intricacies of managing CDH patients on ECMO, an entire chapter in this textbook discusses this topic (see Chapter 18).

Complications

ECMO is a lifesaving tool; however, there are still many potential risks. Nearly 50 on-EC-

Table 17-2. Example of complications and impact on survival in neonates with respiratory failure on ECMO.[4]

Complication	# Reported	% Reported	Survival
Mechanical: Oxygenator failure	1,471	6.0%	53%
Hemorrhagic: Surgical site bleeding	1,539	6.2%	44%
Hemorrhagic: Disseminated intravascular coagulation (DIC)	611	2.5%	40%
Neurologic: Brain death	229	0.9%	0%
Neurologic: Seizures, clinically determined	2,376	9.6%	61%
Neurologic: Seizures, EEG determined	242	1.0%	48%
Neurologic: CNS infarction by US/CT/MRI	1,862	7.5%	54%
Neurologic: CNS hemorrhage by US/CT/MRI	1,697	6.9%	45%
Renal: Creatinine 1.5-3.0	1,744	7.1%	52%
Renal: Dialysis required	796	3.2%	36%
Renal: Hemofiltration required	3,628	14.7%	53%
Cardiovascular: Myocardial stun by ECHO	1,225	5.0%	58%
Pulmonary: Pneumothorax requiring treatment	1,487	6.0%	59%
Pulmonary hemorrhage	1,117	4.5%	43%
Infectious: Culture proven infection	1,490	6.0%	53%

MO complications occur with enough frequency to measure. Unfortunately these complications have an obvious impact on survival; some of the more significant examples are shown in Table 17-2.[4] Complications are categorized into mechanical, hemorrhagic, neurologic, renal, cardiac, infectious, metabolic, and pulmonary.

Neurologic Complications

The most important complication impacting morbidity, as well as survival, in ECMO treated newborns is neurologic insult. This patient population is at particular risk of poor developmental outcome with a reported range of 20% to 40%, although most issues are minor.[72] Both pre-ECMO and on-ECMO events contribute to this situation. Meticulous monitoring and appropriate intervention may help prevent on-ECMO but have no impact on the pre-ECMO events. Patients with neurologic complications on ECMO have decreased survival (Table 17-2) and are at risk of impaired neurodevelopmental outcome. Among neurologic events, ICH has

been the most commonly reported for the last several years (Figure 17-3).[4] The pathogenesis of ICH related to ECMO has been attributed to reperfusion injury, hemodynamic and cerebro-vascular instability, systemic heparinization and increased CVP.[73] Despite research and development, anticoagulation is still a standard requirement for most ECMO circuits. The critically ill hypoxic and acidotic infant requiring ECMO is definitely susceptible to ICH with exposure to anticoagulated blood. This is an additional argument for instituting ECMO in a timely fashion, prior to exposing the infant to extended periods of acidosis, decreased perfusion, and hypoxia.[74] Despite advances in ECMO management, the incidence of intracranial hemorrhage has unfortunately remained significant across the years (Figure 17-4).[4]

Post ECMO head imaging

In addition to serial HUS during the ECMO course, a predischarge CT[75] or MRI of the brain should be performed as a more sensitive measure of injury than the bedside HUS. The frequency of abnormal neuroimaging ranges

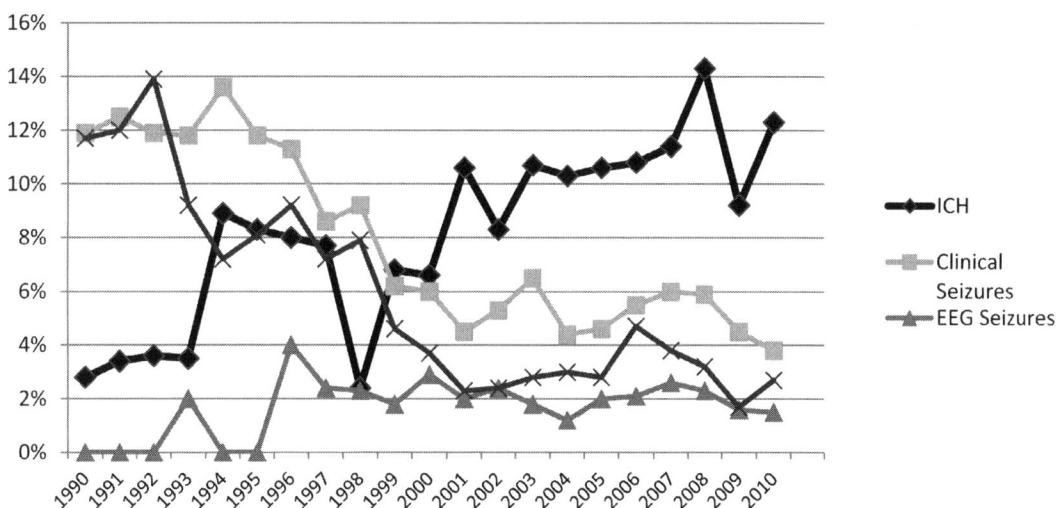

Figure 17-4. Percent reported incidence of central nervous system (CNS) hemorrhage in ECMO-treated neonates with respiratory failure.

from 28-52%, depending on techniques and methods of classification.

Expected Survival

The International Registry reports an 85% ECLS survival and 75% survival to discharge for neonates placed on ECMO for respiratory failure. There are a variety of risk factors for ECMO-treated neonates that increase mortality: primary diagnosis prior to cannulation,[4] need for cardiopulmonary resuscitation,[76] complications during bypass,[4] birthweight,[77] and gestational age.[21] Unfortunately, the annual survival has diminished over the years (Figure 17-5). The overall survival to hospital discharge for neonatal respiratory failure in 2010 was 67%, compared to the peak of 86% in 1989.[4] Patients with meconium aspiration continue to have the best survival compared to all other diagnoses (Table 17-3).[4] This change is due to the inclusion of more critically ill newborns that are refractory to other therapies which were not standard of care in the earlier ECMO years.

Developmental Outcome

Given the severity of illness prior to ECMO treatment and the risks inherent with the procedure, it is important to recognize and monitor the common morbidities that affect the survivors from the neonatal period through childhood. Measures to be followed include nutritional status, pulmonary function, and neurodevelopment.

1. During the newborn period, feeding issues can be a significant problem in this patient population similar to other critically ill newborns. Most children do achieve full oral feedings after a period of time. Home nasogastric feeds may be required by some, but gastrostomy placement is usually not necessary except in those patients with CDH (see Chapter 18). For many post-ECMO neonates, close tracking of nutritional status in the first weeks and, in some cases, months after discharge may be necessary.

2. Significant respiratory sequelae are reported for ECMO survivors during the first two years of life. According to parental report, as many as 25% of ECMO graduates have at least one episode of pneumonia before age two. In a five year cohort reported by Glass, 15% of neonatal ECMO survivors were taking some form of asthma medication at the time of the study, and 10% of the cohort had been hospitalized at least once for asthma (compared to a control

Table 17-3. Survival and ECMO hours per diagnosis.

Diagnosis	# Runs	% Survived	Avg run time (hrs)	Longest run time (hrs)
MAS	7,743	94%	131	1,327
CDH	6,147	51%	248	1,229
Sepsis	2,635	75%	140	1,200
PFC/PPHN	4,043	78%	151	1,176
RDS	1,496	84%	135	1,093
Pneumonia	343	57%	237	1,002
Air Leak	117	74%	167	656
Other	2,146	63%	176	1,277

population with an estimated incidence around 5%).[78]

3. As in other hospitalized newborns, neurodevelopmental outcome is affected by the severity of the ongoing medical condition. The strongest neonatal predictor of handicap in childhood is the extent and severity of abnormality identified by routine cranial ultrasounds during bypass and head CT or MRI scans prior to hospital discharge.[79] Moderate to severe abnormalities occur in approximately 10-15%, with an additional 25% having smaller or more focal lesions. The majority of the lesions are bilateral, with the unilateral lesions distributed equally to both hemispheres.[80] A significant proportion of children who had significant abnormalities on neonatal neuroimaging, however will still have normal IQ scores in childhood.[72] In ECMO survivors, head circumference below the 5th percentile occurs at a higher than expected rate (10%) and is frequently associated with a major handicap at five

years of age, if it occurs in conjunction with a significant brain lesion.[78,81] Macrocephaly has also been reported, which may be due to venous obstruction or late hydrocephalus following intraventricular hemorrhage.[72] In either case, it requires close monitoring and possible interventions. According to Glass, there is a typical pattern of neurodevelopmental sequelae following hospital discharge. By four months of age the typical ECMO-treated neonate is developing in the normal range on formal testing. Residual hypotonia or mild asymmetry persists in 25% of the infants, although the prognosis is generally good for these patients. Early referral and intervention should occur for infants who exhibit more significant problems at this age. By one to two years of age significant neurologic abnormalities are reported in 10 to 15% of the children. A larger proportion (25%) exhibit a more specific delay in either language or visual/perceptual abilities. On entering school, the majority

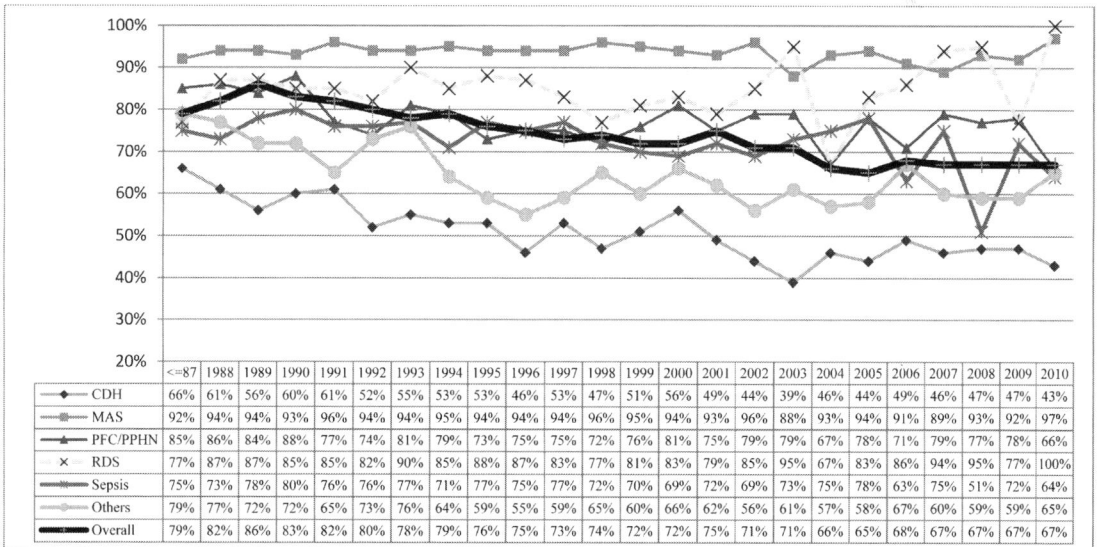

	<=87	1988	1989	1990	1991	1992	1993	1994	1995	1996	1997	1998	1999	2000	2001	2002	2003	2004	2005	2006	2007	2008	2009	2010
CDH	66%	61%	56%	60%	61%	52%	55%	53%	53%	46%	53%	47%	51%	56%	49%	44%	39%	46%	44%	49%	46%	47%	47%	43%
MAS	92%	94%	94%	93%	96%	94%	94%	95%	94%	94%	94%	96%	95%	94%	93%	96%	88%	93%	94%	91%	89%	93%	92%	97%
PFC/PPHN	85%	86%	84%	88%	77%	74%	81%	79%	73%	75%	75%	72%	76%	81%	75%	79%	79%	67%	78%	71%	79%	77%	78%	66%
RDS	77%	87%	87%	85%	85%	82%	90%	85%	88%	87%	83%	77%	81%	83%	79%	85%	95%	67%	83%	86%	94%	95%	77%	100%
Sepsis	75%	73%	78%	80%	76%	76%	77%	71%	77%	75%	77%	72%	70%	69%	72%	69%	73%	75%	78%	63%	75%	51%	72%	64%
Others	79%	77%	72%	72%	65%	73%	76%	64%	59%	55%	59%	65%	60%	66%	62%	56%	61%	57%	58%	67%	60%	59%	59%	65%
Overall	79%	82%	86%	83%	82%	80%	78%	79%	76%	75%	73%	74%	72%	72%	75%	71%	71%	66%	65%	68%	67%	67%	67%	67%

Figure 17-5. Annual survival per diagnosis.

of ECMO neonates are functioning in the normal range on measures of general intelligence, although the mean IQ scores and standard scores on measures of specific neuropsychological functioning are lower than in the normal population. In this age group, Glass reports major disability or handicap in approximately 15% of ECMO-treated neonates. The most common disability is mild to moderate mental retardation. Severe or profound impairment is uncommon (< 5%). Sensorineural hearing loss is reported in the range of 4 to 21% of ECMO-treated neonates by preschool age.[78] There is no evidence that the ECMO procedure itself increases the risk for hearing loss. For many infants this hearing loss is progressive, following normal BAERs in the newborn period.

As these critically ill newborns are at high risk of neurodevelopmental problems, they should be followed and referred for therapy as indicated. The current ELSO recommendation for developmental followup after discharge is for evaluations at the ages of 4 to 6 months, 1 year, 2 years, 3 years, and 5 years.[78] An age appropriate neurodevelopmental evaluation should occur at each of these visits. Behavioral testing, hearing, and language screening are also recommended. For the majority of ECMO-treated neonates, the critical issues are developmental needs and psychosocial support. Comprehensive multidisciplinary followup is essential for ECMO children who have significant medical and developmental issues. A team approach and case management is essential to prioritize the needs of each child.

Long-term cost effectiveness of ECMO in term and late-preterm infants was evaluated and compared to that of conventional management. Information about use of health services during a seven year followup period was analyzed. Based on cost per life-year gained and per disability-free year gained ECMO was shown to be cost-effective.[83]

Family social dynamics

Arranging long-term management and followup is the ECMO team's final responsibility. The team must ease the transition from hospital to home with thorough planning and a detailed "handoff" to those who will continue to care for the patient, particularly the family. The unexpected and acute crisis surrounding ECMO therapy may be devastating for the parents of the neonate and the effects can be long lasting. What is routine to the ECMO team is often overwhelming to the patient's family. This response may be delayed until after the baby is discharged home. Acknowledging the impact of ECMO on the family prior to discharge will help achieve a successful transition to home. Appropriate referral to social services may be helpful.

References

1. Bartlett RH, Roloff DW, Cornell RG, Cornell RG, Andrews AF, Dillon PW, Zwischenberger JB. Extracorporeal circulation in neonatal respiratory failure: a prospective randomized study. Pediatrics. 1985 Oct;76(4):479-87.
2. Firmin RK, Peek GL, Sosnowski AW. Role of extracorporeal membrane oxygenation. Lancet. 1996 Sep 21;348(9030):824.
3. O'Rourke PP, Crone RK, Vacanti JP, Ware JH, Lillehei CW, Parad RB, Epstein MF. Extracorporeal membrane oxygenation and conventional medical therapy neonates with persistent pulmonary hypertension of the newborn: a prospective randomized study. Pediatrics. 1989 Dec;84(6):957-63.
4. ECMO Registry of the Extracorporeal Life Support Organization (ELSO), Ann Arbor, Michigan, Dec, 2011
5. Marway A, Crombleholme TM. The Exit procedure: principles, pitfalls, and progress. Semin Pediatr Surg. 2006 May; 15(2):107-15.
6. Hintz SR, Suttner DM, Sheehan AM, Rhine WD, Van Meurs KP. Decreased use of neonatal extracorporeal membrane oxygenation (ECMO):how new treatment modalities have affected ECMO utilization Pediatrics. 2000 Dec;106(6):1339-43
7. Short BL, Miller MK, Anderson KD. Extracorporeal membrane oxygenation in the management of respiratory failure in the newborn. Clin Perinatol. 1987 Sep;14(3):737-48.
8. Bartlett RH, Andrews AF, Toomasian JM, Haidu NJ, Gazzaniga AB. Extracorporeal membrane oxygenation (ECMO) in neonatal respiratory failure: forty five cases. Surgery. 1982 Aug;92(2):425-33.
9. Van Meurs KP, Hintz SR, Sheehan AM. ECMO for Neonatal Respiratory Failure. Extracorporeal Cardiopulmonary Support in Critical Care, 3rd Edition. 273-295.
10. Schumacher RE. Extracorporeal membrane oxygenation. Will this therapy continue to be as efficacious in the future? Pediatr Clin N Amer. 1993 Oct;40(5):1005-22.
11. Radhakrishnan RS, Lally PA, Lally KP, Cox CS. ECMO for meconium aspiration syndrome: support for relaxed entry criteria. ASAIO J. 2007 Jul-Aug;53(4):489-91.
12. Roy BJ, Cornish JD, Clark RH. The changing demographics of neonatal extracorporeal membrane oxygenation patients reported to the Extracorporeal Life Support Organization (ELSO) Registry. Pediatrics. 2000 Dec;106(6):1334-8.
13. Chapman RL, Perterec SM, Bizzarro MJ, Mercurio MR. Patient selection for neonatal extracorporeal membrane oxygenation: beyond severity of illness. J Perinatol. 2009 Sep;29(9):606-11. Epub 2009 May 21.
14. Hardart GE, Fackler JC. Predictors of intracranial hemorrhage during neonatal extracorporeal membrane oxygenation. J Pediatr. 1999 Feb;134(2):156-9.
15. Rozmiarek AJ, Qureshi FG, Cassidy L, Ford HR, Gaines BA, Rycus P, Hackam DJ. How low can you go? Effectiveness and safety of extracorporeal membrane oxygenation in low-birth-weight neonates. J Pediatr Surg. 2004 Jun;39(6):845-7.
16. Reddy VM. Cardiac surgery for premature and low birth weight neonates. Semin Thorac Cardiovasc Surg Pediatr Card Surg Annu. 2001;4:4:271-6.
17. White JJ, Andrews HG, Risemjberg H, et al. Prolonged respiratory support in newborn infants with a membrane oxygenator. Surgery. 1971 Aug;70(2):288-96.
18. Bartlett RH, Andrews AF, Toomasian JM, Haiduc NJ, et al. Extracorporeal membrane oxygenation for newborn respiratory failure: forty-five cases. Surgery. 1982 Aug;92(2):425-33.
19. Bui KC, LaClair P, Vanderkerhove J,et al. ECMO in premature infants. Review of

factors associated with mortality. ASAIO Trans. 1991 Apr-Jun;37(2):54-9.

20. Hirschl RB, Schumacher RE, Snedecor SN, et al. The efficacy of extracorporeal life support in premature and low birth weight newborns. J Pediatr Surg. 1993 Oct;28(10):1336-40.

21. Hardart GE, Hardart MK, Arnold JH, et al. Intracranial hemorrhage in premature neonates treated with extracorporeal membrane oxygenation correlates with conceptional age. J Pediatr. 2004 Aug;145(2):184-9.

22. Ramachandrappa A, Rosenberg ES, Wagoner S, et al. Morbidity and Mortality in Late Preterm Infants with Severe Hypoxic Respiratory Failure on ECMO. J Pediatr. In Press.

23. Reoma JL, Rojas A, Kim AC, et al. Development of an artificial placenta I: pumpless arterio-venous extracorporeal life support in a neonatal sheep model. J Pediatr Surg. 2009 Jan;44(1):53-9.

24. Ancel PY, Livinec F, Larroque B, et al. Cerebral palsy among very preterm children in relation to gestational age and neonatal ultrasound abnormalities: the EPIPAGE cohort study. Pediatrics. 2006 Mar;117(3):828-35.

25. Mariani E, Scelsa B, Pogliani L, et al. Prognostic value of electroencephalograms in asphyxiated newborns treated with hypothermia. Pediatr Neurol. 2008 Nov;39(5):317-24.

26. Foley DS, Swaniker F, Pranikoff T, Bartlett RH, Hirschl RB. Percutaneous cannulation for pediatric venovenous extracorporeal life support. J Pediatr Surg. 2000 Jun;35(6):943-7.

27. Peek GJ, Firmin RK, Moore HM, Sosnowski AW. Cannulation of neonates for venovenous extracorporeal life support. Ann Thorac Surg. 1996 Jun;61(6):1851-2.

28. Reickert CA, Schreiner RJ, Bartlett RH, Hirschl RB. Percutaneous access for venovenous extracorporeal life support in neonates. J Pediatr Surg.1998 Feb;33(2):365-9.

29. Walker LK, Short BL, Traystman RJ. Impairment of cerebral autoregulation during venovenous estracoreal membrane oxygenation in the newborn lamb. Crit Care Med. 1996 Dec;24(12):2001-6.

30. Skarsgard ED, Salt DR, Lee SK: Extracorporeal Life Support Organization Registry. Venovenous extracorporeal membrane oxygenation in neonatal respiratory failure: does routine, cephalad jugular drainage improve outcome? J Pediatr Surg. 2004 May;39(5):672-6.

31. Anderson HL 3rd, Otsu T, Chapman RA, Barlett RH. Venovenous extracorporeal life support in neonates using a double lumen catheter. ASAIO Trans. 1989 Jul-Sep;35(3):650-3.

32. Fukuda S, Aoyama M, Yamada Y, et al. Comparison of venoarterial versus venovenous access in the cerebral circulation of newborns undergoing extracorporeal membrane oxygenation. Pediatr Surg Int. 1999;15(2):78-84.

33. Hunter CJ, Blood AB, Bishai JM, et al. Cerebral blood flow and oxygenation during venoarterial and venovenous extracorporeal membrane oxygenation in the newborn lamb. Pediatr Crit Care Med. 2004 Sep;5(5):475-81.

34. Ejike JC, Schenkman KA, Seidel K, Ramamoorthy C, Roberts JS. Cerebral oxygenation in neonatal and pediatric patients during veno-arterial extracorporeal life support. Pediatr Crit Care Med. 2006 Mar;7(2):154-8.

35. Fenik JC, Rais-Bahrami K. Neonatal cerebral oximetry monitoring during ECMO cannulation. J Perinatol. 2009 May;29(5):376-81.

36. Van Heijst A, Liem D, Hopman J, Van Der Staak F, Sengers R. Oxygenation and hemodynamics in left and right cerebral hemispheres during induction of veno-arterial

extracorporeal membrane oxygenation. J Pediatr. 2004 Feb;144(2):223-8.

37. Hazelton JL, Balan I, Elmer GI, Kristian T, Rosenthal RE, Krause G, Sanderson TH, Fiskum G. Hyperoxic reperfusion after global cerebral ischemia promotes inflammation and long-term hippocampal neuronal death. J Neurotrauma. 2010 Apr;27(4):753-62.

38. Skippen P, Seear M, Poskitt K, Kestle J, Cochrane D, Annich G, Handel J. Effect of hyperventilation on regional cerebral blood flow in head-injured children. Crit Care Med. 1997 Aug;25(8):1402-9.

39. Short BL, Walker LK, Bender KS, Traystman RJ. Impairment of cerebral autoregulation during extracorporeal membrane oxygenation in newborn lambs. Pediatr Res. 1993 Mar;33(3):289-94.

40. Walker LK, Short BL, Traystman RJ. Impairment of cerebral autoregulation during venovenous estracorporeal membrane oxygenation in the newborn lamb. Crit Care Med. 1996 Dec;24(12):2001-6.

41. Ingyinn M, Rais-Bahrami K, Viswanathan M, et al. Altered cerebrovascular responses after exposure to venoarterial extracorporeal membrane oxygenation: role of the nitric oxide pathway. Pediatr Crit Care Med. 2006 Jul;7(4):368-73.

42. Zahraa JN, Moler FW, Annich GM, Maxvold NJ, Bartlett RH, Custer JR. Venovenous versus venoarterial extracorporeal life support for pediatric respiratory failure: are these differences in survival and acute complications? Crit Care Med. 2000 Feb;28(2):521-5.

43. Ingyinn M, Rais-Bahrami K, Evangelista R, Hogan I, Rivera O, Mikesell GT, Short BL. Comparison of the effect of venovenous versus venoarterial extracorporeal membrane oxygenation on renal blood flow in the newborn lambs. Perfusion. 2004 May;19(3):163-70.

44. Strieper MJ, Sharma S, Dooley KJ, Cornish JD, Clark RH. Effects of venovenous extracorporeal membrane oxygenation on cardiac performance as determined by echocardiographic measurements. J Pediatr. 1993 Jun;122(6):950-5.

45. Cornish JD, Heiss KF, Clark RH, Strieper MJ, Boecler B, Kesser K. Efficacy of venovenous extracorporeal membrane oxygenation for neonates with respiratory and circulatory compromise. J Pediatr. 1993 Jan;122(1):105-9.

46. Buesing KA, Kilian AK, Schaible T, et al. Extracorporeal membrane oxygenation in infants with congenital diaphragmatic hernia: followup MRI evaluating carotid artery reocclusion and neurologic outcome. AJR Am J Roentqenol. 2007 Jun;188(6):1636-42.

47. Chen A, Teruva J. Global hemostasis testing thromboelastography; old technology, new applications. Clin Lab Med. 2009 Jun;29(2):391-407.

48. Evans RA, Thureen P. Early feedings strategies in preterm and critically ill neonates. Neonatal Netw. 2001 Oct;20(7):7-18.

49. Jaksic T, Hull MA, Modi BP, Ching YA, George D, Compher C; American Society for Parenteral and Enteral Nutrition (A.S.P.E.N.) Board of Directors. A.S.P.E.N. Clinical guidelines: nutrition support of neonates supported with extracorporeal membrane oxygenation. JPEN J Parenter Enteral Nutr. 2010 May-Jun;34(3):247-53.

50. Heyland DK, Cook DJ, Guyatt GH. Enteral nutrition in the critically ill patient: a critical review of the evidence. Intensive Care Med. 1993;19(8):435-42.

51. Moore FA, Feliciano DV, Andrassy RJ, McArdle AH, Booth FV, Morgenstein-Wagner TB, Kellum JM Jr, Welling RE, Moore EE. Early enteral feeding, compared with parenteral, reduces postoperative septic complications. The results of a meta-

analysis. Ann Surg. 1992 Aug;216(2):172-83.

52. Okada Y, Klein N, van Saene HK, Pierro A. Small volumes of enteral feedings normalize immune function in infants receiving parenteral nutrition. J Pediatr Surg. 1998 Jan;33(1):16-9.

53. Hanekamp MN, Spoel M, Sharman-Koendjbiharie I, Peters JW, Albers MJ, Tibboel D. Rountine enteral nutrition in neonates on extracorporeal membrane oxygenation. Pediatr Crit Care Med. 2005 May;6(3):275-9.

54. Kurundkar AR, Killingsworth CR, McIlwain RB, Timpa JG, Hartman YE, He D, Karnatak RK, Neel ML, Clancy JP, Anantharamaiah GM, Maheshwari A. Extracorporeal membrane oxygenation causes loss of intestinal epithelial barrier in the newborn piglet. Pediatr Res. 2010 Aug;68(2):128-33.

55. Keszler M, Ryckman FC, McDonald JV Jr, Sweet LD, Moront MG, Boegli MJ, Cox C, Leftridge CA. A prospective, multicenter, randomized study of high versus low positive end-expiratory pressure during extracorporeal membrane oxygenation. 1992 J Pediatr Jan;120(1):107-13.

56. Chen A, Teruya J. Global hemostasis testing thromboelastography: old technology, new applications. Clin Lab Med. 2009 Jun;29(2):391-407

57. Pape KE. Etiology and pathogenesis of intraventricular hemorrhage in newborns. Pediatrics. 1989 Aug;84(2):382-5.

58. Liem KD, Hopman JC, Oeseburg B, et al. Cerebral oxygenation and hemodynamics during induction of extracorporeal membrane oxygenation as investigated by near infrared spectrophotometry. Pediatrics. 1995 Apr;95(4):555-61.

59. Dela Cruz TV, Stewart DL, Winston SJ, Weatherman KS, Phelps JL, Mendoza JC. Risk factors for intracranial hemorrhage in the extracorporeal membrane

oxygenation patient. J Perinatol. 1997 Jan-Feb;17(1):18-23.

60. Hirthler MA, Blackwell E, Abbe D, Doe-Chapman R, LeClair Smith C, Goldthorn J, Canizaro P. Coagulation parameter instability as an early predictor of intracranial hemorrhage during extracorporeal membrane oxygenation. J Pediatr Surg. 1992 Jan;27(1):40-3.

61. Grayck EN, Meliones JN, Kern FH, Hansell DR, Ungerleider RM, Greeley WJ. Elevated serum lactate correlates with intracranial hemorrhage in neonates treated with extracorporeal life support. Pediatrics. 1995 Nov;96(5 Pt 1):914-7.

62. Azzopardi DV, Strohm B, Edwards AD, Dyet L, Halliday HL, Juszczak E, Kapellou O, Levene M, Marlow N, Porter E, Thoresen M, Whitelaw A, Brocklehurst P; TOBY Study Group. Moderate hypothermia to treat perinatal asphyxial encephalopathy. N Engl J Med. 2009 Oct 1;361(14):1349-58.

63. Zanelli S, Buck M, Fairchild K. Physiologic and pharmacologic considerations for hypothermia therapy in neonates. J Perinatol. 2010 Dec 23

64. Massaro A, Rais-Bahrami K, Chang T, Glass P, Short BL, Baumgart S. Therapeutic hypothermia for neonatal encephalopathy and extracorporeal membrane oxygenation. J Pediatr. 2010 Sep;157(3):499-501.

65. Khan AM, Shabarek FM, Zwischenberger JB, Warner BW, Cheu HW, Jaksic T, Goretsky MJ, Meyer TA, Doski J, Lally KP. Utility of daily head ultrasonography for infants on extracorporeal membrane oxygenation. J Pediatr Surg. 1998 Aug;33(8):1229-32.

66. Rais-Bahrami K, Rivera O, Short BL. Validation of a noninvasive neonatal optical cerebral oximeter in veno-venous ECMO patients with a cephalad catheter. J Perinatol. 2006 Oct;26(10):628-35. Epub 2006 Aug 10.

67. Fenik JC, Rais-Bahrami K. Neonatal cerebral oximetry monitoring during

ECMO cannulation. J Perinatol. 2009 May;29(5):376-81. Epub 2009 Jan 22.

68. Nagarajan L, Palumbo L, Ghosh S. Neurodevelopmental outcomes in neonates with seizures: a numerical score of background encephalography to help prognosticate. J Child Neurol. 2010 Aug;25(8):961-8. Epub 2010 Mar 11.

69. Mychaliska GB, Bryner BS, Nugent C, Barks J, Hirschl RB, McCrudden K, Chames M, Gomez-Fifer C, Servin MN, Chiravuri SD Giant pulmonary sequestration: the rare case requiring the EXIT procedure with resection and ECMO. Fetal Diagn Ther. 2009;25(1):163-6. Epub 2009 Mar 17.

70. Kunisaki SM, Barnewolt CE, Estroff JA, Myers LB, Fauza DO, Wilkins-Haug LE, Grable IA, Ringer SA, Benson CB, Nemes LP, Morash D, Buchmiller TL, Wilson JM, Jennings RW. Ex utero intrapartum treatment with extracorporeal membrane oxygenation for severe congenital diaphragmatic hernia. J Pediatr Surg. 2007 Jan;42(1):98-104.

71. Hedrick HL, Flake AW, Crombleholme TM, Howell LJ, Johnson MP, Wilson RD, Adzick NS. The ex utero intrapartum therapy procedure for high-risk fetal lung lesions. J Pediatr Surg. 2005 Jun;40(6):1038-43; discussion 1044.

72. Glass P, ECMO training manual, Chapter 22

73. Volpe JJ. Neurology of the Newborn, 5th ed. Philadelphia, PA: Saunders Elsevier; 2008.

74. Hardart GE, Fackler JC. Predictors of intracranial hemorrhage during neonatal extracorporeal membrane oxygenation. J Pediatr. 1999 Feb;134(2):156-9.

75. Bulas DI, Taylor GA, O'Donnell RM, et al. Intracranial abnormalities in infants treated with extracorporeal membrane oxygenation: update on sonographic and CT findings. AJNR AM J Neuroradiol. 1996 Feb;17(2):287-94.

76. Doski JJ, Butler TJ, Louder DS, et al. Outcome of infants requiring cardiopulmonary resuscitation before extracorporeal membrane oxygenation. J Pediatr Surg. 1997 Sep;32(9):1318-21.

77. Revenis ME, Glass P, Short BL. Mortality and morbidity rates among lower birth weight infants (2000 to 2500 grams) treated with extracorporeal membrane oxygenation. J Pediatr. 1992 Sep;121(3):452-8.

78. Glass P, Wagner AE, Papero PH, et al. Neurodevelopmental status at age five years of neonates treated with extracorporeal membrane oxygenation. J Pediatr. 1995 Sep;127(3):447-57.

79. Glass P, Bulas DI, Wagner AE, et al. Severity of brain injury following neonatal extracorporeal membrane oxygenation and outcome at age 5 years. Dev Med Child Neurol. 1997 Jul;39(7):441-8.

80. Bulas D, Glass P. Neonatal ECMO: neuroimaging and neurodevelopmental outcome. Semin Perinatol. 2005 Feb;29(1):58-65.

81. Walsh-Sukys MC, Bauer RE, Cornell DJ, et al. Severe respiratory failure in neonates: mortality and morbidity rates and neurodevelopmental outcomes. J Pediatr. 1994 Jul;125(1):104-10.

82. Petrou S, Bischof M, Bennett C, Elbourne D, Field D, McNally H. Cost-effectiveness of neonatal extracorporeal membrane oxygenation based on 7-year results from the United Kingdom Collaborative ECMO Trial. Pediatrics. 2006 May;117(5):1640-9.

18

Congenital Diaphragmatic Hernia and ECMO

Phillip A. Letourneau MD, Kevin P. Lally MD MS

Introduction

Congenital diaphragmatic hernia (CDH) is an abnormality of diaphragm development that allows abdominal contents to herniate into the thoracic cavity. CDH was first described in 1679 by Lazarus Riverius, who noted an incidental CDH during an autopsy of a 24 year old patient. In 1701, Sir Charles Holt described the classic clinical and postmortem findings typical of CDH in an infant in the philosophical transactions of the Royal Society of London. In 1761, Giovanni Battista Morgagni described the anterior CDH which now is known as a Morgagni hernia. Finally, in 1848, Victor Bochdalek identified several patients at postmortem with posterolateral diaphragmatic hernias, which now bear his name.

The incidence of CDH is approximately 1 in 2,000 to 4,000 live births. Male children are more commonly affected, with a 1.5:1 male:female ratio. The risk of recurrence for future pregnancies is approximately 2%. These frequencies are consistent in the United States and throughout the world.[1,2] While the pathogenesis of CDH is not fully understood, universally the disease results in a diaphragmatic defect that allows viscera from the abdomen to enter or remain in the thoracic cavity. Roughly 95% of CDH occur in a posterolateral position, with 80% on the left side.[3] CDH likely affects lung development by causing compression of the developing lung by the abdominal organs, causing pulmonary hypoplasia or by acting as a space occupying lesion, and impairing lung growth. Evidence from animal studies has also demonstrated possible lung hypoplasia independent of a mass effect.[4] A recent clinical study demonstrated that low vitamin A (retinol) levels, along with decreased retinol binding protein levels, were associated with patients with CDH. This suggests that the pathogenesis of CDH may be related to dysfunction of vitamin A homeostasis.[5,6] Another complication in children with CDH is pulmonary hypertension secondary to abnormalities in the pulmonary vasculature.[7,8] CDH may also occur along with chromosomal defects and/or cardiac anomalies. This suggests that CDH belongs on a spectrum of problems that include pulmonary hypoplasia, pulmonary hypertension, chromosomal defects, and cardiac anomalies.

Diagnosis

CDH is commonly diagnosed in the prenatal period by ultrasound in up to 50% of the cases.[9] Sonographic findings include bowel loops in the thoracic cavity along with a shift of the heart into the opposite chest. The position of the liver may also help identify CDH and predict disease severity, with significant increases in mortality associated with liver herniation into the chest.[10-12]

If the diagnosis is not made in the prenatal period, clinical signs of CDH may include cyanosis and respiratory distress manifesting after birth. However, the severity of symptoms may range from asymptomatic patients to those that are critically ill. Physical findings reveal a flat or scaphoid abdomen, with decreased breath sounds on the affected side of the thorax (Figure 18-1). A chest radiograph may confirm the presence of bowel loops in the chest (Figure 18-2). Findings include air filled loops of intestine, or a nasogastric tube, that may be visible in the chest. The heart and mediastinum are shifted away from the defect side on chest x-ray.

Other diagnostic tests that are indicated following birth are chromosomal analysis and an echocardiogram, considering the high incidence of chromosomal abnormalities and cardiac defects.

Management

Infants with CDH may demonstrate worsening respiratory distress after birth, with progression to hypoxemia, hypercarbia, and acidosis. Management with endotracheal intubation and mechanical ventilation is usually indicated. Care should be taken to avoid overinflation, even with the initial intubation. A nasogastric

tube should also be placed. Blood pH and gas-exchange status should be assessed with appropriate analysis. Also, preductal (right hand) pulse oximetry is helpful in monitoring infants with CDH. It is prudent to avoid bag-mask ventilation following delivery, as this may cause increased stomach and intestinal air, which could further compromise pulmonary function. The role of continuous positive airway pressure (CPAP) in this setting has not been studied. Medical therapy following delivery may include inotropes for cardiovascular support, as well.

Mechanical ventilation

Infants with CDH can develop hypoxemic respiratory failure (HRF) in varying degrees. The advent of neonatal mechanical ventilation in the 1960s allowed many children with previously fatal CDH to survive following surgical repair of their defect. With increasing knowledge of newborn physiology, neonatal CDH patients with pulmonary hypertension and extra-pulmonary shunting were identified. Studies demonstrated that pulmonary vascular resistance (PVR) could be modulated with manipulation of pH and pCO_2, and the use of hyperventilation strategies became widespread.[13] Although hyperventilation was effective in reducing PVR, this practice resulted in significant ventilator associated lung injury secondary to aggressive ventilation strategies. Wung et

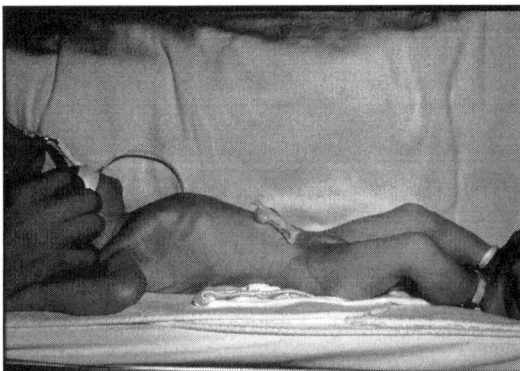

Figure 18-1.

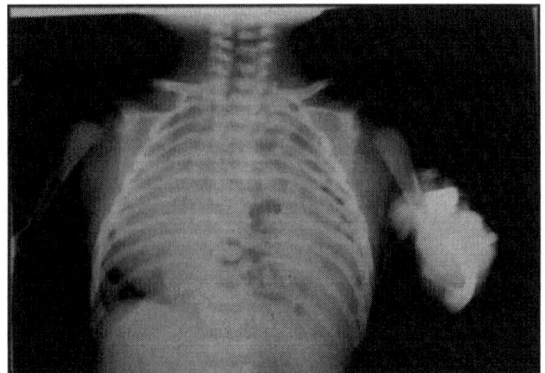

Figure 18-2.

al. demonstrated that in some CDH patients mortality was related to barotrauma induced by mechanical ventilation.[14] Other investigators have advocated gentle ventilation along with permissive hypercapnea as a strategy to reduce mortality.[15] Most ECMO centers utilize a strategy that focuses on minimizing barotrauma by allowing spontaneous ventilation with minimal set respiratory rates, minimal pressure ventilation, permissive hypercapnea, minimal sedation, and avoidance of pharmaceutical paralysis. This strategy has resulted in selected survival rates at some centers near 90%.[16,17] Considering the above, hyperventilation and induced alkalosis as a strategy for infants with CDH has largely been abandoned.

High frequency oscillatory ventilation (HFOV) has been investigated as a ventilation strategy in CDH. HFOV has been demonstrated to be less injurious to lungs in animal models, but evidence in clinical trials has been mixed. Paranka et al. found little benefit from HFOV in CDH using a high-pressure lung recruitment strategy.[18] However, other authors have shown that HFOV can be an effective mode of therapy as an initial treatment for HRF in CDH by avoiding lung overinflation.[19,20] Using historical controls, a European study compared conventional ventilation to HFOV and found improved survival, especially in patients who survived to surgery.[20]

In summary, while the optimal mode of ventilation in CDH is not clear, clinical data suggest that management strategies should be designed to limit lung distention and barotrauma as a strategy to improve survival. A recent review by Logan and Cotton recommended the use setting pressure limits, thus avoiding over distention, and tolerating adequate blood gases as long as cardiac and end organ function remains satisfactory.[21]

Inhaled nitric oxide

Multiple factors contribute to the problem of persistent pulmonary hypertension (PPHN) in patients with CDH. These include decreased area of the pulmonary vascular bed, increased medial thickness of the pulmonary arteries, and blunted oxygen-induced vasodilation.[7] Inhaled nitric oxide (iNO) is a selective pulmonary vasodilator that improves oxygenation and decreases the need for ECMO in infants with respiratory failure secondary to PPHN. However, the data regarding iNO in CDH patients is mixed. When used as a rescue therapy for postoperative patients with CDH and severe respiratory failure, iNO does not improve overall survival or reduce the need for ECMO.[22,23] On the other hand, a recent prospective study of 218 patients over 10 years from the CDH Study Group found that in high-risk infants with diaphragm agenesis there was a trend towards increased iNO utilization (from 30% to 80%) along with decreased ECMO therapy. The authors also reported a trend towards increased survival when comparing the first two years of the study compared to the last two years (47% to 59%).[24] Also, iNO may be useful in patients with CDH after completion of ECMO therapy for treatment of pulmonary hypertension.[25] In many centers iNO is used as an adjuvant therapy in managing right heart failure.

Fetal interventions

Fetal surgery for CDH in humans was first described in 1990 by Harrison et al.[26] Initial attempts at fetal intervention were performed in an open fashion. Both patients with and without liver herniation were selected for intrauterine diaphragm repair. Those with liver herniation proved to have dismal outcomes secondary to compromise of the umbilical vein.[27,28] Subsequent data demonstrated equivalent outcomes from fetal and postnatal intervention in patients without liver herniation.[29] Today, the most commonly performed fetal intervention is tracheal occlusion (TO). A prospective randomized trial was conducted between 1999 and 2001 that compared endoscopic TO to standard postnatal therapy in patients with isolated left sided liver-up CDH. The trial compared 13 standard therapy patients to 11 patients who received TO. The trial was halted as survival was 77% and 73%, respectively.[30] In Europe, the FETO consortium has continued to perform endoscopic TO in greater than 150 cases. In this study group, TO is offered to patients with liver herniation or a lung to head ratio of <1.0 in the third trimester.[31] Utilizing this approach, investigators have reported survival of greater than 50%, which is greater than expected in this high risk group. However, this therapy remains untested in this subset of patients in a randomized fashion and comparisons of TO to conventional therapy remains to be published, hence fetal intervention for CDH should continued to be considered an experimental therapy.

Experience with ex utero intrapartum treatment (EXIT procedure) with ECMO (EXIT to ECMO) for severe cases of CDH (liver herniation and LHR <1.4) has been reported. A six-year retrospective study described 14 patients who underwent EXIT with a trial of ventilation. Three infants passed the ventilation trial and survived, but two required ECMO. Eleven infants received ECMO therapy before delivery. Overall survival was 64% in the EXIT to ECMO group.[32] However, selection criteria have been very imprecise and EXIT to ECMO has not been widely applied or reported. This should be considered an unproven therapy at this time.

Other management options

Other than fetal surgical intervention, medical therapy during the antenatal period has also been investigated. The use of corticosteroids has been studied with mixed results. One small study of three fetuses treated with antenatal betamethasone reported 100% survival, but suffered from small sample size, very large dosing, and no comparison group.[33] On the other hand, a recent randomized trial found no difference in survival when comparing fetuses that received prenatal steroids to those that did not. A cohort study completed concurrently with the randomized trial also confirmed no benefit to steroids in patients treated at the 34th week of pregnancy in this setting.[34]

Surfactant replacement has also been investigated as a postnatal therapy. Evidence of surfactant deficiency related to pool size and kinetics has been demonstrated in children with CDH.[35] Also, a small study demonstrated decreased surfactant phosphatidylcholine synthesis in infants with CDH who required ECMO.[36] However, a large prospective observational study showed worse survival associated with surfactant replacement.[37] Surfactant replacement was also associated with increased complications.[38] Randomized studies exploring this topic are lacking.

ECMO

ECMO for the treatment of CDH was first reported in 1977 by German et al.[39] They described four infants with severe respiratory failure who were placed on ECMO after repair, resulting in one survivor. Since then, ECMO has become widely adopted in infants with CDH. In the 1970s and 1980s CDH was treated as an emergent surgical condition; thus, infants who were placed on ECMO postoperatively often had significant ventilator-induced lung injury. In the late 1980s, the role of pulmonary hypertension in CDH was recognized and clinicians increasingly delayed surgery until the infant was stable or pulmonary hypertension resolved. Some authors have reported improved survival with this strategy, but randomized trials are lacking.[40]

ECMO criteria

ECMO is generally reserved for patients that fail maximal medical management. When incorporated with a strategy of gentle ventilation and permissive hypercapnea, early use of ECMO may allow CDH patients to avoid ventilator related lung injury. Unfortunately, entry criteria that accurately predict high mortality prior to the initiation of ECMO in infants with CDH have not been published. Therefore, a number of different parameters have been used to predict those at highest risk and who may benefit from ECMO (Table 18-1).[41-45] However, none of these criteria have been validated in multicenter studies. As ECMO is currently used, "failure to respond" is a common indication for treatment. Centers use a specific cap on ventilator parameters and move to ECMO if a patient does not respond appropriately with the goal of avoiding lung injury. Limiting peak inspiratory pressure to under 25-27, HFOV to a MAP of 14-15, or if the $PaCO_2$ exceeds 65-70 are examples of criteria used.

The use of ECMO in CDH varies according to the location of providers. A recent report from Brown et al. indicates that ECMO is utilized more frequently in the United States compared to the United Kingdom (30.7% vs. 15.4%, rate ratio, 1.81; 95% CI 1.64-2.00). ECMO survival for CDH infants was 45.8% in the US and 52.9% in the UK. However, overall CDH survival was higher in the US. Multiple confounding factors prevent interpreting the association of ECMO with these outcomes.[46]

Data from the CDH Study group show that a majority of CDH patients who are placed on ECMO undergo ECMO before their CDH repair. When considering the use of ECMO, an earlier report from the CDH Study Group showed that 770 of 2,077 received ECMO therapy, with 15% undergoing cannulation and treatment before surgery. Analysis of trends show that in 1995 ECMO was used postoperatively in 20% of the ECMO cases, with only 5% postoperative use in 2001.[47] Currently, ECMO is primarily used as a component of pre-operative stabilization with most children receiving ECMO before surgical correction of their CDH.[48-50]

Efficacy of ECMO

ECMO provides effective short-term support for respiratory failure. Therefore, reversibility of the underlying disorder is important when considering ECMO therapy. This fundamental selection criterion presents a challenging dilemma when it comes to infants with CDH. The degree of respiratory failure in CDH depends on the severity of the existing pulmonary hypertension and pulmonary hypoplasia, with most cases of ventilator associated lung injury largely avoided by using lung protective strategies. Pulmonary hypertension is potentially

Table 18-1. ECMO Criteria.

Author	Criteria for ECMO
Sebald[41]	OI > 40 for 4 hours or PaO_2 < 40 for 2 hours
Boloker[17]	Preductal O_2 saturation <80% refractory to ventilator manipulation (PIP >30 with convention ventilation, MAP of 20 on HFOV)
Somaschini[42]	OI > 40 or PaO_2 < 40
Nagaya[43]	Emergent: OI > 40 or PaO_2 < 40 or $PaCO_2$ > 100 for 2 hours
	Preventative: FiO_2 > 0.9 or MAP > 12 for 24 hours
Vd Staak[44]	A-aDO_2 > 610 for 8 hours or OI > 40 for 3 of 5 consecutive blood gases
Howell[45]	A-aDO_2 > 610 for 8 hours or OI > 40 for 2 hours

reversible, but may progress in some children to right heart failure. Pulmonary hypoplasia is variably severe amongst infants and will not likely improve over the course of one to two weeks.

These specific problems related to CDH have led to relatively poor outcomes in CDH patients treated with ECMO compared to other diagnoses. The overall survival of infants with CDH reported to the ELSO is approximately 51% and represents the lowest among all etiologies of neonatal HRF requiring ECMO. Furthermore, a recent study by Stevens et al. of the ELSO Registry demonstrated a decrease in overall survival from 64% in 1990 to 52% in 2001.[51] However, other studies have shown an overall improvement in survival with the use of ECMO.[52-54] Two studies that evaluated the efficacy of ECMO demonstrated similar survival rates, but differing rates of use of ECMO, with one study describing a 50% ECMO rate in CDH patients and a 1% utility rate in the other. These data suggest other interventions, other than ECMO may be responsible for improved outcomes.[16,55] A long-term study from Germany recently describes their 20 year experience with ECMO. The authors report 62% overall survival in CDH patients with improved survival associated with referral to an ECMO center in the first 24 hours of life associated with 77% vs. 54% survival.[54]

For preterm infants with CDH the data are mixed. A recently published study from the CDH Registry found that in 1127 infants with CDH, the utilization of ECMO was lower in the preterm group than in term infants (33% vs. 25.6%). In the preterm group ECMO was also associated with increased mortality (25.6% vs. 33.0%) with an OR of 3.13 (95% CI, 2.76-3.55). However, the infants who received ECMO and survived to repair had improved chances of survival.[56]

Patients with right-sided CDH have been identified in one study as requiring increased use of ECMO (54%), but with better than expected survival (80% survival, compared to 63% predicted by CDH Study Group equation). Mortality in this cohort was also linked to the presence of cardiac anomalies.[57]

Considering the above observations, better selection criteria may improve morbidity and mortality related to ECMO in infants with CDH. Pulmonary hypoplasia is thought to be the most important factor affecting outcome of CDH, but represents a difficult condition to assess prenatally. The use of alveolar arterial oxygen gradient, preductal hemoglobin saturations, postductal arterial PaO_2, oxygenation index (OI) and hypercarbia have been utilized by some centers to create algorithms for identification of children with the best chance of survival and who would benefit most from ECMO therapy (Table 18-1).

However, because CDH is a disease with a wide spectrum of severity and stabilization strategies vary among centers, comparing outcomes is difficult and controversial. The CDH Study Group has been working since 1995 to develop treatment-independent risk assessment tools that would allow accurate assessments of outcome between centers according to the severity of disease. Gender, race, birth weight, Apgar scores, immediate distress at birth, CPR, estimated gestational age (EGA), side of CDH, and prenatal diagnosis have been considered. Of these immediately available data, birth weight, and Apgar scores are the most predictive of outcome using logistic regression analysis. Amongst patients in the low-risk group, 74% survival was demonstrated, compared to 16% in the high-risk group.[1] However, other authors have been unable to confirm these results.[58] Furthermore, five minute Apgar scores may not be available in every case if the patient has been intubated immediately.

A recent CDH Study Group report identified predictors of survival in infants with CDH who received ECMO. In ECMO treated patients, survivors were born at a greater estimated gestational age (38 ± 2 weeks vs. 37 ± 2 weeks, p <0.001), had greater birth weights (3.2 ±0.5 vs. 2.9 ± 0.5 kg, p <0.001), were less likely to be diagnosed with CDH pre-natally (53% vs. 63%, p <0.01) and were on ECMO for a shorter length of time (9 ± 5 days vs. 12 ± 5 days, p <0.001).[59]

Other groups have also tried to identify factors that may predict need for ECMO and survival in CDH infants. Concerning predictors of need for ECMO, one group found evidence that lung area to head circumference ratio (LHR < 1.0) and gestational age (GA) at delivery (OR 1.3, 95% CI 1.0-1.6) are significant predictors of the need for ECMO and also survival.[60] While a recent report identified pre-ECMO $PaCO_2$ as a predictor of survival, another group has described difficulty identifying pre-ECMO predictors of survival.[61,62] Larger studies are needed to evaluate this problem.

Mode of ECMO in CDH

Traditionally, infants with CDH requiring ECMO have been placed on venoarterial (VA) ECMO. This practice was based on the assumption that these patients are hemodynamically unstable and could not tolerate venovenous (VV) ECMO. Furthermore, concerns about inadequate venous drainage and insufficient oxygen delivery, when compared to VA ECMO, reinforced the notion that VA ECMO was the mode of choice in CDH. However, several studies have found VV to be an acceptable mode of ECMO for infants with CDH.[63-65] Based on concerns about inadequate venous drainage, there remains a bias in some centers to utilize VA ECMO in infants with right-sided CDH. On the other hand, Dimmitt et al. found no difference between right and left-sided hernias in regard to the failure of VV ECMO and the need for conversion to VA ECMO. Furthermore, infants who did fail VV ECMO and required conversion to VA demonstrated similar outcomes to those placed on VA initially.[65] A recent update from the ELSO in 2009 found that after multivariate regression analysis, mortality and complication rates were equivalent between VA and VV ECMO. Renal complications and inotrope use were more prevalent with VV ECMO, but VA ECMO had higher rates of neurologic morbidity.[66] Considering the above observations, it would be prudent to assume that many infants with CDH can be treated with VV ECMO provided that an adequately sized VV cannula can be placed. Interestingly, Frenckner et al. found that infants with CDH tend to have smaller diameter vessels than other infants, which could make cannula placement for ECMO more difficult.[67] However, it is not clear if vessel size has driven the greater use of VA ECMO in CDH patients. Fisher et al. have described difficulties in right-sided CDH with failure of the venous catheter to pass to the right atrium and two incidences of azygos vein cannulation with one mortality.[68]

CDH surgery on ECMO

The question of optimal surgical timing arose when ECMO became a part of the preoperative stabilization. Operations performed on ECMO are high risk because of the potential for anticoagulation related bleeding complications. Early reports of surgical repair of CDH while on ECMO described significant hemorrhagic complications.[69] These complications resulted in a low survival rate. However, later studies have shown that surgery can be performed safely with little significant bleeding if circuit coagulation status is monitored closely. Aminocaproic acid, an inhibitor of fibrinolysis, has been used in patients undergoing operative repair on ECMO with good results. Downard et al. showed that 5% of infants treated with aminocaproic acid required reexploration for bleeding on ECMO compared to 26% of those patients who did not receive the drug.[70] This has resulted in the increased use of aminocaproic acid along with strict control of circuit coagulation during surgery for CDH on ECMO. Furthermore, Downard et al. found no increased risk of large vessel thrombus or cerebral infarction associated with aminocaproic acid, although there was an increased need for ECMO circuit change.[70]

The optimal timing of repair of CDH on ECMO remains unclear due to inadequate study and variability amongst centers. Data from the CDH Study group shows that of the infants placed on ECMO, 54% underwent surgery on ECMO, 30% had surgery following ECMO, and 16% never underwent repair and all expired. Survival was 83% in patients who had repair after ECMO, compared to 49% in those that had repair on ECMO. The length of hospital stay was shorter (64 vs. 76 days) and need for oxygen therapy lower (56% vs. 64%) in children with CDH repaired after ECMO rather than on ECMO. Considering timing of surgery performed on ECMO, the data are mixed. Operations occurred in the first 24 hours of ECMO, to as long as greater than three weeks into therapy. Not surprisingly, infants who underwent surgery later demonstrated lower survival.[71] A recent update from the CDH Study Group found that after Cox regression analysis, surgical repair of CDH on ECMO was associated with decreased survival (48.2% vs. 77.1%) relative to repair after ECMO therapy (hazard ratio, 1.41, 95% CI 1.03-1.92). This was found to be significant even after controlling for factors associated with severity of CDH.[72] Dassinger et al. have reported a series of 34 infants undergoing early CDH repair on ECMO with 71% survival and 8.8% reexploration rate for bleeding.[73] At Children's Memorial Hermann Hospital (Houston, TX), infants are repaired on ECMO once they have achieved dry weight. If the infants are at or near their dry weights at the time of ECMO initiation, they are repaired within a few days; otherwise the procedure is delayed until adequate diuresis is attained.

Long-term outcome of infants with CDH treated with ECMO

Long-term morbidity among children with CDH has increasingly been recognized over time. Infants with CDH who received ECMO therapy appear to have a higher risk and greater severity of neurological morbidity. An area of growing concern is the observation that infants with CDH treated with ECMO suffer higher rates of neurologic morbidity compared to those who did not receive ECMO and those who received ECMO for other diagnoses. Stolar et al. reported 89% of infants receiving ECMO therapy for non-CDH diagnoses were cognitively normal. On the other hand, only 60% of infants with CDH treated with ECMO had a similar outcome.[74] Another important concern is increased survival at the cost of increased neurologic morbidity. McGahern et al. reported survival of 75%, with 67% of the survivors exhibiting neurologic compromise.[75] Considering these data, it has been argued that poor neurologic outcome may be related to severity of illness, but other independent ECMO factors cannot be excluded.

Gastroesophageal reflux (GER) is also an extremely common condition among CDH patients, and has an incidence of up to 50% in some series. One study has described a patient cohort followed for 10 years with a high incidence of overall nutritional problems. The authors described high rates of GER, failure to thrive, and severe oral aversion requiring gastrostomy tube placement.[76,77] Infants with CDH may also require surgical management of their GER. In one of the previously mentioned studies, 21% of patients required fundoplication, with the highest rate amongst those requiring patch repair of their hernias.[76] Furthermore, hernia recurrence rates have been increasingly reported, with recurrence most prevalent in those patients who underwent patch repair.[77] Fundoplication performed at the same time as

CDH repair has also been described.[78] Although there are no clear studies to support this.

Regarding lung function following ECMO therapy, a recent study prospectively evaluated 14 CDH infants over 12 months. The investigators found that CDH patients who had undergone ECMO had increased functional residual capacity (FRC=32.8, z score= 1.2, 95% CI 0.3-2.1) at 12 months compared to normal values. Forced expiratory flow was within the normal range at this time point. However, only 12 patients were available for followup at 12 months.[79] Another retrospective study found that, in CDH patients following repair, abnormal lung function tests gradually normalized during the first two years of life. The authors found that FRC improved from (z score) -0.84 ± 0.5 to 3.26 ± 2.07 and maximum expiratory flow rate went from -1.63 ± 0.4 to -0.09 ± 0.94.[77]

A study from the UK reported outcomes on patients treated with ECMO between 1991 and 2000. In this report, Davis et al. describe 73 infants with CDH treated with ECMO. Forty-six (63%) were able to be weaned off ECMO, 42 (56%) survived to hospital discharge, and only 27 (37%) lived to one year or longer. Of these 27 survivors, only seven were free of complications.[80] These outcomes are indeed troublesome and further question the utility of ECMO in CDH. Stevens et al. have shown that the incidence of complications has increased over time with the duration of ECMO therapy.[51] While the etiology of this fact is not clear, the authors suggested that improvements in ventilator management has resulted in more severely ill patients being placed on ECMO, resulting in longer duration and increased morbidity.

A recent study from The Netherlands considered the motor and cognitive status at five years of patients who had received ECMO. The CDH cohort demonstrated the lowest survival (58%) and lowest rate of functionally normal children (37.5%, compared to 52.6% in children with meconium aspiration).[81] Another recent study described the use of ECMO as a risk factor for neurodevelopment, psychomotor, and neurocognitive disabilities.[82] Considering these data, practitioners should continue to better define the role of ECMO in the management of CDH. Improved selection criteria would likely improve morbidity and mortality rates, but until these are solidified, the value of ECMO will remain controversial for these patients.

Summary

Infants with CDH may develop severe respiratory failure that is unresponsive to medical treatment and require ECMO therapy for survival. Over time ECMO has evolved into a component of preoperative stabilization as a lung-protective strategy to prevent ventilator associated injury. While advances have been made in ECMO management for infants, these patients remain the most difficult to treat, with the lowest rate of survival. Furthermore, these patients exhibit high rates of long-term morbidity. While some centers have developed selection criteria to identify patients who would benefit most from ECMO, reliable and reproducible algorithms are not yet available. No randomized control trials have been published on this topic, while they certainly are warranted.

References

1. Estimating disease severity of congenital diaphragmatic hernia in the first 5 minutes of life. The Congenital Diaphragmatic Hernia Study Group. J Pediatr Surg, 2001. 36(1): p. 141-5.
2. Narayan H, et al. Familial congenital diaphragmatic hernia: prenatal diagnosis, management, and outcome. Prenat Diagn, 1993. 13(10): p. 893-901.
3. Lally KP. Congenital diaphragmatic hernia. Curr Opin Pediatr, 2002. 14(4): p. 486-90.
4. Babiuk RP, Greer JJ. Diaphragm defects occur in a CDH hernia model independently of myogenesis and lung formation. Am J Physiol Lung Cell Mol Physiol, 2002. 283(6): p. L1310-4.
5. Beurskens LW, et al. Retinol status of newborn infants is associated with congenital diaphragmatic hernia. Pediatrics, 2010. 126(4): p. 712-20.
6. Greer JJ, et al. Etiology of congenital diaphragmatic hernia: the retinoid hypothesis. Pediatr Res, 2003. 53(5): p. 726-30.
7. Mohseni-Bod H, Bohn D. Pulmonary hypertension in congenital diaphragmatic hernia. Semin Pediatr Surg, 2007. 16(2): p. 126-33.
8. Naeye RL, et al. Unsuspected pulmonary vascular abnormalities associated with diaphragmatic hernia. Pediatrics, 1976. 58(6): p. 902-6.
9. Huddy CL, et al. Congenital diaphragmatic hernia: prenatal diagnosis, outcome and continuing morbidity in survivors. Br J Obstet Gynaecol, 1999. 106(11): p. 1192-6.
10. Albanese CT, et al. Fetal liver position and perinatal outcome for congenital diaphragmatic hernia. Prenat Diagn, 1998. 18(11): p. 1138-42.
11. Jani J, et al. Prenatal prediction of survival in isolated left-sided diaphragmatic hernia. Ultrasound Obstet Gynecol, 2006. 27(1): p. 18-22.
12. Mullassery D, et al. Value of liver herniation in prediction of outcome in fetal congenital diaphragmatic hernia: a systematic review and meta-analysis. Ultrasound Obstet Gynecol, 2010. 35(5): p. 609-14.
13. Drummond WH, et al. The independent effects of hyperventilation, tolazoline, and dopamine on infants with persistent pulmonary hypertension. J Pediatr, 1981. 98(4): p. 603-11.
14. Wung JT, et al. Congenital diaphragmatic hernia: survival treated with very delayed surgery, spontaneous respiration, and no chest tube. J Pediatr Surg, 1995. 30(3): p. 406-9.
15. Kays DW, et al. Detrimental effects of standard medical therapy in congenital diaphragmatic hernia. Ann Surg, 1999. 230(3): p. 340-8; discussion 348-51.
16. Wilson JM, et al. Congenital diaphragmatic hernia--a tale of two cities: the Boston experience. J Pediatr Surg, 1997. 32(3): p. 401-5.
17. Boloker J, et al. Congenital diaphragmatic hernia in 120 infants treated consecutively with permissive hypercapnea/spontaneous respiration/elective repair. J Pediatr Surg, 2002. 37(3): p. 357-66.
18. Paranka MS, et al. Predictors of failure of high-frequency oscillatory ventilation in term infants with severe respiratory failure. Pediatrics, 1995. 95(3): p. 400-4.
19. Reyes C, et al. Delayed repair of congenital diaphragmatic hernia with early high-frequency oscillatory ventilation during preoperative stabilization. J Pediatr Surg, 1998. 33(7): p. 1010-4; discussion 1014-6.
20. Cacciari A, et al. High-frequency oscillatory ventilation versus conventional mechanical ventilation in congenital diaphragmatic hernia. Eur J Pediatr Surg, 2001. 11(1): p. 3-7.
21. Logan JW, et al. Mechanical ventilation strategies in the management of congenital diaphragmatic hernia. Semin Pediatr Surg, 2007. 16(2): p. 115-25.

22. Clark RH, et al. Low-dose nitric oxide therapy for persistent pulmonary hypertension of the newborn. Clinical Inhaled Nitric Oxide Research Group. N Engl J Med, 2000. 342(7): p. 469-74.

23. Finer NN, Barrington KJ. Nitric oxide for respiratory failure in infants born at or near term. Cochrane Database Syst Rev, 2006. 18(4): p. CD000399.

24. Lally KP, et al. Treatment evolution in high-risk congenital diaphragmatic hernia: ten years' experience with diaphragmatic agenesis. Ann Surg, 2006. 244(4): p. 505-13.

25. Dillon PW, et al. Nitric oxide reversal of recurrent pulmonary hypertension and respiratory failure in an infant with CDH after successful ECMO therapy. J Pediatr Surg, 1995. 30(5): p. 743-4.

26. Harrison MR, et al. Successful repair in utero of a fetal diaphragmatic hernia after removal of herniated viscera from the left thorax. N Engl J Med, 1990. 322(22): p. 1582-4.

27. Jelin E, Lee H. Tracheal occlusion for fetal congenital diaphragmatic hernia: the US experience. Clin Perinatol, 2009. 36(2): p. 349-61, ix.

28. Harrison MR, et al. Correction of congenital diaphragmatic hernia in utero, V. Initial clinical experience. J Pediatr Surg, 1990. 25(1): p. 47-55; discussion 56-7.

29. Harrison MR, et al. Correction of congenital diaphragmatic hernia in utero VII: a prospective trial. J Pediatr Surg, 1997. 32(11): p. 1637-42.

30. Keller RL, et al. Infant pulmonary function in a randomized trial of fetal tracheal occlusion for severe congenital diaphragmatic hernia. Pediatr Res, 2004. 56(5): p. 818-25.

31. Deprest JA, et al. Changing perspectives on the perinatal management of isolated congenital diaphragmatic hernia in Europe. Clin Perinatol, 2009. 36(2): p. 329-47, ix.

32. Kunisaki SM, et al. Ex utero intrapartum treatment with extracorporeal membrane oxygenation for severe congenital diaphragmatic hernia. J Pediatr Surg, 2007. 42(1): p. 98-104; discussion 104-6.

33. Ford WD, et al. Antenatal betamethasone and favourable outcomes in fetuses with 'poor prognosis' diaphragmatic hernia. Pediatr Surg Int, 2002. 18(4): p. 244-6.

34. Lally KP, et al. Corticosteroids for fetuses with congenital diaphragmatic hernia: can we show benefit? J Pediatr Surg, 2006. 41(4): p. 668-74; discussion 668-74.

35. Cogo PE, et al. Pulmonary surfactant disaturated-phosphatidylcholine (DSPC) turnover and pool size in newborn infants with congenital diaphragmatic hernia (CDH). Pediatr Res, 2003. 54(5): p. 653-8.

36. Janssen DJ, et al. Decreased surfactant phosphatidylcholine synthesis in neonates with congenital diaphragmatic hernia during extracorporeal membrane oxygenation. Intensive Care Med, 2009. 35(10): p. 1754-60.

37. Lally KP, et al. Surfactant does not improve survival rate in preterm infants with congenital diaphragmatic hernia. J Pediatr Surg, 2004. 39(6): p. 829-33.

38. Van Meurs K. Is surfactant therapy beneficial in the treatment of the term newborn infant with congenital diaphragmatic hernia? J Pediatr, 2004. 145(3): p. 312-6.

39. German JC, et al. Management of pulmonary insufficiency in diaphragmatic hernia using extracorporeal circulation with a membrane oxygenator (ECMO). J Pediatr Surg, 1977. 12(6): p. 905-12.

40. Moyer V, et al. Late versus early surgical correction for congenital diaphragmatic hernia in newborn infants. Cochrane Database Syst Rev, 2002. 3(3): p. CD001695.

41. Sebald M, et al. Risk of need for extracorporeal membrane oxygenation support in neonates with congenital diaphragmatic

hernia treated with inhaled nitric oxide. J Perinatol, 2004. 24(3): p. 143-6.

42. Somaschini M, et al. Impact of new treatments for respiratory failure on outcome of infants with congenital diaphragmatic hernia. Eur J Pediatr, 1999. 158(10): p. 780-4.

43. Nagaya M, et al. Analysis of patients with congenital diaphragmatic hernia requiring pre-operative extracorporeal membrane oxygenation (ECMO). Pediatr Surg Int, 1998. 14(1-2): p. 25-9.

44. vd Staak FH, et al. Do we use the right entry criteria for extracorporeal membrane oxygenation in congenital diaphragmatic hernia? J Pediatr Surg, 1993. 28(8): p. 1003-5.

45. Howell CG, et al. Recent experience with diaphragmatic hernia and ECMO. Ann Surg, 1990. 211(6): p. 793-7; discussion 797-8.

46. Brown KL, et al. Extracorporeal membrane oxygenation and term neonatal respiratory failure deaths in the United Kingdom compared with the United States: 1999 to 2005. Pediatr Crit Care Med, 2010. 11(1): p. 60-5.

47. Lally KP. The Congenital Diaphragmatic Hernia Study Group., The use of ECMO for stabilization of infants with Congenital Diaphragmatic Hernia-A Report of the CDH Study Group (Abstract). Surgical Section of the American Academy of Pediatrics, Boston, MA, 2002.

48. Haugen SE, et al. Congenital diaphragmatic hernia: determination of the optimal time for operation by echocardiographic monitoring of the pulmonary arterial pressure. J Pediatr Surg, 1991. 26(5): p. 560-2.

49. West KW, et al. Delayed surgical repair and ECMO improves survival in congenital diaphragmatic hernia. Ann Surg, 1992. 216(4): p. 454-60; discussion 460-2.

50. Tsao K, Lally KP. Surgical Management of the Newborn with Congenital Diaphragmatic Hernia. Fetal Diagn Ther, 2010. 7: p. 7.

51. Stevens TP, et al. Survival in early- and late-term infants with congenital diaphragmatic hernia treated with extracorporeal membrane oxygenation. Pediatrics, 2002. 110(3): p. 590-6.

52. Finer NN, et al. Neonatal congenital diaphragmatic hernia and extracorporeal membrane oxygenation. Cmaj, 1992. 146(4): p. 501-8.

53. D'Agostino JA, et al. Outcome for infants with congenital diaphragmatic hernia requiring extracorporeal membrane oxygenation: the first year. J Pediatr Surg, 1995. 30(1): p. 10-5.

54. Schaible T, et al. A 20-year experience on neonatal extracorporeal membrane oxygenation in a referral center. Intensive Care Med, 2010. 36(7): p. 1229-34.

55. Azarow K, et al. Congenital diaphragmatic hernia--a tale of two cities: the Toronto experience. J Pediatr Surg, 1997. 32(3): p. 395-400.

56. Tsao K, et al. Congenital diaphragmatic hernia in the preterm infant. Surgery, 2010. 148(2): p. 404-10.

57. Bryner BS, et al. Right-sided congenital diaphragmatic hernia: high utilization of extracorporeal membrane oxygenation and high survival. J Pediatr Surg, 2009. 44(5): p. 883-7.

58. Downard CD, et al. Analysis of an improved survival rate for congenital diaphragmatic hernia. J Pediatr Surg, 2003. 38(5): p. 729-32.

59. Seetharamaiah R, et al. Factors associated with survival in infants with congenital diaphragmatic hernia requiring extracorporeal membrane oxygenation: a report from the Congenital Diaphragmatic Hernia Study Group. J Pediatr Surg, 2009. 44(7): p. 1315-21.

60. Odibo AO, et al. Predictors of the need for extracorporeal membrane oxygenation and survival in congenital diaphragmatic hernia:

a center's 10-year experience. Prenat Diagn, 2010. 30(6): p. 518-21.

61. Tiruvoipati R, et al. Predictors of outcome in patients with congenital diaphragmatic hernia requiring extracorporeal membrane oxygenation. J Pediatr Surg, 2007. 42(8): p. 1345-50.

62. Hoffman SB, et al. Predictors of survival in congenital diaphragmatic hernia patients requiring extracorporeal membrane oxygenation: CNMC 15-year experience. J Perinatol, 2010. 30(8): p. 546-52.

63. Cornish JD, et al. Efficacy of venovenous extracorporeal membrane oxygenation for neonates with respiratory and circulatory compromise. J Pediatr, 1993. 122(1): p. 105-9.

64. Heiss KF, et al. Preferential use of venovenous extracorporeal membrane oxygenation for congenital diaphragmatic hernia. J Pediatr Surg, 1995. 30(3): p. 416-9.

65. Dimmitt RA, et al. Venoarterial versus venovenous extracorporeal membrane oxygenation in congenital diaphragmatic hernia: the Extracorporeal Life Support Organization Registry, 1990-1999. J Pediatr Surg, 2001. 36(8): p. 1199-204.

66. Guner YS, et al. Outcome analysis of neonates with congenital diaphragmatic hernia treated with venovenous vs venoarterial extracorporeal membrane oxygenation. J Pediatr Surg, 2009. 44(9): p. 1691-701.

67. Frenckner B, et al. Neonates with congenital diaphragmatic hernia have smaller neck veins than other neonates-An alternative route for ECMO cannulation. J Pediatr Surg, 2002. 37(6): p. 906-8.

68. Fisher JC, et al. Challenges to cannulation for extracorporeal support in neonates with right-sided congenital diaphragmatic hernia. J Pediatr Surg, 2007. 42(12): p. 2123-8.

69. Lally KP, et al. Congenital diaphragmatic hernia. Stabilization and repair on ECMO. Ann Surg, 1992. 216(5): p. 569-73.

70. Downard CD, et al. Impact of AMICAR on hemorrhagic complications of ECMO: a ten-year review. J Pediatr Surg, 2003. 38(8): p. 1212-6.

71. Clark RH, et al. Current surgical management of congenital diaphragmatic hernia: a report from the Congenital Diaphragmatic Hernia Study Group. J Pediatr Surg, 1998. 33(7): p. 1004-9.

72. Bryner BS, et al. Congenital diaphragmatic hernia requiring extracorporeal membrane oxygenation: does timing of repair matter? J Pediatr Surg, 2009. 44(6): p. 1165-71; discussion 1171-2.

73. Dassinger MS, et al. Early repair of congenital diaphragmatic hernia on extracorporeal membrane oxygenation. J Pediatr Surg, 2010. 45(4): p. 693-7.

74. Stolar CJ. What do survivors of congenital diaphragmatic hernia look like when they grow up? Semin Pediatr Surg, 1996. 5(4): p. 275-9.

75. McGahren ED, et al. Neurological outcome is diminished in survivors of congenital diaphragmatic hernia requiring extracorporeal membrane oxygenation. J Pediatr Surg, 1997. 32(8): p. 1216-20.

76. Muratore CS, et al. Nutritional morbidity in survivors of congenital diaphragmatic hernia. J Pediatr Surg, 2001. 36(8): p. 1171-6.

77. Cortes RA, et al. Survival of severe congenital diaphragmatic hernia has morbid consequences. J Pediatr Surg, 2005. 40(1): p. 36-45; discussion 45-6.

78. Guner YS, et al. Anterior fundoplication at the time of congenital diaphragmatic hernia repair. Pediatr Surg Int, 2009. 25(8): p. 715-8.

79. Hofhuis W, et al. Prospective longitudinal evaluation of lung function during the first year of life after extracorporeal membrane oxygenation. Pediatr Crit Care Med, 2010. 24: p. 24.

80. Davis PJ, et al. Long-term outcome following extracorporeal membrane oxygenation

for congenital diaphragmatic hernia: the UK experience. J Pediatr, 2004. 144(3): p. 309-15.

81. Nijhuis-van der Sanden MW, et al. Motor performance in five-year-old extracorporeal membrane oxygenation survivors: a population-based study. Crit Care, 2009. 13(2): p. R47.

82. Danzer E, et al. Neurodevelopmental outcome of infants with congenital diaphragmatic hernia prospectively enrolled in an interdisciplinary follow-up program. J Pediatr Surg, 2010. 45(9): p. 1759-66.

19

ECMO for Pediatric Respiratory Failure

Heidi Dalton MD, James D. Fortenberry MD, Bjorn Frenckner MD PhD, Palle Palmer MD

Pediatric ECLS and ECMO are terms used for extracorporeal life support in children older than one month. This distinction from "neonatal" ECLS is made because of the different pathophysiology and diagnoses encountered in newborns. Conditions treated with ECMO during the first month of life are congenital or acquired at birth, including meconium aspiration syndrome (MAS), pulmonary hypoplasia with or without congenital diaphragmatic hernia (CDH), pneumonia/septicemia, and persistent pulmonary hypertension of the newborn (PPHN). These conditions are characterized by increased pulmonary vascular resistance causing pulmonary hypertension. Since the fetal shunts are still open in newborns, right-to-left shunts with further deterioration in oxygenation are seen when pulmonary pressure exceeds systemic pressure.[1]

Selection Criteria

Strict criteria for the application of ECMO in pediatric respiratory failure are not available. None of the published severity-of-illness markers or clinical parameters have been proven to universally predict outcome but may remain of assistance when trying to identify patients for ECLS support.[2-5]

1. $AaDO_2$:

$$AaDO_2 = FiO_2 \text{ (Barometric Pressure - Water Vapor Pressure)} - PaCO_2/RQ - PaO_2$$

where Barometric Pressure =760 cmH_2O at sea level, Water Vapor Pressure= 47 cmH_2O and RQ assumed to be 1. This marker has been historically used in neonatal respiratory failure. An $AaDO_2$ of >610 for 8 hours correlated to 80% mortality in neonatal respiratory failure by historical controls. Among pediatric patients, an $AaDO_2$ of >470 was noted by Timmons to be 81% predictive of death based on data published in 1991.[6]

2. Oxygenation Index (OI)

$$OI = \frac{FiO_2 \times MAP \ (cmH_2O) \times 100}{PaO_2 \ (mmHg)}$$

OI > 40 predicted mortality of >80%, historically. OI = 25-40 predicted mortality of 50-80%, historically. OI >40 or remaining >25 over multiple hours is associated with high mortality in neonates, pediatric patients, and in adults (especially those following lung transplant).

In pediatric respiratory failure, OI >40 even at 6 hours of ventilation was associated with mortality of 40%, with increasing mortality risk over time, as shown in Figure 19-1.[6]

3. Compliance:

C= ΔVolume/ΔPressure

C= tidal volume/ PIP* - PEEP

*plateau pressure best value to use

Compliance values of <0.5 ml/cmH$_2$O have been used in adult ECLS patient selection

4. Intrapulmonary Shunt > 30-50% on FiO$_2$ >0.6

Shunt has been used as a selection criterion, predominantly in adult ECLS.

5. Murray score:

Murray Score >3

Comprised of PaO$_2$/FiO$_2$, PEEP, Compliance and CXR quadrants involved in disease. Score is between 0-4 and is used in Adult ECLS. This was a criterion for entry into the CESAR trial.

6. Ventilatory failure:

Hypercarbia with persistent pH <7.0 on "high ventilator support" such as PIP >40 cmH$_2$O.

7. PaO$_2$/FiO$_2$

calculated as example, PaO$_2$50 mmHg, FiO$_2$ 100% (1.0)

p/f= 50/1= 50

Values <100 mmHg have been noted predominantly in adult ECLS.

Acute Respiratory Distress Syndrome (ARDS) is defined as a P/F of <200 in most studies while Acute Lung Injury (ALI) is defined as a P/F<300.

While none of these markers have proven to be completely predictive of outcome, having an algorithm that includes serial evaluation of some of these markers may allow centers to identify potential ECLS candidates more readily.

Patient Population

The major categories of pediatric respiratory failure from the Extracorporeal Life Support Registry who have received ECLS are shown in Table 19-1.[7] Viral pneumonia, bacterial pneumonia, ARDS, and aspiration are the most common

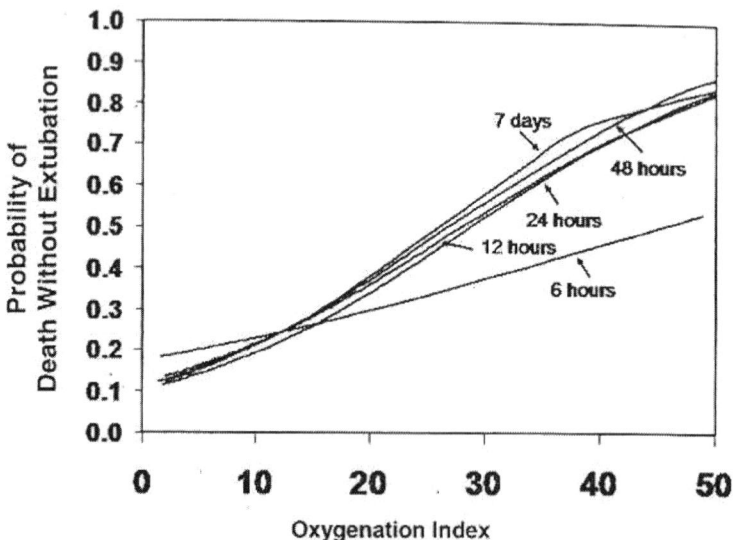

Figure 19-1. Oxygenation Index and Outcome in Pediatric Respirtory Failure. Adapted from Trachsel D, McCrindle BW, Nakagawa S, Bohn D. Oxygenation index predicts outcome in children with acute hypoxemic respiratory failure. Am J Respir Crit Care Med 2005;172:206-11.

diagnoses encountered. Survival has increased slightly over time; the first third of the 2,810 ECLS runs were reported before 1994 with a mean survival of 52%, while the following two-thirds had survivals of 58% and 57%, respectively. This is a significant difference (based on Chi square analysis), but it is not possible to conclude if this is because of patient selection or improved ECLS survival. Survival is highest in cases of aspiration pneumonia (67%), viral pneumonia (63%), and postoperative or post-traumatic ARDS (59%). Many patients have conditions that are rare and are difficult to place into these large categories. Consequently, many pediatric patients in the ELSO Registry are reported as having "other" diagnoses. Efforts to more easily specify diagnosis without needing to look up each associated ICD-9 code will be enhanced by the changes which have been and are being made to the ELSO registry.

As experience with ECLS has grown, the expansion to patient populations avoided in the past is nowhere as clearly seen as pediatric patients. The "old days" when a healthy child would contract overwhelming pneumonia and be rescued with ECLS support are now few, as most pediatric ECLS patients today have underlying comorbidities in addition to their acute critical illness.[8-15]

The most recent Registry review of over 3,000 pediatric respiratory failure patients between 1993 and 2007 provides valuable information regarding experience and indications (Table 19-2).[16] Survivors had a lower median body weight (9 vs 9.9 kg), with a similar median age to non-survivors (Table 19-3). Older children (aged 10-18 years) had lower survival (50%) compared to infants (57%), toddlers (61%), and children (55%). In this review, while survival changed little over the time period, patients with comorbidities increased from 19% in 1993 to 47% of overall ECMO patients in 2007. Renal failure, chronic lung disease and congenital heart disease (two ventricle) formed the bulk of underlying comorbid conditions. While comorbidities exist in many patients, it is also true that patients who do NOT have this additional burden have better outcomes. In this same ELSO review, children without comorbidities were noted to have improved survival over time, from 57% in 1993 to 72% in 2007 (Figure 19-2). Another important factor reported in this summary is that no significant decline in survival was noted until patients reached a duration of ventilation prior to ECMO of >14 days (Figure 19-3). This is a large change from prior reports, which found that duration of ventilation for >7 days was associated with worsening outcome. The impact of ventilator mode was also assessed. The use of high frequency ventilation was noted in 38% of patients and did not change over the period

Table 19-1. ELSO Survival in Pediatric Respiratory Failure 1985-July 2011. Adapted from the International Extracorporeal Life Support Registry, Ann Arbor, MI.

	Total Runs	Mean Run Time (hours)	Mean Longest Run (hours)	Survived (%)
Viral pneumonia	1,014	321	1372	649 (53%)
Bacterial Pneumonia	550	284	1411	318 (58%)
Pneumocystis	31	363	1144	15 (48%)
Aspiration	206	270	2437	137 (67%)
ARDS, postop/trauma	123	249	935	73 (59%)
ARDS, not postop/trauma	411	310	2026	216 (53%)
Acute resp. failure, non-ARDS	861	250	1483	442 (51%)
Other	1,903	219	2968	981 (52%)

Table 19-2. Survival by Patient Age Group and Diagnosis 2000-2010. Adapted from Zabrocki L et al. Crit Care Med 2011; 39: 364-370

Primary Diagnosis	n (%)	Survival
Neonatal	9086	68.6
MAS	2239 (24.6)	92.9
RDS	203 (2.2)	85.2
PPHN/PFC	1820 (20.0)	75.9
Air Leak Syndrome	16 (0.2)	75.0
Sepsis	252 (2.8)	70.2
Other	1785 (19.7)	65.5
CDH	2767 (30.5)	46.7
Pneumonia	4 (0.04)	25.0
Pediatric	2992	55.7
Aspiration	13 (0.43)	69.2
Bacterial	134 (4.48)	62.7
ARDS, postop/trauma	80 (2.7)	60.0
Acute Respiratory Failure, not ARDS	306 (10.2)	56.5
Pneumocystis	16 (0.53)	56.3
Other	2246 (75.1)	55.1
ARDS, not postop/trauma	185 (6.2)	54.1
Viral	12 (0.4)	50.0
Adult	1921	56.0
Viral	35 (1.8)	74.3
Aspiration	7 (0.4)	71.4
Bacterial	156 (8.1)	62.8
ARDS, postop/trauma	143 (7.4)	60.1
Acute Respiratory Failure, non ARDS	102 (5.3)	57.8
Other	1266 (65.9)	55.4
ARDS, not postop	212 (11.0)	47.2

Table 19-3. Demographics of Pediatric Respiratory Failure ECMO (1993-2007). Adapted from Zabrocki L et al. Crit Care Med 2011; 39: 364-370

Variable	Survivors (n=1824)	Nonsurvivors (n=1389)	Survival	p
Gender [n (%)]				.784
Male	890 (49)	695 (50)	56%	
Female	896 (49)	666 (48)	57%	
Missing	38 (2)	28 (2)	58%	
Weight, kg (median, interquartile range)	9 (4-17)	9.9 (4.3-23)		.003
Age group [n(%)]				.001
30 days-1 yr	880 (48)	661 (48)	57%	
1-5 yrs	513 (28)	329 (24)	61%	
5-10 yrs	165 (9)	133 (10)	55%	
10-18 yrs	266 (15)	266 (19)	50%	

1993-2007. Survival was not different between modes of ventilation. Patients who received high frequency oscillation, however, did have a longer period of ventilation before ECMO than those who received conventional mechanical ventilation (4.6 vs 3 days).

In regard to markers of severity of illness, non-survivors had a higher median OI (48 vs. 42) and lower pH (7.27 vs. 7.31) than survivors.

Pre-ECMO pH was progressively lower in both survivors and non-survivors as the years progressed. Of note, a pre-ECMO pH < 7.29 was an independent risk factor for mortality. This decline in pH was accompanied by a trend for increasing $PaCO_2$ over time, which may indicate that "permissive hypercapnia" as a means of limiting ventilator induced lung injury has become accepted medical practice. Another

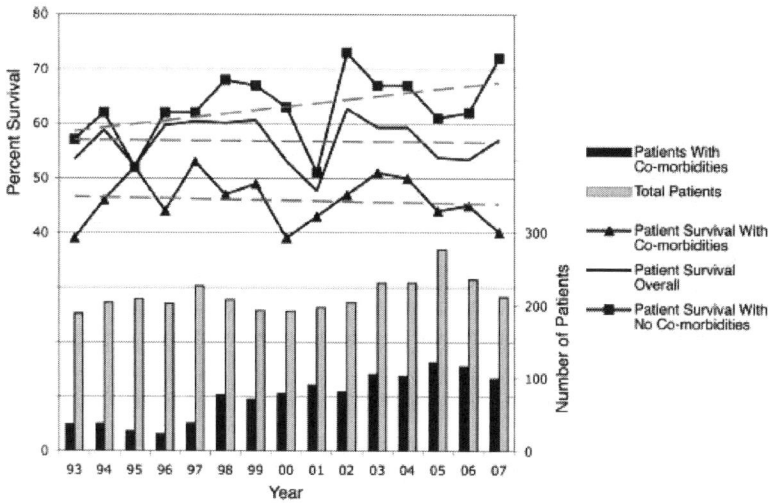

Figure 19-2. Survival with co-morbidities over Time. Adapted from Zabrocki L et al. Crit Care Med 2011; 39: 364-370

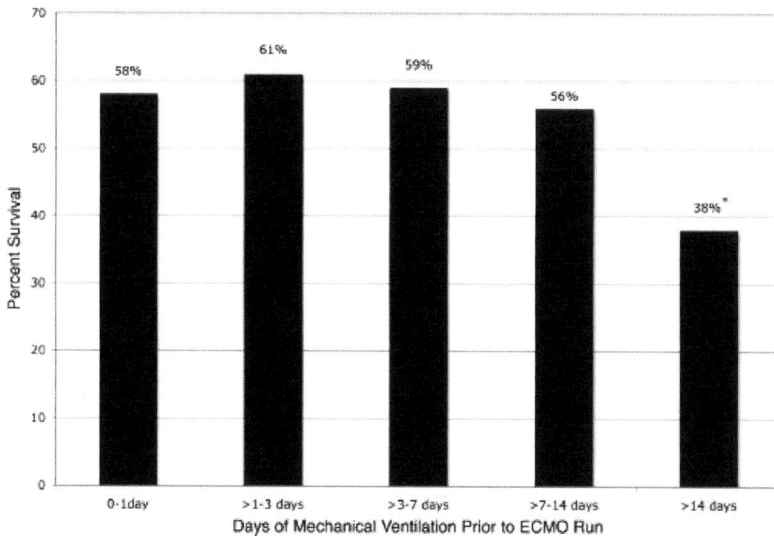

Figure 19-3. Survival by Days of Mechanical Ventilation Prior to ECMO. Adapted from Zabrocki L et al. Crit Care Med 2011; 39: 364-370

small review of ECMO in a recent time period also noted changes in pH and pCO_2 over time (Figure 19-4).[17]

In the ELSO review, patients with ARDS related to sepsis had increased mortality as compared to patients with underlying bacterial or viral pneumonia, influenza, or ARDS that was related to trauma or surgery. Patients with pertussis or fungal pneumonia had increased odds of death. In contrast, patients with asthma, respiratory syncytial virus, or aspiration had decreased odds of death. Other parameters associated with risk of death are shown in Table 19-4. Other reports have outlined the use of ECMO in patients with cancer, solid organ transplant, immunodeficiencies, and burns.[11,13]

One report of 107 children with a hematologic malignancy (72) or a solid tumour (34) found that 42% who received ECMO were weaned off support with 35% surviving to hospital discharge.[9] This has fostered an increasing practice of considering ECMO for these children if their underlying cancer or immune defect is felt amenable to a good long-term outcome. Perhaps even more representative of how the philosophy of ECLS has changed is the application of ECLS for cardiorespiratory support in patients who are recently postoperative, following trauma, who have intracranial bleeding and in those who are recipients of bone marrow transplant.[8,11,18] Despite the concerns that these types of patients would have complications of bleeding, infection, or other problems which would make use of ECMO futile, survival has been attained. In pediatric patients, there are no randomized studies comparing ECLS treatment with conventional treatment. In a retrospective multicenter study involving 331 patients from 32 hospitals, ECLS was compared with conventional treatment. In 53 diagnosis- and risk-matched pairs, there was a significantly lower mortality among the ECLS patients (26% vs. 47%).[19] The authors concluded that ECLS was responsible for the

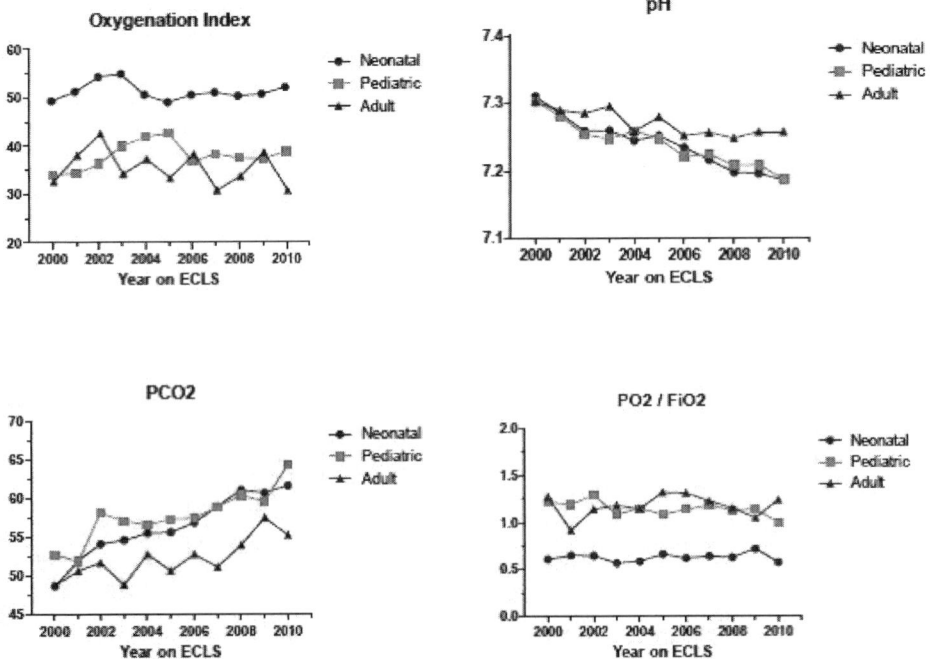

Figure 19-4. Severity Indices and blood gas data by major diagnostic category (2000-2010). Dalton HJ, Garcia-Filion P, unpublished data, with permission.

improved survival, as there was no association of outcome with the use of other tertiary technologies.

Unique Patient Populations for ECLS Use:

Selective CO_2 Removal

For status asthmaticus and other conditions in which $PaCO_2$ is very high, reducing the $PaCO_2$ gradually to avoid acid-base imbalances or cerebral complications is advisable. A suggested rate of decreasing $PaCO_2$ is 20 mm/Hg/hr.

Table 19-4. Odds Ratios of Selected Variables and ECMO Survival. Adapted from Zabrocki L et al. Crit Care Med 2011; 39: 364-370

Variable	Adjusted Odds Radio	95% Confidence Interval
Diagnosis[a]		
Asthma	0.37	0.18-0.75
Submersion	0.50	0.23-1.10
Pulmonary hemorrhage	0.56	0.28-1.12
Aspiration	0.59	0.42-0.83
Respiratory syncytial virus	0.63	0.50-0.81
ARDS, other	0.93	0.32-2.68
Pneumocystis	1.20	0.49-2.90
Acute respiratory failure	1.29	1.04-1.61
Other	1.29	0.95-1.75
ARDS, sepsis	1.53	1.11-2.11
Pertussis	1.71	1.05-2.77
Fungal pneumonia	5.88	1.18-29.32
Comorbidity		
Renal failure	2.20	1.68-2.89
Primary immunodeficiency	2.35	1.30-4.25
Cardiac arrest	2.25	1.35-3.74
Cancer	2.56	1.55-4.23
Liver failure	4.33	1.95-9.62
Pre-ECMO characteristics		
Treatment before 2001	1.22	1.03-1.44
Age > 10 yrs	1.37	1.10-1.71
Ventilation > 14 days	2.55	1.90-3.42
Pre-ECMO blood pH		
<7.19	1.53	1.24-1.88
7.19-7.29	1.34	1.11-1.62
>7.29	1	Reference group
Pre-ECMO P/F	.997	0.996-0.999
ECMO support		
Venovenous ECMO	.66	0.56-0.77
Venoarterial ECMO	1	Reference group

ARDS, acute respiratory distress; ECMO, extracorporeal membrane oxygenation; P/F, PaO_2/FIO_2 ratio
[a]Reference group = bacterial pneumonia+other viral pneumonia+ARDS-trauma/postoperative+influenza (n=1060).
Model characteristics: n=2926, Nagelkerke R^2=.60

When selective CO_2 removal is used to treat permissive hypercapnia and to achieve rest lung settings in ARDS, CO_2 can be normalized at acceptable rest lung settings with low blood flow (20% of cardiac output). If the lung failure is severe, this can result in major hypoxemia. If the cardiac output and hemoglobin concentration are normal, arterial saturation as low as 75% is safe and well tolerated. However, increasing extracorporeal blood flow to improve oxygenation is preferable to increasing ventilator pressure or FiO_2 when selective CO_2 removal is used.[10]

Support of the Tracheobronchial Tree

ECMO may be extremely useful in providing airway support during or following surgical repair of the tracheobronchial tree. It allows adequate carbon dioxide removal and oxygenation at low levels of mechanical ventilator support. Use of ECLS may also eliminate the need for endotracheal intubation and mechanical ventilation altogether. This may enhance the ease of surgical repair and subsequently facilitate healing without concern for rupturing suture lines from applied positive pressure.

Mediastinal Masses

ECLS may be applied in conditions where anterior mediastinal masses cause airway compression and high risk of death during endotracheal intubation.[20] Application of ECLS under local anesthesia or light sedation with the patient in the upright position may avoid acute death in situations where loss of negative pressure from spontaneous breathing results in collapse of compressed airways which cannot be reexpanded with conventional tracheal intubation.

Pulmonary Embolism

Many patients with primary or secondary ARDS will have small (segmental) pulmonary emboli on contrast CT or angiography. Such emboli do not require any specific treatment aside from the heparinization which accompanies ECLS. When major or massive pulmonary embolism is the cause of respiratory/cardiac failure, venoarterial (VA) ECLS can be very successful if cannulation and extracorporeal support can be instituted before brain injury occurs. After VA access and successful ECLS is established, the extent of pulmonary embolism can be documented by appropriate imaging studies.[14,21] Massive pulmonary emboli will usually resolve or move into segmental branches within 48-72 hours of ECLS support. The patient can be weaned from ECLS then and managed with ongoing prophylaxis against further pulmonary embolism. Almost all such patients are managed with placement of an inferior vena caval filter. If heart/lung function has not recovered within two days, or if there is a secondary reason to get the patient off ECLS (e.g., gastrointestinal bleeding), the patient should undergo pulmonary thrombectomy with cardiopulmonary bypass support. When thrombectomy is done it is usually necessary to continue ECLS for days until lung function is normal.

ARDS with Secondary Lung Injury (Following Shock, Trauma, Sepsis, etc.)

Once the patient is on ECLS support for stability, adequate repair of secondary organ damage must be performed. If surgical repair of organ injury is required (e.g., pancreatic resection and drainage for necrotizing pancreatitis, fasciotomy and/or amputation for compartment syndromes and gangrene, excision and drainage of abscesses), these procedures may be adequately performed during ECMO support. Due to concern about increased bleeding, pulmonary failure after major trauma was previously considered a contraindication for ECLS. Encouraging results with adult trauma patients have stimulated centers to use ECLS for pediatric trauma patients when they meet traditional ECLS criteria. In a recently published report, five children were treated with ECLS after motor vehicle accidents and major injuries, of which four required major surgery. The PaO_2/FiO_2 ratio before ECLS was 23-109. Of the five children, four survived to hospital discharge.[8]

Pulmonary Hemorrhage

Pulmonary hemorrhage is a rare but potentially fatal condition when treated with conventional treatment. In spite of anticoagulation and impaired homeostasis due to the extracorporeal circulation, the ECLS survival is good. Good outcomes have been reported in neonates and adults, including one patient with profuse bleeding from several mycotic aneurysms leading to hypovolemic shock. In a report of eight children with pulmonary hemorrhage and a PaO_2/FiO_2 ratio between 33 and 70 on mechanical ventilation, all survived to hospital discharge after venovenous (VV) or venoarterial (VA) ECLS.[22] Further more, a case series by Kolovos et al. in 1999 demonstrated excellent survival in patients with pulmonary/renal syndromes who had failed conventional ventilator management. ECLS allowed time for appropriate therapy to be initiated and recovery with pulmonary healing to occur.[24]

Pertussis

Severe *Bordetella pertussis* infection in infants is associated with extremely high mortality. Initial reports of ECLS treatment were disappointing and the value of ECLS treatment of patients with pertussis infection was questioned. In a single-center series of 12 infants there were 7 deaths.[23] The authors concluded that in spite of the high mortality, ECLS support should be offered to infants with severe pertussis meeting conventional ECLS criteria. A retrospective chart review of the ELSO Registry revealed a total of 61 children with pertussis placed on ECLS support between 1990 and 2002. The mean age of the patients was 88 days, and the overall mortality was 70%. Mortality was significantly higher in infants younger than 6 weeks (84%) compared to children older than 6 weeks (61%).[24]

Pneumocystis jiroveci

Pneumocystis jiroveci (formerly *Pneumocystis carinii*) pneumonia mainly occurs during immunosuppressive treatment in patients with malignancies and is a severe complication with a poor prognosis if mechanical ventilation is required. In the ELSO Registry, only 22 cases have been reported, out of which 9 (41%) survived. A single-center experience was more encouraging, with 3 of 4 patients surviving.[11]

Other Rare Conditions

ECLS has been used for rare causes of pulmonary failure with variable success. When considering ECLS for a specific diagnosis for the first time in any given center it may be helpful to consult the ELSO registry for the worldwide experience with that condition. Examples are vasculitis, autoimmune lung disease, bronchiolitis obliterans, Goodpasture syndrome, and rare bacterial, fungal or viral infections.[25,26]

ECLS in Sepsis

One difficulty in interpreting ELSO data is that many patients who are currently receiving ECLS have a combination of respiratory and cardiac failure—thus, assigning them to the three major groups in the ELSO Registry (respiratory, cardiac, or emergency CPR) is difficult. This skews the ability to accurately report results and is one major area where the ELSO registry is being refined. Without data on severity of illness beyond the respiratory indices previously discussed, identifying risk factors for outcome or complications is difficult. One such example of this issue is in children with septic shock. These patients often have both respira-

tory and cardiac dysfunction as well as injury to other organs.[27] The ELSO registry notes that 12% of pediatric respiratory failure patients have coexisting sepsis. Outcome of patients in septic shock is believed to be lower than in patients with single organ failure, although good comparisons on a large scale have not been conducted. One early report from 1997 noted that although children with sepsis had lower survival (37% vs 52% in non-septic patients), sepsis alone was not a multivariate predictor of outcome when compared with other pre-ECMO variables such as age, pH, presence of renal failure, or ventilator settings.[28] Septic patients, however, were noted to have increased seizures and other neurologic complications. In another report of 82 patients from a single center, while only 12 had ECMO initiated for septic shock alone (50% survival), 40% had sepsis as a coexisting diagnosis. Another point of interest from this series was that among patients with significant inotropic requirement, 35% were supported with venovenous cannulation and 36% with venoarterial support. Vasoactive support was able to be weaned in the first 24 hours of support in the majority of patients. The ability of VV cannulation to support patients with hemodynamic compromise prior to ECMO is another changing aspect of ECMO care that requires more investigation.[29] Better refinement of organ failure and severity of illness by the ELSO Registry may allow more sophisticated analyses of these complex patients in the future.

The recognition of ECMO support for sepsis is highlighted by groups such as the American College of Critical Care Medicine. The 2007 guidelines from this group for hemodynamic support in infants and children with septic shock now recommend consideration of ECMO as an option in patients who remain in shock following fluid resuscitation, vasoactive infusions, and corticosteroids.[30-32] However, the guidelines do not provide any specific markers to use in patient selection, excepting hypotension. Some variables which may be useful to follow to help identify potential patients include:[33]

1. Plasma lactate persistently >5 mmol/L
2. SvO2 <55% at an estimated Cardiac Index of at least 2.1
3. Severe ventricular dysfunction
4. Intractable arrhythmia with hemodynamic compromise
5. Cardiac Arrest
6. Inotrope score >50 for 1 hour or >45 for 8 hours. IE= Dopamine (mcg/kg/min) + Dobutamine (mcg/kg/min) + 100 x Epinephrine (mcg/kg/min). Modified Inotrope/Vasoactive Score= Dopamine (mcg/kg/min) + Dobutamine (mcg/kg/min) + 100 x Epinephrine (mcg/kg/min)+ 100 x Norepinephrine (mcg/kg/min) + Milrinone (mcg/kg/min) x 10 (15 is also used by some clinicians) + 10,000 x vasopressin dose (mcg/kg/min)
7. Failure to wean from cardiopulmonary bypass (see Chapter 28 on Sepsis)

More recent reports of ECMO in sepsis have found much improved outcomes than in years past. Of interest to many has been the report of improved survival in patients who initially were supported with peripheral cannulation techniques but who were converted to mediastinal support or had primary mediastinal cannulation due to access difficulties. Of the 23 patients in this report, 22 had 3 or more organ system failures, 23 were requiring >2 inotropes, 8 suffered a cardiac arrest prior to ECMO, and overall survival was 74%. Pre-ECLS lactate levels were higher in non-survivors (11.7 vs 6, p=0.007).[31] When these 23 patients were analyzed, a significantly higher blood flow during the first 24 hours of ECLS was associated with improved outcome. Patients with central cannulation were noted to have increased blood flow during ECLS. The authors speculated that the increased oxygen delivery from the higher blood flow improved organ recovery and thus, survival. Another small report found that in 13 patients with enteroviral infection, central cannulation was performed with successful weaning from ECMO in 77% and 60% survival to discharge with "good" neurologic outcome.[34] When compared to the prior cohort of patients with similar infection but who were not treated with ECMO, survival was only 30% and none of the survivors were described as having "good" neurologic outcome.

The H1N1 epidemic of 2009 also provided a unique opportunity to evaluate ECLS in patients with multiple organ failure related to influenza. Success in supporting these patients generated great discussion on the use of ECLS, especially among adult patients.[35-38]

Contraindications

Given the increasingly reported success with conditions once considered incompatible with ECMO, few absolute contraindications exist for considering children with respiratory failure for ECMO support. Assessment is best made on an individual patient basis. Conversation is recommended with the referral ECMO center before making a final decision on eligibility for support to allow for the complexities of these patients. ECMO center staff often discuss difficult patients as a group to determine a consensus. Long term outcome from underlying comorbidities are often the most important considerations when deciding whether to implement ECLS or not. Risks, benefits, resource use and availability are also practical issues to consider.

The Pediatric ECLS Circuit:

Cannulation Modes and Methods of Support:

Despite the differences in pathophysiology between neonatal and pediatric patients, the basic principles of ECLS are the same.[39] Desaturated blood is withdrawn from a central vein or the right atrium and pumped through a membrane oxygenator and a heat exchanger before it is returned to the patient. In the oxygenator, the blood is oxygenated and carbon dioxide is removed. If the blood is returned to a major artery, the process is referred to as VA ECMO, whereas if the blood is returned to a major vein, the bypass is referred to as VV ECMO. The specific cannulation techniques are described in detail in other chapters, as is the physiology and advantages of the different modes of ECLS.

Similar to the lack of specific ECMO initiation criteria in children, there is also little complete standardization of ECMO circuit design, cannulation techniques, and patient management, although general principles remain fairly constant. Guidelines for ECMO center training, equipment selection, patient selection, and management have recently been developed by expert consensus and are posted on the ELSO website www.elso.med.umich.edu. While the guidelines are fairly general, they may enable greater standardization of practice in the future across centers.

Specific Points in Pediatric Cannulation

Traditionally VA ECLS has been the most frequently utilized mode of ECLS in children for both respiratory and cardiac failure, accounting for the majority of pediatric respiratory failure cases in the ELSO Registry.[1] However, there is an increasing trend toward the use of VV bypass. In 2004, only half of the pediatric respiratory ECLS cases used VA ECLS. VV support has been increasingly used, and several reports have found improved survival in patients supported with VV ECMO. As the ELSO registry gives little detail on severity of illness before ECMO, interpretation of outcome comparisons between VA and VV ECMO can be difficult, but the consistent difference in survivals with VV

use bears strong consideration of VV use given ongoing improvement in cannulae and patient management experience.

Newer cannulas now allow use of VV ECLS in patients from newborn through adult using a single surgical site.[40] One device is the Avalon® catheter, which is a wire wrapped single cannula which has two venous drainage ports that sit in the SVC/RA and IVC/RA junctions with the inflow (arterial return) port directed at the tricuspid valve when the cannula is correctly placed. The cannulas range in size from 13 Fr to 31 Fr and have markedly less recirculation than other cannulas. Despite these features, the cannula is somewhat difficult to place without fluoroscopic or echocardiographic guidance. Older versions of double lumen, single cannulas have had some problems with collapse of the venous return lumen with centrifugal pumps and problems with kinking—a problem which seems poised to be resolved with newer production models soon to be in clinical trials. Percutaneous kits which do not require surgical cutdown and improved dilator systems for easier placement of cannulas have also improved cannulation for ECLS patients. A recent review of 1200 patients supported with ECMO at eight large childrens' hospitals found that venovenous support has risen in all age groups in the ELSO registry over the last two years (Figure 19-5).[17]

For patients who are receiving extracorporeal cannulation, it is essential that the drainage capacity is adequate, as this determines the maximum extracorporeal blood flow attainable and thereby influences how much support is provided. The venous cannula must be of adequate size and placed in the correct position. If venous drainage remains inadequate despite volume replacement and optimal catheter position, an additional venous cannula may be required. This is easily connected to the drainage tubing with a Y-connector.

In VA ECLS, the oxygenated blood is returned to the patient through a cannula inserted into a major artery. The common carotid artery has traditionally been the largest artery used for access. While some centers ligate the vessel and some repair it at decannulation, long term outcomes in terms of stroke or neurologic compromise later in life are still unclear.[41-44] Nonetheless, avoidance of the carotid artery is often suggested in older patients due to the potential for adverse neurologic events.

Non-cervical Cannulation

For children who are >15 kgs, the femoral artery is usually large enough to be accessed for oxygenated blood return. Due to the relatively sparse collateral circulation at the femoral site, this usually requires distal cannulation to provide perfusion of the limb. Despite the use of distal perfusion cannulas, however, limb ischemia leading to neurovascular compromise or amputation can occur.[45,46] Similarly, cannulation of the femoral vein can lead to distal venous engorgement and compartment syndrome. Careful monitoring of neurovascular integrity if femoral vessels are used for ECLS support is mandatory. Another disadvantage of femoral artery cannulation is that oxygenated blood is delivered far from the aortic root (Figure 19-6). For patients with severe respiratory failure, the upper half of the body, including the head and heart, will be perfused by desaturated blood ejected from

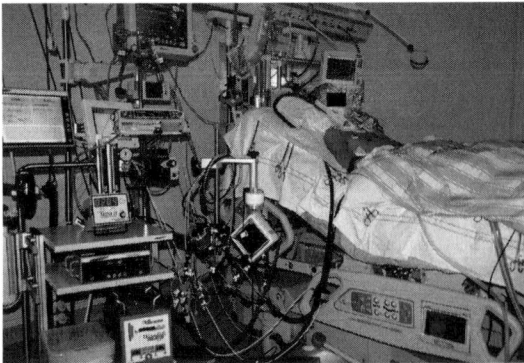

Figure 19-5. Adolescent Male on VV ECLS for Sepsis/Respiratory Failure

the left ventricle. Unless the extracorporeal circuit drains nearly all blood returned to the right atrium, this can lead to the "blue upper body, red lower body" phenomenon. If there is concern for adequate oxygen delivery to the upper body, as evidenced by myocardial ischemia, impaired neurologic performance by clinical symptoms, or near-infrared spectroscopy or other monitoring techniques, one solution is to insert a cannula in the internal jugular to the right atrium (VAV ECMO) and divert some of the oxygenated return from the ECLS circuit into this cannula to increase oxygenation to the right atrium (and thus to the left ventricle and ascending aorta). Another possibility is to use a very long femoral cannula and to position the tip in the aortic root; however, the flow resistance of this long cannula will be high and may limit arterial return.

Cannulation of the subclavian or axillary artery can also be performed, although similar limb ischemia problems may occur.[47] Direct cannulation of the aortic root requires an open thoracotomy and is not the preferred method of ECLS for respiratory support without concomitant cardiac dysfunction.

Conversion from VV to VA

VA ECLS can be converted to VV ECLS and vice versa during the run. If a patient on VA ECLS improves but the run is estimated to continue for a considerable time, this may be an indication for conversion to VV, as the risk of complications on VV ECLS is lower. For example, the consequences of an accidental embolus from the circuit are considerably more serious if the patient is on VA bypass. On the other hand, a patient initially put on VV bypass may need conversion to VA bypass if the support is found to be inadequate. Increased pulmonary vascular resistance, pulmonary hypertension, and right heart failure may also be indications for conversion from VV to VA bypass. In the ELSO Registry, 6% of pediatric patients were converted from VV to VA (of which 45% survived); very few were converted from VA to VV. In adult patients, 11% were converted from VA to VV (of which 82% survived) and 7% converted from VV to VA (none survived).[48]

As soon as the cannulas are in position and have been adequately secured, they are connected to the ECLS circuit. Air must be evacuated carefully, after which the extracorporeal circulation is started. If venous return is adequate, the venous cannula is likely in the correct position. If the venous return is inadequate, the cannula may be incorrectly placed. Chest radiograph and/or ultrasound will provide the desired information, as well as information regarding the position of the arterial cannula in cases of VA ECMO. Echocardiography remains the optimal means of assessing cannula placement especially in cervical cannulation.[49] If cervical arterial cannulation is used, the cannula

should be positioned so that it is not directed at the aortic valve to avoid damaging the valve or interfering with left ventricular emptying.

Oxygenator

The silicone rubber membrane oxygenator has been the traditional device used in pediatric respiratory failure ECMO and has proven suitable for long term extracorporeal use. Although its gas exchange is not as efficient in terms of gas exchange per square meter (m^2) as the more modern hollow fiber membranes, it is a true membrane with no plasma leakage from the blood to the gas phase during long-term use. This membrane oxygenator remains the only device approved by the FDA for long-term use. AVECOR oxygenators, most commonly used, are available in sizes from 0.4 to 4.5 m^2; however, membranes smaller than 0.8 m^2 are not

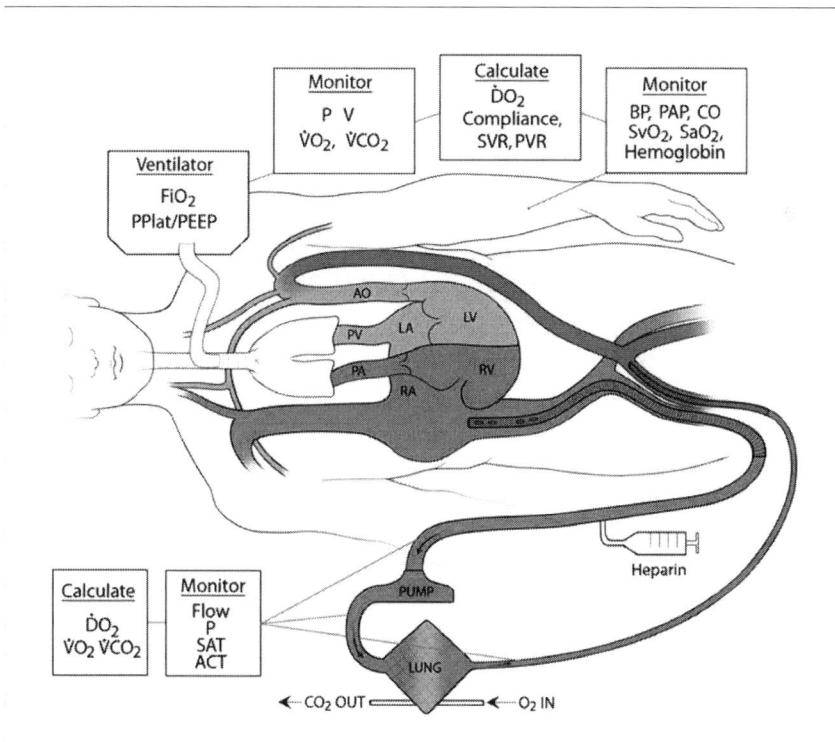

Figure 19-6. Blood flow from Femoral Venoarterial ECMO. With permission from R. Bartlett MD.

recommended for standard ECLS. In children greater than 30 kg, and in adults, dual 4.5 m² oxygenators are generally necessary. These can be assembled in parallel or in series. A parallel circuit will yield a lower pre-oxygenator circuit pressure and allow the oxygenators to be changed without interrupting the ECLS flow. The smallest oxygenators are equipped with 1/4-inch connectors while the larger ones have 3/8-inch connectors.

Newer polymethyl pentene fiber technology has led to new oxygenators that are rapidly becoming the standard for pediatric respiratory failure support. The oxygenators are highly efficient in gas exchange, low resistance, and ease of priming. At this writing, the Quadrox D and iD are the major PMP oxygenators used in the US, while other countries have a variety of other hollow fiber oxygenators. These newer devices have not had the same association with plasma leakage and short lifespans as older models.

Pumps

While roller head, semiocclusive pumps have been the predominant means of ECLS support for many years, a new series of centrifugal pumps have become available which are also having a major impact on ECMO support. Recent ELSO information estimates that over 70% of ECLS support is now provided with centrifugal devices. These pumps have smaller priming volumes and work for days to weeks without requiring replacement. The combination of these new pumps and oxygenators now allow circuits to be primed in minutes with small priming volumes and can be applied from neonates through adults. Such systems are being used for transport, for initiation during cardiac arrest, and for routine support (Figure 19-7). There are also theoretical considerations that these systems may cause less hemolysis, require less anticoagulation and generate less inflammatory response, although these facts have not yet been clinically

proven in a rigorous, studied fashion.[50] There are several small single center reports, however. One study compared two groups of ECMO patients: those from 1998-2001(Biomedicus pump and Scimed oxygenator) and those from 2002-2006 (Jostra pump and Quadrox pmp, hollow fiber oxygenator).[51] Patient survival to hospital discharge improved from 24 to 49% in the later group (Jostra pump and Quadrox), mechanical complications per 10,000 hours fell from 70 to 50, pump heads used per 10,000 hrs fell from 160 to 110, and oxygenators used per 10,000 hrs fell from 130 to110. Another recent report using the same setup (Jostra pump and Quadrox) noted less bleeding complications and sanguineous chest tube drainage in postoperative ECMO patients compared to patients receiving "standard" ECMO with a roller-head/silicone membrane circuit.[52]

Despite all these good points, however, centrifugal pumps can be dangerous, generating high levels of negative pressure on the venous inlet side, resulting in cavitation and hemolysis or propagating air throughout the circuit (and potentially into the patient) if it gets past the centrifugal head and is not captured by the oxygenator. To lessen the risk of cavitation

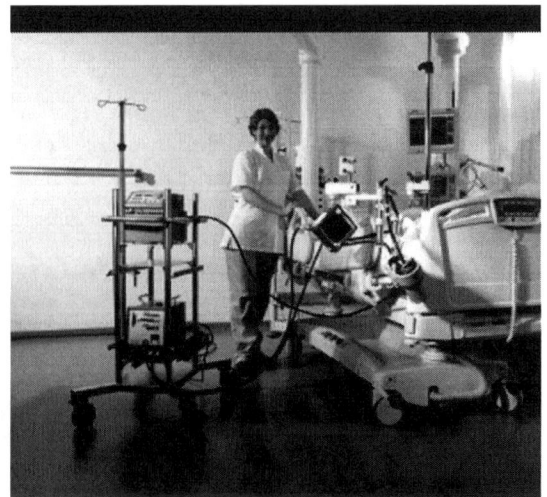

Figure 19-7. Centrifugal pump and hollow fiber oxygenator

from excessive negative pressure, many centers employ a reservoir device such as the Better Bladder® that can help regulate pump function if the negative pressure limit is reached and lessen "peaks and valley" pressure swings at the inlet and outlet of the centrifugal head. Such devices may also help trap air bubbles prior to reaching the centrifugal head. Many centers also employ pressure monitoring devices which can provide servo regulation to slow down or stop the ECMO circuit, temperature monitoring sites, sampling sites for medication infusion or blood sampling or continuous readouts of blood gases, venous saturation, hemoglobin, or other available parameters, and as sites where adjunct support systems such as renal replacement or plasma exchange devices can be integrated. The advantages of these aspects of ECMO circuit components must be weighed against the risks of inadvertent air entry at potential sites of high negative pressure, blood loss if on the "high" pressure return side of the circuit, or potential infection from accessing ports within the circuit over time. Centers vary in their circuit design, with some eliminating all access ports on the drainage side of the pump head to limit risk of air entrainment and some allowing no access ports at all. While limiting access ports may make the circuit simpler, less sites for access also limits the amount of pressure monitoring or other safety parameters that can also be useful during ECLS. In patients with limited or no venous access, circuit ports can also be an important route for medication administration and blood sampling. The optimal circuit design may be different in varying circumstances and determination of a universally agreed upon circuit may be an unachievable goal.

ECLS Circuit Management/Monitoring:

Currently, the ECLS patient is monitored by a bedside ECLS specialist 24 hours a day. The ECLS specialist must be familiar with the principles of ECLS and must have an indepth knowledge of the technical equipment and management of patients on ECLS. The ECLS specialist must also be capable of managing emergency situations until an ECLS-trained physician is available. In many ECMO centers, the specialist is an ICU nurse, nurse anesthetist, respiratory therapist, or perfusionist, has been trained inhouse, and is referred to as the "ECLS specialist" or "ECMO technician."

In addition to technical support, continuous clinical observation of the patient is essential. Visual observation of the color of the blood (i.e., the light red blood entering the patient and the dark color of blood drained) is a simple bedside test that the patient is being oxygenated by the ECLS machine. In some centers the ECLS specialist is also responsible for general patient care, but in the majority of ECLS centers, a separate ICU nurse will have the responsibility for general patient care. In all instances, the ECLS specialist is responsible for the continuous surveillance of the ECLS machine and the extracorporeal support. As circuitry becomes more miniaturized and technology continues to advance, the need for 24/7 monitoring of the ECLS circuit may become similar to that of renal replacement therapy or ventricular assist devices.

The technical aspects of the ECLS circuit including the devices used in Pediatric ECLS are covered in detail in Chapter 8 and provide an excellent reference for the equipment presently utilized worldwide in ECLS management and care.

Patient Management

The goal of ECLS is to provide adequate tissue oxygenation and cardiorespiratory support. Following markers such lactate, venous saturation, metabolic acidosis, and arterial oxygen saturation is helpful in assessing adequacy of oxygen delivery. Clinical examination can provide important clues for assessing the patient's state as well—vital signs, urine output, perfusion state, neurologic response.

Patients placed on ECLS, especially for respiratory failure, have often suffered from some period of hypoxemia which may have affected the myocardium. Many patients have required inotropic drugs before initiation of ECLS. As soon as the patient is on bypass, oxygenation will immediately improve and, unless the myocardium has suffered irreversible damage, cardiac performance will improve allowing inotropic support to be gradually withdrawn. Severe cardiac dysfunction on ECLS will result in a low pulse pressure and low cardiac output (referred to as "cardiac stun").

VV ECLS generally yields a higher saturation in the coronary arteries than VA ECLS, as oxygenated blood is infused in the right atrium or the inferior vena cava. The best coronary oxygenation in VV ECLS will occur with femoro-atrial bypass (i.e., venous drainage from femoral vein and reinfusion into right atrium) or when a double lumen cannula is used and the infusion line is directed correctly toward the tricuspid valve.[53] However, VV ECLS obviously does not directly support cardiac function, and patients on VV bypass may initially need inotropic support while on bypass. If myocardial performance is still inadequate, conversion to VA bypass may be necessary. VA ECLS supports both cardiac and pulmonary function; however, the coronary arteries are perfused with blood at low saturation in patients with respiratory dysfunction as long as blood is ejected from the left ventricle.[54]

Ventilator Management

ECLS alone does not cure the underlying pulmonary disease, instead, it provides gas exchange until pulmonary recovery occurs. Therefore, it is important to provide optimal pulmonary therapy during the ECLS course. There is little scientific data concerning pulmonary management on ECLS and the current strategy is based mostly on clinical experience.

Prior to bypass, patients have been managed with high ventilator settings, including high pressure and oxygen concentration. These conditions are injurious to the lungs and cause further damage if continued. As soon as ECLS has started, it is essential to decrease oxygen concentration and peak pressure to nontraumatic levels. The oxygen concentration is reduced to approximately 40% and peak inspiratory pressures should be limited to 20 cmH_2O in infants and 30 cmH_2O in older children. High PEEP (8-14 cmH_2O) has been shown to reduce lung opacification after initiation of ECLS in neonates and the length of the ECLS run in general.[55] Many centers advocate a high PEEP (10-15 cm H2O) in older children as well to maintain some lung expansion.[56] Although some patients will have been transitioned to ECLS while on high frequency ventilation, continuing this mode of ventilator support is not common and patients can be placed back on conventional support during ECLS. High frequency ventilation limits the ability to perform frequent pulmonary toilet, makes it difficult to assess tidal volume and often requires high levels of sedation, especially in patients outside the neonatal period.

Pulmonary toilet must be performed properly while the patient is on ECLS. If secretions are abundant, suctioning should be done frequently. Instillation of saline in the endotracheal tube may facilitate evacuation of mucus. Generally, the suction catheter should not pass beyond the endotracheal tube in order to avoid injury to the trachea and bleeding. Bronchoscopy can be performed easily when the patient is on bypass and should be done if there is any suspicion of bronchial obstruction from mucus or other material.

It may be advantageous to keep patients on spontaneous pressure supported ventilation by increasing $PaCO_2$ or decreasing pH if the patient is alkalotic. This approach requires the patient to be awake or only mildly sedated (see Chapter 34). Although not scientifically proven, pressure supported spontaneous ventilation seems beneficial compared to standard positive pressure ventilation. Further studies are needed to determine the optimal mode to ventilate patients on ECLS. Recovery of lung function is often heralded by increasing tidal volume, improved elimination of carbon dioxide from the native lung, clearing of the chest radiograph and increased arterial oxygen saturations (at stable ECLS support).

Sedation

Pediatric patients who need extracorporeal support have usually been ventilated for some period. At initiation of ECLS, they are normally sedated and often paralyzed. Most children require significant sedation and analgesics for the first days on bypass. Pharmacological paralysis is only rarely needed. After the first few days, the need for sedation varies. The general management of pain and sedation during ECLS is outlined in a later chapter. As in all ICU patients, usual causes of anxiety must be considered before routine sedation is given. Pain is best controlled with analgesics. Hypercarbia and hypoxemia should ideally be alleviated by adjusting ECLS flow and gas flow to the oxygenator. Establishing a close relationship between staff and the patient may decrease the need for pharmacological sedation. Gentle patient care, frequent verbal communication, and physical contact are often effective sedatives. For most children it is essential to have a parent at bedside most of the time. Storytelling and book reading can help calm the patient. Many children prefer to be entertained with television or games. Most children will only require mild pharmacological sedation by the end of the ECLS run and are able to communicate to some extent with parents and staff. When needed, opiates and benzodiazepines are frequently used for pharmacological sedation in these patients and for pain management.

While the traditional approach to ECMO management in the US has been to keep patients heavily sedated with narcotics or benzodiazepines to prevent inadvertent cannula dislodgement and other concerns, this is not the case in other areas of the world. Prolonged use of such medications, often at escalating doses due to dependence and resistance that develops over time, has been associated with increased risk of ventilator associated pneumonia and skin breakdown from lack of "normal" movement. Further, prolonged hospitalization related to treatment of drug withdrawal occurs among ECMO patients and is a major adverse event. Working with some of our Swedish and European colleagues to move towards less dependence on sedation and more "awake" states offers many advantages for patient care and outcome. Some centers in the US are making strides in this direction but further work needs to be done to make this an "accepted" and standard practice. Recent videos and reports of ECLS patients completely awake, walking, talking, and interacting with family and staff members may indicate that dependence on heavy sedation is waning.

Nutrition

Total parenteral nutrition (TPN) with amino acids, fat, and glucose has been used frequently in ECLS patients. In neonates, there has been concern that enteral feeding might increase the risk for necrotizing enterocolitis. The possibility that there has been prior ischemic insult to the gut in combination with use of vasopressors has led to concerns regarding enteral feeding in older patients. These critically ill patients may also have gastrointestinal dysmotility resulting in adynamic ileus. Nevertheless, absence of enteral feeding and support of the patient with total parenteral nutrition will result in hypoplasia of intestinal villi, risk for bacterial translocation, and risk for TPN associated cholestasis. Many centers currently advocate enteral feeding, even at trophic amounts to maintain gut integrity. Allowing full enteral feedings should be a goal.[21] Placement of enteral feeding tubes into the duodenum or jejunum can be helpful if gastric motility is impaired. These tubes can be placed safely despite the heparinization of the patient.

Renal

As previously noted, patients placed on ECLS often have capillary leakage and have received copious fluid resuscitation in order to maintain an adequate blood volume and pressure. Early in the ECLS course, patients may need large volumes of fluid to maintain adequate venous return, and they may develop edema or anasarca. When capillary leakage subsides, extracellular fluid returns to the vascular compartment and diuresis will increase. In general, maintaining patients with balanced fluid intake and output is recommended. ECLS offers the opportunity to treat massive fluid overload easily. Adequate renal perfusion through native cardiac output or ECLS support can maintain renal function. As long as renal perfusion is adequate, pharmacologic diuresis can be instituted and maintained even in septic patients with active capillary leak. Continuous hemofiltration may be added to the circuit if pharmacologic diuresis is inadequate. The hourly fluid balance goal should be set and maintained until normal extracellular fluid volume is reached (no systemic edema, within 5% of "dry" weight). Use of renal replacement therapy to enhance fluid removal and allow adequate nutritional support is often performed. Despite the literature surrounding fluid overload (>10%) as a risk factor for death, review of the ELSO Registry also finds that use of renal replacement therapy is also associated with worse overall outcome.[57,58] This likely represents the fact that underlying acute kidney injury (AKI) is a key risk factor for death in ECMO. Even if AKI occurs with

ECLS, resolution in survivors occurs in >90% of patients without need for long-term dialysis. More specific data collection regarding whether renal replacement is applied for renal insufficiency or merely fluid balance may help guide prognostication for patients in the future.

Skin Integrity and Positioning

As in other ICU patients, it is beneficial to change the patient's position in order to facilitate drainage of different parts of the lungs. Development of decubiti during ECLS is a constant risk if the duration of ECLS is long and the patient maintained immobile. Prevention of decubiti is important to prevent wound infection and morbidity. Repositioning, letting the patient awaken and move spontaneously may help prevent decubiti. Prone positioning may be used in order to recruit lung tissue and improve ventilation-perfusion matching. When the patient's position is changed, great attention must be paid to the cannulas so that bleeding from the cannulation site or accidental decannulation does not occur. In a study of 95 pediatric ECMO patients, 63 received intermittent prone positioning. There were no complications from this practice and survival was 82%.[59,60]

Antibiotic Therapy

The majority of patients will be already receiving antibiotics for suspected or confirmed infection prior to ECLS. Treatment for confirmed infection should be continued but the use of long term prophylactic antibiotics is not recommended.

Complications

Bleeding and thrombosis remain the scourge of ECLS support today. Mechanical thrombosis within the ECLS circuit or components is reported in 26% of pediatric patients while 34% of patients have bleeding complications such as surgical site bleeding, GI hemorrhage, or cannulation site bleeding. Hemolysis occurs in 10% of patients. Neurologic complications such as seizures (7%), CNS infarction (1.5%), or CNS hemorrhage (4%) are serious events during ECLS which can result in adverse outcomes. Infection occurs in roughly 18% of pediatric ECLS patients. In a recent evaluation of eight large childrens' hospitals who are part of the Collaborative Pediatric Critical Care Research Network (CPCCRN), 1215 ECLS patients (62% neonatal) were assessed and complications were noted in 88% (n=1075).Up to or over three complications were noted in 65% of the patients and the presence of complications correlated with decreased survival (49% vs 85%;p<0.01).[17] In this review, leading complications included the need for inotropes (69%; n=739) and occurrence of bleeding (49%; n=595). Over the study years (2005-2009), overall and bleeding complication rates decreased 25% (p_{linear}<0.01) and 8% (p_{linear}=0.035), respectively. Complications were more frequent in pediatric than neonatal (92% vs 87%; p=0.01) patients; a similar difference was noted for bleeding complications (43% vs 33%; p<0.01). Bleeding complications included bleeding at cannulation (25%; n=228 events) and surgical (22%; n=198 events) sites, as well as intracranial hemorrhage (17%; n=152 events), and hemolysis (14%; n=125 events). Risk factors for complications were pre-ECLS cardiac arrest (p=0.002), low pH (p=0.01), and high pCO_2 (p=0.01). For bleeding, risk factors were ECPR support (p=0.03), pre-ECLS cardiac arrest (p<0.01), low pH (p<0.01), and high $PaCO_2$ (p<0.01). In this review, cardiac support was the most frequent indication (50%) for ECLS in pediatric patients (n=459). Common diagnoses were respiratory illness (21%), cardiomyopathy (7%), and HLHS (6%). Pediatric survival increased over study years (51% to 59%; p_{linear}<0.01) but did not differ by diagnostic indication (p=0.07). Complications were noted in 97% of pediatric patients; 70% had ≥3. High pH (7.3 vs 7.2; p=0.03), low PaO_2 (50 vs 58;

p<0.01), high $PaCO_2$ (51 vs 55; p=0.06), and no complications (77% vs 49%; p<0.01) differentiated survivors in the pediatric cohort.

The impact of new technology and patient management techniques on reduction of complications and improving outcomes will require more investigation.

Weaning and Decannulation

As soon as the patient is stable on bypass, ventilator settings are decreased to non-injurious levels. After cannulation, lung compliance is extremely low; decreasing the ventilator pressures will diminish the tidal volume significantly, in many cases close to zero. At the onset of ECLS, there is often increased capillary leakage, the patient may need substantial fluid replacement, and will exhibit poor urinary output. General body and pulmonary edema will often increase during the first days on ECLS. Pulmonary radiographs will demonstrate increased atelectasis and only small segments of the lungs will be aerated. Measurements of end tidal CO_2 will show values close to zero as the alveoli are essentially unventilated and there is very little gas exchange taking place.

Increased diuresis may be one sign of clinical improvement, and will be followed by resolving edema. Ideally, at this time, compliance will increase, and the volume will increase either on ventilator induced breaths or on spontaneous pressure-supported breaths. Breath sounds can be heard by auscultation. End tidal CO_2 measurement will show increasing values, indicating that there is gas exchange. Tidal volume measurement from improving lung expansion may also be evident. Improvement will also be visible on a chest radiograph, although this is often delayed at least 24 hours following signs of clinical improvement. Pulmonary improvement will be reflected by an increased mixed venous saturation and may also be evident from increased arterial oxygen saturation or partial pressure of oxygen (assuming that ECLS flow and oxygen delivery remain constant). At a constant circuit flow rate, an increased mixed venous saturation (SvO_2) means decreased extracorporeal oxygen delivery, as the delivered oxygen is directly proportional to Q x $(1 - SvO_2 \div 100)$, where Q is the extracorporeal flow rate. Assuming that the total oxygen consumption of the patient is not changed, decreased extracorporeal oxygen delivery means increased oxygen uptake by the lungs.

Once pulmonary function improves, the extracorporeal flow may be decreased. When the patient is on VA bypass, the decrease in extracorporeal flow may be regulated by monitoring the SvO_2. The latter reflects hemoglobin bound oxygen which has not been extracted by the tissue when the arterial blood passes through the capillaries to the venous side. An $SvO_2 > 65-70\%$ indicates that there is adequate oxygen delivery. The extracorporeal flow can be decreased in small increments as long as the SvO_2 is kept above 65-70%. In lengthy ECLS runs where the patient is difficult to wean, lower values of SvO_2 may need to be tolerated until improvement is seen. After further improvement in pulmonary function, and when the ECLS machine is contributing only minimally to the patient's gas exchange (i.e., the flow rate is down to $\approx$ 20-30 cc/kg/min for small children, $\approx$10 cc/kg/min in older children), the patient is probably ready for discontinuation of ECLS.

There are several options for discontinuation of VA bypass:[61]

- The patient is decannulated if the ECLS run has been fairly short, the weaning process has been uneventful and if the patient is stable after several hours on minimal ECLS flow.
- If there has been a long ECLS run or if there is uncertainty whether the patient will tolerate removal from ECLS, the circuit may be disconnected, the cannulas connected with short pieces of tubing through a roller pump, and blood is circulated through this AV shunt at a minimal flow rate.
- Similar to the situation above, some centers cut away the circuit and keep the cannulas patent by infusing a heparinized solution.
- If a bridge is used between the arterial and venous lines in the circuit, the cannulas can be clamped, filled with a heparinized solution, and the bridge opened. The blood is then circulated through the circuit now isolated from the patient. The catheters are "flashed" to prevent clot formation.

The last three alternatives leave the cannulas in place while ECLS is discontinued. In this way, a trial off ECLS may be carried out for up to 24 hours before decannulation. If this is not tolerated, the patient is easily placed back on bypass. Prolonged trial off ECLS with the cannulas in place, however, do expose the patient to an increased risk of thrombosis despite continued use of heparin or flushing of cannulas.

Patients on venovenous bypass do not require weaning flow to such minimal levels. The oxygen concentration can simply be reduced to the oxygenator and if adequate gas exchange and hemodynamics are maintained in the patient, support can be discontinued. Patients on VV bypass may have falsely high venous saturation readings on the ECLS circuit due to drainage of oxygenated blood returning from the ECLS circuit into the venous drainage line. Some of the newer venovenous cannulas have very minimal recirculation. The accuracy of the venous saturation from the ECLS circuit can be assessed by comparing venous saturation levels at a site distant from the cannula where the recirculation effect is not present. Other parameters to assess tolerance of weaning may also be followed, such as: arterial blood gases, vital signs, tidal volumes, compliance, and end tidal CO_2. When the patient is on minimal support and is ready for a trial off ECLS, this is accomplished by disconnecting the gas supply to the oxygenator. Cannulas inserted with a percutaneous or a semi-percutaneous technique can be simply removed without a surgical procedure. Bleeding is controlled by a skin suture and simple pressure at the cannulation site. Cannulas inserted with an open technique require a surgical procedure for removal. The majority of patients receive sedation and neuromuscular blockage during surgical decannulation. However, some patients have improved pulmonary performance when decannulated with spontaneous breathing modalities and decannulation is, therefore, performed using only sedation and a local anesthetic. During removal of a venous cannula in the upper body, care should be taken to avoid negative intrathoracic pressure as the cannula is withdrawn to avoid air embolus. This can be easily prevented by doing an "inspiratory hold" on the ventilator to maintain intrathoracic pressure or by asking the patient to hold their breath during cannula removal.[31]

Patients who experience severe lung injury from necrotizing pneumonia, or from very high plateau pressures prior to ECLS will have the physiologic syndrome of very high alveolar level dead space. This is characterized by adequate oxygenation on low FiO_2 but CO_2 retention, respiratory acidosis, the need for hyperventilation (either spontaneous or via the ventilator) to maintain $PaCO_2$ under 60, and an emphysematous (honeycomb) appearance on chest x-ray or CT scan. Although this condition has the characteristics of chronic irreversible obstructive lung disease, it may reverse to normal within 1-6 weeks. These conditions heal by contracture, eliminating the alveolar level dead space.

Outcome and Followup

The overall survival of pediatric respiratory failure patients remains around 55% according to the ELSO registry. Outcome for major patient groups has already been discussed. Most reports, however, only provide details on short term outcome to the point of discharge. Among pediatric patients, little long term outcome data are available. This area represents one of the most needed areas for continued research. All patients should have a thorough neurologic evaluation, including imaging with a CT or MRI scan, done prior to hospital discharge. Correlating imaging findings, neurologic exam, and outcome may provide valuable information in the future. A followup plan that involves a minimum of yearly patient assessment should also be developed. Following progress in normal developmental milestones, school performance, and subsequent hospitalizations post-ECMO should be a part of every post-ECMO follow up plan.

While there is little specific data for pediatric respiratory failure patients in terms of long term outcome, it is important to note that roughly 50% of children supported for cardiac dysfunction have abnormal neurodevelopmental outcomes.[62-65] The impact of their underlying disease and pre-ECLS factors on morbidity is unknown and many of these patients are recovering following repair of congenital heart defects or have suffered cardiac arrest. Neonatal ECLS survivors also have significant morbidity, although longer term studies finds that developmental abnormalities may improve over time and few have severe dysfunction. In older children, as few centers maintain followup clinics or standardized evaluations, the assessment of the patient as they leave the hospital is often equated to their outcome. Children are described as with "good" or "abnormal" outcome. Thus, while optimism for long term prognosis can be realistic, much more work needs to be done before accurate outcome from pediatric ECLS can be established. Of note, among adults supported with ECLS for respiratory failure, however, there is considerable morbidity, although few have severe dysfunction. Even among patients with ARDS who do NOT receive ECLS, however, adult reports of long term morbidity find that, although patients often do not return to normal, they are yet able to lead functional lives.[66] As evaluating the quality of life and cost/benefit related to respiratory failure and supportive techniques such as ECLS is important to the health care community, more efforts to collaborate with other centers and collect data on longer term outcome past survival from the hospital should be an ongoing goal.

ECLS Termination

Unfortunately, not all ECLS runs are successful. Termination of ECLS may be necessary because of various complications. Cerebral hemorrhage or infarction may lead to cerebral edema and subsequent brain death, making further ECLS pointless. Life threatening bleeding complications which cannot be controlled surgically may also prompt discontinuation of ECLS and if this occurs when the patient is totally dependent on ECLS, death will be unavoidable. If lung function is present, it may be possible to transition off ECLS to high ventilator settings. If necessary, ECLS may be reinstituted when bleeding has been controlled.

Determining the duration of respiratory failure ECLS in the absence of improvement in lung function remains a controversial question. The cause of severe respiratory failure may be unknown when the patient is started on ECLS. Although lung biopsy is the next step in diagnosis, it is potentially dangerous in patients on ECLS with anticoagulation. If pulmonary function is not improving after several weeks, the primary diagnosis has not been established by bronchoscopy or other means and the status of lung recovery uncertain, open lung biopsy on ECLS has been suggested to determine if the lungs show irreversible damage.[67] Lung biopsy is best done by thoracotomy (or thoracoscopy) rather than transbronchially because of the risk of major hemorrhage into the airway with transbronchial biopsy.

However, this procedure cannot be performed without at least some risk for bleeding. Evaluation of pulmonary prognosis from a single biopsy specimen is also problematic.

The difficulty of discontinuing ECLS is further illustrated by Green et al.[19] who, in a multicenter study of 382 patients treated with ECLS, found that the probability of survival was the same in children with ECLS courses >2 weeks compared with those treated for shorter periods. ECLS was terminated in some patients for pulmonary futility at durations of ECLS associated with survival in a substantial number of patients in whom ECLS was continued. Nevertheless, if lung function does not improve, termination of ECLS must be considered at some point unless pulmonary transplantation is feasible. Growing experience with ECMO as a bridge to lung transplant is being reported, but the approach presents many ethical and practical issues.[68] The possibility that a patient's lungs will not recover while on support should ideally be discussed with the parents before initiation of ECLS.

Summary

Pediatric ECLS refers to extracorporeal support in children beyond the neonatal period. A different pathophysiology is encountered compared to neonates. The basic principles of ECLS are the same as in neonates and in adults. Desaturated blood is withdrawn from a central vein or the right atrium and pumped through a membrane oxygenator and a heat exchanger before it is returned to a major artery (VA ECLS) or to a central vein (VV ECLS). The size of the different components of the circuit is determined by the weight of the patient and thereby the anticipated extracorporeal flow. The patients may be cannulated through an open cut down procedure, by a semi-percutaneous procedure or by a percutaneous technique.

Pulmonary care and treatment of the underlying disease is of utmost importance as ECLS per se does not cure the patient. A successful outcome relies upon adequate pulmonary recovery during the extracorporeal support. The overall survival of pediatric respiratory failure ECLS patients seems to be increasing slightly over time, despite some evidence that patients are more complex and "sicker" than in earlier years. There are no prospective randomized studies in the pediatric age group comparing survival with ECLS vs. conventional treatment, but in a retrospective multicenter study, ECLS survival was 47% compared to 26% in the matched control group. Survival is highest in aspiration pneumonia, viral pneumonia, and posttraumatic ARDS. Future research should focus on long-term outcome of patients receiving ECLS and efforts to make ECLS safer and more efficient should continue.

References

1. Short BL, Pearson GD. Neonatal extracorporeal membrane oxygenation: A review. J Inten Care Med 1986;1:48.
2. Beck R, Anderson KD, Pearson GD, Cronin J, Miller MK, Short BL. Criteria for extracorporeal membrane oxygenation in a population of infants with persistent pulmonary hypertension of the newborn. J Pediatr Surg 1986;21:297-302.
3. Bartlett RH, Gazzaniga AB, Wetmore NE, Rucker R, Huxtable RF. Extracorporeal membrane oxygenation (ECMO) in the treatment of cardiac and respiratory failure in children. Trans Am Soc Artif Intern Organs 1980;26:578-81.
4. Mehta NM, Turner D, Walsh B, et al. Factors associated with survival in pediatric extracorporeal membrane oxygenation--a single-center experience. J Pediatr Surg 2010;45:1995-2003.
5. Marsh TD, Wilkerson SA, Cook LN. Extracorporeal membrane oxygenation selection criteria: partial pressure of arterial oxygen versus alveolar-arterial oxygen gradient. Pediatrics 1988;82:162-6.
6. Timmons OD, Dean JM, Vernon DD. Mortality rates and prognostic variables in children with adult respiratory distress syndrome. J Pediatr. 1991;119:896-9.
7. ECMO Registry of the Extracorporeal Life Support Organization, Ann Arbor, Michigan. July 2011.
8. Fortenberry JD, Meier AH, Pettignano R, Heard M, Chambliss CR, Wulkan M. Extracorporeal life support for posttraumatic acute respiratory distress syndrome at a children's medical center. J Pediatr Surg 2003;38:1221-6.
9. Gow KW, Heiss KF, Wulkan ML, et al. Extracorporeal life support for support of children with malignancy and respiratory or cardiac failure: The extracorporeal

life support experience. Crit Care Med 2009;37:1308-16.
10. Hebbar KB, Petrillo-Albarano T, Coto-Puckett W, Heard M, Rycus PT, Fortenberry JD. Experience with use of extracorporeal life support for severe refractory status asthmaticus in children. Crit Care 2009;13:R29.
11. Linden V, Karlen J, Olsson M, et al. Successful extracorporeal membrane oxygenation in four children with malignant disease and severe Pneumocystis carinii pneumonia. Med Pediatr Oncol 1999;32:25-31.
12. O'Rourke PP, Crone RK. Pediatric applications of extracorporeal membrane oxygenation. J Pediatr 1990;116:393-4.
13. Sheridan RL, Schnitzer JJ. Management of the high-risk pediatric burn patient. J Pediatr Surg 2001;36:1308-12.
14. Szocik J, Rudich S, Csete M. ECMO resuscitation after massive pulmonary embolism during liver transplantation. Anesthesiology 2002;97:763-4.
15. Thiagarajan RR, Roth SJ, Margossian S, et al. Extracorporeal membrane oxygenation as a bridge to cardiac transplantation in a patient with cardiomyopathy and hemophilia A. Intensive Care Med 2003;29:985-8.
16. Zabrocki LA, Brogan TV, Statler KD, Poss WB, Rollins MD, Bratton SL. Extracorporeal membrane oxygenation for pediatric respiratory failure: Survival and predictors of mortality. Crit Care Med 2011;39:364-70.
17. Dalton HJ, Garcia-Filion P. Unpublished data.
18. Cordell-Smith JA, Roberts N, Peek GJ, Firmin RK. Traumatic lung injury treated by extracorporeal membrane oxygenation (ECMO). Injury 2006;37:29-32.
19. Green TP, Timmons OD, Fackler JC, Moler FW, Thompson AE, Sweeney MF. The impact of extracorporeal membrane oxygenation on survival in pediatric patients with acute respiratory failure. Pediatric Critical Care Study Group. Crit Care Med 1996;24:323-9.

20. Frey TK, Chopra A, Lin RJ, et al. A child with anterior mediastinal mass supported with veno-arterial extracorporeal membrane oxygenation. Pediatr Crit Care Med 2006;7:479-81.

21. Tulenko DR. An update on ECMO. Neonatal Netw 2004;23:11-8.

22. Kolovos NS, Schuerer DJ, Moler FW, et al. Extracorporal life support for pulmonary hemorrhage in children: a case series. Crit Care Med 2002;30:577-80.

23. Pooboni S, Roberts N, Westrope C, et al. Extracorporeal life support in pertussis. Pediatr Pulmonol 2003;36:310-5.

24. Kolovos NS, Schuerer DJ, Moler FW, Bratton SL, Swaniker F, Bartlett RH, Custer JR, Annich GM: Extracorporeal Life Support for Pulmonary Hemorrhage in Children: A Case Series. Crit Care Med 30:577-580, 2002.

25. Daimon S, Umeda T, Michishita I, Wakasugi H, Genda A, Koni I. Goodpasture's-like syndrome and effect of extracorporeal membrane oxygenator support. Intern Med 1994;33:569-73.

26. Blasco V, Leone M, Xeridat F, Albanese J, Martin C. [Lemierre's syndrome from necrotizing pneumonia treated with extracorporeal CO2 removal]. Ann Fr Anesth Reanim 2008;27:244-8.

27. Beca J, Butt W. Extracorporeal membrane oxygenation for refractory septic shock in children. Pediatrics 1994;93:726-9.

28. Meyer DM, Jessen ME. Results of extracorporeal membrane oxygenation in children with sepsis. The Extracorporeal Life Support Organization. Ann Thorac Surg 1997;63:756-61.

29. Pettignano R, Fortenberry JD, Heard ML, et al. Primary use of the venovenous approach for extracorporeal membrane oxygenation in pediatric acute respiratory failure. Pediatr Crit Care Med 2003;4:291-8.

30. Kissoon N, Orr RA, Carcillo JA. Updated American College of Critical Care Medicine--pediatric advanced life support guidelines for management of pediatric and neonatal septic shock: relevance to the emergency care clinician. Pediatr Emerg Care 2010;26:867-9.

31. Maclaren G, Butt W, Best D, Donath S, Taylor A. Extracorporeal membrane oxygenation for refractory septic shock in children: one institution's experience. Pediatr Crit Care Med 2007;8:447-51.

32. MacLaren G, Butt W, Best D, Donath S. Central extracorporeal membrane oxygenation for refractory pediatric septic shock. Pediatr Crit Care Med 2011;12:133-6.

33. Gaies MG, Gurney JG, Yen AH, et al. Vasoactive-inotropic score as a predictor of morbidity and mortality in infants after cardiopulmonary bypass. Pediatr Crit Care Med 2010;11:234-8.

34. Jan SL, Lin SJ, Fu YC, et al. Extracorporeal life support for treatment of children with enterovirus 71 infection-related cardiopulmonary failure. Intensive Care Med 2010;36:520-7.

35. Davies A, Jones D, Bailey M, et al. Extracorporeal Membrane Oxygenation for 2009 Influenza A(H1N1) Acute Respiratory Distress Syndrome. JAMA 2009;302:1888-95.

36. Morris AH, Hirshberg E, Miller RR, 3rd, Statler KD, Hite RD. Counterpoint: Efficacy of extracorporeal membrane oxygenation in 2009 influenza A(H1N1): sufficient evidence? Chest 2010;138:778-81; discussion 82-4.

37. Park PK, Dalton HJ, Bartlett RH. Point: Efficacy of extracorporeal membrane oxygenation in 2009 influenza A(H1N1): sufficient evidence? Chest 2010;138:776-8.

38. Kumar A, Zarychanski R, Pinto R, et al. Critically ill patients with 2009 influenza A(H1N1) infection in Canada. JAMA 2009;302:1872-9.

39. Custer JR. The evolution of patient selection criteria and indications for extracorporeal life support in pediatric cardiopulmonary

failure: Next time, let's not eat the bones. Organogenesis 2011;7:13-22.

40. Javidfar J, Brodie D, Wang D, et al. Use of bicaval dual-lumen catheter for adult venovenous extracorporeal membrane oxygenation. Ann Thorac Surg 2011;91:1763-8; discussion 9.

41. Karl TR, Iyer KS, Sano S, Mee RB. Infant ECMO cannulation technique allowing preservation of carotid and jugular vessels. Ann Thorac Surg 1990;50:488-9.

42. Adolph V, Bonis S, Falterman K, Arensman R. Carotid artery repair after pediatric extracorporeal membrane oxygenation. J Pediatr Surg 1990;25:867-9; discussion 9-70.

43. Crombleholme TM, Adzick NS, deLorimier AA, Longaker MT, Harrison MR, Charlton VE. Carotid artery reconstruction following extracorporeal membrane oxygenation. Am J Dis Child 1990;144:872-4.

44. Jacobs JP, Goldman AP, Cullen S, et al. Carotid artery pseudoaneurysm as a complication of ECMO. Ann Vasc Surg 1997;11:630-3.

45. Bisdas T, Beutel G, Warnecke G, et al. Vascular complications in patients undergoing femoral cannulation for extracorporeal membrane oxygenation support. Ann Thorac Surg 2011;92:626-31.

46. Greason KL, Hemp JR, Maxwell JM, Fetter JE, Moreno-Cabral RJ. Prevention of distal limb ischemia during cardiopulmonary support via femoral cannulation. Ann Thorac Surg 1995;60:209-10.

47. Moazami N, Moon MR, Lawton JS, Bailey M, Damiano R, Jr. Axillary artery cannulation for extracorporeal membrane oxygenator support in adults: an approach to minimize complications. J Thorac Cardiovasc Surg 2003;126:2097-8.

48. International Registry of the Extracorporeal Life Support Organization, Ann Arbor, Michigan. July 2011.

49. Thomas TH, Price R, Ramaciotti C, Thompson M, Megison S, Lemler MS. Echocardiography, not chest radiography, for evaluation of cannula placement during pediatric extracorporeal membrane oxygenation. Pediatr Crit Care Med 2009;10:56-9.

50. Yee S, Qiu F, Su X, et al. Evaluation of HL-20 roller pump and Rotaflow centrifugal pump on perfusion quality and gaseous microemboli delivery. Artif Organs 2010;34:937-43.

51. Sivarajan VB, Best D, Brizard CP, et al. Improved outcomes of paediatric extracorporeal support associated with technology change. Interact Cardiovasc Thorac Surg 2010;11:400-5.

52. McMullan DM, Emmert JA, Permut LC, et al. Minimizing bleeding associated with mechanical circulatory support following pediatric heart surgery. Eur J Cardiothorac Surg 2011;39:392-7.

53. Rich PB, Awad SS, Crotti S, Hirschl RB, Bartlett RH, Schreiner RJ. A prospective comparison of atrio-femoral and femoro-atrial flow in adult venovenous extracorporeal life support. J Thorac Cardiovasc Surg 1998;116:628-32.

54. Dalton HJ, Rycus PT, Conrad SA. Update on extracorporeal life support 2004. Seminars in Perinatology 2005;29:24-33.

55. Lequier L. Extracorporeal Life Support in Pediatric and Neonatal Critical Care: A Review. Journal of Intensive Care Medicine 2004;19:243-58.

56. Keszler M, Subramanian KN, Smith YA, et al. Pulmonary management during extracorporeal membrane oxygenation. Crit Care Med 1989;17:495-500.

57. Paden ML, Warshaw BL, Heard ML, Fortenberry JD. Recovery of renal function and survival after continuous renal replacement therapy during extracorporeal membrane oxygenation. Pediatr Crit Care Med 2011;12:153-8.

58. Hoover NG, Heard M, Reid C, et al. Enhanced fluid management with continuous venovenous hemofiltration in pediatric

respiratory failure patients receiving extracorporeal membrane oxygenation support. Intensive Care Med 2008;34:2241-7.

59. Kavanagh BP. Prone positioning in children with ARDS: positive reflections on a negative clinical trial. JAMA 2005;294:248-50.

60. Raoof S, Goulet K, Esan A, Hess DR, Sessler CN. Severe hypoxemic respiratory failure: part 2--nonventilatory strategies. Chest 2010;137:1437-48.

61. Cronin J. Cycling: An alternative method for weaning for ECMO. CNMC National ECMO Symposium, Breckinridge, CO 1990:p. 69.

62. Hervey-Jumper SL, Annich GM, Yancon AR, Garton HJ, Muraszko KM, Maher CO. Neurological complications of extracorporeal membrane oxygenation in children. J Neurosurg Pediatr 2011;7:338-44.

63. Adolph V, Ekelund C, Smith C, Starrett A, Falterman K, Arensman R. Developmental outcome of neonates treated with extracorporeal membrane oxygenation. J Pediatr Surg 1990;25:43-6.

64. Hofkosh D, Thompson AE, Nozza RJ, Kemp SS, Bowen A, Feldman HM. Ten years of extracorporeal membrane oxygenation: neurodevelopmental outcome. Pediatrics 1991;87:549-55.

65. Raymond TT, Cunnyngham CB, Thompson MT, Thomas JA, Dalton HJ, Nadkarni VM. Outcomes among neonates, infants, and children after extracorporeal cardiopulmonary resuscitation for refractory inhospital pediatric cardiac arrest: a report from the National Registry of Cardiopulmonary Resuscitation. Pediatr Crit Care Med 2010;11:362-71.

66. Herridge MS, Tansey CM, Matte A, et al. Functional disability 5 years after acute respiratory distress syndrome. N Engl J Med 2011;364:1293-304.

67. Bond SJ, Lee DJ, Stewart DL, Buchino JJ. Open lung biopsy in pediatric patients on extracorporeal membrane oxygenation. J Pediatr Surg 1996;31:1376-8.

68. Garcia JP, Iacono A, Kon ZN, Griffith BP. Ambulatory extracorporeal membrane oxygenation: a new approach for bridge-to-lung transplantation. J Thorac Cardiovasc Surg 2010;139:e137-9.

20

Pediatric Cardiac Extracorporeal Life Support

David S. Cooper MD MPH, Jennifer C. Hirsch MD MS, Jeffrey P. Jacobs MD FACS FACC FCCP

Introduction

Mechanical circulatory support is an invaluable tool in the care of children with severe refractory cardiac and/or pulmonary failure.[1] There are two forms of mechanical circulatory support currently available to neonates, infants, and smaller children: extracorporeal membrane oxygenation (ECMO) and ventricular assist device (VAD), with each technique having unique advantages and disadvantages. The intraaortic balloon pump is a third form of mechanical support that has been successfully used in larger children, adolescents, and adults, but has limited applicability in smaller children.[1] The use of ECMO to provide support for circulatory failure arose as a natural followup to work in the 1970s that established the efficacy of ECMO in the treatment of respiratory failure. Baffes and colleagues are credited with the first use of prolonged extracorporeal circulation for congenital heart disease.[2] The duration of support was relatively brief for the patients in this study; however, significant innovations were introduced, including the use of an ECMO circuit for resuscitation after cardiac arrest and for perioperative stabilization at the time of palliative cardiac procedures. The first reported use of ECMO for extended periods in a pediatric heart patient was supplied by Soeter and colleagues who described the successful use of ECMO to support a 4 year old girl with severe hypoxemia after repair of tetralogy of Fallot.[3] The patient was weaned from support within 48 hours, extubated two days later, and discharged on postoperative day 13.

As the field of mechanical circulatory support has evolved in children, the indications for use have expanded and outcomes have improved. When combined with an active transplantation program, mechanical circulatory support can have a significant impact on survival. The majority of the pediatric experience consists of use of ECMO.[4] The July 2011 Extracorporeal Life Support Organization (ELSO) Summary[5] reported 9,798 neonatal and pediatric cardiac failure cases (24% of cases) since 1989. For neonatal and pediatric cardiac failure, survival to separation from ECMO is 62% and survival to discharge is 43%. Despite recent advances in VAD technology, ECMO remains the most common circulatory assist system in use for pediatric patients. The advantages of ECMO include its familiarity among practitioners, ability to provide biventricular support and respiratory support, universal availability across all pediatric age groups, and relative low cost. Unlike adults in whom pure left ventricular failure is the common indication for mechanical support, cardiopulmonary support is more commonly required in children due to a combination of pulmonary dysfunction, pulmonary hyperten-

293

sion, and right ventricular dysfunction. This is particularly true in the immediate postoperative period. Extracorporeal life support is obviously the mechanical support of choice for rapid deployment during cardiopulmonary arrest. There are a number of disadvantages, including the need for a dedicated team of specialists, immobilization, intensive care monitoring, risks of bleeding, thrombosis, infection, and multiorgan failure. These attendant disadvantages increase over time and hamper the use of ECMO for long term support. Over the last few years, substantial progress has been made in pediatric mechanical support.[6] Ventricular assist devices are being used with increasing frequency in children with cardiac failure refractory to medical therapy for primary treatment as a long-term bridge to recovery or transplantation and will be discussed in detail Chapter 24.[7] In this chapter, we focus our discussion on the technical aspects, indications, and outcomes of ECMO in patients with critical cardiac disease. Additionally, ECMO in patients with functionally univentricular circulation and in the setting of cardiopulmonary resuscitation will be discussed.

Technical Aspects

Circuit Selection

Systems for extracorporeal membrane oxygenation generally consist of an oxygenator (silicone membrane, hollow fiber or polymethylpentene), a heat exchanger, a bladder, and a roller or centrifugal pump and have been covered in Chapter 8. Hollow fiber oxygenators combine highly efficient gas exchange with easy priming, especially important when ECMO is used as a resuscitation tool following cardiac arrest.[8] A significant historical limitation of hollow fiber devices was plasma leakage across the oxygenator, which required the device to be replaced frequently.[9] Although many centers continue to use roller pumps, centrifugal pumps,

which maintain venous inflow independent of gravity drainage, allow the patient to be maintained at any height relative to the pump and may even be clamped directly to the bed, substantially reducing tubing length. Centrifugal pumps may be especially useful in larger patients to maintain adequate venous return at higher flows.[10-13] An additional advantage of the centrifugal pump is that occlusion of arterial outflow from the pump does not generate excessive arterial line pressure, reducing the risk of rupture of the arterial limb of the circuit. The chief disadvantage of the centrifugal pump is the high negative pressure that may be generated on the venous side of the circuit, potentially leading to cavitation, hemolysis, and air entrainment with circuit disruption on the venous side.[14]

Cannulation

Venoarterial ECMO is usually required, since the majority of patients need cardiac support. Cannulation is transthoracic, with direct cannulation of the right atrium and aorta via a median sternotomy, cervical with cannulation of the right internal jugular vein and right carotid artery, or rarely the femoral approach is used (>15 kg). The approach to cannulation should be flexible and based on the underlying need for ECMO. Transthoracic cannulation of the right atrial appendage and the ascending aorta is most appropriate for cases that require intraoperative support due to failure to wean from cardiopulmonary bypass (CPB). In the immediate postoperative period, reopening the sternal wound with direct cardiac cannulation provides the most expeditious route to institute support, especially in patients who suffer cardiac arrest. Adequate venous drainage and excellent arterial perfusion are assured by chest cannulation; however, significant hemorrhage and risk of mediastinitis remain major disadvantages of chest cannulation, making peripheral cannulation preferable in most other settings.

Venovenous (VV) ECMO may currently be an underutilized modality in pediatric cardiac patients.[15,16] While circulatory support is not achieved directly with VV ECMO, elimination of hypoxia along with decreased pulmonary vascular resistance may improve right ventricular function resulting in a substantial circulatory benefit. An interesting approach is the assistance respiratoire extra-corporelle (AREC) system which provides single cannula VV ECMO using a nonocclusive rotary pump with tidal flow in the circuit provided by alternating clamps.[17] This system has been successfully used in pediatric cardiac patients with hypoxia and pulmonary hypertension as the primary indication for ECMO support.[16,18]

Distension of the left heart can impede myocardial recovery and inadequate decompression of the left-sided cardiac chambers during ECMO support is common in cases of profound cardiac dysfunction. Steps should be taken to prevent pulmonary edema and further distension injury of the left ventricle. Left-sided distension is usually managed by increasing ECMO flow to empty the right heart, minimizing pulmonary blood flow, and decreasing pulmonary venous return to the left heart.[19] Careful evaluation to detect distension of the left atrium and ventricle is achieved with echocardiography and direct measurement of left atrial pressure when available. Although increasing ECMO flow is usually effective, persistent distension of the left-sided cardiac chambers may require further intervention, either by balloon atrial septostomy,[20] or by placement of an additional drainage catheter in the left atrium that can be placed by the percutaneous[21] or transthoracic route.

Anticoagulation

The whole blood activated clotting time (ACT) is used to monitor anticoagulation. Achieving an ACT of 180-200 seconds with a continuous heparin infusion maintains the circuit with a minimal risk of significant thrombosis.[11,12,15] Platelets are maintained above 100,000/dL and, in patients requiring postoperative support where bleeding is a critical problem, above 150,000/dL. Clotting factors are supplied with infusions of fresh frozen plasma or cryoprecipitate to maintain fibrinogen levels above 100 mg/dL. Instituting the heparin infusion may be safely deferred for several hours until the ACT drifts downward in the bleeding postoperative patient. Heparin-bonded hollow fiber oxygenators and heparin-bonded tubing have been utilized to further delay the institution of heparin therapy (up to 24 hours) and in an attempt to decrease the amount of systemic heparin that is required.[9] Epsilon aminocaproic acid (Amicar) may be used to diminish the risk of postoperative hemorrhage.[15,22,23] Amicar is usually administered as an initial bolus, followed by a continuous IV infusion for 48 hours, and then discontinued. Maintaining the infusion for longer periods is usually unnecessary, as postsurgical bleeding subsides while circuit thrombosis resulting from prolonged administration becomes a greater concern. A review of nearly 300 patients treated with Amicar during ECMO failed to demonstrate decreased rates of intracranial hemorrhage; however, surgical site bleeding was reduced, particularly in cardiac surgical patients.[24]

General Principles of Management

While on extracorporeal membrane oxygenation, adequacy of systemic perfusion should be continuously assessed using the usual parameters such as urine output, acid-base status, mixed venous oxygen saturation, serum lactate, serum creatinine, and liver enzymes. As previously stated, one should evaluate for adequate left atrial decompression using serial chest radiographs and bedside echocardiography. Every effort should be made to minimize afterload using vasodilators such as milrinone and nipride. When using a membrane oxygenator, ventilator settings should be optimized to prevent lung injury but avoid atelectasis. In order to assess the neurologic state, every attempt should be made to avoid neuromuscular blockade. In infants with an open fontanelle, daily ultrasonic examinations of the head should be performed for the first two to three days to evaluate for intracranial hemorrhage. Daily blood cultures should be obtained from the circuit to monitor for infection. If there is no significant myocardial recovery over three to five days, the patient should be evaluated for cardiac transplantation or implantation of a ventricular assist device should be considered for long term support as a bridge to transplantation/recovery.

Indications and Outcomes

The indications for ECMO can be divided into two groups, those involving or not involving cardiac surgery. The indications related to cardiac surgery include preoperative stabilization, failure to wean from CPB, low cardiac output syndrome in the postoperative period, and cardiopulmonary arrest. The indications in the absence of cardiac surgery include cardiopulmonary arrest, myocarditis and cardiomyopathy, pulmonary hypertension, intractable arrhythmias, and respiratory indications. In either group, the importance of early ECMO support cannot be overemphasized and should occur before prolonged periods of low cardiac output result in end-organ damage.

As the use of ECMO for cardiac patients has increased, clinical features considered to be contraindications have evolved. It is universally understood that certain conditions constitute absolute contraindications, including incurable malignancy, advanced multisystem organ failure, extreme prematurity, and severe central nervous system damage.[11,15,25] Patients who are not transplant candidates should be considered for support only in carefully selected cases, as any patient placed on ECMO may ultimately require cardiac transplantation for recovery.[11]

A number of conditions previously thought to be at high risk for further complications with ECMO support, including those with functionally univentricular physiology, have recently been treated with ECMO with modest success. The ability to provide mechanical circulatory support is now considered an important adjunct in the treatment of these patients.[15,19,25-29] In general, rigid contraindications for mechanical support, other than those mentioned above, have not been developed. Instead, each case should be evaluated individually.

Preoperative Stabilization

Mechanical circulatory support is occasionally required in neonates who present with profound cyanosis, and or cardiogenic shock. Examples include patients with obstructed total anomalous pulmonary venous connection or Tetralogy of Fallot with absent pulmonary valve syndrome. Such patients may present close to death and require preoperative stabilization with extracorporeal membrane oxygenation. Pulmonary hypertension refractory to conventional therapy can occur in neonates with d-transposition of the great arteries and there are several reports of the successful use of ECMO for preoperative stabilization.[30,31] Another example is the neonate with severe Ebstein's malformation of the tricuspid valve and functional pulmonary atresia with ductal-dependent flow of blood to the lungs that has a circular shunt from a wide open duct. Such a patient will benefit from extracorporeal life support while pulmonary vascular resistance declines.[32]

Postcardiotomy Support

The role of ECMO to provide postcardiotomy support for children with severe cardiopulmonary dysfunction after surgery for congenital cardiac disease is well established. Mechanical circulatory support may be required in the postoperative period, either due to the inability to separate from cardiopulmonary bypass, or a progressive low cardiac output syndrome due to a number of factors, such as ventricular dysfunction, pulmonary hypertension, or intractable arrhythmias. In this group of patients, it is imperative to rule out residual anatomic reasons with echocardiography and, if necessary, cardiac catheterization. Booth and colleagues[33] have demonstrated that cardiac catheterization can be safely performed in children while on extracorporeal life support. The majority of patients requiring ECMO immediately after cardiopulmonary bypass remain cannulated via the median sternotomy with an atrial cannula and an arterial cannula in the aorta. Patients requiring support later in their postoperative course are more likely to be cannulated via the right internal jugular vein and right carotid artery. Bleeding is a major complication of ECMO after cardiac surgery. Reexploration of the mediastinum is often necessary when transthoracic cannulation is used, increasing the risk of displacement of the cannulae and infection.

Numerous publications have documented the experiences in individual centers.[15,25,34-39] The combined experiences of these centers demonstrate that ECMO can allow survival of many children with congenitally malformed hearts and refractory cardiopulmonary dysfunction, with between 33-60% of patients surviving. Walters and colleagues[25] reviewed 73 children with congenitally malformed hearts placed on ECMO. The patients were analyzed in three groups, those receiving support preoperatively, those who could not be weaned from cardiopulmonary bypass and were converted to support immediately after repair, and those cannulated postoperatively after an initial period of clinical stability. Overall survival for all patients was 58%. Survival to discharge was only 23% in patients who could not be weaned from cardiopulmonary bypass, compared to 69% in patients who were cannulated postoperatively after an initial period of clinical stability. These results support the theory that ECMO is most

effective if initiated at some interval after being successfully weaned from cardiopulmonary bypass. Morris and colleagues[39] reported on the use of ECMO in 137 children seen from January 1995 to June 2001, with an overall survival to discharge of 39%. In this series, 66% required ECMO in the postoperative period. In this cohort, risk factors for mortality were age below one month, male gender, longer duration of mechanical ventilation before support, and development of renal or hepatic dysfunction while on support. Functionally univentricular physiology and failure to separate from cardiopulmonary bypass were not associated with an increased risk of mortality. Cardiac physiology and the indications for support were not associated with the incidence of death.

Extracorporeal Cardiopulmonary Resuscitation (E-CPR)

As the familiarity and experience with ECMO has grown, new indications have evolved, including emergent resuscitation. This utilization has been termed extracorporeal cardiopulmonary resuscitation (E-CPR). del Nido and colleagues[40] initially described the use of rapid resuscitation with ECMO after cardiopulmonary arrest. Limitations in available therapeutic modalities, combined with the effectiveness and familiarity of ECMO, have compelled most pediatric centers to use a conventional setup for cardiac support and emergency resuscitation. Although effective in providing pulmonary support, conventional ECMO may not be the best method of providing postcardiotomy or emergent cardiopulmonary support. Extended times for cardiopulmonary resuscitation are a limiting factor in the effectiveness of any rescue during acute cardiac and/or pulmonary failure, though prolonged effective cardiopulmonary resuscitation does not preclude survival and favorable neurologic outcomes.[41] In these populations, ECMO has several limitations, including the prolonged time to set up the equipment, varying from 45 to 60 minutes, the large volumes needed for priming, from 450 to 800 milliliters, the increased postoperative loss of blood, and its unwieldiness during transport. In a retrospective study by Dalton and colleagues,[11] all patients with times of cardiopulmonary resuscitation less than 15 minutes survived, while only just over half survived when those times were greater than 42 minutes. Some centers have resorted to maintaining pre-primed circuits for allotted periods of time in an attempt to overcome the problem of prolonged setup. Use of these pre-primed circuits accepts the added risk of infection should the circuit become contaminated, and the expense of not using the circuit during the allotted time span.

Due to the limitations of conventional circuits, some centers have developed novel systems for cardiopulmonary support. Duncan and colleagues[42] described a fully portable circuit that is maintained vacuum- and carbon dioxide-primed at all times. When needed, the circuit is primed with crystalloid, and can be ready for use within 15 minutes. In their experience of 11 children suffering full cardiopulmonary arrest, the median duration of resuscitation duration was 55 minutes, with 66% surviving to discharge. Ojito and colleagues[43] developed a modified miniaturized system suitable for neonates. The circuit was designed to accelerate the setup, reduce the priming volume, eliminate the need for priming with blood even in neonates, and simplify transport. This system consists of a preassembled completely heparin coated (Carmeda® Bio-Active Surface) circuit, a centrifugal blood pump, a Minimax® hollow fiber oxygenator, a Bio-Probe flow probe, and a BioTrend Oxygen Saturation and Hematocrit Monitor, which can be assembled and primed in less than five minutes. Complete Carmeda® coating reduces the requirements for heparin in an effort to reduce postoperative loss of blood and the need for aggressive heparinization in the immediately post-resuscitated patient. Studies

by Jacobs and colleagues,[44] and Hannan and colleagues,[45] have demonstrated the safe and effective implementation of this technology, with lower hemorrhagic complications involving the central nervous system, and survival to discharge of 48% and 54%, respectively. The potential disadvantages with this system include a limited durability for the oxygenator and an increased potential for air embolism. Advantages over conventional ECMO for children with congenital malformed hearts and refractory cardiopulmonary dysfunction include rapid set-up time with a bloodless prime, decreased postoperative loss of blood, and simplified transport.

The literature supporting emergent cardiopulmonary support is mounting.[38,46-48] The outcomes after initiation of support during active compressions of the chest following in-hospital cardiac arrest was reported by Morris and colleagues.[46] One-third of their cohort survived to discharge, with neither age, weight, or duration of compressions before E-CPR correlating with survival. No patient who received greater than 30 minutes of resuscitation without extracorporeal cardiopulmonary support survived, while 33% of those receiving greater than 30 minutes of CPR survived with the use of extracorporeal support. Early neurologic assessment was unchanged compared to admission in half of the survivors, even when the duration of resuscitation was prolonged to greater than 60 minutes. In this series, children with isolated cardiac disease were more likely to survive following support than children with other medical conditions. A recent study by Alsoufi and colleagues[47] presented a retrospective review of 80 consecutive children with a median age of 150 days, ranging in age from 1 day to 17.6 years, who were treated with venoarterial E-CPR for cardiac arrest refractory to conventional cardiopulmonary resuscitation. The authors report that 30% of their cohort had favorable outcomes, defined as hospital survival with grossly intact neurological state. Neither age, weight, sex, cardiac versus noncardiac etiology, duration of CPR, site of cannulation site, nor timing, or location of ECMO proved to be a significant predictor of favorable outcome. The authors concluded "Lack of predictors of poor outcome support aggressive attempts to initiate extracorporeal cardiopulmonary resuscitation in all patients followed by subsequent assessment of organ salvage." [47] A study by Allen and colleagues[48] reviewed the use of emergent cardiopulmonary support in patients undergoing cardiac catheterization over a period of eight years. Indications for support included catheter induced complication, severe low cardiac output syndrome and hypoxemia. During cannulation, almost 90% of their patients were undergoing chest compressions, with a median duration of cardiopulmonary resuscitation of 29 minutes. Just over 80% survived to discharge, with 5 needing cardiac transplantation. Of 19 patients who received cardiopulmonary resuscitation during cannulation, 80% survived to discharge, but almost 50% sustained neurologic injury. There was no significant difference between survivors and non-survivors in terms of age, weight, duration of cardiopulmonary resuscitation, duration of ECMO support, pH, or lactate levels.

Myocarditis and Cardiomyopathy

Children with acute fulminant myocarditis can benefit greatly from mechanical circulatory support with eventual myocardial recovery. Similar to the experience in adults, survival is also excellent in children. Hence in children with acute myocarditis, persistent low cardiac output syndrome despite escalating inotropic support should be an indication for mechanical circulatory support. The Extracorporeal Life Support Organization reports that survival with myocarditis is highest for any diagnostic group, with almost 60% being successfully weaned from ECMO.[5] ECMO is the mechanical support of choice in these patients because of the speed with which it can be instituted and its

easy reversibility. In this subgroup of patients, ECMO may be used as a bridge to recovery, transplantation, or VAD. In a retrospective study by Duncan and colleagues,[49] the technique was used in 12 patients with clinical, laboratory or endomyocardial biopsy proven myocarditis as a bridge to recovery or transplantation, with just over 80% surviving. Deaths in this cohort of patients were secondary to post support nosocomial infections. In more heterogeneous groups, Chen and colleagues[50] and Asaumi and colleagues[51] demonstrated a survival to discharge of almost 75% for patients with fulminant myocarditis treated with ECMO.

ECMO can also be used as a bridge to transplantation in children with irreversible myocardial dysfunction.[52-54] This includes patients with dilated cardiomyopathy, restrictive cardiomyopathy, endstage congenital cardiac disease, and chronic graft dysfunction after transplantation. ECMO can also be used after heart transplantation. Indications for support in this setting include failure to separate from CPB and progressive low cardiac output syndrome in the immediate postoperative period, along with circulatory collapse due to rejection or graft vasculopathy later in the course.[55,56] Right heart failure and/or pulmonary hypertension are often responsible for the inability to separate from cardiopulmonary bypass, and hence extracorporeal membrane oxygenation is the mechanical support of choice. Galantowicz and colleagues[57] examined the role of the technique as an adjunct to pediatric cardiac transplantation, using it as a bridge to transplantation in 20% of patients, in 40% to facilitate resuscitation of the cardiac allograft in the immediate postoperative period, while in just under 33%, it complemented therapy for severe rejection in the late postoperative period. Of the patients, 60% survived, all demonstrating normal function of the cardiac allograft. The Extracorporeal Life Support Organization has reported an overall survival of from 33-66% for this population.[5]

Pulmonary Hypertension Refractory to Medical Therapy

Select patients with pulmonary hypertension refractory to medical therapy will benefit from extracorporeal life support.[58] A classic example is preoperative stabilization of obstructed total anomalous pulmonary venous connection when the patient is close to death, and in the postoperative period when the pulmonary vascular resistance may be transiently elevated. In this group of patients, it is important to rule out any residual pulmonary venous obstruction as a cause of pulmonary hypertension. Mechanical support is controversial for patients with irreversible pulmonary hypertension, such as primary pulmonary hypertension, as the likelihood of survival as a bridge to lung transplantation or heart-lung transplantation is minimal.

Intractable Arrhythmias with Hemodynamic Compromise

In select patients with malignant tachyarrhythmias and bradyarrhythmias, a short trial of mechanical support may be warranted to prevent circulatory collapse while medical therapy is being optimized, or prior to an attempt at radiofrequency ablation. Patients who have benefited from the use of mechanical support for this indication include those with lethal arrhythmias secondary to acute myocarditis or cardiomyopathy, supraventricular tachycardia, junctional ectopic tachycardia or ventricular tachycardia after cardiac surgery, and recalcitrant supraventricular tachycardia in the setting of Ebstein's malformation.[59-61] It is important to rule out residual lesions or coronary ischemia in the postcardiotomy patients. ECMO has mostly been used for this indication, though there are occasional reports of the effective use of ventricular assist device as well.[61]

Respiratory Failure

Patients with congenital cardiac disease can develop respiratory failure due to parenchymal lung disease from viral infections such as respiratory syncytial virus, adenovirus and so on, or due to severe tracheobronchomalacia as seen in the severest form of tetralogy of Fallot with absent pulmonary valve syndrome. Patients with cyanotic disease who develop parenchymal lung disease can be supported with venovenous ECMO as a bridge to recovery or surgical palliation.[62] ECMO can also be used to provide short term ventilatory support to allow time for definitive tracheal surgery in infants and children, in whom it would otherwise not be possible to achieve adequate gas exchange because of major airway disease as seen with long segment tracheal stenosis.[63]

ECMO in Patients With Functionally Univentricular Circulation

Many centers previously considered a functionally univentricular circulation to be a contraindication to ECMO, but improved results have been achieved recently with this complex subset of patients.[28] Indications for extracorporeal life support in these children include inability to separate from cardiopulmonary bypass, low cardiac output refractory to conventional therapy, cardiopulmonary arrest, thrombosis of the shunt, and elective support. Techniques for oxygenation often require modifications in these patients. Jaggers and colleagues[64] among others have clearly demonstrated that the aortopulmonary shunt can be left open, as long as the flows are adjusted to maintain adequate systemic blood pressure, tissue perfusion, and gas exchange. Importantly with this strategy, patients may require increased flow through the pump of 150 to 200 mL/kg/min due to a significant runoff via the shunt to the pulmonary bed. In these patients, it is often possible to isolate the membrane and thus utilize the circuit as a ventricular assist device. Mechanical ventilator support and/or sweep gas should be adjusted to maintain adequate gas exchange.

The ELSO Registry recently reported the outcome of extracorporeal life support used in neonates for cardiac indications from 1996 to 2000.[65] Of the 740 neonates who were placed on extracorporeal life support for cardiac indications, 118 had hypoplastic left heart syndrome. There was no significant difference in survival between these patients and those with other defects. For patients with hypoplastic left heart syndrome, placement on extracorporeal life support at greater than 15 days of age and shorter duration of extracorporeal life support, was significantly associated with better survival. Allan and colleagues[66] reviewed their experience with the support of infants with shunted functionally univentricular circulations. Almost 50% survived to discharge. Patients cannulated for hypoxemia, particularly with thrombosis of the shunt, had markedly improved survival compared with those supported primarily for hypotension or cardiovascular collapse. Survival did not differ depending on anatomic diagnosis. Ravishankar and colleagues[67] examined the use of ECMO following the first stage of reconstruction for hypoplastic left heart syndrome and its variants. Almost 40% of their cohort survived to hospital discharge. Non-survivors had longer CPB time, need for support less than 24 hours after the initial reconstruction, and longer duration of support. All those with an acutely thrombosed shunt were early survivors. Half of their early survivors remained alive at a median followup of 20 months. Initiation of "non-elective" mechanical support in the early postoperative period after Norwood reconstruction is associated with poor outcome. This is likely secondary to irreversible myocardial ischemia, and or residual hemodynamic issues such as obstruction in the aortic arch. Extracorporeal life support, nonetheless, can be lifesaving in infants with a functionally univentricular circulation with otherwise fatal conditions. It is particularly useful in potentially reversible conditions such as acute thrombosis of the shunt and transient depression of ventricular function.

Ungerleider and colleagues have reported a role for use of "routine" mechanical ventricular assist device after the Norwood reconstruction in an attempt to simplify postoperative management and improve hospital survival.[68] They used a ventricular assist device after modified ultrafiltration, using the cardiopulmonary bypass cannulae in the right atrium and neoaorta. Mean duration of mechanical support was 3 days, and almost 90% survived to discharge. They also reported an improved early neurodevelopmental outcome. Routine mechanical support after the Norwood operation is a novel approach that addresses the increased cardiac output demands in the immediate postoperative period, and simplifies postoperative care, albeit with increased complexity and that it will likely increase cost and the need for additional personnel.

There is very limited experience with mechanical support in patients with cavopulmonary connections.[11,69] The ELSO registry reported survival of 25% for patients with this physiology. In the largest retrospective study, Booth and colleagues[29] reported on their institutional experience following bidirectional Glenn and Fontan operations. Only one patient with a bidirectional Glenn anastomosis survived, albeit with severe neurological damage. In those with the Fontan circulation, 50% survived to discharge, and 33% are alive at followup. Their report highlights some of the technical difficulties in this challenging group of patients. Patients with cavopulmonary connections are difficult to resuscitate effectively with conventional cardiopulmonary resuscitation. During resuscitation, the increase in intrathoracic pressure may restrict effective blood flow to the lungs and thereby limit oxygenation, as well as increasing cerebral venous pressure that may further limit cerebral perfusion. The cannulation of the patient with a bidirectional Glenn shunt is particularly challenging because of the separation of the systemic venous drainage, thus requiring placement of multiple venous cannulae. It is particularly important to achieve adequate and early decompression of the superior vena cava to maximize cerebral perfusion pressure, and thus potentially improve neurological outcome. Rood and colleagues analyzed data from the ELSO Registry on patients requiring ECMO after the Fontan operation to identify the in-hospital mortality and factors associated with mortality in these patients.[70] The overall survival to hospital discharge was 35% with greater utilization and improved survival over time. In this cohort, neurologic injury, surgical bleeding and renal failure were associated with increased odds of mortality. Mortality was not associated with demographic, pre-ECMO support or ECMO support variables suggesting that ECMO complications are particularly problematic in these patients and may limit their survival outcomes.

Outcome and Risk Factors for Death

Variable survival statistics have been reported for pediatric cardiac ECMO. In 2000, cumulative survival for cardiac ECMO in the ELSO Registry was 42%.[71] Interestingly, ten years later, the cumulative survival rate remains similar despite advances in management.[5] Analysis of the ELSO Registry by Meliones and colleagues listed ongoing cardiac failure (37%) and major central nervous system damage (15%) as the most common causes of mortality.[72] Cardiac failure and complications arising from low cardiac output are, likewise, the most commonly reported causes of death in numerous other reports.[12,19,29,66,67,70] Thus, attempts to improve results achieved with pediatric cardiac ECMO should address optimization of ventricular function, avoidance of extended periods of low cardiac output, and minimization of other end organ dysfunction. Prompt institution of ECMO support achieves these goals by preserving myocardial, central nervous system, and visceral perfusion. Allowing patients to remain in a low cardiac output state on increasing dosages of inotropic and vasoconstrictive agents prior to ECMO may lead to end-organ damage that may not be reversible after circulatory support has been established. Once ECMO is initiated, meticulous patient management is required to limit infectious complications that may progress to multisystem organ failure. For the salvage of continuing severe cardiac dysfunction, an early and aggressive approach to cardiac transplantation may be the only life-saving therapy available.

Lack of return of ventricular function within 48-72 hours in postcardiotomy patients, confers a poor prognosis.[15] Return of ventricular function is defined as the return of a pulsatile waveform on the peripheral arterial trace on maximal levels of support (80% of normal cardiac output provided by the device). The return of a pulsatile waveform on the arterial line trace by 72 hours of support was seen in 24 of 25 non-transplanted ECMO survivors (96%). These data have been used as additional prognostic information, as postcardiotomy patients without return of ventricular function within 48-72 hours of support are currently considered for transplantation or termination of support when transplantation is contraindicated. Delaying this decision while awaiting return of ventricular function beyond the first 48-72 hours of support is not justified based on these results. Due to the scarcity of pediatric organ donors, early consideration for transplantation optimizes the chances of successful organ procurement. While return of ventricular function occurs early or not at all for ECMO supported patients after cardiac surgery, patients with myocarditis may require prolonged periods of mechanical circulatory support with ultimate complete recovery of ventricular function.[49,73-76]

Long Term Followup

Data regarding neurodevelopmental outcome[77,78] of long-term survivors of ECMO are emerging. Ibrahim and colleagues[78] reported on 37 children who survived mechanical circulatory support, 26 with ECMO and 11 with a ventricular assist device, who were followed for an average of more than four years. Only one patient died in either group. Eighty percent of children in both groups were reportedly in excellent general condition and ventricular function by echocardiographic evaluation was normal in all the survivors of ECMO and 90% of those surviving after use of the assist device. More than 60% of children supported with ECMO had moderate to severe neurologic impairment, whereas only 20% of those surviving after ventricular assist device support demonstrated the same degree of neurologic impairment. These results may suggest an advantage for use of the ventricular assist device, possibly because of decreased requirements for anticoagulation, with less risk for intracranial hemorrhage. These results must be interpreted with caution, as the group supported with ECMO had a greater proportion of critically ill neonates, with more complex underlying cardiac conditions. Costello and colleagues assessed the quality of life of pediatric cardiac ECMO survivors.[79] This was done by parent proxy reporting and was compared to that of a general U.S. population and other cardiac populations with the purpose of identifying factors associated with lower quality of life. They found that the physical component of health related quality of life is lower than that of the general population but similar to that of patients with complex cardiac disease, whereas psychosocial quality of life is similar to that of the general population and of other pediatric cardiac populations. Older children and adolescents who previously required cardiac ECMO perceived their quality of life to be quite good.

Conclusions

A variety of forms of mechanical circulatory support are available for children with cardiopulmonary dysfunction refractory to conventional management. These devices require extensive resources, both human and economic. Extracorporeal membrane oxygenation can be effectively used in a variety of settings to provide support to critically ill patients with cardiac disease. The approach for children with complex cardiac disease has required the development of innovative measures to help ensure successful outcomes. Careful selection of patients and timing of intervention remains challenging. Special consideration should be given to children with cardiac disease with regard to anatomy, physiology, cannulation, and circuit management. The principles employed presently in the application of ECMO to support the failing circulation in children will serve as the foundation for developing innovative circulatory support techniques for the future.

References

1. Jacobs JP. Pediatric Mechanical Circulatory Support. In: Pediatric Cardiac Surgery, 3rd Edition, Chapter 45, Pages 778 - 792. Mavroudis C and Backer CL, editors, Mosby Inc., An affiliate of Elsevier, Philadelphia, Pennsylvania, 2003.

2. Baffes TG, Fridman JL, Bicoff JP, Whitehill JL. Extracorporeal circulation for support of palliative cardiac surgery in infants. Ann Thorac Surg 1970; 10:354-363.

3. Soeter JR, Mamiya RT, Sprague AY, McNamara JJ. Prolonged extracorporeal oxygenation for cardiorespiratory failure after tetralogy correction. J Thorac Cardiovasc Surg 1973; 66:214-218.

4. Duncan BW. Pediatric Mechanical Circulatory Support. ASAIO 2005; 51: ix-xiv.

5. The July 2011 Extracorporeal Life Support Organization (ELSO) Extracorporeal Life Support (ECLS) Registry Report International Summary. Ann Arbor, Michigan, Extracorporeal Life Support Organization, 2011.

6. Duncan BW. Pediatric Mechanical Circulatory Support in the United States: Past, Present, and Future. ASAIO 2006; 52:525-9.

7. Blume ED, Naftel DC, Bastardi HJ et al. Outcomes of children bridged to heart transplantation with ventricular assist devices: a multi-institutional study. Circulation. 2006 May 16; 113(19): 2313-9.

8. Willms DC, Atkins PJ, Dembitsky WP, et al. Analysis of clinical trends in a program of emergent ECLS for cardiovascular collapse. ASAIO J 1997; 43:65-68.

9. del Nido PJ. Extracorporeal membrane oxygenation for cardiac support in children. Ann Thorac Surg 1996; 61:336-339.

10. Black MD, Coles JG, Williams WG, et al. Determinants of success in pediatric cardiac patients undergoing extracorporeal membrane oxygenation. Ann Thorac Surg 1995; 60:133-138.

11. Dalton HJ, Siewers RD, Fuhrman BP, et al. Extracorporeal membrane oxygenation for cardiac rescue in children with severe myocardial dysfunction. Crit Care Med 1993; 21:1020-1028.

12. Kanter KR, Pennington DG, Weber TR, et al. Extracorporeal membrane oxygenation for postoperative cardiac support in children. J Thorac Cardiovasc Surg 1987; 93:27-35.

13. Klein MD, Shaheen KW, Whittlesey GC, et al. Extracorporeal membrane oxygenation for the circulatory support of children after repair of congenital heart disease. J Thorac Cardiovasc Surg 1990; 100:498-505.

14. Hirschl RB. Devices. In: Zwischenberger JB, Bartlett RH, eds. ECMO: Extracorporeal cardiopulmonary support in critical care. 2 ed. Ann Arbor, Michigan: ELSO, 1995:150-190.

15. Duncan BW, Hraska V, Jonas RA et al., Mechanical circulatory support in children with cardiac disease. J Thorac Cardiovasc Surg 1999; 117: 529–542.

16. Trittenwein G, Furst G, Golej J, et al. Preoperative ECMO in congenital cyanotic heart disease using the AREC system. Ann Thorac Surg 1997; 63:1298-1302.

17. Chevalier JY, Couprie C, Larroquet M, Renolleau S, Durandy Y, Costil J. Venovenous single lumen cannula extracorporeal lung support in neonates. ASAIO J 1993; 39:M654-658.

18. Trittenwein G, Golej J, Burda G, et al. Neonatal and pediatric extracorporeal membrane oxygenation using nonocclusive blood pumps: the Vienna experience. Artif Organs 2001; 25:994-999.

19. Ziomek S, Harrell JE, Fasules JW, et al. Extracorporeal membrane oxygenation for cardiac failure after congenital heart operation. Ann Thorac Surg 1992; 54:861-868.

20. Koenig PR, Ralston MA, Kimball TR, et al. Balloon atrial septostomy for left ventricular decompression in patients receiv-

ing extracorporeal membrane oxygenation for myocardial failure. J Pediatr. 1993; 122:S95-9.

21. Aiyagari R, Rocchini A, Remenapp R, et al. Decompression of the left atrium during extracorporeal membrane oxygenation using transseptal cannula incorporated into the circuit. Crit Care Med 2006; 34: 2603-06.

22. Wilson JM, Bower LK, Fackler JC, et al. Aminocaproic acid decreases the incidence of intracranial hemorrhage and other hemorrhagic complications of ECMO. J Pediatr Surg 1993; 28:536-541.

23. Horwitz JR, Cofer BR, Warner BH, et al. A multi-center trial of 6-aminocaproic acid (Amicar) in the prevention of bleeding in infants on ECMO. J Pediatr Surg 1998; 33:1610-1613.

24. Downard CD, Betit P, Chang RW, et al. Impact of AMICAR on hemorrhagic complications of ECMO: a ten-year review. J Pediatr Surg 2003; 38:1212-1216.

25. Walters HL, Hakimi M, Rice MD, et al. Pediatric cardiac surgical ECMO: Multivariate analysis of risk factors for hospital death. Ann Thorac Surg 1995; 60:329-337.

26. Aharon AS, Drinkwater DC, Jr., Churchwell KB, et al. Extracorporeal membrane oxygenation in children after repair of congenital cardiac lesions. Ann Thorac Surg 2001; 72:2095-101.

27. Darling EM, Kaemmer D, Lawson DS, et al. Use of ECMO without the oxygenator to provide ventricular support after Norwood Stage I procedures. Ann Thorac Surg 2001; 71:735-736.

28. Pizarro C, Davis DA, Healy RM, et al. Is there a role for extracorporeal life support after stage I Norwood? Euro J Cardiothorac Surg 2001; 19:294-301.

29. Booth KL, Roth SJ, Thiagarajan RR, et al. Extracorporeal membrane oxygenation support of the Fontan and bidirectional Glenn circulations. Ann Thorac Surg 2004; 77:1341-1348.

30. Chang AC, Wernovsky G, Kulik T et al. Management of the neonate with transposition of the great arteries and persistent pulmonary hypertension. Am J Cardiol 1991; 68: 1253-55.

31. Luciani GB, Chang AC, Starnes VA. Surgical repair of transposition of great arteries in neonates with persistent pulmonary hypertension. Ann Thorac Surg 1996; 61:800-05.

32. Di Russo GB, Clark BJ, Bridges ND et al. Prolonged extracorporeal membrane oxygenation as a bridge to cardiac transplantation. Ann Thorac Surg. 2000; 69: 925-927.

33. Booth KL, Roth SJ, Perry SB et al. Cardiac catheterization of patients supported by extracorporeal membrane oxygenation. J Am Coll Cardiol. 2002; 40:1681-6.

34. Alsoufi B, Shen I, Karamlou T, et al. Extracorporeal Life Support in Neonates, Infants and Children after repair of Congenital Heart Disease: Modern Era Results in a Single Institution. Ann Thorac Surg 2005; 80:15-21.

35. Hoskote A, Bohn D, Gruenwald C, et al. Extracorporeal life support after staged palliation of a functional single ventricle: Subsequent morbidity and survival. J Thorac Cardiovasc Surg 2006; 131:1114-21.

36. Aharon AS, Drinkwater DC, Churchwell KB et al. Extracorporeal membrane oxygenation in children after repair of congenital cardiac lesions. Ann Thorac Surg 2001; 72: 2095-2101.

37. Kolovos NS, Bratton SL, Moler FW et al. Outcome of pediatric patients treated with extracorporeal life support after cardiac surgery. Ann Thorac Surg 2003; 76: 1435-1441; discussion 1441-1442.

38. Thourani V, Kirshborm P, Kanter P, et al. Venoarterial Extracorporeal Membrane Oxygenation (VA-ECMO) in Pediatric Cardiac Support. Ann Thorac Surg 2006; 82: 138-45.

39. Morris M, Ittenback R, Godinez R, et al. Risk factors for mortality in 137 pediatric cardiac intensive care unit patients managed with extracorporeal membrane oxygenation. Crit Care Med 2004:32:1061-1069.

40. del Nido PJ, Dalton HJ, Thomson AE, et al. Extracorporeal membrane oxygenator rescue in children during cardiac arrest after cardiac surgery. Circulation 1992; 86: II 300-304.

41. Posner JC, Osterhoudt KC, Mollen CJ, et al. Extracorporeal membrane oxygenation as a resuscitative measure in the pediatric emergency department. Pediatr Emerg Care. 2000; 16(6):413-5.

42. Duncan BW, Ibrahim AE, Hraska V, et al. Use of rapid-deployment extracorporeal membrane oxygenation for the resuscitation of pediatric patients with heart disease after cardiac arrest. J Thorac Cardiovasc Surg 1998; 116:305-11.

43. Ojito JW, McConaghey T, Jacobs JP, et al. Rapid pediatric cardiopulmonary support system. J Extra Corpor Technol 1997; 29:96-99.

44. Jacobs JP, Ojito JW, McConaghey T, et al. Rapid Cardiopulmonary Support for Children with Complex Congenital Heart Disease. Ann Thorac Surg 2000; 70:742-749.

45. Hannan R, Ojito J, Ybarra M, et al. Rapid Cardiopulmonary Support in Children with Heart Disease: A Nine Year Experience. Ann Thorac Surg 2006; 82:1637-42.

46. Morris M, Wernovsky G, Nadkarni V, et al. Survival outcomes after extracorporeal cardiopulmonary resuscitation instituted during active chest compressions following refractory in-hospital pediatric cardiac arrest. Pediatr Crit Care Med 2004; 5:440-46.

47. Alsoufi B, Al-Radi OO, Nazer RI, et al. Survival outcomes after rescue extracorporeal cardiopulmonary resuscitation in pediatric patients with refractory cardiac arrest. J Thorac Cardiovasc Surg 2007 Oct; 134(4):952-959.

48. Allan C, Thiagarajan R, Armsby L, et al. Emergent use of extracorporeal membrane oxygenation during pediatric cardiac catheterization. Pediatr Crit Care Med 2006; 7:212-9.

49. Duncan B, Bohn D, Atz A, et al. Mechanical circulatory support for the treatment of children with acute fulminant myocarditis. J Thorac and Cardiovasc Surg 2001; 122:400-8.

50. Chen Y, Yu H, Huang S, et al. Experience and Result of Extracorporeal Membrane Oxygenation in Treating Fulminant Myocarditis with Shock: What Mechanical Support Should be considered first? J Heart Lung Transplant 2005; 24: 81-7.

51. Asaumi Y, Yasuda S, Morii I, et al. Favourable clinical outcome in patients with cardiogenic shock due to fulminant myocarditis supported by percutaneous extracorporeal membrane oxygenation. European Heart Journal 2005; 26: 2185-92.

52. del Nido PJ, Armitage JM, Fricker FJ, et al. Extracorporeal membrane oxygenation support as a bridge to pediatric heart transplantation. Circulation 1994; 90: II66–II69.

53. Fiser W, Yetman A, Gunselman R, et al. Pediatric Arteriovenous Extracorporeal Membrane Oxygenation (ECMO) as a bridge to Cardiac Transplantation. J Heart Lung Transplant 2003; Vol. 22: No. 7.

54. Gajarski R, Mosca R, Ohye R, et al. Use of Extracorporeal Life Support as a Bridge to Pediatric Cardiac Transplantation. J Heart Lung Transplant 2003; 22:28-34.

55. Kirshbom PM, Bridges ND, Myung RJ, et al. Use of extracorporeal membrane oxygenation in pediatric thoracic organ transplantation. J Thorac Cardiovasc Surg 2002; 123: 130-136.

56. Hoffman TM, Spray TL, Gaynor JW, et al. Survival after acute graft failure in pediatric

thoracic organ transplant recipients. Pediatr Transplant 2000; 4:112-117.

57. Galantówicz ME, Stolar CJ. Extracorporeal membrane oxygenation for perioperative support in pediatric heart transplantation. J Thorac Cardiovasc Surg 1991; 102:148-51.

58. Dhillon R, Pearson GA, Firmin RK, et al. Extracorporeal membrane oxygenation and the treatment of critical pulmonary hypertension in congenital heart disease. Eur J Cardiothorac Surg 1995; 9: 553-556.

59. Walker GM, McLeod K, Brown KL et al. Extracorporeal life support as a treatment of supraventricular tachycardia in infants. Pediatr Crit Care Med. 2003; 4: 52-54.

60. Cohen MI, Gaynor JW, Ramesh V et al. Extracorporeal membrane oxygenation for patients with refractory ventricular arrhythmias. J Thorac Cardiovasc Surg. 1999; 118: 961-63.

61. Pastuszko P, Gruber PJ, Wernovsky G et al. Thoratec left ventricular assist device as a bridge to recovery in a child weighing 27 kilograms. J Thorac Cardiovasc Surg. 2004; 127:1203-04.

62. Imamura M, Schmitz, ML, Watkins B, et al. Venovenous Extracorporeal Membrane Oxygenation for Cyanotic Congenital Heart Disease. Ann Thorac Surg 2004; 78:1723-7.

63. Goldman AP, Macrae DJ, Tasker RC, et al. Extracorporeal membrane oxygenation as a bridge to definitive tracheal surgery in children. J Pediatr 1996; 128: 386-388.

64. Jaggers J, Forbess J, Shah A, et al. Extracorporeal Membrane Oxygenation for Infant Postcardiotomy Support: Significance of Shunt Management. Ann Thorac Surg 2000; 69:1476-83.

65. Hintz S, Benitz W, Colby C, et al. Utilization and outcomes of neonatal cardiac extracorporeal life support: 1996-2000. Pediatr Crit Care Med 2005; 6:33-38.

66. Allan C, Thiagarajan R, del Nido P, et al. Indication for initiation of mechanical circulatory support impacts survival of infants with shunted single-ventricle circulation supported with extracorporeal membrane oxygenation. J Thorac Cardiovasc Surg 2007; 133: 660-7.

67. Ravishankar C, Dominguez T, Kreutzer J, et al. Extracorporeal membrane oxygenation after stage I reconstruction for hypoplastic left heart syndrome. Pediatr Crit Care Med 2006; 7:319-23.

68. Ungerleider RM, Shen I, Yeh T, et al. Routine mechanical ventricular assist following the Norwood procedure—improved neurologic outcome and hospital survival. Ann Thorac Surg 2004; 77:18-22.

69. Klein MD, Shaheen KW, Whittlesey GC, et al. Extracorporeal membrane oxygenation for the circulatory support of children after repair of congenital heart disease. J Thorac Cardiovasc Surg 1990; 100:498-505.

70. Rood KL, Teele SA, Barrett CS, et al. Extracorporeal membrane oxygenation support after the Fontan operation. J Thorac Cardiovasc Surg 2011 Sep; 142 (3): 504-10.

71. Duncan BW. Mechanical circulatory support in infants and children with cardiac disease. In: Zwischenberger JB, Bartlett RH, eds. ECMO Extracorporeal Cardiopulmonary Support in Critical Care. Ann Arbor, Michigan: ELSO, 2000.

72. Meliones JN, Custer JR, Snedecor S, et al. Extracorporeal life support for cardiac assist in pediatric patients. Circulation 1991; 84:168-172.

73. Frazier EA, Faulkner SC, Seib PM, et al. Prolonged extracorporeal life support for bridging to transplant. Perfusion 1997; 12:93-98.

74. Holman WL, Bourge RC, Kirklin JK. Circulatory support for seventy days with resolution of acute heart failure. J Thorac Cardiovasc Surg 1991; 102:932-934.

75. Kato S, Marimoto S, Hiramitsu S, et al. Use of percutaneous cardiopulmonary support of patients with fulminant myocarditis and

cardiogenic shock for improving prognosis. Am J Cardiol 1999; 85:623-625.

76. Kawahito K, Murata S, Yasu T, et al. Usefulness of extracorporeal membrane oxygenation for treatment of fulminant myocarditis and circulatory collapse. Am J Cardiol 1998; 82:910-911.

77. Hamrick S, Gremmels D, Keet C, et al. Neurodevelopmental Outcome of Infant Supported with Extracorporeal Membrane Oxygenation after Cardiac Surgery. Pediatrics 2003; 111:671-5.

78. Ibrahim A, Duncan B, Blume E, et al. Long-Term Follow-up of Pediatric Cardiac patients requiring mechanical circulatory support. Ann Thorac Surg 2000; 69:186-92.

79. Costello JM, O'Brien M, Wypij D, et al. Quality of life of pediatric cardiac patients who previously required extracorporeal membrane oxygenation. Pediatr Crit Care Med 2012; 13:000–000.

21

Adult Respiratory ECMO

Giles J Peek MD FRCS CTh, Chris Harvey MB ChB MRCS, Gail Faulkner RSCN

Introduction

After the initial success of Hill and coworkers in 1971[1] the failure of the NIH adult ECMO study[2] led to a global loss of interest in ECMO for respiratory support in adults. Fortunately a few tenacious investigators understood the flaws in the NIH study and persevered with their efforts to make ECMO an effective strategy of support for adults with severe but potentially reversible respiratory failure.[3,4] In this chapter we will discuss the evidence base for, case selection, treatment protocols, and results of adult respiratory ECMO support.

Evidence base

There are three randomized controlled trials (RCTs) and a number of cohort studies which are relevant to adult ECMO, these will be addressed in chronological order. This is not an exhaustive review of the literature, but an attempt to select those studies that proved a turning point in the argument for or against ECMO use.

Hill et al.[1]

Case report of first successful adult respiratory ECMO use. A 24 year old man supported on venoarterial (VA) ECMO for 75 hours with ARDS after repair of a transected aorta following a motorcycle accident. This paper was proof of concept, and interestingly included the concept of "lung rest," reducing peak airway pressures from 60 cmH_2O to 35–40. Sadly the importance of this manoeuvre was not appreciated by the NIH ECMO providers.

Zapol et al.[2]

1970s NIH sponsored RCT. Ninety patients randomized to continued high pressure ventilation or continued high pressure ventilation plus VA ECMO support in 9 US medical centers. Survival 8.3 and 9.5% in control and ECMO arms respectively, not significantly different. This study is commonly cited by sceptics as showing that ECMO does not work for adults. However there are major differences between this study and modern practices; patients had been ventilated for a mean of 9.6 days prior to randomization to ECMO, they suffered continued lung damaging ventilation and had massive ongoing hemorrhage while on ECMO due to primitive cannulation techniques and heparin management. All ECMO was VA. The analyses of the reasons for failure of this study lead us to the concepts of lung rest and venovenous (VV) ECMO.

Gattinoni et al.[3]

This cohort study of venovenous extracorporeal CO_2 removal (VV $ECCO_2R$) with 49% survival in 43 patients demonstrated that ventilation and oxygenation were separable. Removal of CO_2 by the low flow venovenous circuit allowed "apnoeic" oxygenation to be achieved with low frequency ventilation, in turn causing less lung injury. This study was proof of concept of VV support and is the first step towards lung protective ventilation.

Morris et al.[5]

This study was an RCT of VV $ECCO_2R$ vs computer directed, pressure controlled inverse ratio ventilation (PCIRV). Forty patients were randomized, survival was 33% and 42% (not significantly different p=0.8) in treatment and control groups respectively. The PCIRV results were much better than expected when compared with historical controls. The authors concluded that $ECCO_2R$ was ineffective and should not be used outside RCTs. However, in this study the team was unable to achieve apnoeic oxygenation in the $ECCO_2R$ group and responded by increasing the airway pressure to reverse hypoxia. In addition, the study team was inexperienced in the use of ECLS and had significant problems with bleeding and circuit clotting, necessitating the removal of patients from support. This study demonstrated the limitation of $ECCO_2R$ (low flow ECLS) in patients who require high flow ECLS (i.e., ECMO) to support oxygenation as well as CO_2 removal. It also shows the importance of experience in delivering effective ECLS and the utility of PCIRV.

Bartlett[4]

This cohort study of 30 adults with respiratory and 10 with cardiac failure, supported with predominantly VV ECMO in the respiratory patients with 45% overall survival was the first description of the modern recipe for successful adult ECMO. The concepts of case selection before irreversible ventilator induced lung injury has developed, provision of full nutrition, normal haematocrit, lung rest, and VV support are all enumerated in this landmark paper.

Case Series[6,7]

These case series of 100 patients from the University for Michigan and 50 patients from Leicester, UK with 54% and 66% survival respectively showed proof of concept that the technology and treatment protocols were reliable. They paved the way for the CESAR Trial.

CESAR[8]

This pragmatic British National RCT of **C**onventional Ventilation or **E**CMO for **S**evere **A**dult **R**espiratory Failure, randomized 180 patients from 68 medical centers to either continued conventional treatment or transfer to Glenfield Hospital in Leicester for consideration of ECMO. ECMO was only available in the UK as part of the study protocol. The primary end point was survival without severe disability at 6 months was 63% vs 47% in treatment and control arms respectively (p=0.03), equivalent to saving an additional patient for every 6 patients treated. The ECMO team managed to treat 1/5 of their patients without ECMO, and used significantly more lung protective ventilation and steroids than the control group. The concurrent economic evaluation showed a predicted lifetime cost per quality-adjusted life year (QALY) of £19,252, equivalent in cost efficacy to lung transplantation. The study was hampered by resistance of the UK intensive care community to agree on a protocol for conventional treatment or to collaborate in collection of extensive data. Although CESAR is slightly limited by these shortcomings, it is safe to conclude that the outcome in adults with severe respiratory failure in the UK NHS was better when patients were transferred to the care of a team specializing in such patients where ECMO was part of the treatment algorithm. In the post-CESAR/H1N1 era it would be ethically impossible to design another RCT of ECMO in any age group where death was the end point in the control arm and ECMO was denied.

Case Selection

The key to successful case selection is to identify patients who are at high risk of death due to non-response to conventional treatment, who are suffering from a potentially reversible disease, and who do not have contraindications. These three aspects will be addressed separately. Patients must pass all three levels before becoming candidates for ECMO support, illness severity or impending death alone are not sufficient justification. It is futile to support a patient with ECMO who has no chance of recovery!

Severity of illness & failure of conventional treatment

For patients with Type 1 (hypoxic) respiratory failure a Murray lung injury score[9] of ≥ 3.0 is used as an indication of sufficiently severe illness to warrant ECMO support. The Murray Lung Injury Score (MLIS) is determined by a compilation of respiratory support measures as well as chest radiologic findings that are given specific scoring (Figure 21-1). For example a patient has a PaO_2 of 49.5 mmHg on 100% oxygen, and this results in a PaO_2/FiO_2 ratio of < 100 giving a score of 4 for this parameter of the MLIS. The chest x-ray of this patient has consolidation and infiltration in 3 out of 4 quadrants giving a score of 3 for this parameter. They are on a PEEP of 10 cmH_2O which gives a score of 2 and the PIP is measured at 38 cmH_2O with a tidal volume of 420 mL. The PIP-PEEP difference is 28 and the compliance is therefore calculated at 420/28=15 for a score of 4. This patient's MLIS is therefore 13/4=3.3 and is con-

sistent with Type 1 (hypoxic) respiratory failure warranting consideration for ECMO support.

Patients with Type 2 (hypercapnic) respiratory failure do not score highly under the Murray system and are considered when the pH ≤ 7.2. Patients must also have failed conventional management, this is a subjective assessment based on locally available resources and expertise as well as the history and stability of the patient. For example, a patient who has been ventilated for 2 days with aspiration pneumonia, who has a Murray score of 3.8, and a positive fluid balance of 12 liters will almost certainly improve with diuresis and may not need ECMO. It is not mandatory to insist on a trial of high frequency oscillatory ventilation (HFOV) and/ or inhaled nitric oxide (iNO) in all patients prior to ECMO. Although these modalities can sometimes be useful, it is important to remember that unlike ECMO, neither of these treatments has been shown to improve survival in adult respiratory failure. Sometimes the treatment pathway prior to ECMO referral will have resulted in a

Score Values

- PaO_2/FiO_2: ≥300 = 0, 225-299 = 1, 175-224 = 2, 100-174 = 3, <100 = 4
- CXR: normal = 0, 1 point per quadrant infiltrated.
- PEEP: ≤5 = 0, 6-8 = 1, 9-11 = 2, 12-14 = 3, ≥15 = 4.
- Compliance (ml/cmH₂O): ≥80 = 0, 60-70 = 1, 40-59 =2, 20-39 = 3, and ≤19 = 4.

The compliance may be calculated as follows:

$$\frac{TV}{PIP-PEEP}$$

Where TV is Tidal Volume, and PIP is Peak Inspiratory Pressure

Figure 21-1.

vicious spiral that is impossible to break out of without resorting to ECMO. Use of extreme levels of PEEP (i.e., >20) can precipitate one of these spirals. Fluid is necessary to combat the associated hypotension as are inotropes. More pulmonary oedema is the result, requiring more PEEP, more fluid, etc. In these circumstances, hemodynamic instability can be the trigger that mandates ECMO earlier in the disease, prior to having a Murray score exceeding 3.0.

Potentially reversible disease

Approximately half of the patients referred for ECMO will be suffering from either viral or bacterial pneumonia (including atypical pneumonias). The other half will have some kind of acute respiratory distress syndrome (ARDS). A small number will have diseases such as Wegeners Granulomatosis, alveolar lipoproteinosis, or severe asthma. As long as the disease process is potentially reversible the patient has a chance of recovery and ECMO can be considered. In general terms pneumonia associated with bone marrow failure in the context of chemotherapy or bone marrow transplantation carries a grave prognosis and should be considered irreversible in most patients. This is also the case with ARDS as the first presentation of HIV disease.

Contraindications

Contraindications can be thought of as those related to premorbid condition of the patient and those related to the treatment of the current illness.

i) Premorbid Condition: Recovery from respiratory failure severe enough to need ECMO requires considerable physiological reserve. Certain infections, (such as Panton-Valentine Leukocidin [PVL] staph is a toxic substance produced by some strains of *Staphylococcus aureus* and is associated with an increased ability to cause disease), can cause significant permanent lung injury and those with preexist-

ing lung parenchymal disease may not have sufficient reserve to survive. For most patients it is their premorbid level of function that should be the determinant of their fitness as an ECMO candidate. For example; a 50 year old man with COPD who cycled 8 miles to work each day before he was knocked down by a car and suffered bilateral lung contusions would be a reasonable candidate. Alternatively; a 50 year old man with COPD, on home oxygen, wheelchair bound, still smoking, breathless while combing his hair, will not survive pneumonia severe enough to warrant ECMO and should not be considered a candidate. Certain conditions should prompt the ECMO-ologist to take up a default position of "no" rather than the usual default position of "yes." Patients with most types of active cancer, patients with interstitial lung disease, patients with severe kyphoscoliosis, those who are wheelchair bound, and patients with Cystic Fibrosis should be recognized as patients with less chance of reaching meaningful survival.

ii) Current Illness: A prolonged course of high pressure and high FiO_2 ventilation, i.e., more than 7 days with a peak airway pressure >30 cmH_2O and/or an FiO_2 >0.8, results in significant ventilator induced lung injury (VILI) and is a contraindication to ECMO. Older patients may be at risk for VILI earlier in the time course than 7 days. This relationship is shown in Figure 21-2.[6]

During the 2009 H1N1 pandemic our group was referred a number of young adult patients who had received more prolonged ventilation, as they were young, previously fit, many having just delivered a baby, we gave them the benefit of the doubt and supported them with ECMO. Unfortunately, however, the outcome was disappointing for patients who had been ventilated for more than 7 days (Figure 21-3).

Contraindications to anticoagulation can be a contraindication for ECMO. Any active intracranial bleeding is an absolute contraindication, although the patient may become a candidate if they survive the acute phase and the bleeding stops. After 5-6 days, the intracranial clot will stabilize sufficiently so that anticoagulation, and therefore ECMO, is possible. Most other bleeding complications are only relative contraindications. It is preferable to stop the patient bleeding, deferring ECMO for a period of time when possible. Pulmonary hemorrhage can actually improve once on ECMO. Ventilation can be reduced and bleeding can be controlled. This can be seen as an indication rather than a contraindication to ECMO.

Transport

A patient has been referred and accepted for ECMO and must be successfully transported to your ECMO center. It is possible to transport the patient on ECMO but this is resource intensive and may not be practical in all health care systems. In the UK, distances are small compared to Australia and North America, and

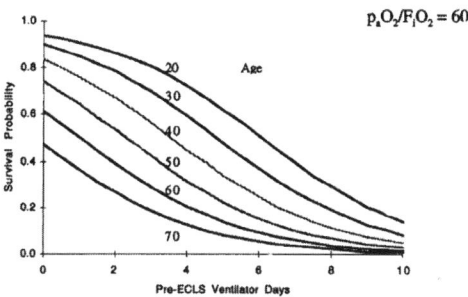

Figure 21-2.

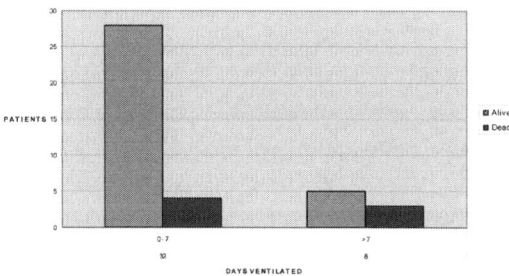

Figure 21-3

it is possible to transport most patients using conventional transport ventilators. The transport team must be experienced, slick, and authoritative in order to safely transport these precarious patients. During the CESAR Trial[8] the Leicester ECMO transport team moved 62 patients (24 by air, 38 by ground) from around the UK to Glenfield Hospital using conventional transport methods. The longest transport was 469 miles from Inverness to Leicester and required a ground ambulance, a Lockhead Hercules airplane, and a Westland Sea King Helicopter. Two patients died in transit. One died when the gas supply failed in the ambulance (not due to exhaustion of the supply) and the other from an exsanguinating pulmonary hemorrhage. It is unlikely that either of these deaths would have been prevented if mobile ECMO had been used instead of conventional transport methods. It is our practice to use mobile ECMO to retrieve patients if they will not stabilize on the transport ventilator, if they will not convert back from HFOV to conventional ventilation, if they are hemodynamically unstable, or if logistics preclude a rapid retrieval in an unstable patient. In the last year, our team transported 127 adults using mobile ECMO for 10 (7.9%) patients. During the 2009 H1N1 pandemic mobile ECMO retrieval was the norm for the Australian teams.[10]

Cannulation

Our practice is to always use VV cannulation for adults with respiratory failure irrespective of the level of inotropic support or the echo appearance of ventricular function prior to ECMO. Once VV support is established, ventilating pressures can be reduced, inotropes wean off quickly and ventricular function improves. Our group currently uses a bicaval double lumen cannula (Avalon Elite) placed via the right jugular vein under fluoroscopic guidance. In patients who require more flow than can be obtained from the double lumen cannula with a venous line pressure of -70 mmHg, an additional femoral venous cannula can be inserted to increase the venous drainage. For patients in whom the right jugular vein is unusable, venous access is established by using 2 or 3 single lumen cannula placed via the femoral and left jugular vein.[11]

Circuit design

The use of polymethyl pentene oxygenators has resulted in a marked reduction in priming volume and transfusion requirement when compared to silicone devices.[12] Following the CESAR trial we switched from a roller pump/bladder box system to a smaller circuit with a centrifugal pump and no bridge. In patients in excess of 100 kg it may be necessary to use two oxygenators in parallel.

Treatment Protocols

The most important goal is to support gas exchange with ECMO while achieving lung rest. Additional goals are supporting nutritional requirements, diuresis to dry weight, transfusion to a normal hematocrit, treatment of underlying disease processes, prevention of bleeding, early tracheostomy, and minimization of sedation.

Respiratory Management

Lung rest is achieved by reducing the ventilation pressure and decreasing inspired oxygen. This is commonly done using pressure control mode and PEEP of 10-15 cmH_2O. Peak airway pressures are PEEP+10. FiO_2 = 0.3 and respiratory rate of 10 bpm. These rest settings will commonly yield a tidal volume of 60-100 ml in most adults. In patients with severe air leak or pulmonary hemorrhage HFOV is used with a mean airway pressure of 10-13 cmH_2O in order to reduce the volutrauma even further. It usually takes 6-12 hours to wean the patient down to rest settings. If the patient has not been successfully weaned by this time, it is usually an indication that more extracorporeal flow is needed. Frequent bronchoscopy is employed for bronchial toilet, DNAse or perfluorocarbon lavage is employed if secretions are particularly tenacious and cannot be removed with bronchoscopy and saline lavage alone. Pneumothoraces are drained to achieve full lung expansion and surgery is undertaken to control bleeding, remove intrathoracic hematoma, release incarcerated lung segments, repair bronchopleural fistulae, or resect necrotic lobes that are sources of bleeding or air leaks. In patients who are not septic, a Meduri steroid protocol is employed starting at a dose of 1mg/kg methylprednisolone per day by continuous infusion, gradually weaning off over the subsequent four weeks.[13] In patients whose lung parenchyma does not recover after several weeks of support, a high dose steroid pulse is used (methylprednisolone 30mg/kg) this has proven effective in a number of cases. Muscle relaxation is discontinued, sedation is weaned off, and tracheostomy is employed to facilitate this. Tracheostomy may be either percutaneous or open depending on the patient's anatomy. The amount of sedation considered necessary is subjective and dependent on the sedation culture in your hospital. We are in the process of trying to change from a culture of heavy sedation to a strategy similar to that used at the ECMO Centrum Karolinska, Stockholm, Sweden. The Karolinska approach is one where patients are supported fully awake. Karolinska has reported a 76% survival in adult ECMO patients where the sedation goal is one that allows an awake, alert, interactive patient.[14] In the majority of our cases, prone positioning for 16/24 hours is used. Exceptions are patients who improve rapidly, patients who remain hemodynamically unstable, patients who are actively bleeding, or who have pressure sores from previous proning. Although prone positioning has yet to be proven to improve outcome on its own, there is good physiological evidence[15] for its use and a suggestion that the degree of benefit is proportional to the duration of proning. In patients whose lungs remain consolidated despite several weeks of ECMO support and prone positioning, we have found HFOV can be useful in recruiting the lungs.

ECMO Management and Weaning

On ECMO we aim for sufficient flow to maintain a target PaO_2 of 45-60 mmHg and adjust the sweep to keep a $PaCO_2$ of 30-45 mmHg, the ventilation is not adjusted once rest settings are achieved. Heparin is infused to maintain an ACT (Maxact, Actalyte) of 140-160 seconds, transfusion of blood and products is undertaken to maintain a Hb 12-14g/dl, INR <1.5, platelets > 75 x10^9/L, and an albumin concentration of >30 g/L. In patients who are bleeding the platelet target is increased to >150 x10^9/L, fibrinogen > 2 g/L, and the heparin infusion is reduced to 10 u/kg/hr. Aprotinin, although removed from many of the world's markets, remains available in some settings. A loading dose of Aprotinin of 1x10^6 units is given over one hour and an infusion is commenced at a dose of 0.5x10^6 units/hr. Surgical treatment is undertaken, when possible, to control hemorrhage. Amicar (aminocaproic acid) is another option for management of bleeding. Amicar inhibits fibrinolysis. A typical strategy for Amicar is a loading dose (100 mg/kg) given over 60 minutes followed by a maintenance dose (20-30 mg/kg/hr with adjustment for renal failure). It is important to continue a typical ACT target (160-200 secs) while using an Amicar infusion to minimize the risk of circuit thrombosis. Novoseven (90 mcg/kg) may be given if these measures are ineffective. This is not an approved indication for Novoseven use but can be effective. The incidence of thromboembolic complication is 4.5% in our hospital (4/90 patients) for adults and children given Novoseven for all reasons. Eight of these patients were on ECMO with one instance of fatal thrombosis in a child on ECMO.[16] This child had disseminated intravascular coagulation (DIC) in the setting of a prosthetic mitral valve and very poor LV function with stasis of blood in the left ventricle. It has been our practice to avoid using Novoseven in this situation since then. In rare instances it may be necessary to stop the heparin infusion altogether for 6-12 hours to get control of bleeding. Flow is kept up above 2 L/min during this period; if the circuit shows evidence of thrombosis, another circuit is primed and kept on standby. Patients who develop heparin induced thrombocytopenia (HIT) are anticoagulated using the direct thrombin inhibitor Lepirudin at a dose of 0.12 mg/kg/hr, aiming for an APTT >1.5 times normal.

Extracorporeal support is reduced as the lungs recover. Lung mechanics improve as does the appearance of the chest x-ray. Once the flow has fallen to 1 L/min the patient may be ready to trial off ECMO. The ventilation is increased, usually in pressure control mode, up to a maximum PIP of 29 cmH$_2$0, PEEP is set to maximize saturation at a level above the lower inflection point on the expiratory limb of the pressure-volume curve, the FiO$_2$ is increased to a maximum of 0.6 and the sweep is disconnected. The minimum length of a trial off is 2 hours, but in patients where there is a degree of uncertainty about their readiness for decannulation, the trial off can be extended overnight. Once stable blood gases with a PaO$_2$ over 60 mmHg and a PaCO$_2$ of 30-45 mmHg are obtained on the lung protective ventilator settings above, the patient is ready for decannulation. This is often performed with the patients anaesthetized and occasionally paralyzed. A mattress suture is placed around the cannula, which is clamped and swiftly withdrawn while the suture is tied. There is risk of air embolism with decannulation secondary to the negative intrathoracic pressure. Reverse Trendelenburg positioning when removing the dual lumen cannula can minimize this risk. It is not necessary to hold pressure on the wound as the suture is sufficient to control bleeding from the vein. There is some concern that holding pressure can promote vein occlusion with thrombus. After decannulation all the venous and arterial lines are changed, antibiotic coated lines are used whenever possible.

Cardiac Management

Inotropes are weaned according to the improvement in the patients' hemodynamics. All patients undergo a detailed echocardiogram to exclude structural congenital or acquired heart disease. Other cardiac conditions are investigated and treated on their merits. It is not our practice to convert adult respiratory patients to VA ECMO if they do not respond to VV support. In our experience, the outcome after converting from VV to VA for respiratory failure in adults has been uniformly fatal, albeit several weeks later.

Neurological Management

Minimizing sedation should be the standard. Sedation and analgesia should be offered as indicated. The patient should be awake enough to interact with care providers and family. The goal should be an "animated" patient as long as the patient is not a risk to him/herself and the care givers. There is significant evidence that ICU sedation has long-term consequences. As with all ICU patients on mechanical ventilators, daily "wakeups" and "spontaneous breathing trials" should be the norm. "Daily wakeups" help determine the necessary level of sedation per patient, minimizing the risk related to over-sedation. "Spontaneous breathing trials" remind the care providers of the importance of assessing the patient's support needs frequently. Getting rid of the "unnecessary" as soon as possible should be the focus. Having patients awake and active should take place as soon as practical. This strategy of ICU management, shifting towards the awake and active patient, is a paradigm shift when compared to the ICU of 20 years ago. This same philosophy can be safely applied to the respiratory failure patient on ECMO.

Musculoskeletal Management

Passive movement of all major joints is performed by the physiotherapists on a daily basis to try and prevent contractures forming. Splints are made to prevent footdrop. In patients with skeletal trauma requiring immobilization or traction, these are continued until they are off ECMO. Once off ECMO, definitive procedures, such as internal fixation or nailing, is undertaken as indicated.

Renal Management

Diuresis to dry weight is achieved by using diuretics or continuous renal replacement therapy (CRRT). CRRT is can be established by accessing the ECMO circuit or by using standard vascular access techniques. Once a patient is heparinized and on ECMO, the addition of central venous access has inherent risks. High flux CRRT can also be used in patients who are septic.

Liver Management

Patients who develop hepatic impairment due to progression of their multiorgan failure are supported with MARS (Molecular Albumin Recirculating System, Gambro, UK). Ultrasound imaging of the biliary tree is used to exclude a treatable obstructive cause. These studies typically show biliary stasis and sludge in the gallbladder. Once treatable causes have been excluded, MARS can be offered. MARS is indicated when the plasma bilirubin exceeds 200 umol/L. MARS is continued until the MARS circuit fails or the bilirubin stops decreasing.[17] Up to 4 treatments are given. We believe that this strategy reduces the mortality in patients with hepatic failure by around 50%.

Nutritional/GI Management

The aim is to provide full nutrition as soon as possible. Ileus is common in the volume overloaded, hypoxic, hypotensive, respiratory failure patient. Initiation of ECMO and reduction of airway pressure improves oxygen delivery and reduces venous congestion allowing the gut to recover. This may take several days so in patients with ileus. Total parenteral nutrition (TPN) is started in this circumstance, along with low volume "trophic" enteral feed. Once the ileus has resolved and full enteral feeding is tolerated, TPN is discontinued. TPN can be given by a dedicated central line/lumen or via the circuit. All patients receive ranitidine as prophylaxis for stress ulceration.

Adrenal Management

When the patient is admitted a blood sample is sent for random cortisol estimation. Patients who are not receiving steroids and are demonstrated to be adrenal insufficient, receive a replacement dose of hydrocortisone (300mg/day). Once the plasma cortisol is > 414 units nmol/L[18] the hydrocortisone is stopped.

Management of Sepsis

Prophylactic antibiotics are used to cover surgical procedures, including cannulation. Surveillance cultures of blood, sputum, urine, and surgical wounds are sent three times per week. White cell count, C-reactive protein, and sweep gas increases can suggest possible infection with sepsis. Patient temperature is typically controlled via the ECMO system, often taking away temperature as a clinical sign of infection. Antibiotics are used according to culture results and clinical suspicion. All patients receiving antibiotics receive prophylactic antifungal coverage with fluconazole. Efforts are made to exclude and eradicate septic foci if possible. Patients are kept euglycemic between 4.4 and 8.3 mMol/L in accordance to the "surviving sepsis campaign" guidelines (www.sccm/org/). It is not our practice to use activated protein C while patients are on ECMO because of the risk of hemorrhage. Activated protein c was used for septic ECMO patients without using heparin.[19]

The ECMO Specialist and Nursing Care

In the Heartlink ECMO Center in Leister, all ECMO specialists are trained to manage ECMO patients under the direction, guidance, and supervision of the ECMO physician and ECMO coordinator. Our ECMO specialists are most typically registered nurses who have a background in adult, pediatric, or neonatal intensive care. However, respiratory therapists, perfusionists, and operating room practitioners can also perform the role of an ECMO specialist. The primary function of the ECMO specialist is to provide care to the patient requiring ECMO support. The specialist is responsible for managing the ECMO circuit and associated technology and must be capable of recognizing and addressing problems. The specialist works in conjunction with the bedside nurse. These bedside care providers should work together as a team, delivering care to the uniquely complex ICU patient supported with ECMO.

The ECMO specialist is trained to troubleshoot, problem solve, and initiate emergency care for the patient on ECMO. The ECMO coordinator acts as a clinical resource to all team members. The ECMO coordinator is responsible for the education and training of all specialists. Communication is paramount to the success of the nurse/specialist partnership. The nursing and medical care requires input from all members of the multidisciplinary team. Collaboration between all members of the ECMO team is essential for the smooth running and operation of the service. Some centers in Europe and Australia have used a single caregiver approach. In this model, the intensive care nurse also manages the circuit. In order for this to be done safely the ECMO circuit needs to be very simple, usually comprising a centrifugal pump, oxygenator, and no access to the circuit. All drugs are given to the patient and the nurse is not required to manipulate the circuit except in an emergency.

Results

The following data are drawn from the ELSO annual report released in January 2010 and therefore contains few patients with H1N1. Adult respiratory support is becoming an increasingly used form of ECLS, reminiscent of neonatal ECLS in the early 1990s. Approximately half the patients have some type of pneumonia, with the other half suffering from ARDS and a smattering of miscellaneous diagnoses such as Wegener's granulomatosis and asthma. The overall survival to hospital discharge is around 50%. We can see the increased use of the new VVDL ECMO cannula 2010 ECLS Registry Report, which is included.

Conclusion

The key to successful adult ECMO is a seamless integration of good case selection, slick retrieval, trouble free cannulation, lung protective ventilation, and attention to the detail of nutrition, sedation, transfusion, diuresis, positioning, and organ support. ECMO is a "team sport" and collaboration between a team of experienced and skilled health care professionals will ensure the best outcome possible for adults with severe potentially reversible respiratory failure.

ECLS Registry Report
International Summary
January, 2012

Extracorporeal Life Support Organization
2800 Plymouth Road
Building 300, Room 303
Ann Arbor, MI 48109

Overall Outcomes

	Total Patients	*Survived ECLS*		*Survived to DC or Transfer*	
Neonatal					
Respiratory	25,267	21,337	84%	18,846	75%
Cardiac	4,579	2,770	60%	1,807	39%
ECPR	749	473	63%	288	38%
Pediatric					
Respiratory	5,220	3,382	65%	2,901	56%
Cardiac	5,708	3,649	64%	2,751	48%
ECPR	1,477	786	53%	587	40%
Adult					
Respiratory	2,893	1,823	63%	1,572	54%
Cardiac	1,896	1,003	53%	733	39%
ECPR	648	243	38%	183	28%
Total	48,437	35,466	73%	29,668	61%

Centers

Centers by Year

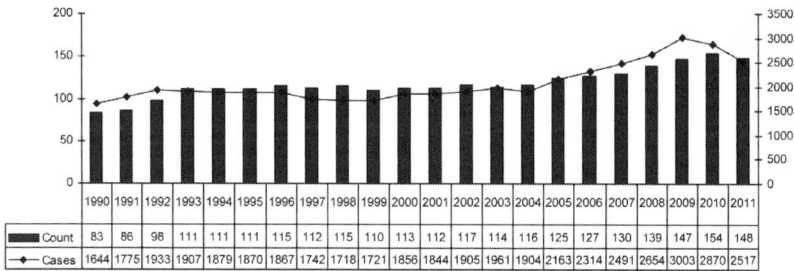

	1990	1991	1992	1993	1994	1995	1996	1997	1998	1999	2000	2001	2002	2003	2004	2005	2006	2007	2008	2009	2010	2011
Count	83	86	98	111	111	111	115	112	115	110	113	112	117	114	116	125	127	130	139	147	154	148
Cases	1644	1775	1933	1907	1879	1870	1867	1742	1718	1721	1856	1844	1905	1961	1904	2163	2314	2491	2654	3003	2870	2517

International Summary - January, 2012

Adult Respiratory Runs by Diagnosis

	Total Runs	*Avg Run Time*	*Longest Run Time*	*Survived*	*% Survived*
Viral pneumonia	115	277	1357	76	66%
Bacterial pneumonia	503	232	1585	302	60%
Aspiration pneumonia	75	202	1663	47	63%
ARDS, postop/trauma	232	240	1656	121	52%
ARDS, not postop/trauma	415	299	5014	203	49%
Acute resp failure, non-ARDS	192	238	1317	105	55%
Other	1,409	202	3018	741	53%

Run time in hours. Survived = survival to discharge or transfer based on number of runs

Adult Respiratory Support Mode

Cumulative

Past Year

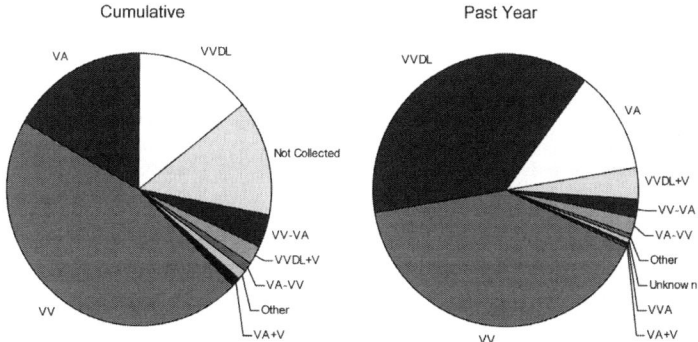

319

References

1. Prolonged Extracoproeal oxygenation for post-traumatic respiratory failure (Shock-Lung Syndrome). Hill JD, O'Brien TG, Murray JJ, Dontigny LL, Bramson ML, Osborn JJ & Gerbode F. 629-634: New England J Med, 1972, Vol. 286.
2. Extracorporeal membrane oxygenation in severe acute respiratoryfailure. A randomized prospective study. Zapol WM, Snider MT, Hill JD, et al: JAMA, 1979, Vols. 242:2193–6.
3. Low-frequency positive-pressure ventilation with extracorporeal CO_2 removal in severe acute respiratory failure. Gattinoni L, Pesenti A, Mascheroni D et al. 881-6: JAMA, 1986, Vol. 256.
4. Extracorporeal Life Support for Adult Cardio-respiratory failure. Anderson H III, Steimle C, Shapiro M, Delius R, Chapman R, Hirschl R & Bartlett RH. 164-73: Surgery, 1993, Vol. 114.
5. Randomized clinical trial of pressure-controlled inverse ratio ventilation and extracorporeal CO_2 removal for adult respiratory distress syndrome. Morris AH, Wallace CJ, Menlove RL, Clemmer TP, Orme JF, WeaverLK, Dean NC, Thomas F, East TD, Pace NL: Am J Resp Crit Care Med, 1994, Vols. 149:295-305.
6. Extracorporeal life support for100 adult patients with severe respiratory failure. Kolla S, Awad SS, Rich PB, Schreiner RJ, Hirschl RB, Bartlett RH: Ann Surg, 1997, Vols. 226:544–64; discussion 565–6.
7. Extracorporeal membrane oxygenation for adult respiratory failure. Peek GJ, Moore HM, Moore N, Sosnowski AW, Firmin RK: Chest, 1997, Vols. 112:759–64.
8. Efficacy and economic assessment of conventional ventilatory support versus extracorporeal membrane oxygenation for severe adult respiratory failure (CESAR): a multicentre randomised controlled trial.

Peek GJ, Mugford M, Tiruvoipati R et al. 1351 - 1363: Lancet, 2009, Vol. 374.
9. An expanded definition of the adult respiratory distress syndrome. Murray JF, Matthay MA, Luce JM, Flick MR: Am Rev Resp Dis, 1988, Vols. 138:720-723.
10. Extracorporeal membrane oxygenation for 2009 influenza A(H1N1) acute respiratory distress syndrome. Investigators., ANZICS H1N1 ECMO Study (Australia and New Zealand Extracorporeal Membrane Oxygenation Influenza): JAMA, 2009, Vols. 302:1888-95.
11. Modifying a venovenous extracorporeal membrane oxygenation circuit to reduce recirculation. Ichiba S, Peek GJ, Sosnowski AW et al. 69:298-299: Annals of Thoracic Surgery, 2000.
12. Early Experience with a Polymethyl Pentene Oxygenator for Adult Extracorporeal Life Support. Peek, Giles J., et al. 480-482: ASAIO Journal, 2002, Vol. 48:5.
13. Methylprednisolone infusion in early severe ARDS: Results of a randomized controlled trial. Meduri UG, Goklen E, Freire AX, et al: Chest 2007; 131:954-963
14. High survival in adult patients with acute respiratory distress syndrome treated by extracorporeal membrane oxygenation, minimal sedation, and pressure supported ventilation . Linden V, Palmer K,Reinhard J, Westman R, Ehren H, Granholm T & Freckner B. 1630-1637: Intensive Care Medicine, 2000, Vol. 26:11.
15. Efficacy of prone ventilation in adult patients with acute respiratory failure: A meta analysis. Tiruvoipati R, Bangash M, Manktelow B, Peek GJ. 101–110: Journal of Critical Care, 2008, Vol. 23.
16. Fatal thrombosis with activated factor VII in a paediatric patient on extracorporeal membrane oxygenation . Chalwin RP, Tiruvoipati R & Peek GJ. sl: European Journal of Cardio-Thoracic Surgery, 2008, Volume

34, Issue 3, September 2008, Pages 685-686 .

17. Modular Extra-corporeal Life Support for Multi-Organ Failure Patients. Peek GJ, Killer HM, Sosnowski MA, Firmin RK: Liver, 2002, Vols. 22(Suppl. 2):69–71.

18. Corticosteroids for severe sepsis and septic shock: a systematic review and meta-analysis. Annane D, Bellissant E, Bollaert PE, Briegel J, Keh D, Kupfer Y: BMJ, Vol. 329:480.

19. Combined use of extracorporeal membrane oxygenation and activated protein C for severe acute respiratory distress syndrome and septic shock. Lamarche Y, Cheung A, Walley K, Dodek P: J Thorac Cardiovasc Surg 2009, Vol 138:246-247.

22

Adult Cardiac Support

Jonathan Haft MD, Richard Firmin MD

Introduction

Cardiogenic shock occurs in a multitude of clinical scenarios. By far, the most common cause is acute myocardial infarction (MI), in which 5-10 percent of patients will develop cardiogenic shock. Chronic heart failure is a growing worldwide epidemic. Whether from ischemic or nonischemic etiology, the natural progression of the disease is one of gradual decline in systolic function. A precipitating event, frequently infectious, incites acute decline in a patient with previously well compensated heart failure, resulting in profound shock. Other less common but no less dramatic causes of heart failure include fulminant viral myocarditis, postcardiotomy shock, peripartum cardiomyopathy, and myocardial depression associated with sepsis. While these conditions may differ in etiology, presentation, and natural course, they all have one similar basic feature: impairment of satisfactory myocardial systolic function resulting in inadequate end organ oxygen delivery.

Conventional treatments include optimal fluid resuscitation, inotropes, vasoconstrictors, and revascularization when appropriate. However, when shock persists despite these measures, mortality rate is extremely high.[1] Intraaortic balloon counter-pulsation can be an extremely effective tool in restoring hemodynamic stability. By increasing diastolic pressure, coronary perfusion is enhanced, potentially improving both systolic and diastolic function. By reducing afterload, the intraaortic balloon pump can improve cardiac output even in the nonischemic setting by as much as 15%. However, a balloon pump cannot be used in extreme tachycardia or during malignant ventricular dysrhythmias. In this setting, mechanical circulatory support should be considered.

Mechanical blood pumps used to support the failing circulation have undergone dramatic evolution over the last several decades. Implantable ventricular assist devices (VADs) are now routinely used as a bridge to heart transplantation (BTT) in eligible but decompensating patients,[2] and as destination therapy (DT) in those that are ineligible for transplant.[3] Contemporary devices such as the HeartMate II and HeartWare (Figure 22-1) are highly sophisticated, engineered to be durable for years, and biocompatible to reduce thrombotic complications. These devices are extremely expensive (~$100,000 U.S.) and require complex systems of care. As such, they are typically only inserted in highly specialized centers, and rarely in patients in profound shock. However, temporary mechanical circulatory support using external blood pumps can be instituted simply in many hospitals using less expensive and complex technology. The pumps are connected to the circulation either directly into the cardiac chambers or via peripheral vessels, and can be applied either as short term VADs or as a component in Extracorporeal Membrane Oxygenation (ECMO). How temporary support is initiated and applied depends upon the clinical circumstances, the experience of the physicians and center, and the technology available. These approaches will be discussed, along with frequently seen complications.

Options for Temporary Mechanical Circulatory Support

Surgical Temporary Extracorporeal VADs

A variety of extracorporeal blood pumps can be connected directly to the heart after median sternotomy. Support can be applied for isolated left ventricular failure as a left VAD (LVAD) or for right ventricular failure (RVAD), or both (BiVADs). For drainage in right-sided support, cannulation can be via the right atrium, superior or inferior vena cava (SVC or IVC), or the right ventricle (Table 22-1). Infusion is either by cannulation of the pulmonary artery (PA), or via a graft sewn onto the PA. For LVAD support, drainage can be from the right superior pulmonary vein, the dome of the left atrium between the SVC and aorta, the left atrial appendage, or the left ventricular apex. Infusion is directed

into the ascending aorta either by cannulation or via a graft sewn onto the ascending aorta. In unusual circumstances, LVAD support can be initiated via left thoracotomy by draining the left atrial appendage or the left ventricular apex and infusing into the descending thoracic aorta.

As noted previously, a variety of extracorporeal blood pumps can be used as a temporary VAD.[4,5] In the US, two are specifically approved by the Food and Drug Administration (FDA) and marketed for these purposes. The Abiomed AB5000 (Abiomed Inc., Danvers, MA) (Figure 22-2A) is a pneumatic pulsatile pump with polyurethane inflow and outflow valves to ensure unidirectional flow. These pumps require full anticoagulation to prevent thrombus formation, particularly in the sinus regions of the valves. The console can be programmed either to operate in a fixed mode with a specified output, or in an automatic mode, in which flow rate adjusts to the rate of venous return by actuating ejection at the completion of VAD filling. The Levitronix CentriMag (Thoratec, Inc., Pleasanton, CA) (Figure 22-2B) is a magnetically levitated and actuated centrifugal design pump without bearings or seals. There is less heat generation and minimal stagnant

Table 22-1. Potential cannulation sites for temporary ventricular assist devices.

Source	Location
Right sided drainage	Right internal jugular
	Femoral vein
	Right atrial appendage
Right sided infusion	Pulmonary artery
	Right ventricular outflow tract
Left sided drainage	Right superior pulmonary vein
	Interatrial groove
	Left atrial dome
	Left atrial appendage
	Left ventricular apex
Left sided infusion	Ascending aorta
	Descending thoracic aorta
	Femoral artery
	Axillary artery

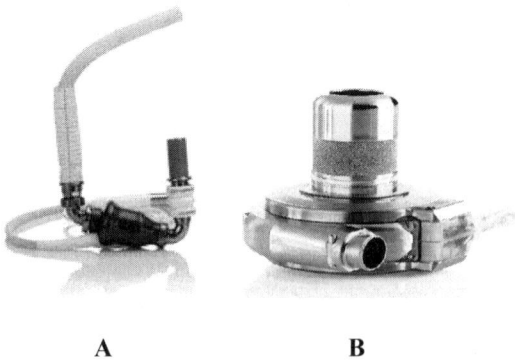

A **B**

Figure 22-1. A: HeartMate II (Image courtesy of Thoratec Inc.). B: HeartWare (Image courtesy of HeartWare Inc.).

zones, making this pump more advantageous than other centrifugal design pumps and substantially more biocompatible than the pulsatile pumps. The CentriMag operates at a fixed rotational speed and unlike the pulsatile Abiomed, requires manual interface to increase flow when venous return allows.

Surgically placed temporary VADs with direct cannulation of the cardiac chambers provide two distinct advantages. Large bore cannulae can be utilized, maximizing flow potential and minimizing sheer forces with cellular injury. Furthermore, satisfactory cardiac decompression reduces the likelihood of left ventricular distension and pulmonary edema, as will be described later in the chapter. In addition, cardiac decompression seems to facilitate recovery and restoration of native function. The drawback is the need for sternotomy and the

potential for substantial postoperative bleeding complications. Temporary extracorporeal VADs seem to be ideal for postcardiotomy shock, when sternotomy has already been performed.[6]

Percutaneous VADs

TandemHeart (Cardiac Assist Inc., Pittsburgh, PA)

The TandemHeart System consists of an extracorporeal centrifugal design blood pump, a controller, and a unique venous drainage cannula. This cannula is designed to be placed in the left atrium percutaneously from the femoral vein by crossing the interatrial septum (Figure 22-3). The blood is then returned to the systemic circulation into the femoral artery. In this configuration, the system is capable of delivering up to 5 L/min. The centrifugal pump uses a hydrodynamic bearing generated by a continuous infusion of saline injected directly into the motor compartment. This fluid cools

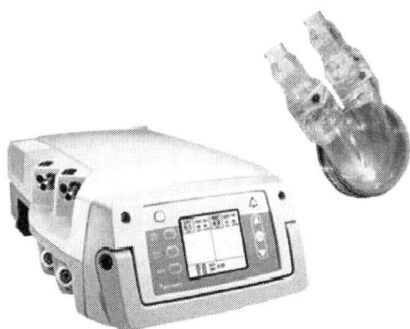

Figure 22-2A. Abiomed AB5000 Ventricular Assist Device (Image courtesy of Abiomed Inc.).

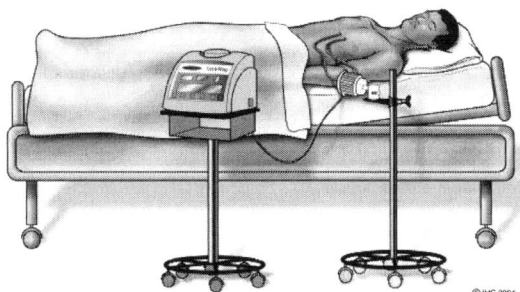

Figure 22-2B. CentriMag (Image courtesy of Levitronix Inc.).

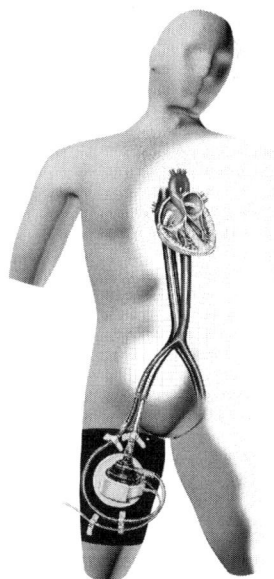

Figure 22-3. TandemHeart percutaneous ventricular assist system (Image courtesy of Cardiac Assist Inc.).

and lubricates the bearing, reducing risks of hemolysis and thrombus formation. Although the pump can be used in a temporary surgical VAD configuration, its current FDA approval is limited to six hours of support in the US. Despite this, it is frequently used off label in a broader application.[7] Advantages of the TandemHeart include its direct left sided decompression and the percutaneous nature of support. Disadvantages include limitations to left sided support and the need for fluoroscopically guided placement by a physician skilled in transeptal puncture techniques.

Impella (Abiomed Inc., Danvers, MA)

The Impella devices are microaxial flow blood pumps designed to be positioned across the aortic valve (Figure 22-4), actively pumping blood from the left ventricle into the ascending aorta. A variety of devices are available, depending on the individual needs. The Impella 2.5 is the smallest version at only nine French in maximum diameter, and can be placed percutaneously via the femoral artery. As its

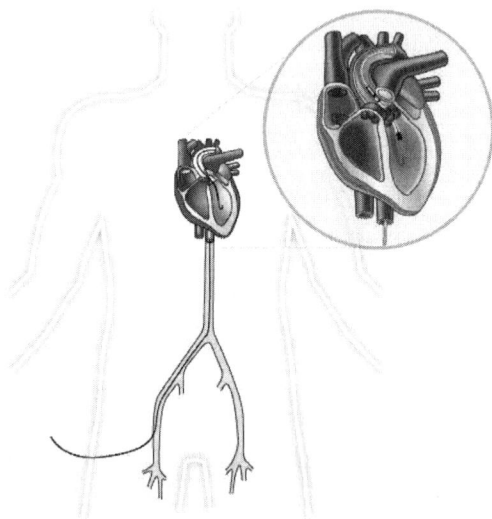

Figure 22-4. Impella microaxial left ventricular assist device (Image courtesy of Abiomed, Inc.).

name implies, it delivers up to 2.5 L/min of blood flow. The Impella 5.0 delivers up to 5 L/min of flow and has a maximum diameter of 21 French, requiring direct surgical exposure of the femoral or axillary artery for insertion. A third version, the Impella LD, is designed to be implanted directly into the ascending aorta, and is also capable of pumping 5L/min. Like the TandemHeart, the Impella pumps are approved in the US by the FDA for only six hours of support but are often used for longer duration of support.[8,9] The pumps are all easy to insert and the small catheter size minimizes lower extremity ischemic complications. They also only currently provide left sided support, limiting their utility to patients without severe biventricular failure.

VA ECMO

VA ECMO is partial cardiopulmonary bypass, draining the venous circulation and infusing into the systemic circulation. It can be applied for cardiac failure centrally by directly cannulating the cardiac chambers, or peripherally using the femoral artery and vein. ECMO provides biventricular support and will exchange respiratory gases that can be beneficial if there is significant pulmonary edema. ECMO is the preferred treatment for refractory cardiogenic shock when there is severe biventricular failure, cardiopulmonary arrest, recurrent malignant ventricular dysrhythmias, or cardiac failure coexistant with severe respiratory dysfunction. Equipment utilized for VA ECMO, techniques of cannulation, and basic management strategies of ECMO have been discussed elsewhere in this book. However, several important complications can occur in patients on VA ECMO for adults in cardiac failure which require prompt identification and correction. These include left ventricular distension, aortic root thrombus, and cerebral hypoxia.

Left ventricular distension. Unlike any of the other modalities available to mechanically support patients in cardiogenic shock, ECMO does not directly decompress the left ventricle. Because no venous reservoir is used in an ECMO circuit, some venous blood continues to enter the right ventricle and thus is delivered through the pulmonary circulation into the left ventricle. In addition, bronchial circulation and thebesian veins will also deliver blood into the left ventricle. This blood must be ejected through the aortic valve and into the arterial circulation. Without satisfactory ejection, blood will accumulate under pressure, until it eventually equalizes with systemic arterial pressure. The left ventricle will not eject if it is fibrillating or if its systolic function is too poor to overcome afterload.

Without urgent recognition and correction, severe pulmonary edema will ensue, followed by fatal pulmonary hemorrhage. The best treatment for this problem is prevention. The left ventricle must be encouraged to eject, by maintaining inotropes and minimizing afterload (blood pressure). An intraaortic balloon pump can be instrumental by reducing afterload. The arterial waveform should be monitored closely for pulsatility, confirming ejection. Liberal use of echocardiography can be helpful in demonstrating routine opening of the aortic valve and allowing measurement of left ventricular dimensions. A pulmonary artery catheter can also be helpful by noting a progressive rise in left sided filling pressures. If the left ventricle is distended despite inotropes, afterload reduction, and balloon counterpulsation, it must be vented. Temporary decompression can be afforded by external cardiac massage intermittently until a more durable solution. An atrial septostomy can be performed percutaneously with balloon dilation after transeptal atrial puncture (Figure 22-5). This will allow left atrial blood to drain across the septal defect into the ECMO drainage catheter and pumped back into the systemic circulation.

Aortic root thrombus. When ECMO is provided via the femoral vessels, blood travels in a laminar fashion retrograde up the descending thoracic aorta until it meets blood ejected from the left ventricle. When there is minimal left ventricular ejection, blood flow from the ECMO circuit terminates abruptly at the closed aortic valve. Some degree of stagnation will occur, and despite the moderate degree of anticoagulation employed in ECMO support, thrombus will begin to form (Figure 22-6). This clot hazards stroke or other embolic complications, particularly during cardiac recovery. This complication can be avoided if the left ventricle routinely ejects, creating turbulence and washing of the aortic root. If thrombus is detected echocardiographically, anticoagulation should be aggressively increased as tolerated.

Cerebral hypoxia. A frequently overlooked complication of VA ECMO support is cerebral hypoxia. Fully saturated blood from the ECMO circuit will meet blood ejected from the native ventricle. The location of this mixing point depends upon the amount of ECMO support provided and the degree of left ventricular ejection. If there is severe myocardial dysfunction, the mixing point will typically be in the proximal ascending aorta or aortic root. As myocardial function improves, the mixing

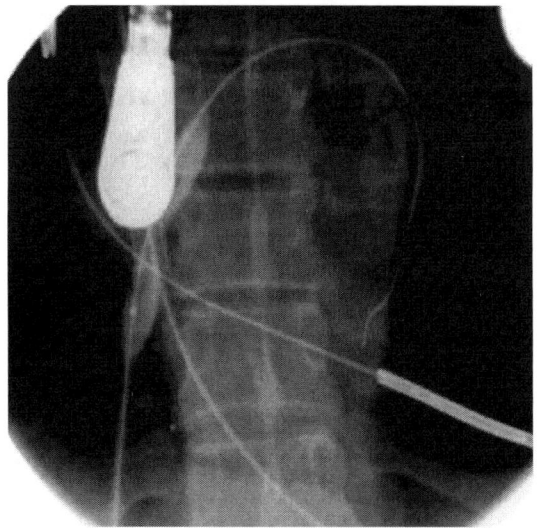

Figure 22-5. Interatrial balloon septostomy.

point may migrate more distally into the aortic arch. Blood ejected by the left ventricle relies upon adequately functioning lungs for oxygenation. If significant pulmonary edema is present, hypoxic blood may perfuse the proximal aortic branches, including the coronaries and the innominate artery (Figure 22-7). The patient's head will appear blue, while the lower extremities will be pink. Arterial blood gases sampled from a femoral arterial line will reveal fully saturated blood, while blood sampled from the right radial artery will be hypoxic. Because of the misconception that the lungs are unimportant while the patient is "on bypass," ventilator settings are frequently reduced or patients may be extubated. This complication must be diagnosed by always measuring saturations in the right hand or sampling arterial blood gases from the right radial artery. Treatment typically includes only modest ventilator adjustments including increased supplemental oxygen, positive end expiratory pressure, or pulmonary recruitment.

Weaning

Myocardial recovery should be suspected when there is increased pulsatility in the arterial circulation and improvement in the echocardiographic appearance of systolic function. Flow can be gradually decreased to 1 L/min, and hemodynamics assessed. If blood pressure and cardiac output can be maintained on reasonable doses of inotropic infusions, decannulation should be considered. If revascularization was performed, we routinely perform coronary angiography to confirm satisfactory coronary flow. Femoral cannulae are removed either by direct surgical exposure and repair, or by direct removal with manual compression. If hemodynamics are more tenuous, cannulae can be left in and continuously infused with a low dose heparin solution for up to 24 hours.

If there is no evidence of adequate myocardial recovery, long term cardiac replacement will be required either in the form of transplantation or implantable and durable circulatory support. However, patients with severe irrevers-

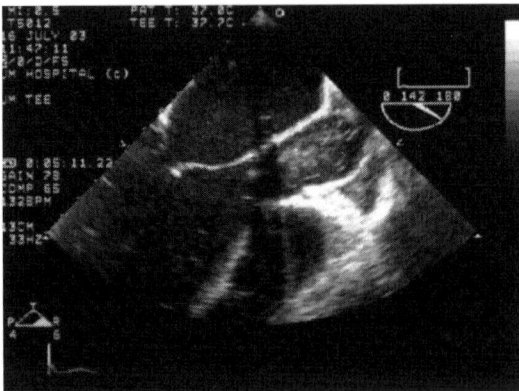

Figure 22-6. Thrombus within the aortic root and left ventricular outflow tract.

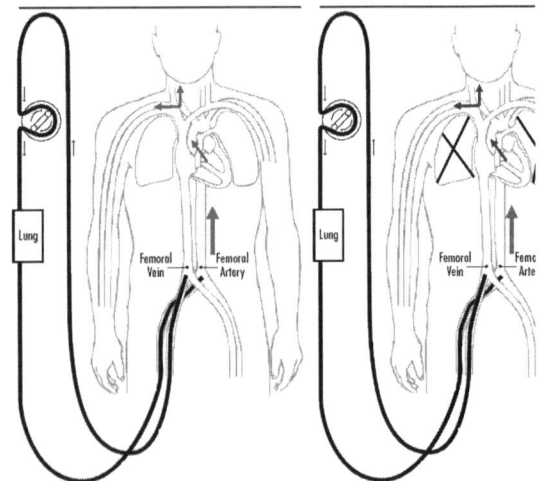

Figure 22-7. Cerebral hypoxia on VA ECMO via the femoral artery in the setting of pulmonary dysfunction.

ible organ dysfunction (i.e., cirrhosis, advanced emphysema, disabling stroke), poor medical compliance, or compromising social situations may not be ideal candidates for implantable VAD or heart transplantation. This can make an extremely frustrating scenario in which a patient with end stage heart failure is well supported and neurologically intact on temporary mechanical support with no viable exit strategy. This can often be avoided by critically considering the endpoint prior to initiation temporary mechanical support for patients in shock. If there is unrealistically low likelihood of myocardial recovery, temporary support including ECMO should only be offered if there are no obvious conditions that would preclude heart transplantation or VAD implantation.

Results

Unlike neonatal or adult respiratory failure, there are no large prospective randomized trials demonstrating efficacy of ECMO for adults in cardiac failure. Evidence comes from single institution retrospective reports and from the ELSO Registry. Pagani and coworkers reported an experience of 25 patients with cardiogenic shock supported with ECMO.[10] Four patients had cardiac recovery and were successfully decannulated, and eight patients were transitioned to implantable VAD. Overall survival to hospital discharge was 36%. Smedira from Cleveland Clinic reported on 202 patients supported on ECMO for cardiac failure, half of whom required support for post cardiotomy shock.[11] Thirty day survival was 38% and advanced age was an independent predictor of death. Jaski et al. described 150 patients treated placed on ECMO, many of which were actively receiving cardiopulmonary resuscitation.[12] Patients that arrested in the cardiac cath lab had better outcomes, presumably because of more rapid initiation of support. Overall survival was 26%. The 2010 ELSO Registry report included 1,131 patients categorized as "Adult Cardiac"

and an additional 408 adults placed on ECMO during cardiopulmonary resuscitation (ECPR). Survival for adult cardiac was 34% and 27% for ECPR, both consistent with single institution retrospective reviews.

Summary

Temporary mechanical support can restore blood flow to vital organs in the setting of cardiogenic shock. A variety of approaches and technology can be used, each with advantages and limitations. ECMO provides biventricular support and exchanges respiratory gases if necessary. Left ventricular distension, aortic root thrombus, and cerebral hypoxia must be avoided. Surviving patients will either be bridged to myocardial recovery, heart transplantation, or implantable VAD. Survival rates of 20-40% are typically expected.

References

1. Reynolds HR, Hochman JS. Cardiogenic shock: current concepts and improving outcomes. Circulation 2008;117:686-97.

2. Frazier OH, et al. Multicenter clinical evaluation of the HeartMate Vented Electric ventricular assist system in patients awaiting heart transplantation. J Thorac Cardiovasc Surg 2001; 122:1186-95.

3. Slaughter MS, et al. Advanced heart failure treated with continuous-flow left ventricular assist device. New Engl J Med 2009; 361:2241-51.

4. Samuels LE, Kaufman MS, Thomas MP, Holmes EC, Brockman SK, Wechsler AS. Pharmacological criteria for ventricular assist device insertion following postcardiotomy shock: experience with the Abiomed BVS system. J Card Surg 1999;14:288-93.

5. John R, et al. Outcomes of a multicenter trial of the Levitronix CentriMag ventricular assist system for short-term circulatory support. J Thorac Cardiovasc Surg 2001; 141:932-9.

6. Haft JW, Pagani FD, Romano MA, Leventhal CL, Dyke DB, Matthews JC. Short- and long-term survival of patients transferred to a tertiary care center on temporary extracorporeal circulatory support. Ann Thorac Surg 2009;88:711-7.

7. Idelchik GM, Simpson L, Civitello AB, et al. Use of the percutaneous left ventricular assist device in patients with severe refractory cardiogenic shock as a bridge to long-term left ventricular assist device implantation. J Heart Lung Transplant 2008;27:106-11.

8. Engstrom A, Sjauw K, Baan J, et al. Long-term safety and sustained left ventricular recovery: long-term results of percutaneous left ventricular support with Impella LP2.5 in ST-elevation myocardial infarction. Eurointervention 2011; 6:860-5.

9. Granfeldt H, Hellgren L, Dellgren G, et al. Experience with the Impella recovery axial-flow system for acute heart failure at three cardiothoracic centers in Sweden. Scand Cardiovasc J 2009; 43:233-9.

10. Pagani FD, Aaronson KD, Swaniker F, Bartlett RH. The use of extracorporeal life support in adult patients with primary cardiac failure as a bridge to implantable left ventricular assist device. Ann Thorac Surg 2001;71:S77-81.

11. Smedira NG, Moazami N, Golding CM, et al. Clinical experience with 202 adults receiving extracorporeal membrane oxygenation for cardiac failure: survival at five years. J Thorac Cardiovasc Surg 2001;122:92-102.

12. Jaski BE, Ortiz B, Alla KR, et al. A 20-year experience with urgent percutaneous cardiopulmonary bypass for salvage of potential survivors of refractory cardiovascular collapse. J Thorac Cardiovasc Surg 2010; 139:753-7.

23

Extracorporeal Cardiopulmonary Resuscitation: ECPR

Kate L Brown MPH MRCPCH, Heidi J Dalton MD FCCM

Definition

ECPR (extracorporeal cardiopulmonary resuscitation) is the use of ECLS for patients in cardiac arrest when conventional resuscitative measures have failed. ECPR is defined as extracorporeal support initiated during conventional resuscitation, or when repetitive arrest events occur without return of spontaneous circulation (ROSC) for >20 minutes. In the past, patients may have been entered into the ELSO Registry as receiving ECPR, despite return of circulation with an ongoing low cardiac output state, but this technically should not be defined as ECPR. Patients in such a condition should be listed as having a pre-ECLS cardiac arrest, but not entered into the ECPR category. In a similar fashion, if the call for ECLS goes out due to an arrest event, but the patient recovers spontaneous circulation and then deteriorates and requires ECLS several hours later, this is not ECPR. Adherence to these definitions and refinement of more specific data elements in the ECPR portion of the registry is needed to allow more accurate understanding of patients receiving ECLS for ECPR.

The ECPR category in the ELSO Registry exists as a subset under the neonatal, pediatric, and adult sections.[1] As of January 2010, neonatal ECPR numbered 537 registrations, of which 38% survived. Pediatric ECPR was noted in 1003 entries with 39% survival, while adult ECPR had 408 entries with 27% survival. Again, patients who suffer cardiac arrest and have ROSC prior to ECMO are entered into the ELSO Registry according to their other diagnostic and age-related features (not as ECPR cases), but are noted to have had a pre-ECLS cardiac arrest.

Recently published guidelines for resuscitation during cardiac arrest make the following comment on the use of ECPR:

"Extracorporeal Life Support (ECLS) Extracorporeal life support (ECLS) is a modified form of cardiopulmonary bypass used to provide prolonged delivery of oxygen to tissues. Consider early activation of ECLS for a cardiac arrest that occurs in a highly supervised environment, such as an ICU, with the clinical protocols in place and the expertise and equipment available to initiate it rapidly. ECLS should be considered only for children in cardiac arrest refractory to standard resuscitation attempts, with a potentially reversible cause of arrest (Class IIa, LOE C). When ECLS is employed during cardiac arrest, outcome for children with underlying cardiac disease is better than the outcome for children with noncardiac disease. With underlying cardiac disease, long-term survival when ECLS is initiated in a critical care setting has been reported even after >50 minutes of standard CPR."[2]

Patient Selection

In a recent evaluation from the National Registry of Cardio Pulmonary Resuscitation (NRCPR), ECLS was employed in 3.2% of 6288 reported pediatric cardiac arrests.[3] Survival to hospital discharge was 44%. Of the 87 survivors, neurologic assessment by the Pediatric Cerebral Performance Category (PCPC) was available in 59 patients and was recorded as normal in 95%. Multivariate analysis noted that pre-arrest renal insufficiency, presence of metabolic or electrolyte abnormalities at the time of arrest, and the use of sodium bicarbonate during resuscitation were associated with impaired outcome. After adjustment for confounding factors, patients with cardiac disease prior to arrest had improved survival. An ELSO Registry study of ECPR in patients under 18 years published in 2007 noted that of 26 242 ECMO uses reported, 695 (2.6%) were for ECPR and survival to discharge was 38%.[4] This study found that worse acidosis, renal dysfunction, pulmonary hemorrhage, and neurological injury were adverse risk factors, whereas cardiac disease was a protective factor in comparison to other conditions.

Pediatric Cardiac Patients

The majority of published studies documenting the use of ECPR are skewed towards children with congenital or acquired cardiac disease, who suffered cardiac arrest in a highly supervised environment such as the intensive care unit,[5-19] operating suite,[20,21] or catheterization laboratory.[22,23] The majority of the patients included in these reports are postoperative congenital cardiac cases that suffered cardiac arrest as a complication of cardiac surgery. These studies indicate that in these specific circumstances, ECPR does improve early outcome with the assumption that the patients included were in sustained cardiac arrest refractory to conventional resuscitation methods and would have died without ECPR. The proportion of

survivors with favorable outcome at the time of hospital discharge varied from 30% to 75%.

The selection of patients for ECPR does vary somewhat from center to center, based on institutional philosophy. For example, a report from Asia highlighted the inclusion of certain cardiac arrest cases such as those with oncologic disease that may have been deemed futile in other locations.[15,24] Based on a large case series of cardiac ECPR (N= 492, 42% survival) reported to the ELSO Registry between 1992 and 2005, there is some evidence to suggest that patients with more complex cardiac disease and more severe metabolic acidosis prior to ECPR are less likely to benefit.[25] In this study, there were 196 patients with single ventricles (35% survival), 186 biventricular patients (48% survival), and 110 heart muscle disease patients (45% survival) included. Patients with single ventricles had worse outcome (p=0.03) after adjustment for other factors. Patients with worse pre-ECMO acidemia (p=0.01) and more complex surgery based on the RACHS score (p=0.02) also had worse outcome from ECPR. Carotid artery cannulation was associated with a lower risk of death (p=0.03) in children with cardiac disease undergoing ECPR, which was a surprise to the authors since these patients are more likely to have had closed chest CPR. The reasons for this are uncertain but may include greater stability prior to arrest, performance of better CPR as no interruption for chest-opening during CPR was required, surgical expertise, or other issues related to institutional experience and practices.

Non-ICU Patients (Children)

There are a small number of pediatric reports of ECPR based outside of the specialized conditions of the ICU, catheterization lab, or operating room. One report of two patients from the emergency room was equivocal[26] since one patient died and the other patient sustained multiple episodes of short cardiac arrests. In a further emergency department report including both adults and children,[27] all of the three children included died. A case report of ECPR in the general medical operating room[28] reported major neurological damage leading to death. Therefore, at present, published evidence does not support the use of ECPR in children outside the specialized environment of the ICU or similar areas, other than cases of hypothermic-induced cardiac arrest which are discussed below. One potential explanation for this lower survival is that outside of the ICU, catheterization lab, and operating room, patients may have a period of less-optimal CPR and monitoring prior to initiation of ECLS, which may adversely affect the outcome of ECPR.

Patients with Non-Cardiac Conditions (Children)

Studies that included children with medical conditions other than heart disease tended to indicate an unfavorable or equivocal outcome. A large single center series of ECPR by Morris in 2004[6] indicated early survival in 2 out of 21 children with other underlying conditions apart from heart disease. A further large single center study by Alsoufi in 2007[14] indicated a favourable outcome for only 1 out of 9 children with non-cardiac diagnoses that had ECPR. This topic was also addressed by the report from the ELSO Registry by Thiagarajan.[4] In this study there were 43 pediatric respiratory patients who had ECPR (21% survival), 54 children with sepsis and ECPR (22% survival), and 52 with other diagnoses and ECPR (23% survival). Surprisingly, 17/34 (50%) neonatal respiratory failure ECPR cases survived, but given the Registry's 20,993 non-ECPR neonatal respiratory failure cases, this very small number must be interpreted with caution. Other important aspects from this review included the finding that death within 72 hours of ECPR was associated with brain death in 85% of patients, while 61% of patients were noted to have a pH lower than 6.9 prior to ECPR flow initiation. Among non-survivors who died > 72 hours following ECPR initiation, brain death was noted in 15% and pH<6.9 in 39%. In a series by Prodhan from 2009, 5 out of 6 general PICU or NICU ECPR cases survived to discharge,[16] that is a more positive finding than previous studies, albeit with very small numbers. A further report in 2011 of 42 children treated with ECPR found 40% overall survival to discharge, with no difference in outcome between patients with underlying cardiac disease from those with other medical conditions.[5] This report noted that longer duration of CPR and need for multiple inotropes at high dose prior to arrest were associated with mortality. Of the 42 patients, 37 were cannulated through the mediastinum. Of note, sternal cannulation has also recently been associated with improved outcome in patients with severe septic shock or arrest by clinicians in Australia with 74% survival in 23 patients.[29]

Factors which may explain the lower survival rates in non-cardiac ECPR patients have not been clearly identified. Some authors comment that non-cardiac patients may have multiple organ failure and high severity of illness, there may also be difficulties with oxygenation during more prolonged periods of CPR due to severe lung disease. Other authors have cited the potential disparity in access of ECPR between cardiac and non-cardiac ICUs in terms of surgical cannulation availability or implementation procedures. Currently, careful assessment and continued evaluation of ECPR use in non-cardiac patients is prudent.

Out of hospital cardiac arrest (OHCA) and hypothermia (Children)

There are a small numbers of reports of pediatric patients undergoing ECPR or emergency cardiopulmonary bypass for severe hypothermia and cardiac arrest. Scaife reported the results of a clear and detailed protocol for use of ECMO in cases of hypothermia with non-perfusing rhythm.[30] Two of four children who met inclusion criteria survived but both were reported to have some degree of long-term neurological impairment. Walpoth[31,32] reported late neurological follow up of 15 of 32 survivors, including both adults and children, from emergency cardiopulmonary bypass as treatment for OHCA with hypothermia. All patients were leading a full life and none had more than minor abnormalities found at testing. Wollenek[33] reported a case series of emergency cardiopulmonary bypass for children who had OHCA with hypothermia, including three cases in his experience and nine further cases from the literature. All 12 children suffered hypothermia secondary to submersion or exposure and were treated with either femoral-femoral or open chest bypass. Of ten survivors, one was described as normal, five to have clear neurological deficits although the nature of these abnormalities was not stated, and three to have possible neurological deficits. Eich[34] reported a case series of 12 hypothermic children from drowning with OHCA treated with emergency cardiopulmonary bypass, following a protocol between 1987 and 2005. Five of 12 (42%) survived, two with good neurological outcome but three in a vegetative state (PCPC 5).

Adults

Use of ECPR in adults with cardiac arrest is reported infrequently in the United States. The ELSO Registry notes 476 adults who have received ECPR with 29% surviving to hospital discharge.[1] In a recent meta-analysis of studies of adult ECPR spanning the time period 1990-2007, 135 patients were analyzed with survival to discharge of 40%.[35] Of note, this analysis included patients in whom spontaneous circulation had been restored but who remained in a low cardiac output state, which, as noted above, should not be classified as ECPR. Data available on 21 patients in whom CPR was ongoing during cannulation noted 48% survival.

The average duration of CPR prior to ECLS (n=102 patients) was 40 minutes (range 1-180 minutes), with patients having CPR for <30 minutes having improved survival (OR 1.9, 95% CI 0.9-4.2). Median ECLS duration was 54 hours (range 0-3881). Females had slightly shorter duration of ECLS (p=0.04). Patients were also evaluated by age group, with those patients 17-40 years of age having slightly better outcomes than older age groups, although this was not statistically significant. The majority of adult ECPR occurred in the ICU environment, with survival of 24%. Patients cannulated in the cardiac catheterization laboratory (n=23) had survival of 43% and 60% of patients receiving ECLS in the Emergency Department (n=5) survived.

Other adult reports have also found ECPR to be useful. Reports of resuscitation following prolonged hypothermia, especially in the Alps, note that ECPR or cardiopulmonary bypass is the preferred mode of rewarming in this population. In one interesting report, standard extracorporeal re-warming versus ECMO was compared in 59 patients between the years 1987-2006.[36] Overall, ROSC was achieved in 54% of patients, with 20% surviving to discharge. In patients rewarmed with bypass alone, severe pulmonary edema was noted in 64% of non-survivors, while none of the ECMO patients died from this complication. Rewarming with ECMO had a 6.6 fold increase in chance for survival versus extracorporeal rewarming alone. Patients suffering asphyxia-related arrest from avalanches or drowning had poor outcome. In Japan and other Asian centers, specialized emergency departments providing care to cardiac patients report the ability to initiate ECPR via femoral cannulation within several minutes of a patient's arrival in the ED.[37,38] Fluoroscopy allows for emergent diagnosis of coronary artery occlusion and rapid therapy can thus be instituted. In a recent meta-analysis of Japanese ECPR, 105 reports between 1983 and 2008 identified out-of-hospital arrests in 1282 patients.[38] In

516 ECPR patients, 27% survival to discharge was reported. In-depth evaluation of 139 cases noted good recovery in 48% of survivors, mild disability in 3%, severe disability in 2%, and vegetative state in 37%. Currently, an adult project entitled SAVE-J, evaluating the use of ECMO during cardiac arrest in adults with ventricular fibrillation in Japan, is underway and may provide more specific and in-depth information on this modality in the future. Recent articles have also found ECPR of benefit using propensity statistical design to compare patients resuscitated with ECPR to those receiving only conventional CPR. Propensity scoring tries to balance baseline characteristics and selected variables which may affect outcome to allow interpretation of effects of a therapy or procedure (ECPR in this case) on another group without performing a strict randomized, controlled trial. In one recent report of 120 matched patients, the odds ratio for survival with minimal neurologic impairment was 0.17 (95% CI 0.29-0.77, p=0.003) for ECPR versus conventional CPR. When subgroup analysis of cardiac patients was performed, ECPR also had a survival benefit observed (OR=0.19, 95% CI0.33-0.97, p=0.038).[38]

Technical Issues

Published studies stress the importance of protocols as being integral to the ECPR process, including resident or rapidly available staff for decision making, ECMO cannulation, and starting ECMO.

Cannulation

The majority of pediatric and neonatal patients receive venoarterial cannulation. For patients <2 years of age, cervical access is most commonly initiated, with the alternative being open chest cannulation. Older patients may have cannulation of femoral vessels (usually vein and artery) done via percutaneous or open procedures during CPR. For patients who have recently had cardiac surgery, the sternotomy incision can be easily reopened and cannulation of the right atrium and aorta can occur directly. Cessation of continuous CPR during cannulation to facilitate the procedure should be limited, as lack of adequate CPR is a major factor in poor outcome. As mentioned above, mediastinal cannulation for patients without preexisting sternotomy has also been associated with relatively good outcome in some recent reports.[5,39] This is an intriguing finding that requires further evaluation, as it adds potentially more complexity to the surgical expertise and equipment required to initiate ECPR. The evidence is also confusing, since the ELSO Registry data on ECPR found either no advantage with either cervical or thoracic cannulation[4] or benefit from cervical cannulation.[25] While some authors have noted that venovenous access can be applied during CPR and cardiac function improved when the myocardium receives improved oxygenation and blood flow with ECLS initiation, this approach is not common.

Circuit

Components used for ECPR vary between centers. Some maintain a pre-primed roller pump, silicone membrane lung system while others employ a centrifugal pump, hollow fiber oxygenator system that can be primed and operational within a few minutes. The advantages of the centrifugal/hollow fiber system include low priming volumes, easy portability and fast priming rates. As centrifugal pumps create active suction without the need for gravity drainage noted in roller head devices, position of the pump head can be at any level related to the patient, which may also allow a decrease in overall tubing length and priming volume. Hollow fiber oxygenators have less resistance to blood flow which also may be advantageous. Together, these features may also allow for less heparin usage and less bleeding complications, which are major complications, especially in postoperative patients. While there are currently no direct comparison trials between roller pump/silicone membrane systems and centrifugal pump/hollow fiber setups, many centers are switching to the latter combination, especially for ECPR, due to its ease of priming and ability to support patients of a wide variety of weights. Whether centrifugal systems are "better" than roller pump systems will require ongoing evaluation. Some preliminary reports are promising in terms of improved survival and reduction of blood product exposure.[39,40]

Team Composition

Another important factor in ECPR is the type of team approach used to provide this service. The optimal ECPR program would have 24/7 availability onsite of attending-level ICU personnel, surgical cannulating personnel, ECLS initiation specialists, a prepared or quickly primed circuit, and patient-specific blood available, and these factors are in place in many centers which provide ECPR. Centers who require surgical, ICU and/or ECLS personnel to come in from off-site locations to provide ECPR initiation have reported reasonable outcomes, despite the fact that delay in initiation in such sites might seem a limitation.[12] In fact, the majority of centers who report ECPR to the ELSO registry do not have 24/7 capability in all areas of ECPR initiation, and measures such as a prepared standby circuit have been described to reduce response times.[41] The impact of different approaches to ECPR team composition and access to outcome has not been evaluated in-depth.

Duration of CPR

Clearly the quality of CPR provided is important in determining the outcome of ECPR, and this may be one reason why the successful reports of ECPR are skewed towards in-hospital

cardiac arrests, in particular from the ICU. Most practitioners would agree that the goal is to minimize the duration of cardiac arrest and advocate shorter periods of CPR as being optimal,[6,13,15,16,18,19,42] but it is unclear whether there is an upper limit beyond which survival is very unlikely. Protocols regarding patient selection, cannulation, and readiness of the ECLS circuit are all essential in order to minimize ECPR times. A study by Huang from 2008[15] suggested that longer CPR times had a negative effect on survival, and a study by Prodhan from 2009[16] showed equivocal evidence that CPR > 60 minutes was a risk factor for death. A 2011 study by Sivarajan of 116 children found a significantly increased risk of death with CPR times longer than 30 minutes.[19] However, there are a small number of survivors in case series with ECPR times of around 90 minutes or even longer.[43] There is evidence from studies of both ECPR and non-ECMO cardiac arrest patients that ECPR patients tolerate longer CPR times.[44,45] Possible explanations for this include selection of better risk patients for ECPR, better quality perfusion in patients with cardiac arrest due to primary cardiac disease, and the advantages of better perfusion with ECMO after cardiac arrest.

Outcomes

Favorable early outcomes of ECPR reported in single-center studies range from 30% to 65%,[14] or even 75% in one report.[16] The ELSO Registry indicates early survival rates of 39% in children, and 27% in adults. A review of the ELSO Registry focusing on ECPR in children[4] indicated that the use of ECPR appears to be increasing over time (p<0.001) but the proportion discharged alive remained constant at 30-40% per year (p=0.96). Cardiac and neonatal respiratory failure diagnoses were linked to greater chance of survival (p<0.001). Non-white race (p=0.01) and severity of acidemia before ECLS (p<0.001), CNS injury (p=0.001), renal failure (p=0.009), and pulmonary hemorrhage (p=0.02) were associated with reduced chance of survival. The approach to cannulation (open chest versus peripheral) was not linked to survival in this study.

It is important to consider that the majority of favorable studies reporting ECPR indicated neurological outcome based on a clinical examination at discharge and a small number of studies did not include any data on neurology at all. The ELSO Registry-based studies only reported certain defined neurological abnormalities based on the database, such as evidence of cerebral bleeds or seizures, rather than a clinical evaluation of the patient's neurology.46,47 A Registry study by Cengiz47 has shown that cardiac arrest (all types) is an adverse risk factor for neurological events in the ECMO population. The small number of late follow up studies of ECPR indicate that early outcome measures do not necessarily correlate with long-term neurological outcome, in particular if detailed testing is performed on survivors. There are only a small number of studies that contain data about long-term assessment of ECPR survivors. These appear to identify a certain amount of late morbidity: Huang15 included 27 ECPR patients with 41% early survival and 63% survivors intact, Ibrahim18 included 21 ECPR with 48% early survival and 38% long term survivors intact, Lequier48 included 12 ECPR cases with 46% early survival and 38% survivors intact, Prodhan49 included 34 ECPR cases with 74% early survival and 75% of survivors with no change in neurological status. This issue is an important caution when interpreting favorable early results. Neurological issues in survivors with heart disease, who represent the majority of ECPR patients, may also be linked with the underlying heart condition and subsequent surgeries. Congenital heart disease itself is recognized to carry significant risk of neurodevelopmental problems49 and this further confounds attempts to establish and delineate the links between ECPR and outcome. It is therefore of great importance that survivors of ECPR undergo neurodevelopmental followup, such that appropriate supportive therapies can be initiated in a timely fashion.

Future Directions

With the advent of new, miniature ECLS systems, improved cannulation techniques and experience in successful outcomes for patients cannulated during arrest, it is likely that this group will continue to increase as an ECLS population. Recent interest in application of ECLS to adults in US emergency departments is also occurring, although some clinicians involved in this effort seem to have little interest in allying efforts with established groups such as ELSO. It is hoped that collaboration in the use of ECPR between all sites, US and abroad, will continue to provide much needed data to further define appropriate patient selection, management techniques and long-term information on outcome.

References

1. International ECLS Registry 2011, Extracorporeal Life Support Organization, Ann Arbor MI. ELSO. Registry of the Extracorporeal Life Support Organisation. Michigan: Ann Arbor;2011.

2. Kleinman ME, de Caen AR, Chameides L, et al. Part 10: Pediatric basic and advanced life support: 2010 International Consensus on Cardiopulmonary Resuscitation and Emergency Cardiovascular Care Science With Treatment Recommendations. Circulation. Oct 19 2010;122(16 Suppl 2):S466-515.

3. Raymond TT, Cunnyngham CB, Thompson MT, Thomas JA, Dalton HJ, Nadkarni VM. Outcomes among neonates, infants, and children after extracorporeal cardiopulmonary resuscitation for refractory inhospital pediatric cardiac arrest: a report from the National Registry of Cardiopulmonary

Resuscitation. Pediatr Crit Care Med. May 2010;11(3):362-371.

4. Thiagarajan RR, Laussen PC, Rycus PT, Bartlett RH, Bratton SL. Extracorporeal membrane oxygenation to aid cardiopulmonary resuscitation in infants and children. Circulation. Oct 9 2007;116(15):1693-1700.

5. Delmo Walter EM, Alexi-Meskishvili V, Huebler M, et al. Rescue extracorporeal membrane oxygenation in children with refractory cardiac arrest. Interact Cardiovasc Thorac Surg. Jun 2011;12(6):929-934.

6. Morris MC, Wernovsky G, Nadkarni VM. Survival outcomes after extracorporeal cardiopulmonary resuscitation instituted during active chest compressions following refractory in-hospital pediatric cardiac arrest. Pediatr Crit Care Med. Sep 2004;5(5):440-446.

7. del Nido PJ. Extracorporeal membrane oxygenation for cardiac support in children. Ann Thorac Surg. Jan 1996;61(1):336-339; discussion 340-341.

8. del Nido PJ, Dalton HJ, Thompson AE, Siewers RD. Extracorporeal membrane oxygenator rescue in children during cardiac arrest after cardiac surgery. Circulation. 1992 Nov 1992;86(suppl)(5):II300-II304.

9. Dalton HJ, Siewers RD, Fuhrman BP, et al. Extracorporeal membrane oxygenation for cardiac rescue in children with severe myocardial dysfunction. Crit Care Med. Jul 1993;21(7):1020-1028.

10. Duncan BW, Ibrahim AE, Hraska V, et al. Use of rapid-deployment extracorporeal membrane oxygenation for the resuscitation of pediatric patients with heart disease after cardiac arrest. J Thorac Cardiovasc Surg. Aug 1998;116(2):305-311.

11. Thourani VH, Kirshbom PM, Kanter KR, et al. Venoarterial extracorporeal membrane oxygenation (VA-ECMO) in pediatric cardiac support. Ann Thorac Surg. Jul 2006;82(1):138-144; discussion 144-135.

12. Ghez O, Fouilloux V, Charpentier A, et al. Absence of rapid deployment extracorporeal membrane oxygenation (ECMO) team does not preclude resuscitation ecmo in pediatric cardiac patients with good results. ASAIO J. Nov-Dec 2007;53(6):692-695.

13. Baslaim G, Bashore J, Al-Malki F, Jamjoom A. Can the outcome of pediatric extracorporeal membrane oxygenation after cardiac surgery be predicted? Ann Thorac Cardiovasc Surg. Feb 2006;12(1):21-27.

14. Alsoufi B, Al-Radi OO, Nazer RI, et al. Survival outcomes after rescue extracorporeal cardiopulmonary resuscitation in pediatric patients with refractory cardiac arrest. J Thorac Cardiovasc Surg. Oct 2007;134(4):952-959 e952.

15. Huang SC, Wu ET, Chen YS, et al. Extracorporeal membrane oxygenation rescue for cardiopulmonary resuscitation in pediatric patients. Crit Care Med. May 2008;36(5):1607-1613.

16. Prodhan P, Fiser RT, Dyamenahalli U, et al. Outcomes after extracorporeal cardiopulmonary resuscitation (ECPR) following refractory pediatric cardiac arrest in the intensive care unit. Resuscitation. Oct 2009;80(10):1124-1129.

17. Hoskote A, Bohn D, Gruenwald C, et al. Extracorporeal life support after staged palliation of a functional single ventricle: subsequent morbidity and survival. J Thorac Cardiovasc Surg. May 2006;131(5):1114-1121.

18. Ibrahim AE, Duncan BW, Blume ED, Jonas RA. Long-term follow-up of pediatric cardiac patients requiring mechanical circulatory support. Ann Thorac Surg. Jan 2000;69(1):186-192.

19. Sivarajan VB, Best D, Brizard CP, Shekerdemian LS, d'Udekem Y, Butt W. Duration of resuscitation prior to rescue extracorporeal membrane oxygenation impacts outcome in children with heart disease.

Intensive Care Med. May 2011;37(5):853-860.

20. Aharon AS, Drinkwater DC, Jr., Churchwell KB, et al. Extracorporeal membrane oxygenation in children after repair of congenital cardiac lesions. Ann Thorac Surg. Dec 2001;72(6):2095-2101; discussion 2101-2092.

21. Yamasaki Y, Hayashi T, Nakatani T, et al. Early experience with low-prime (99 ml) extracorporeal membrane oxygenation support in children. ASAIO J. Jan-Feb 2006;52(1):110-114.

22. Allan CK, Thiagarajan RR, Armsby LR, del Nido PJ, Laussen PC. Emergent use of extracorporeal membrane oxygenation during pediatric cardiac catheterization. Pediatr Crit Care Med. May 2006;7(3):212-219.

23. Cochran JB, Tecklenburg FW, Lau YR, Habib DM. Emergency cardiopulmonary bypass for cardiac arrest refractory to pediatric advanced life support. Pediatr Emerg Care. Feb 1999;15(1):30-32.

24. Wu ET, Li MJ, Huang SC, et al. Survey of outcome of CPR in pediatric in-hospital cardiac arrest in a medical center in Taiwan. Resuscitation. Apr 2009;80(4):443-448.

25. Chan T, Thiagarajan RR, Frank D, Bratton SL. Survival after extracorporeal cardiopulmonary resuscitation in infants and children with heart disease. J Thorac Cardiovasc Surg. Oct 2008;136(4):984-992.

26. Posner JC, Osterhoudt KC, Mollen CJ, Jacobstein CR, Nicolson SC, Gaynor JW. Extracorporeal membrane oxygenation as a resuscitative measure in the pediatric emergency department. Pediatr Emerg Care. Dec 2000;16(6):413-415.

27. Younger JG, Schreiner RJ, Swaniker F, Hirschl RB, Chapman RA, Bartlett RH. Extracorporeal resuscitation of cardiac arrest. Acad Emerg Med. Jul 1999;6(7):700-707.

28. Al-Takrouri H, Martin TW, Mayhew JF. Hyperkalemic cardiac arrest following succinylcholine administration: The use of

extracorporeal membrane oxygenation in an emergency situation. J Clin Anesth. Sep 2004;16(6):449-451.

29. Maclaren G, Butt W, Best D, Donath S. Central extracorporeal membrane oxygenation for refractory pediatric septic shock. Pediatr Crit Care Med. Mar 2011;12(2):133-136..

30. Scaife ER, Connors RC, Morris SE, et al. An established extracorporeal membrane oxygenation protocol promotes survival in extreme hypothermia. J Pediatr Surg. Dec 2007;42(12):2012-2016.

31. Walpoth BH, Locher T, Leupi F, Schupbach P, Muhlemann W, Althaus U. Accidental deep hypothermia with cardiopulmonary arrest: extracorporeal blood rewarming in 11 patients. Eur J Cardiothorac Surg. 1990;4(7):390-393.

32. Walpoth BH, Walpoth-Aslan BN, Mattle HP, et al. Outcome of survivors of accidental deep hypothermia and circulatory arrest treated with extracorporeal blood warming. N Engl J Med. Nov 20 1997;337(21):1500-1505.

33. Wollenek G, Honarwar N, Golej J, Marx M. Cold water submersion and cardiac arrest in treatment of severe hypothermia with cardiopulmonary bypass. Resuscitation. 2002;52(3):255-263.

34. Eich C, Brauer A, Timmermann A, et al. Outcome of 12 drowned children with attempted resuscitation on cardiopulmonary bypass: an analysis of variables based on the "Utstein Style for Drowning". Resuscitation. Oct 2007;75(1):42-52.

35. Cardarelli MG, Young AJ, Griffith B. Use of extracorporeal membrane oxygenation for adults in cardiac arrest (E-CPR): a meta-analysis of observational studies. ASAIO J. Nov-Dec 2009;55(6):581-586.

36. Ruttmann E, Weissenbacher A, Ulmer H, et al. Prolonged extracorporeal membrane oxygenation-assisted support provides improved survival in hypothermic patients

with cardiocirculatory arrest. J Thorac Cardiovasc Surg. Sep 2007;134(3):594-600.

37. Morimura N, Sakamoto T, Nagao K, et al. Extracorporeal cardiopulmonary resuscitation for out-of-hospital cardiac arrest: A review of the Japanese literature. Resuscitation. Jan 2011;82(1):10-14.

38. Shin TG, Choi JH, Jo IJ, et al. Extracorporeal cardiopulmonary resuscitation in patients with inhospital cardiac arrest: A comparison with conventional cardiopulmonary resuscitation. Crit Care Med. Jan 2011;39(1):1-7.

39. Sivarajan VB, Best D, Brizard CP, et al. Improved outcomes of paediatric extracorporeal support associated with technology change. Interact Cardiovasc Thorac Surg. Oct 2010;11(4):400-405.

40. McMullan DM, Emmert JA, Permut LC, et al. Minimizing bleeding associated with mechanical circulatory support following pediatric heart surgery. Eur J Cardiothorac Surg. Mar 2011;39(3):392-397.

41. Karimova A, Robertson A, Cross N, et al. A wet-primed extracorporeal membrane oxygenation circuit with hollow-fiber membrane oxygenator maintains adequate function for use during cardiopulmonary resuscitation after 2 weeks on standby. Crit Care Med. Jul 2005;33(7):1572-1576.

42. Dalton HJ, Siewers RD, Fuhrman BP, et al. Extracorporeal membrane oxygenation for cardiac rescue in children with severe myocardial dysfunction. Crit Care Med. 1993 Jul 1993;21(7):1020-1028.

43. Kelly RB, Porter PA, Meier AH, Myers JL, Thomas NJ. Duration of cardiopulmonary resuscitation before extracorporeal rescue: how long is not long enough? ASAIO J. Sep-Oct 2005;51(5):665-667.

44. de Mos N, van Litsenburg RR, McCrindle B, Bohn DJ, Parshuram CS. Pediatric in-intensive-care-unit cardiac arrest: incidence, survival, and predictive factors. Crit Care Med. Apr 2006;34(4):1209-1215.

45. Morris MC, Wernovsky G, Nadkarni VM. Survival outcomes after extracorporeal cardiopulmonary resuscitation instituted during active chest compressions following refractory in-hospital pediatric cardiac arrest. Pediatr Crit Care Med. Sep 2004;5(5):440-446.

46. Barrett CS, Bratton SL, Salvin JW, Laussen PC, Rycus PT, Thiagarajan RR. Neurological injury after extracorporeal membrane oxygenation use to aid pediatric cardiopulmonary resuscitation. Pediatr Crit Care Med. Jul 2009;10(4):445-451.

47. Cengiz P, Seidel K, Rycus PT, Brogan TV, Roberts JS. Central nervous system complications during pediatric extracorporeal life support: incidence and risk factors. Crit Care Med. Dec 2005;33(12):2817-2824.

48. Lequier L, Joffe AR, Robertson CM, et al. Two-year survival, mental, and motor outcomes after cardiac extracorporeal life support at less than five years of age. J Thorac Cardiovasc Surg. Oct 2008;136(4):976-983 e973.

49. Gaynor JW, Gerdes M, Nord AS, et al. Is cardiac diagnosis a predictor of neurodevelopmental outcome after cardiac surgery in infancy? J Thorac Cardiovasc Surg. Dec 2010;140(6):1230-1237.

24

Ventricular Assist Devices in Children

David S. Cooper MD MPH, Ravi R. Thiagarajan MBBS MPH, Christopher S. Almond MD, Christina J. VanderPluym MD, Holger Buchholz MD, Jeffrey P. Jacobs MD FACS FACC FCCP

Introduction

Mechanical circulatory support is an invaluable tool in the care of children with severe refractory cardiac and/or pulmonary failure.[1] There are two forms of mechanical circulatory support currently available to neonates, infants, and smaller children: extracorporeal membrane oxygenation (ECMO) and ventricular assist device (VAD), with each technique having unique advantages and disadvantages. The intraaortic balloon pump is a third form of mechanical support that has been successfully used in larger children, adolescents, and adults, but has limited applicability in smaller children.[1] As the field of mechanical circulatory support has evolved in children, the indications for use have expanded and outcomes have improved. When combined with an active transplantation program, mechanical circulatory support can have a significant impact on survival. The majority of the pediatric experience consists of use of ECMO.[2] The July 2011 Extracorporeal Life Support Organization (ELSO) Summary[3] reported 9,798 neonatal and pediatric cardiac failure cases (24% of cases) since 1989. For neonatal and pediatric cardiac failure, survival to separation from ECMO is 62% and survival to discharge is 43%. Despite recent advances in VAD technology, ECMO remains the most common circulatory assist system in use for pediatric patients. The advantages of ECMO include its familiarity among practitioners, ability to provide biventricular support and respiratory support, universal availability across all pediatric age groups, and relative low cost. Unlike adults in whom pure left ventricular failure is the common indication for mechanical support, cardiopulmonary support is more commonly required in children due to a combination of pulmonary dysfunction, pulmonary hypertension, and right ventricular dysfunction. This is particularly true in the immediate postoperative period. Extracorporeal life support is obviously the mechanical support of choice for rapid deployment during cardiopulmonary arrest. There are a number of disadvantages, including the need for a dedicated team of specialists, immobilization, requirement for intensive care monitoring, risks of bleeding, thrombosis, infection, and multiorgan failure. These attendant disadvantages increase over time and hamper the use of ECMO for long term support. The advantages of VAD include less trauma to blood cells (lack of membrane oxygenator) thus decreasing the need for anticoagulation, and decreased risk of infection compared to ECMO where the system is more open with multiple access ports. Implantable assist devices allow greater mobility for cardiac rehabilitation and have chronic support capability as a bridge to transplantation. Their disadvantages include the need for transthoracic cannulation, while ECMO can be initiated with peripheral cannulation. In addition, biventricular support with ventricular assist devices requires four cannulas, whereas extracorporeal membrane oxygenation provides biventricular support with two cannulas.

Although ECMO has become a standard of care for many pediatric centers, its utility is limited to those patients who require only short-term cardiopulmonary support. Mechanical support devices have become standard therapy for adults with heart failure refractory to maximal medical management. Several devices are readily available in the United States for the adult population, but there are fewer options available to children. Over the last few years, substantial progress has been made in pediatric mechanical support.[4] Ventricular assist devices are being used with increasing frequency in children with cardiac failure refractory to medical therapy for primary treatment as a long-term bridge to recovery or transplantation.[5] Mechanical circulatory support should be anticipated and every attempt must be made to initiate support "urgently" rather than "emergently" before the presence of end organ dysfunction or circulatory collapse. In an emergency these patients can be resuscitated with ECMO and subsequently transitioned to a long-term VAD after a period of stability. Destination therapy, defined as intracorporeal VAD implantation with the goal of "permanent support", is currently not an option in the pediatric population. In this chapter, we focus our discussion on the types of VADs available and current experience in children, bridge to cardiac transplantation using ECMO and VADs and anticoagulation for VAD patients.

Types of Ventricular Assist Devices

Axial Flow Devices

Although the pediatric experience with these ventricular assist devices is limited, they have been used successfully in children ages 5-16 years with body surface area of $\geq 0.7m^2$. Advantages of axial flow pumps include their small size, relatively easy implant/explant procedures, low infection rates, and continuous flows that minimize thrombus formation. Disadvantages include nonpulsatile flow, size limitation for pediatric patients and larger sized ventricular apical cannulation. The MicroMed DeBakey VAD® was designed as a miniaturized heart pump to provide blood flow up to 10 L/min. The implantable axial flow pump weighs less than four ounces and contains only one moving part, the inducer/impeller. In the United States, the MicroMed DeBakey VAD® was approved in February 2004 under the humanitarian device exemption and has been used to successfully bridge several pediatric patients to cardiac transplantation.[6] The Jarvik-2000 is a similar intravascular assist device made of titanium, measuring 25mm in diameter and 55mm in length. The impeller rotates at 8,000-12,000 revolutions per minute, generating a flow rate of 3-6 L/min. It is currently under evaluation in pediatric animal models.[7]

Pulsatile Devices

Experience in pediatric long term pulsatile devices is growing.[8-11] These devices offer univentricular or biventricular support. Children do not require mechanical ventilation and are able to mobilize out of the intensive care unit on relatively low levels of anticoagulation. Some disadvantages include thromboembolic complications, infection, and cost. The MEDOS-HIA VAD, another paracorporeal, pneumatically driven blood pump, is available in Europe in three left ventricular sizes (10, 25, and 60 mL stroke volumes), and three right ventricular sizes (9, 22.5 and 54 mL stroke volumes). This system has also been successfully used for long-term support and bridge to transplantation.[12] The Thoratec Ventricular Assist System, Abiomed's AB5000 Circulatory Support System and Heart-mate are pulsatile assist devices that can be used in larger children and adolescent patients.[13] Due to device size, these ventricular assist systems are not practical for use in children with a body surface area <0.8 m[2]. Sharma et al. reviewed their experience with pulsatile ventricular assist devices as a bridge to heart transplantation in 18 patients over a 15 year time period.[14] Diagnoses included dilated cardiomyopathy, myocarditis, and postcardiotomy ventricular failure. Ten children underwent insertion of biventricular assist devices and eight had implantation of a left ventricular assist device only. The mean support duration was 57 days with successful transplantation in 14 patients (77%). Complications included bleeding requiring reoperation, stroke and device related infection. Survival at 1 and 5-years after orthotopic heart transplantation was 83%.

The Berlin Heart *EXCOR® Pediatric* is an extracorporeal pneumatically driven pulsatile VAD that was initially developed and approved for clinical use in Europe and has garnered the most experience in the pediatric population to date.[15] It was granted CE Mark approval in 1992 with growing worldwide experience ensuing over the next decade.[5,9,16,17] In August 2000, the *EXCOR® Pediatric* emerged in North America as an alternative for children requiring mechanical circulatory support. The application of this device grew under Humanitarian Use regulated by the FDA Office of Orphan Products and the Special Access Regulations by Health Canada. By 2007, 97 children in the US had received the device, with each implantation approved on a case-by-case basis after completing the process for a compassionate use protocol for bridge to transplantation. A clinical IDE trial centered on

assessing safety and efficacy of the *EXCOR® Pediatric* as a bridge to transplantation is now completed, with the results to be published shortly. This device was approved by the FDA in December of 2011.

Berlin Heart EXCOR® Pediatric

The Berlin Heart *EXCOR® Pediatric* is available in 10-, 25-, 30-, 50-, 60- and 80 mL sizes, with the smallest pump size suitable for infants weighing up to 3 to 9 kg. Children with weight up to 25 kg are optimally supported with 25- or 30 mL pumps.[18] The pump has a transparent polyurethane housing, which is separated into an air chamber and a blood chamber by a triple layer membrane. Graphite powder is located between the membrane layers in order to minimize friction. The blood chamber has an inflow and an outflow stub to which the inflow and outflow cannulas are connected via a titanium connector fitted around the stubs. Mounted within the inflow and outflow pump stubs are trileaflet polyurethane valves. Pump sizes greater than 50 mL are fitted with mechanical tilting disc valves. To reduce thrombus formation, the interior surface of the pump is heparin coated with a *Carmeda®BioActive Surface*. The blood pump chamber is equipped with a nipple used for deairing the blood chamber when the pump is commissioned for use. The air chamber of the pump is equipped with a driving tube connector through which air is pumped from the *Ikus* stationary driving unit. The *Ikus* generates the suction and driving pressures required to move the blood pump membrane. Three different types of cannulas are available in varying configurations and sizes. All cannulas are designed to exit the body though the upper abdominal wall. The cannulas are made of tissue friendly silicone with polyester-velour suture rings enabling expedient and safe anastomosis of the cannulas. The midsection of the cannula is enveloped with a Dacron velour cover that promotes tissue growth and provides a biological barrier against ascending skin infections. Conventional LVAD support consists of inflow and outflow cannulation via the left ventricle apex and the ascending aorta respectively. Left atrial cannulation is generally only reserved for patients with restrictive cardiomyopathy, in which LV apical cannulation would not permit sufficient volume unloading and predispose to thromboembolic events. RVAD cannulation consists of right atrial inflow and pulmonary artery outflow cannulas. The inflow or atrial cannula is angled at the tissue contacting end and designed with various head lengths, all of which terminate in a basket that protrudes into the atrium after placement. For apical inflow cannulation, the cannula configuration does not incorporate an angled head at its tissue contacting end. Like the inflow cannula, the outflow or arterial cannulas are also angled with the polyester-velour sewing ring allowing for end to side anastomosis to either the aorta or the pulmonary artery. The pulsatile electropneumatic Stationary Driving Unit named "Ikus" drives the pumps. The casing of the driving unit contains the pneumatic and electronic components as well as a laptop computer that serves as an interface to the operator (Figure 24-1). *Ikus* has three pneumatic systems that operate independently of each other. One

pneumatic system is required for each blood pump, with the third serving as an emergency backup. Each pneumatic system includes a compressor, pressure and suction limiters, pressure and vacuum cylinders, control electronics and control valves. The compressor and the pressure and suction limiters create constant pressure conditions in the pressure and vacuum cylinders. The control valves at the outlet of each cylinder allow optimum adjustment of the positive and negative (suction) values. The *Ikus* system has two control processors operating independently of each other. If there is no working *Ikus* available, the manual pump mounted on *Ikus* can be used temporarily to drive the blood pump(s). The Mobile Driving System *Excor* is a component of the *EXCOR Pediatric* VAD cardiac assist system. *Excor* may only be used to drive *EXCOR* blood pumps of the 60- and 80 mL size. *Excor* may only be used in followup therapy for patients formerly supplied by the stationary driving unit *Ikus*. *Excor* may not be used for initially starting the *EXCOR Pediatric* blood pumps in the operative or perioperative setting. *Excor* is intended exclusively for supporting mobile patients with stable hemodynamic parameters. *Excor* is a piston pump designed to achieve a full stroke volume provided that the

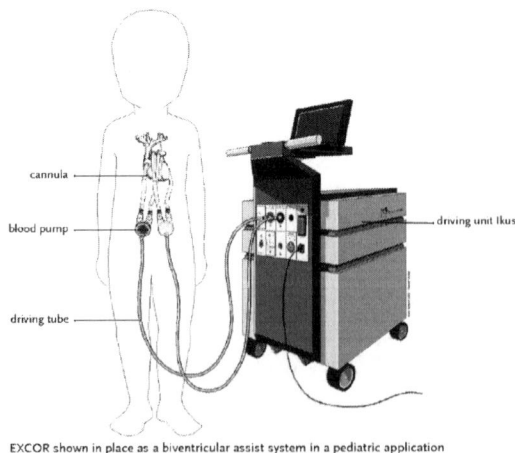

EXCOR shown in place as a biventricular assist system in a pediatric application

Figure 24-1. Berlin Heart EXCOR Pediatric with Stationary Driving Unit Ikus.

inflow and outflow conditions permit this. The drive unit pressures are adapted automatically, provided that they do not reach the set limits. A pressure limit is particularly necessary for the suction pressure in order to keep the pump's filling volume matched to the inflow conditions.

EXCOR® Pediatric Worldwide Experience

The EXCOR® Pediatric is now used at 122 pediatric heart centers in 32 countries. It has been shown to be reliable in providing stable circulatory support from infants weighing as little as 2.9 kg to teenagers.[5,16,17] The most recent worldwide clinical experience reported by Berlin Heart GmbH describes a total of 840 implantations with a cumulative time of 175.2 years on device with a mean of 76.2 days (range 0-977 days).[19] Left ventricle support (LVAD) has predominated with 56% of cases, followed by biventricular support (BiVAD) at 43% and only 1% with right ventricular (RVAD) support in isolation. The greatest experience with implantations has been in neonates with weight less than 10 kg (Figure 24-2). Etiologies of end stage cardiac failure necessitating EXCOR support include dilated cardiomyopathy (50%), congenital heart disease (20%), myocarditis (13%), restrictive cardiomyopathy (4%), and postcardiotomy (2%). Overall survival to transplantation is 61% and successful weaning from device in 10% (Figure 24-3). Better survival outcomes have been reported in a variety of studies, with the German Heart Institute Berlin demonstrating 78% survival to discharge.[20] These more favorable outcomes most likely reflect the refinements in pre- and postimplantation management strategies that have evolved over decades of EXCOR® experience in the single largest implantation center.

ECMO to Bridge Children to Cardiac Transplantation

ECMO is a commonly used mechanical circulatory support modality used to bridge children to transplantation (BTT).[21,22] The use of ECMO as a mechanical circulatory support modality to bridge children to transplantation arises from the extensive clinical experience available with the use of ECMO as a circulatory support modality in general. In children with congenital heart disease with severe postoperative cardiac dysfunction or those with acute fulminant myocarditis, ECMO is often the first mechanical circulatory modality of choice because of the

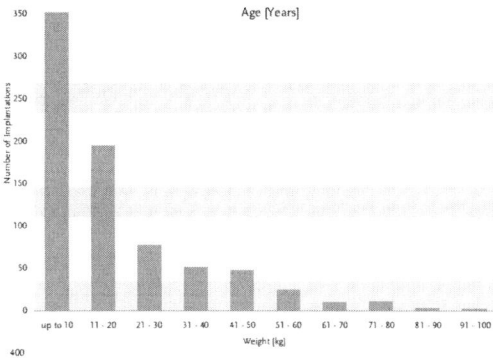

Figure **24-2.** Total number of Berlin Heart EXCOR Pediatric implantations distributed across patient weight (kg) (Reproduced with permission of Berlin Heart GmbH, Wiesenweg).

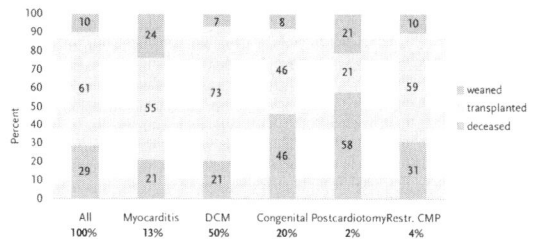

Figure **24-3.** Outcomes for Berlin Heart EXCOR Pediatric in patients analyzed according to underlying diagnosis. DCM; dilated cardiomyopathy, congenital; congenital heart disease, Restr. CMP; restrictive cardiomyopathy.

vast clinical experience with ECMO and ease of circulatory support deployment with the goal of providing mechanical circulatory support until myocardial recovery. However, in some children myocardial recovery does not occur in the expected time frame (usually 5-7 days), and these children require cardiac transplantation for survival. These children may be considered candidates for transplantation if end-organ function is preserved and the family wishes to pursue transplantation. In these situations, ECMO may then be used to bridge children to transplantation. Children supported with ECMO as a bridge to cardiac transplantation have poor outcomes with increased mortality waiting for, as well as after, transplantation.

Almond et al. evaluated factors associated with waiting list mortality in 3098 children listed for cardiac transplantation during 1999-2006 using data reported to the United Network for Organ Sharing (UNOS).[21] They found that both the use of ECMO (hazard ratio for mortality 3.1) and mechanical ventilation (hazard ratio for mortality 1.9) were associated with increased risk for mortality (Figure 24-4). The increased risk of mortality in children using ECMO as a bridge to transplantation may be related to the fact that ECMO can only provide a short duration of complication free mechani-

cal circulatory support (complications usually increase beyond 14 days of ECMO support), which is much shorter than the average organ waiting time. Furthermore, children on ECMO in intensive care units remain on mechanical ventilation, are heavily sedated and immobile resulting in muscle wasting, are often provided with inadequate nutrition resulting in nutritional debilitation, have multiple risk factors for healthcare acquired infections, and may have end-organ injury as result of disease and pharmacological therapies resulting in poorer posttransplant outcomes.

Using data from both the ELSO registry and the UNOS data report on outcomes for children supported with ECMO as BTT, Almond et al. identified 773 children who were bridged using ECMO and found that 272 (35%) died on ECMO and 348 (45%) died while waiting for transplantation.[22] The median duration of ECMO support was 22 days. Transplantation wait list mortality was associated with a diagnosis of congenital heart disease (Odds ratio [OR]=1.8), need for CPR prior to ECMO (OR=1.4), and severe renal dysfunction on ECMO (OR=2.7). In those who were successfully bridged to transplantation, posttransplant mortality was increased in those supported with ECMO for longer than 14 days (OR=3.3) and those initially supported with ECMO with the expectation of recovery (OR=3.2). Infection, bleeding, and neurological injury were common complications in patients supported with ECMO as BTT. Based on these data, one can say that although ECMO provides lifesaving circulatory support during critical illness, its use as a BTT support modality is associated with significant waiting list and posttransplant mortality. Children requiring mechanical circulatory assistance as BTT may have improved outcomes on other devices such as VADs, or early transition from ECMO to VAD when myocardial recovery and weaning off circulatory support is not possible. The following paragraphs discuss these important issues.

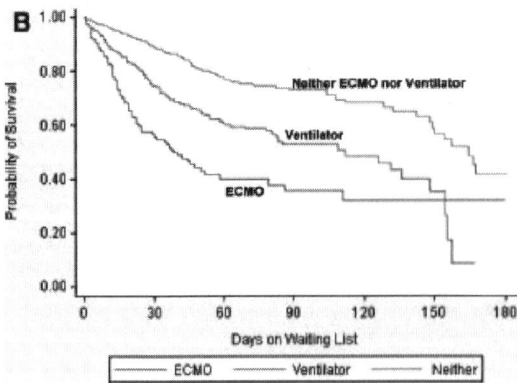

Figure 24-4. Waiting List mortality for children supported listed for transplantation.

ECMO versus VAD as Initial Device for Bridge to Transplantation

There are no large studies directly comparing the efficacy of VAD with ECMO for successful bridge to transplantation and posttransplant survival. A report by Imamura et al. from a single center comparing patients supported with the Berlin Heart VAD (n = 21) and those supported with ECMO (n =21) to bridge children to cardiac transplantation, found that those supported with the Berlin Heart VAD had better survival to and following cardiac transplantation (Figure 24-5).[23] The Berlin Heart VAD provided longer duration of mechanical circulatory support without a significant increase in neurologic complications. The majority of patients supported with VAD and ECMO in this series were children with cardiomyopathy and the cohort had few patients with congenital heart disease. Although matched for age and weight, severity of illness at the time of VAD implantation or ECMO deployment was not evaluated. Thus whether poor outcomes for ECMO patients were influenced by level of illness at ECMO deployment is hard to evaluate. In a 2006 report of VAD use in children, Blume et al. reported that congenital heart disease was a significant risk factor for poor outcomes in children supported with VAD (Figure 24-6).[5] Given that ECMO is frequently used to support children in the postoperative period after surgery for congenital heart disease, one can say that VAD implantation for BTT may be more suitable than ECMO to bridge patients with cardiomyopathies to cardiac transplantation, however future studies focused on comparing VAD and ECMO as BTT devices in children with congenital heart disease are needed.

Transition of ECMO patients to VAD

As previously mentioned, ECMO complications including organ and surgical bleeding, neurologic and end-organ injury, and healthcare acquired infections increase with increasing ECMO duration (particularly >2 weeks of ECMO). Additionally, organ availability for transplantation is limited, unpredictable, and waiting times vary by region and generally exceed the complication free ECMO support duration, resulting in poor BTT outcomes when ECMO is used to provide mechanical circulatory support. Furthermore, the morbidity acquired during the course of ECMO may decrease post-transplant survival in those bridged successfully

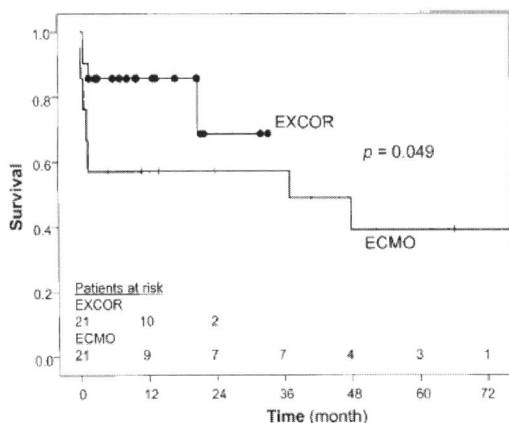

Figure 24-5. Survival to Cardiac Transplantation and post-transplantation in children supported with the Berlin Heart VAD and ECMO.

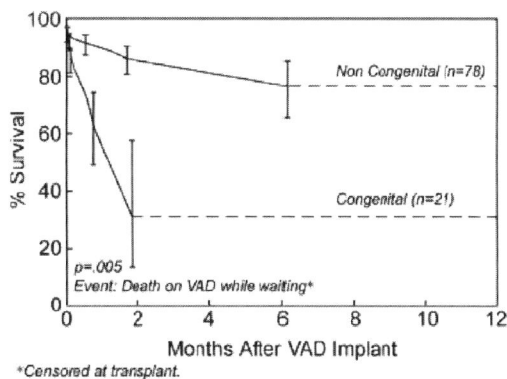

Figure 24-6. Risk of mortality is increased in children with congenital heart disease supported with VAD.

using ECMO. For both these reasons, transitioning ECMO patients to mechanical circulatory assist devices such as VADs that can provide longer duration support with lower incidence of complications, allow patients to be extubated from mechanical ventilation, promote physical and nutritional rehabilitation is desirable to improve posttransplant survival. However, the type of patient (age, size, diagnosis) and the timing of transition from ECMO for patients initially supported with it but requiring cardiac transplantation is unclear. We speculate that patients with acute cardiogenic shock initially supported with ECMO with the intention of recovery should be considered candidates for VAD as soon as all hope of myocardial recovery is exhausted, providing they are eligible candidates for cardiac transplantation. A proposed schema for timing of transition to VAD from ECMO based on the experience at Children's Hospital Boston is shown in Figure 24-7. Transition to VAD after the onset of end-organ injury such as renal failure is unlikely to produce successful bridging to transplantation and may also impact posttransplant survival.

In a recent report by Morales et al. describing outcomes in 73 children supported with the Berlin Heart VAD, 22 (31%) of children placed on VAD as BTT were transitioned to VAD after initial support with ECMO.[24] Prior use of ECMO was not associated with increased mortality on the waiting list. In another retrospective case series (using an administrative database) of children (n=187) supported with VAD, Morales et al. showed that use of ECMO prior to VAD implantation was associated with increased odds of mortality prior to hospital discharge (OR=35).[8] Given that transition to VAD from ECMO is often undertaken in children bridged to cardiac transplantation, future research should focus on selecting appropriate ECMO candidates and timing of transition to improve outcomes for these children.

Ventricular Assist Device Use in Single Ventricle Patients

The use of mechanical assist devices for the treatment of endstage heart failure in children awaiting transplant has been increasing as

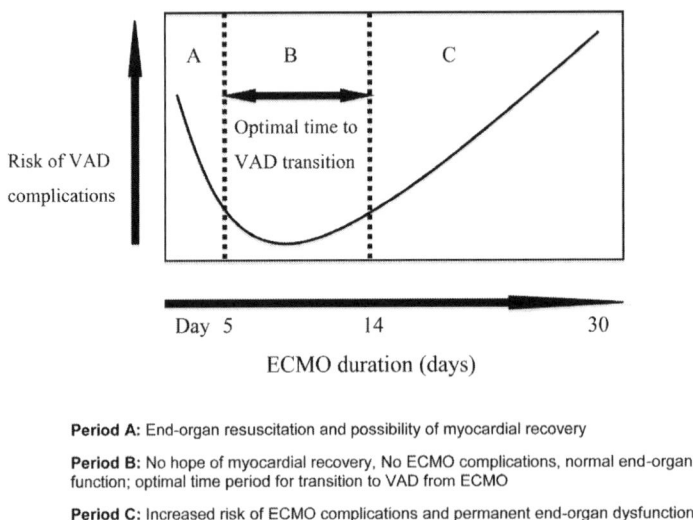

Period A: End-organ resuscitation and possibility of myocardial recovery

Period B: No hope of myocardial recovery, No ECMO complications, normal end-organ function; optimal time period for transition to VAD from ECMO

Period C: Increased risk of ECMO complications and permanent end-organ dysfunction

Figure 24-7. Theoretical schema proposing optimal transition time to VAD from ECMO.

device design allowed smaller pump volumes. Patients with single ventricle anatomy and physiology are at high risk for myocardial failure at any stage of palliation and accordingly the applicability of VAD support in this challenging patient population has been questioned. Patients with shunt dependent circulation can be adequately supported; however, parallel circulation usually requires increased pump flow rates (200 mL/kg/min) to accommodate the need for both pulmonary and systemic perfusion and to maintain adequate oxygenation and oxygen delivery. A larger pump size may be needed to meet these end-organ oxygen demands. There are several challenges associated with single ventricle VAD support. These patients have reconstructed aortas and often ventricles with no clear apex, making cannulation difficult. Additionally, they likely require a "redo" sternotomy, with all of its inherent risks and complications. In patients following bidirectional Glenn and Fontan operations, there may also be issues with pulmonary vascular resistance (PVR) and systemic venous hypertension. Primary ventricular dysfunction can be addressed with single pump VAD support. However, increased PVR may require an additional pump within the pulmonary circulation to address systemic venous hypertension. The implantation of a pulmonary VAD requires

revision of the Fontan pathway for separation of the systemic venous and pulmonary circulations and in the event of pump failure or a necessary pump change, complete cessation of pulmonary flow and cardiac output would occur.

Ungerleider et al. investigated the routine use of mechanical ventricular assist following the Norwood procedure for hypoplastic left heart syndrome as a means to attenuate the low cardiac output syndrome that occurs during the immediate postoperative period.[25] Patients were placed on a VAD in the operating room using the CPB cannulas in the right atrium and the neoaorta. VAD flows were maintained at ~200mL/kg/min to compensate for the shunted physiology. There were two cases of postoperative bleeding (11.1%) requiring reexploration and one case of mediastinitis (5.5%). Patient survival was 89% and neurodevelopmental testing was normal for all infants tested. Despite these data, the routine application of VADs for this indication in this patient population has not been utilized. With regard to VAD utilization in the setting of single ventricle myocardial failure, data are limited to case reports (Table 24-1).[26] In examining these reports, the median age at support was 4 years (1.3-14 years) with a median support of 11 days (5-179 days). There were morbidities (renal failure, neurologic injury)

Table 24-1. VAD utilization in pediatric patients with single ventricle anatomy (adapted from [26])

Case Reports	Age (y)	Surgical Procedure	Device	Duration of Support (days)	Outcome
Matsuda (1988)	10	Fontan	Toyobo	7	Death
Sadeghi (2000)	3	BT shunt	Toyobo	5	Death
Frazier (2005)	10	Fontan	Berlin Heart	7	Transplantation
Nathan (2006)	8	Fontan	BVS 5000	8	Transplantation
Calvaruso (2007)	4	Glenn	Berlin Heart	13	Death
Chu (2007)	4	Fontan	Berlin Heart	28	Transplantation (Death due to graft failure)
Russo (2008)	14	Fontan	Centrifugal pump + HeartMate I	45	Transplantation (ARF, HIT)
Pearse (2009)	1.3	BT shunt	Berlin Heart	49	Transplantation
Cardarelli (2009)	1.5	Fontan	Berlin Heart	179	Recovery (Neurologic injury)
Irving (2009)	2.9	Glenn	Berlin Heart	7	Transplantation

and a mortality rate of 40%. The application of VADs in the single ventricle population will continue to be explored.

Ventricular Assist Device Anticoagulation

Clinically significant thromboembolic events continue to be a devastating complication during VAD support. It remains difficult to characterize the true incidence of thromboembolic or hemorrhagic events with the multitude of different VAD systems, be they pulsatile or continuous flow pumps.[27-29] Despite monumental advances in mechanical circulatory support technology, the monitoring and management of coagulation in the presence of substantial foreign material remains an ongoing challenge. Furthermore, the peculiarity of hemostasis in children places these patients at increased risk of devastating complications even in the presence of standard anticoagulation regimes. For all patients, sepsis and other inflammatory states can greatly affect coagulation profiles, necessitating vigilant monitoring and adjustments of anticoagulation/antiplatelet (AC/AP) regimes. Current monitoring of AC/AP therapy has expanded

past activated clotting time (ACT) traditionally used for ECMO, to include antifactor Xa for unfractionated heparin levels, International Normalized Ratio (INR), Thromboelastograph (TEG®), and Platelet Mapping™. These tests are instrumental in providing the necessary information to monitor and adjust unfractionated heparin (UFH), low molecular weight heparin (LMWH), and antiplatelet therapy.

Preexisting coagulation abnormalities due to renal and hepatic dysfunction exacerbated by depletion of clotting factors secondary to cardiopulmonary bypass and altered rheological states all conspire to increase bleeding in the perioperative period. These considerations must be weighed with the risk of clot formation and thromboembolic events over time. As such, there have been a multitude of different algorithms for initiation and continuation of anticoagulants in VAD patients. Outlined below is a brief overview of the current recommendations for anticoagulation in four of the more commonly used pediatric and adult VADs including the Berlin Heart *EXCOR® Pediatric*, the HeartMate II, the Levitronix PediVAS® and CentriMag®, and the HeartWare (Table 24-2).

Table 24-2. Anticoagulation for VADs

Device	Anticoagulation	Anticoagulation Monitoring	Timing of Anticoagulation
Berlin Heart EXCOR Pediatric	Perioperative: UFH Long term: LMWH or warfarin and antiplatelet	UFH: antifactor-Xa level 0.35-0.5 U/ml LMWH: antifactor-Xa level 0.6-1 U/ml Warfarin: INR 2.5-3 Antiplatelet: TEG® monitoring	0-24 hrs: no anticoagulation >24-48 hrs: UFH >48 hrs: transition to LMWH or vitamin K antagonist* and ASA >4 days: dipyridamole ◊
HeartMate II	Perioperative: UFH Long term: warfarin and antiplatelet	UFH: aPTT 55-65s or 1.5-1.8 times normal Warfarin: INR 1.5-2	0-24 hrs: no anticoagulation >24 hrs: UFH >48 hrs: antiplatelet (ASA) Transition to warfarin
Levitronix	Heparin	aPTT 1.5-2 times normal ACT 180-200s	>6-12 hrs post-op and for duration of support
Heartware	Perioperative: UFH Long term: warfarin and antiplatelet	UFH: Warfarin: INR 2-2.5 Antiplatelet: TEG® monitoring	0-24 hrs: no anticoagulation >24 hrs: UFH >48 hrs: antiplatelet (ASA) No post op bleeding and enteral feeding, change to warfarin

UFH; unfractionated heparin, LMWH; low molecular weight heparin, ASA; acetylsalicylic acid,
* Vitamin K antagonist (warfarin) only used in children >1 year old with stable enteral nutrition
◊ Dipyridamole started if hemostatically stable, platelet count > 40,000/μL

Anticoagulation in Berlin Heart EXCOR®
Pediatric

The Edmonton Anticoagulation and Platelet Inhibition Guidelines for Pediatric VADs© is currently applied to the North American FDA Berlin Heart EXCOR® Pediatric trial. The guideline suggests no anticoagulation for the first 24 hours postimplantation, followed by the initiation of age appropriate dosing of intravenous UFH at 24 to 48 hours once bleeding has resolved and platelet count is >20,000/μl (Table 24-3). At 48 hours following surgery, a hemostatically and hemodynamically stable patient may be transitioned from UFH to LMWH (Enoxaparin™) (Table 24-4). In patients older than 12 months of age, oral anticoagulation therapy with a vitamin K antagonist can be initiated (target INR 2.7-3.5) once they are hemodynamically stable and receiving adequate enteral feeds. Patients younger than 12 months of age are unstable on oral anticoagulation regimes due to difficulties monitoring the warfarin effect secondary to multiple drug and diet interactions. Based on results of TEG® and Platelet Mapping™, acetylsalicylic acid may be started at 48 hours and dipyridamole at 4 days postimplantation if the patient is hemodynamically stable, with no bleeding and a platelet count greater than 40,000/μl (Table 24-5).

Despite adherence to these guidelines, there remains a significant risk of thromboembolic or hemorrhagic events. As such, not only is strict monitoring of coagulation profiles necessary, but vigilant surveillance of the pump and cannulas. In the initiation and transition stages of AC/AP therapy, frequent checking of the pump with a flashlight for any fibrin or clot formation must be done every few hours. Once the patient has stabilized, pump and cannula inspection

Table 24-3. Unfractionated Heparin (UFH) dosing at 24-48 hours post EXCOR Pediatric insertion

	≤ 12 months	≥ 12 months
Initial Dose[1]	15 IU/kg/hour	10 IU/kg/hour
After 6 hours[2]	28 IU/kg/hour	20 IU/kg/hour

[1]Criteria for UFH initiation
- Platelet count >20,000/μl
- Normal function on Platelet Mapping™ studies
- Minimal bleeding (<2ml/kg/day)

[2]6 hours after increase to therapeutic dose, obtain a PTT and anti-factor Xa level (desired range 0.35-0.7 U/ml or aPTT 1.5-2.5 times baseline if PTT correlates with anti-factor Xa, secondary target: TEG R_k 8-15 minutes)

Table 24-4. Low Molecular Weight Heparin (LMWH) at 48 hours post EXCOR Pediatric insertion

	≤ 3 months	≥ 3 months
LMWH dosing[1, 2]	1.5 mg/kg sc	1 mg/kg sc

[1]Criteria for LMWH initiation
- No bleeding
- Patient is hemodynamically stable
- Normal renal function (normal creatinine and urea)

[2]Stop UFH and administer subcutaneous (sc) LMWH with antifactor Xa 4 hours after second dose (therapeutic range 0.6-1 U/ml, secondary target: TEG R_k 8-15 mins)

can be completed twice daily. In the event of significant fibrin or clot formation, additional anticoagulation dosing may be given and consideration must be given to changing the pump depending on the location and size of the clot. Fibrin and clot formation tends to occur in areas of blood stasis and as such the valve leaflets are a nidus for growth. For LVADs, the presence of a clot in the pump dictates frequent neurologic monitoring and decreases the threshold for a pump change. Pump changes can be done quickly with relatively low risk in the intensive care unit under sedation, without the need for ventilatory support.

Anticoagulation for the HeartMate II

The HeartMate II is a continuous flow LVAD that has gained widespread acceptance due to its small size and ease of implantation. Furthermore, initial clinical results from the HeartMate II Pivotal BTT trial demonstrated survival rates of 75% at 6 months and 68% at 1 year.[30] The HeartMate II Pivotal BTT trial outlined an anticoagulation strategy that consisted of UFH within 12 to 24 hours following implantation. UFH was titrated using a goal PTT

of 45-50 seconds for the first 24 hours, 50-60 seconds for the second 24 hours and then 55-65 seconds thereafter. Antiplatelet therapy is initiated on postoperative day 2-3 with aspirin 81 mg and dipyridamole 75 mg three times daily. Following removal of thoracostomy tubes on postimplantation day 3-5, the UFH can be discontinued and transitioned to warfarin with target INR of 2-3.

The higher than expected frequency of hemorrhagic events, especially gastrointestinal bleeds, has resulted in reexamination of the anticoagulation regime.[31] Boyle et al. examined the risk of thromboembolic and hemorrhagic events in relation to the INR.[32] In the 331 patients discharged, thrombotic events occurred in only 3%, while bleeding related complications were present in 17.5%. The highest incidence of hemorrhagic events were at INR>2.5, with the lowest risk of thromboembolic events with INR> 1.5. The authors concluded that lowering the target INR to 1.5-2.5 might decrease the risk of devastating hemorrhagic complications while attenuating the risk for thromboembolism. Further insights into the effect of continuous flow devices on the coagulation cascade suggest that these changes to the anticoagulation

Table 24-5. Antiplatelet therapy post EXCOR Pediatric insertion

	Acetylsalicylic Acid	Dipyridamole
First Dose timing	> 48 hours	> 4 days
Dosing	1 mg/kg/day divided into 2 doses[1]	4 mg/kg/day divided into 4 doses[2]

[1]Criteria for Acetylsalicylic acid initiation
- No bleeding and hemodynamically stable
- Platelet Mapping™ does not show significantly decreased platelet function: net ADP G ≥ 4 and AA inhibition >70%
- Platelet count >40,000/μl
- TEG® MA >56 from a CKH sample

[2]Criteria for Dipyridamole initiation
- Platelet Mapping™ shows platelet inhibition in the presence of net ADP G > 4
- TEG® MA ≥ 72 mm from a CKH sample

regime alone may be insufficient. Acquired von Willbrand syndrome has been universally demonstrated in patients supported with continuous flow devices and predisposes them to increased morbidity during support and at time of transplantation.[33]

Anticoagulation for the Levitronix

The Levitronix CentriMag® and PediVAS® systems are continuous flow devices that can be used for left, right, and biventricular support in adults and children. The device is generally used for short to intermediate term support as a bridge to decision or bridge to bridge with the exchange to a longer term VAD. Furthermore, Levitronix can function as part of an ECMO circuit with the placement of an oxygenator. The suggested anticoagulation guidelines consist of UFH infusion starting 6-12 hours after cardiopulmonary bypass for implantation, in the presence of thoracostomy tube drainage less than 50 mL/hr or 2mL/kg/hr for 2-3 hours. Anticoagulation is titrated to maintain target ACTs 160-180 seconds and aPTT 1.3-1.6 times baseline. The target ACT and aPTT is increased by 5% per day to ACT of 190-210 and aPTT 1.5-1.8 times baseline by postimplantation day 4. An antiplatelet agent can be initiated after four days depending on the hemostatic conditions of the patient and the pump.

Anticoagulation for the HeartWare

The HeartWare is one of the newest mechanical circulatory support devices, with the purported advantages of being smaller and more durable than previous LVADs.[34] With a pump weight of only 140 grams, it is implanted within the pericardial space. The pump is a continuous flow impeller with communication to the external power and control panel via the driveline that is externalized through the abdominal wall. Similar to the HeartMate II, continuous anticoagulation is recommended and can be

tailored to specific patient risk factors. The initial multicenter evaluation of the HeartWare used an anticoagulation regime that consisted of UFH in the postoperatively once bleeding had decreased.[35] The UFH is titrated to increase aPTT to target of 50-60 seconds or an ACT of 140-160 seconds. Once the patient is hemodynamically stable and tolerating enteral nutrition, warfarin therapy is started with the discontinuation of UFH to maintain target INRs of 2-3. Antiplatelet therapy can be initiated with aspirin or clopidogrel. The initial clinical experience of 50 patients using this anticoagulation therapy demonstrated a relatively low incidence of thromboembolic events (two ischemic strokes) and higher frequency of bleeding complications (four hemorrhagic stroke, three deaths).[35] Bleeding events occurred most frequently in the perioperative setting and all were observed less than 30 days post implantation.

Conclusion

A variety of forms of mechanical circulatory support are available for children with cardiopulmonary dysfunction refractory to conventional management. These devices require extensive resources, both human and economic. Extracorporeal membrane oxygenation can be effectively used in a variety of settings to provide support to critically ill cardiac patients, particularly those with complex anatomy and/or univentricular circulation, and for rapid resuscitation. Careful patient selection and timing of intervention remain challenging. Special consideration should be given to pediatric cardiac patients with regard to anatomy, physiology, cannulation, and circuit management. Mechanical circulatory support in children has undergone a dramatic evolution with the advent of smaller VADs. Furthermore, the time dependent increase in complications associated with ECMO support and decade long plateau in cardiac allograft donor availability, coupled with emerging data of the superiority of VADs as long term support devices for recovery or bridge to transplant, vitalizes the need for continued and progressive application of this technology in critically ill patients with cardiac failure. In addition, ongoing research and refinement of anticoagulation strategies are necessary to prevent or limit the complications associated with VAD therapy.

References

1. Jacobs JP. Pediatric Mechanical Circulatory Support. In: Pediatric Cardiac Surgery, 3rd Edition, Chapter 45, Pages 778 - 792. Mavroudis C and Backer CL, editors, Mosby Inc., An affiliate of Elsevier, Philadelphia, Pennsylvania, 2003

2. Duncan BW. Pediatric Mechanical Circulatory Support. ASAIO 2005; 51: ix-xiv.

3. The July 2011 Extracorporeal Life Support Organization (ELSO) Extracorporeal Life Support (ECLS) Registry Report International Summary. Ann Arbor, Michigan, Extracorporeal Life Support Organization, 2011.

4. Duncan BW. Pediatric Mechanical Circulatory Support in the United States: Past, Present, and Future. ASAIO 2006; 52:525-9.

5. Blume ED, Naftel DC, Bastardi HJ et al. Outcomes of children bridged to heart transplantation with ventricular assist devices: a multi-institutional study. Circulation. 2006 May 16; 113(19):2313-9.

6. Fraser CD, Jr., Carberry KE, Owens WR, et al. Preliminary experience with the MicroMed DeBakey pediatric ventricular assist device. Semin Thorac Cardiovasc Surg Pediatr Card Surg Annu 2006; 9:109–114.\

7. Kilic A, Nolan TD, Li, T, et al. Early In Vivo Experience With the Pediatric Jarvik 2000 Heart. ASAIO 2007; 53:374-378.

8. Morales DL, Zafar F, Rossano JW, et al. Use of ventricular assist devices in children across the United States: analysis of 7.5 million pediatric hospitalizations. Ann Thorac Surg. 2010; 90(4): 1313-8; discussion 8-9.

9. Hetzer R, Potapov EV, Stiller B et al. Improvement in survival after mechanical circulatory support with pneumatic pulsatile ventricular assist devices in pediatric patients. Ann Thorac Surg. 2006; 82(3):917-24; discussion 924-5.

10. Arabia FA, Tsau PH, Smith RG, et al. Pediatric bridge to heart transplantation: application of the Berlin Heart, Medos and Thoratec ventricular assist devices. J Heart Lung Transplant. 2006; 25:16-21.

11. Schmid C, Debus V, Gogarten W, et al. Pediatric assist with the Medos and Excor systems in small children. ASAIO J. 2006; 52:505-8.

12. Kaczmarek I, Sachweh J, Groetzner J, et al. Mechanical circulatory support in pediatric patients with the MEDOS assist device. ASAIO J. 2005; 51:498-500.

13. Reinhartz O, Stiller B, Eilers R, et al. Current clinical status of pulsatile pediatric circulatory support. ASAIO 2002; 48:455-9.

14. Sharma M, Webber S, Morell V, et al. Ventricular Assist Device Support in Children and Adolescents as a Bridge to Heart Transplantation. Ann Thorac Surg 2006; 82:926-33.

15. Warnecke H, Berdjis F, Hennig E, et al. Mechanical left ventricular support as a bridge to cardiac transplantation in childhood. Eur J Cardiothorac Surg 1991; 5:330-3.

16. Hetzer R, Alexi-Meskishvilli V, Weng Y et al. Mechanical cardiac support in the young with the Berlin Heart EXCOR pulsatile ventricular assist device: 15 years' experience. Semin Thorac Cardiovasc Surg Pediatr Card Surg Ann 9:99-108, 2006.

17. Stiller B, Weng Y, Hubler M, et al. Pneumatic pulsatile ventricular assist devices in children under 1 year of age. Eur J Cardiothorac Surg 28:234–239, 2005.

18. Kirklin J. Mechanical Circulatory support as a bridge to Pediatric Cardiac Transplantation. Semin Thorac Cardiovasc Surg Pediatr Card Surg Ann 11:80-85, 2008.

19. EXCOR® Pediatric Clinical Update. Clinical Experience with EXCOR® Pediatric. Berlin Heart GhmB. January 2011.

20. Stiller B, Lemmer J, Schubert S, et al. Management of pediatric patients after implantation of Berlin Heart EXCOR ventricular assist device. ASAIO J. 2006 Sep-Oct; 52(5): 497-500.

21. Almond CS, Thiagarajan RR, Piercey GE, et al. Waiting list mortality among children listed for heart transplantation in the United States. Circulation. 2009; 119(5): 717-27.

22. Almond CS, Singh TP, Gauvreau K, et al. Extracorporeal Membrane Oxygenation for Bridge to Heart Transplantation Among Children in the United States. Analysis of Data From the Organ Procurement and Transplant Network and Extracorporeal Life Support Organization Registry. Circulation. 2011; 123: 2975-2984.

23. Imamura M, Dossey AM, Prodhan P, et al. Bridge to cardiac transplant in children: Berlin Heart versus extracorporeal membrane oxygenation. Ann Thorac Surg. 2009; 87(6): 1894-901; discussion 901.

24. Morales DL, Almond CS, Jaquiss RD, et al. Bridging children of all sizes to cardiac transplantation: the initial multicenter North American experience with the Berlin Heart EXCOR ventricular assist device. J Heart Lung Transplant. 2011; 30(1): 1-8.

25. Ungerleider RM, Shen I, Yeh T, et al. Routine Mechanical Ventricular Assist Following the Norwood Procedure—Improved Neurologic Outcome and Excellent Hospital Survival. Ann Thorac Surg 2004; 77:18-22.

26. VanderPluym CJ, Rebeyka IM, Ross DB, et al. The use of ventricular assist devices in pediatric patients with univentricular hearts. J Thorac Cardiovasc Surg 2011; 141:588-90.

27. Kirklin JK, Naftel DC, Kormos RL, et al. Third INTERMACS Annual Report: The evolution of destination therapy in the United States. J Heart Lung Transplant 2011; 30:115-23.

28. Goldstein DJ, Beauford RB. Left ventricular assist devices and bleeding: adding insult to injury. Ann Thorac Surg 2003; 75(6 Suppl): S42-7.

29. Reilly MP, Wiegers SE, Cucchiara AJ, et al. Frequency, risk factors and clinical outcomes of left ventricular assist device-associated ventricular thrombus. Am J Cardiol 2000; 86:1156-9, A10.

30. Miller LW, Pagani FD, Russell SD et al. Use of a continuous-flow device in patients awaiting heart transplantation. N Engl J Med 2007;357:885-96.

31. Crow S, John R, Boyle A, et al. Gastrointestinal bleeding rates in recipients of nonpulsatile and pulsatile left ventricular assist device. J Thorac Cardiovasc Surg 2009; 137:208-15.

32. Boyle AJ, Russell SD, Teuteberg JJ, et al. Low Thromboembolism and Pump Thrombosis With The HeartMate II Left Ventricular Assist Device: Analysis of Outpatient Anti-Coagulation. J Heart Lung Transplant 2009; 28:881-7.

33. Uriel N, Pak S, Jorde UP, et al. Acquired von Willebrand Syndrome After Continous-Flow Mechanical Deice Support Contributed to a High Prevalence of Bleeding During Long-Term Support and at the Time of Transplantation. J Am Coll Cardiol 2010; 56:1207-13.

34. Larose JA, Tamez DL, Ashenuga M, Reyes C. Design concepts and principle of operation of the HeartWare ventricular assist system. ASAIO J 2010; 56:285-9.

35. Strueber M, O'Driscoll G, Jansz P, et al. Multicenter Evaluation of an Intrapericardial Left Ventricular Assist System. J Am Coll Cardiol 2011; 57:1375-82.

Chapter 25

Plasmapheresis

Jeffrey B. Sussmane MD, Shayan Vyas MD

Introduction

Plasmapheresis is a term used interchangeably for a variety of clinical applications that refer to the removal, exchange, modification, or filtration a circulating blood component. This may be done with or without the returning of a blood component. The term "aphaeresis" is derived from the Greek work "to take away." The goal of plasmapheresis is to modify or remove unique circulating substances in blood.

Therapeutic Plasma Exchange (TPE) is the most frequent "pheresis" immunomodulatory therapy performed. The therapy is provided to improve a clinical condition by concomitantly removing and replacing the circulating plasma. Therapeutic cytapheresis is the removal of a specific circulating cellular component. Erythrocytapheresis is the removal of red blood cells and the return of predetermined replacements fluid, most commonly donor RBCs. Plateletpheresis (thrombocytopheresis) is the therapeutic removal of platelets. Leukopheresis is the removal of white blood cells and includes Leukodepletion which is employed for the removal of pathologic numbers of circulating white blood cells. Leukopheresis also commonly refers to peripheral pleuripotential stem cell collection which is performed to remove specific CD +34 progenitor monocytes from peripheral blood for the storage and reinfusion during the process of bone marrow transplantation (TPE). The application of TPE includes autoimmune/rheumatic, infection, inflammatory, metabolic, neurological, oncologic, toxicologic, or renal diseases.[1-7] In this chapter, we will discuss the theory, science, and practice of different therapeutic apheresis therapies available. We will also discuss the application as it applies to ECMO.

Historical Perspective

Huang Di, the "Yellow Emperor" of China, in the middle of the third millennium BCE, first introduced the concept of balancing circulating "forces" within the body to promote health and treat disease in perhaps the greatest text on Internal Medicine "The Huangdi Neijing" or "The Inner Canon of the Yellow Emperor".[8] The Yellow Emperor is believed to have lived until the age of 100, attained immortality after his physical death, and is the Father of Traditional Chinese Medicine.[8]

Hippocrates, known as the "Father of Modern Medicine," also believed in balancing forces. He taught that health is good when the four humours; blood, yellow bile, black bile, and phlegm, are in balance. He taught that these fluids occur in naturally equal proportion (pepsis) in healthy adults. [9,10] The Greek physician Galen also believed that when the four humours were not in balance, a person would become ill and therapy was directed towards restoring this balance.[11]

Therapeutic techniques dealing with blood-letting were mastered by the barber-surgeons, during the Middle Ages (500-1500 ACE), while classic surgeons shunned away from this practice.[12] In fact, the barber's pole is a symbol which represents the stick which was gasped by the patient to promote bleeding. The white stripe represents the white tourniquet and red strip represents the blood flowing out of the patient.[13] Bloodletting was considered one the oldest medical practices among the records of Western ancient people including the Meso-potamians, Egyptians, Greeks, and Mayans.[13] Historians believe that America's first president, George Washington died of sepsis and dehydra-tion while undergoing bloodletting and suffer-ing from mercury toxicity (calomel treatment) while his physician was trying to cure him of what most likely was laryngotrachetitis or pos-sibly even epiglottitis.[13,14] Regardless of the historical origins of either balancing "forces" or "humours" or bloodletting, the basic concepts of modifying circulating blood components have been in promoted by the founders of medical practice for at least 4000 years.

Plasmapheresis finally entered the world of modern medicine and was recorded by John J Abel's "Plasma Removal with return of cor-puscles (Plasmapheresis)" in 1914.[15] He aptly described the process of separating and col-lecting large amounts of plasma from a donor dog's blood and returning red blood cells to the donor dog. In 1944, Co Tui et al, showed that frequent plasmapheresis of donors could meet the demand for plasma to cope with wartime emergencies.[16] The first therapeutic plasmapher-esis trial in the United States occurred in 1952 to control the hyperviscosity associated with multiple myeloma.[17]

In 1965, a collaboration between the IBM corporation and the National Cancer Institu-tion gave rise to the first continuous flow cell separator. This development occurred shortly after Judith Pool discovered cryoprecipitate or Factor VIII concentration, which allowed for the commercialization of fresh frozen plasma.[18] By the mid 1970s plasmapheresis was used to effectively treated Goodpasture's Disease and Myasthenia Gravis.[19,20] During the mid 70s to the late 1980s, almost any disorder with an immune component, over 90 diseases, was treated with plasma exchange.[21-23] During the late 1980s, Great Britain attempted to correct their national blood product shortage with the introduction of automated apheresis machine donation programs.[24] Modern technologies now allow plasmapheresis to be in every intensive care unit (ICU) and become a practical con-sideration in appropriate clinical situations.[25-28]

We began aggressive immunomodulatory therapy for the establishment of homeostasis, for sepsis with plasmapheresis in 1994.[29] Plasma-pheresis for sepsis has been well described.[30,34] The recently renamed peak concentration theory of sepsis now nicely frames the application of plasmapheresis.[35] This 4000 year old theory of partially removing soluble mediators of inflammation has gained renewed widespread attention because the mortality from sepsis for hospitalized children in the United States is still >10 percent.[36] We have provided over 275 plasmapheresis treatments during the five days of acute illness with a mortality of <1%.[29]

Physiology

The goal of plasmapheresis is the removal of immune-modulating molecules from the plasma such as pathogenic autoantibodies, im-mune complexes, cryoglobulins, myeloma light chains, endotoxin, and cholesterol-containing lipoproteins.[3,29,37-41] The apheresis removal of molecules, dependant on the therapeutic mo-dality, relies on the molecular size, volume of distribution, rate of synthesis and metabolism. The acute rate of removal of intravascular molecules during apheresis must exceed the rate of acute synthesis and metabolism of that molecule. The extravascular space serves as a reservoir for these molecules and contributes to the total body concentration. The plasma volume may be calculated (estimated plasma volume, or EPV) from the patient's weight and hematocrit using the formula,

$$EPV = (0.065 \times weight (kg)) \times (1\text{-hematocrit})$$

The removal of plasma volume molecules may be estimated by the application of first order kinetics:

$$X_1 = X_0 e^{-VeEPV}$$

Where X_1 equals the final concentration, X_0 equals the initial concentration, V_e equals the volume exchanged[42], or more simply,

$$\text{Residual volume concentration} = e^{-v/V}$$

Where v equals the total volume exchanged and V equals the patient's plasma volume.[43] Any calculation will be off by up to 10% based on the partial recirculation of a double lumen catheter. A single exchange model will decrease concentrations by 63% and a 1.4 exchange is calculated to reduce concentrations by 75%.[40-43] While the ancient concept of apheresis remains clear, science is just beginning to quantify the mechanisms of action. TPE is a rational therapeutic choice if the substance to be removed has a sufficiently long half-life, so that extracorporeal removal is much more rapid than endogenous clearance pathways, and must be acutely toxic and resistant to conventional therapy, so that the rapid elimination from the extracellular fluid by TPE is indicated.[41-44]

The efficacy of treatment may be measured by a reduction in concentration of pathologic and toxic substances such as proinflammatory cytokines.[41-45] The majority of immunoglobulin M, D, and fibrinogen (75%) remain in the intravascular space, thus a larger proportion of the body's IgM and fibrinogen will be removed with apheresis. Albumin, immunoglobulin G, A, and C_3 complement are equally found in the intravascular and extravascular space (47%-60%), thus less will be proportionally removed during an individual treatment.[41-43] The volume of distribution based on molecule size will also contribute to the amount of molecules removed. Based on a single-volume of the estimated plasma exchange and the continuous apheresis method (approximately 40mL/kg), 63% of the IgM and IgG levels from the intravascular compartment will be removed whereas whole body IgM and IgG will be reduced 47% and 28%, respectively. If the plasma exchange is increased to 1.5 times the estimated intravascular plasma volume, IgM and IgG levels will fall by 78%, while whole body IgM levels will fall to 59% and IgG 35% per treatment.[41-43] The extravascular to intravascular equilibration of a large molecular weight substance is relatively slow (approximately 1% to 3% per hour),[41-43] thus serum and total body levels of target substances such as IgM and IgG can be predicted to reach complete equilibration between the extravascular space and intravascular space within a 48 hr period from each plasmapheresis treatment. A 70% absolute reduction for a pathologic autoantibody requires at least three treatments, whereas four cycles of repetitive single-exchange plasma would be required to deplete whole body IgM, and 6-7 cycles to deplete whole body IgG. If the exchange volume is increased to 1.5 volume exchanges then 3-5 cycles are needed to remove 85-90 % of intravascular and whole body IgM and IgG. Intravascular targets are thus more readily removed whereas solutes in the extravascular space require somewhat larger exchange volumes and increased cycles.[46,47] Intravascular molecules present during the onset of the therapy will have a reduced immunomodulatory effect with a lower volume and fewer cycles compared to molecules that are primarily extravascular.[46,47]

Apheresis Procedure

In general, the apheresis machine utilizes a pump to pull the patient's blood from the venous circulation, and a second pump to immediately mix the blood with anticoagulant before it enters the separation system. The blood is than separated into components based on density or filtered by molecular size. The separated substances can either be removed or modified before the blood is returned to the patient (Figure 25-1). The technique varies by each condition, which will determine specific therapies and will vary based on the type of machine. The specific therapy will determine what is removed, what is modified and the fluid or donor blood product that is chosen to be used as a replacement.

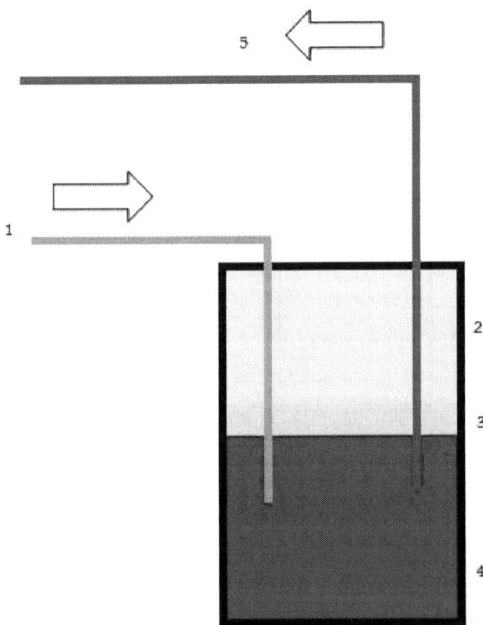

Figure 25-1. Plasmapheresis. Whole blood enters the centrifuge (1) and separates into plasma (2), leukocytes (3), and erythrocytes (4). Depending on the process, selected components are then returned to the patient (5). Remaining components are removed from the patient.

Apheresis machines use either a centrifuge or a semipermeable filter membrane for separation. The centrifuge cell separator device is the most commonly used in most institutions in the US and Canada. Whereas in Asia and Europe, membrane filter apheresis is more common.[48-53]

Continuous centrifugation apheresis uses a blood separator that relies on the different densities and specific gravities of each blood component. The centrifugation process separates the plasma by densities. Whole blood constituents are layered into plasma (specific gravity (SG) 1.025-1.109), platelets (SG 1.040), lymph (SG 1.070), granulocytes (SG 1.087-1.082), and red blood cells (SG 1.093-1.069). The patient blood is withdrawn and is driven into a semi-rigid, ring-shaped plastic tubing pack. These tubing packs are specific for each individual therapy. Each tubing pack is specifically designed to collect unique components of the blood. The tubing pack is placed in a centrifuge which applies a centrifugal force to the blood. This centrifugal force separates the blood into layers, primarily as a consequence of specific gravity. The heaviest blood component, erythrocytes, are forced to the outside layer. Cushioned in the middle is the lighter cell and particulate layer, the "buffy coat" primarily composed of leukocytes, and the lightest blood component, plasma, layers into the inside of the separation chamber. Each therapeutically unique tubing pack collects these elements separately for therapeutic manipulation. Common components of blood with their densities and molecular sizes are listed in Table 25-1.

Centrifugal TPE utilizes optical sensors to detect each layer interface, minimizing contamination of each cell and fluid layer. The desired components are automatically removed to collection bags and the remaining blood components, along with appropriate replacement fluids, are returned to the patient. Rotary peristaltic pumps automatically control the amount of blood pumped from the patient, the amount of the component sent to the collection bag, the specific amount of anticoagulant, and (when programmed) the appropriate constitution of reinfused fluids. Warmers can be added to the circuit to warm replacement fluid and prevent hypothermia. This is generally unnecessary with a functioning heat exchanger during ECMO, as these fluids are entered preheat exchanger. Most apheresis machines also have the capability of selecting the percentage of fluids for automatic reinfusion. This is done in direct proportion to the percentage of fluid removed, thus decreasing the possibility of the patient developing hypovolemia or hypervolemia. Multiple audiovisual alarms alert the operator to potential problems.

Discontinuous centrifugation apheresis is a less commonly used apheresis procedure. In this technique, blood is pumped from the patient into a balloon-like processing unit. Inside the processing unit, a transparent bell-shaped bowl rotates to produce a centrifuge. As the blood components separate by density, plasma is separated away from the bowl and red blood cells accumulate in the bowl. The standard bowl has a capacity of 350 ml. Once the bowl is filled with red blood cells, the processing stops and the red blood cells are returned to the patient. Bowl capacity sizes can be changed to accommodate special circumstances. Patients with cardiovascular instability, in particular, cannot tolerate these large changes in intravascular blood volumes during collection.

Apheresis can also occur utilizing a semipermeable filter membrane which separates whole blood from plasma based on the difference in solute size. The semipermeable filter is composed of hollow porous fibers that are wrapped in a plastic cylinder. The filter's pores vary in size from to 0.6 µm to as small as 0.2 µm. This allows all liquid blood products to pass through except for plasma's cellular components (see Table 25-1). This technique performs well for specific plasma filtration scenarios but is reliant upon the filter pore size.[54,55]

Table 25-1. Blood Components. (Kaplan AA: A Practical Guide to Therapeutic Plasma Exchange, Blackwell Science, Maiden MA 1999)

Protein	Concentration (mg/dl)	MW x 103 d	Intravascular (%)	Fractional Turnover Rate (%/d)	Half-life (d)
IgG	12	150	45	7	22
IgM	0.9	950	78	19	5
IgA	2.5	160	42	25	6
IgE	0.0001	190	45	94	2.5
Albumin	45	66	44	11	17
C3	1.4	240	67	41	2
Fibrinogen	3-4	340	81	24	4.2
Factor VIII	0.1	100-340	71	150	0.6
Antithromin III	0.2	56-58	45	55	2.4
Lipoprotein Cholesterol	1.5-2.0	1300	>90	*	35
Endotoxin	3.25x10-7	100-2400	>50	*	*
Immune Complexes	>300	>50	*	*	*
Tumor necrosis factor	3-5 x 10-7	50	<50	*	6-20min

*Highly variable

This semipermeable filter technique relies on adequate blood flow from the patient, which necessitates the use of central venous access. The filter's pores are limited and can only resist certain transmembrane pressure forces. When the pores exceed maximum transmembrane pressure force, the pores rupture, causing separated blood components to mix with the filtered plasma components. Depending on molecular size, very large immune-complexes may not get filtered by the pores. All of these techniques can be added in-line with any extracorporeal therapy, such as ECMO or CRRT (continuous renal replacement therapy). Affinity columns can be added inline with these techniques. The separated plasma passes through the affinity columns that contain specific proteins that have a high affinity to certain antigens within the plasma. These antigens are trapped and removed from the plasma. There are two types of affinity columns approved by the FDA though they are not currently being manufactured in the U.S.

Apheresis techniques require the replacement of the fluids that are being removed. The replacement fluids include normal saline, donated blood products such as fresh frozen plasma, albumin, or red blood cells, e,g., patients with sickle cell anemia commonly require red blood cell exchange. These patient's predominantly sickled red blood cells are filtered out and retransfused with donor, sickle cell-free, red blood cells.

Vascular Access

Adequate vascular access is a prerequisite during apheresis. The choice of vascular catheters depends upon the type of pheresis procedure. For example, access flows of only 35-50 mL/min are required for the centrifugal exchange and can be obtained from a large-bore peripheral venous catheter. Apheresis using the semipermeable membrane technique requires blood flow >100 mL/min. This requires larger central venous access in most patients. Intermittent or discontinuous apheresis techniques require single large venous cannulation whereas continuous apheresis requires two large peripheral catheters or a double lumen catheter. Pheresis catheters may be the same catheter used for dialysis or CRRT. We recommend an age-appropriately sized double lumen hemodialysis catheter for continuous apheresis placed in the femoral vein (Table 25-2). Multiple manufacturers make catheters of different size and length. In regards to the length of the catheter, the closer the tip to the right atrium, the better the flow.

We traditionally use the femoral vein for central venous access in the pediatric population due to the highest success rate for insertion, lowest rate of complications, and largest acceptable vein site for small children. One may also use the subclavian or internal jugular veins for access, especially in larger or heavily sedated patients.

Table 25-2. Central Femoral Venous Catheter size for patient's weight.

Patient Weight	Size of Apheresis/Hemofiltration Catheter
<10 kg	4 or 5 French double-lumen
10-15 kg	6.5-7 French double-lumen
15-23 kg	8 French double-lumen
24-49 kg	10-11.5 French double-lumen
>50 kg	12 French double-lumen

Circuit Priming

The fluid status of the patient needs to be carefully evaluated. The goal is to leave the patient in a fluid balance range between 75-125% of calculated baseline. Introducing more or less than 25% of the circuit volume may have cardiovascular consequences. The Cobe Spectra® machine default volume level is 100% baseline (no net increase or decrease). Older Cobe ® Spectra circuits require 345 ml to prime. The circulating internal volume is 150 ml and the residual or rinse-back volume is 195 ml. Crystalloid prime is often used for children larger than 45 kg. Colloid prime is recommended for children 20 to 45 kg. Blood prime may be ordered by the physician for any child. Children less than 20 kg often require one unit of crossmatched, CMV negative, irradiated, leukodepleted blood to prime the apheresis circuit. The 20 kg child may have approximately 14% dilution from the circuit volume, which may consequently be primed with blood to minimize the dilutional effects of priming. These packed red blood cells will prevent further dilution of the hematocrit and anemia, as well as possible hypovolemia. There are newer circuits primed with less than 100 ml and circulating less than 50 ml. These circuits may allow crystalloid priming for children greater than 10 kg.

The calculation of fluid utilized for priming (blood priming) is dependent on physician preference. Blood priming with reconstituted blood (fresh frozen plasma [FFP] with RBCs) may be considered. This should be considered when the extracorporeal volume is large relative to the patient, such as a neonate, and when the hematocrit is desired to be higher than baseline. Blood priming is not a consistently reliable method for keeping the hematocrit normal or high, or to maintain coagulation factor levels. Managing the hematocrit for an anemic, fluid-overloaded, or volume intolerant patient, may require RBCs and become the component of choice for priming. If rinse-back is given when the procedure is programmed to leave the patient at 100% balance, then the patient will be an additional 195 cc positive at the end of the procedure. One should not rinse-back at the end of a procedure unless there is a need to increase the patient's volume or to return RBCs. The recorded values can be subtracted from final run values to measure total volume given.

The decision to utilize FFP or fractionated human albumin as priming and replacement fluid should be made clinically, based on the immunologic, protein, pulmonary, and cardiovascular condition of the child. Crystalloid solutions (normal saline) and colloid solutions (albumin or FFP) may be utilized alone or in combination. The risk of transfusion and physiologic complications increases with the use of foreign protein, but children with unstable or suboptimal physiology often benefit from the use of a combination of FFP and fractioned human albumin. Fresh frozen plasma is the replacement of choice if coagulation factors are depleted; however, administration requires immunologic compatibility and carries an increased risk of exposure to foreign protein. Albumin is less immuno-reactive than FFP and will not lower the colloid oncotic pressure during repeated therapies. Crystalloid alone should be reserved for larger patient and conditions that do not require repeated courses of apheresis. In patients undergoing multiple runs, albumin, colloid oncotic pressure, and Ig G should be measured as a minimum.

Anticoagulation

Anticoagulation is required in the apheresis process to prevent the extracorporeal circuit from clotting. The most common anticoagulant used is buffered acid-citrate-dextrose (ACD) or Anticoagulant Citrate Dextrose Solution for centrifuge apheresis. Unfractionated heparin is the most common anticoagulant used for the membrane plasma separation method. The anticoagulation agent used is added to the patient's blood as it enters the extracorporeal circuit and most of it is removed during the apheresis process, thus reducing the systemic anticoagulation effect.

The half-life of citrate is 30 minutes and it is readily metabolized in the liver. Citrate (trisodium citrate) anticoagulation proprieties occur by acting as a mild chelating agent on free circulating ionized calcium, thus lowing extracorporeal ionized calcium levels. Calcium functions as a cofactor required to form tenase and prothrombinase complexes. It also mediates the binding of the complexes via the terminal gamma-carboxy residues on factor X and factor IXa to the phospholipids surface expressed on platelets. Non-protein bound calcium or normal ionized calcium's levels are 1.1–1.4 mmol/L. Citrate will cause metabolic acidosis if the citrate metabolism is reduced in the liver or an excess is given.

Heparin is most commonly used for membrane plasma separation techniques but may be used in centrifuged apheresis. Heparin produces its major anticoagulant effect by activating antithrombin III, thus reducing the conversion of prothrombin to thrombin. Heparin also activates factor Xa through an antithrombin-dependent mechanism. When using heparin, activated clotting time (ACT) levels or partial thromboplastin times (PTT) are monitored. A goal of maintaining ACT levels between 160 and 180 seconds is adequate using an iSTAT ® device. Apheresis removes most protein-bound and free heparin. Our institution uses ACD when the patient is not on ECMO.

Platelet consumption or reduced activity of circulating platelets may occur with repeated plasmapheresis therapies. Close monitoring of the platelet count, PT, PTT, magnesium, ionized calcium, fibrinogen, antithrombin III, and heparin levels are important as the number of exchanges and exchanged plasma volume increases. One must be aware of the side effects associated with anticoagulation. Patients undergoing apheresis are often very sick and have an increased risk of bleeding. The risk of bleeding vs. clotting the extracorporeal circuit must always be balanced. The ECMO patient is systemically anticoagulated and additional anticoagulation is not needed during plasmapheresis, but careful monitoring and the increase risk for bleeding is inherent.

Selected Indications for Plasmapheresis

See Table 25-3.

Apheresis in the ECMO patient

For the patient on ECMO, TPE is performed in the ICU by individuals who are ECMO-certified or under the direct supervision of an ECMO specialist. The direct supervision of a qualified ECMO physician is also necessary. The patient's weight, sex, height, hematocrit, and procedure-specific information are programmed into the machine software and the machine is wheeled next to the ECMO circuit. A unique TPE circuit is loaded into a centrifugal machine for each therapy. The appropriate prescribed fluids are connected to the TPE and the circuit is primed automatically by the specific software program chosen for each therapy. Alternatively, commercial CRRT machines with plasma filters may be used. Replacement fluids, anticoagulant, and priming solutions are dependent on the patient's size and underlying illness. Newborns and smaller children <20 kgs will require blood priming. Access to the systemic circulation is drawn directly from the ECMO circuit without interruption or alteration of ECMO flow. One common configuration is where venous access is connected to the prebladder/venous/prepump ECMO circuit via a pigtail connection, and the arterial return line is connected after the venous access and before the bladder/pump via a pigtail connection although, similar to CRRT and ECMO, there is no one correct circuit configuration. Once the TPE circuit is connected to the ECMO circuit, blood is pumped into the machine via the peristaltic pumps. Additional anticoagulant may be automatically calculated and added as the blood enters the centrifuge. In some centers, the systemic anticoagulation provided by the heparin in the ECMO circuit suffices and no further anticoagulant is needed. A fully heparinized ECMO circuit may negate the need for additional anticoagulation. Heparin-bonded or other coated ECMO circuits may affect the anticoagulation necessary for the TPE circuit. The need for additional or alternative anticoagulation should be evaluated for each patient and each therapy.

Apheresis is indicated when there is an acute clinical need to separate blood components. Once maintained, the parallel apheresis circuit does not affect ECMO circuit flows. Once therapy is stabilized the ECMO flows will

Table 25-3. Indications for Plasmapheresis (ASFA: American Society for Apheresis)

Disease	ASFA Category	Disease	ASFA Category
ABO Incompatible Hematopoetic Progenitor Cell Transplantation	II	Heart Transplant Rejection	III
ABO Incompatible Solid Organ Transplantation	II (kidney, heart [infants]) III (liver)	Hemolytic Uremic Syndrome; Thrombotic Microangiopathy; and Transplant Associated Microangiopathy	III (aHUS, TMA, TAM) IV (Pediatric, diarrheal)
Acute Disseminated Encephalomyelitis	III	Hyperleukocytosis	I (Leukostasis)
Acute Liver Failure	III	Hypertriglyceridemic Pancreatitis	III
Acute Inflammatory Demyelinating Polyneuropathy (Guillain-Barré Syndrome)	I	Idiopathic Thrombocytopenic Purpura	IV
ANCA-Associated Rapidly Progressive Glomerulonephritis (Wegener's Granulomatosis)	II	Malaria	II (severe)
Anti-Glomerular Basement Membrane Disease (Goodpasture's Syndrome)	I	Multiple Sclerosis	II (Acute CNS inflammatory demyelinating disease)
Autoimmune Hemolytic Anemia (Warm Autoimmune Hemolytic Anemia; Cold Agglutinin Disease)	III WAIHA III CAD	Myasthenia Gravis	I
Catastrophic Antiphospholipid Syndrome	III	Overdose and Poisoning	II (mushroom poisoning) III (other compounds)
Chronic Inflammatory Demyelinating Polyradiculoneuropathy	I	Paraneoplastic Neurologic Syndromes	III
Cryoglobulinemia	I	Sepsis	III
Focal Segmental Glomerulosclerosis	III (primary) II (recurrent)	Thrombotic Thrombocytopenic Purpura	I

remain unchanged. The initial "total" ECMO circuit compliance and capacitance may transiently change during the initiation of apheresis. If the ECMO venous drainage is unrecognized as borderline or marginal, the venous pressure alarm may sound ("chirp"), suggesting an acute decrease in venous return. The servo regulation of the pump may also suddenly reduce ECMO flow. This may require additional volume boluses during initiation of apheresis. The apheresis circuit will also add 195 ml of dilution to the existing circuit, which may affect circulating levels of therapeutic drugs in small volume circuits for small babies. The apheresis protocol and software from the manufacturer should be followed for continued maintenance of the separation therapy. Unique conditions may require manual programming of the device, or overriding specific parameters. The scope and nature of every unique scenario is beyond the scope of this chapter. If these occur, it may be best to acquire additional expertise from the manufacturer or a more experienced center before beginning therapy.

Provider Responsibilities

- Verify procedure with apheresis/ECMO specialist, physician, and family
- Assist in explaining indication, procedure, and risks to family
- Record patient height, weight, hematocrit, and indication
- Send baseline preprocedure labs- CBC, iCa, and electrolytes (notify physician of results).
- Labs for specific procedures (notify physician of results).
- TSM (red cell exchange)
- CD34+, disease markers and HIV (need consent), for peripheral blood stem cell harvest
- Specific disease markers and HIV (need consent)
- Antiinflammatory panels

- Extra labs for multiple procedures (notify physician of results)
- Mg & PO4 & iCa
- PT/PTT
- FDP, Fibrinogen
- IgG
- Standby emergency replacement fluid (PRBC's, Albumin, FFP, NS)
- Connect apheresis access line (using sterile and airless technique) to venous pigtail close to patient (pre-bladder)
- Connect apheresis return line (using sterile and airless technique) to any of the venous pigtails downstream from access line and pre-raceway
- Halfway through procedure, or if symptomatic for hypocalcaemia, send iCa (notify physician of results)
- Monitor ACTs; if decision to utilize citrate, adjustments in heparin may be necessary
- If patient deteriorates, stop apheresis immediately, notify physician STAT and follow ECLS protocol.
- When procedure is completed, disconnect apheresis access and return line (using sterile and airless technique) and flush pigtails with 1 cc NS and place port cap on site
- Postprocedure send: iCa, Mg , electrolytes, and PT/PTT postprocedure prn (notify physician of results)
- Antiinflammatory panel

Specific humoral considerations of Therapeutic Apheresis

The manipulation of removing, diluting, and returning foreign plasma components initiates an immune response which can be seen in the elevation of all major circulating immune complexes 1-3 hours post treatment. There is an immediate serum elevation of complement, including C3a, C4a, C5a, and an increase in the total number of circulating granulocytes and macrophages within the first two treatments. Lymphocytes increase in treatment three and the

T helper/suppressor ratio increase in treatment four. The aggressive use of IgG concomitant with TPE has been widely reported for pre-transplant patients and for blood group incompatibilities incurred with transplantation and rejection.[56] The progressive decrease in serum concentrations of circulating normal immunomodulatory molecules must be considered for all extended therapies. The significant reduction of circulating immunoglobulins during repeated procedures utilizing only albumin as replacement deserves specific attention. Circulating inflammatory mediators are widely recognized as contributing to the morbidity and mortality of certain clinical conditions. This is the predominant pathophysiologic condition during sepsis and the application of plasmapheresis has been directly shown to improve outcome in select patient populations and reduce the "humoral" imbalance.[9,56-63] Apheresis also appears to mobilize CD34[+] cells from extravascular depots in peripheral blood stem/progenitor cell (PBSC) donors, resulting in collection of more than twice as many CD34[+] cells than estimated based on preapheresis peripheral blood cell count.[64] This may play a role in the acute inflammatory response.

Care of the apheresis patient

TPE treatments are usually from one to three hours in duration. They may be ordered once a day or every other day, for a period of 3-14 days. The number of treatments is dependent upon patient response and can usually be established after the completion of the first two treatments. Improved lab values and clinical status will become apparent for the rapid responder within the first 24 hours. Repeated therapies for conditions that are slowly responding should be cycled every four to seven treatments with a day or two without TPE. This will minimize the depletion of endogenous healthy circulating cofactors. Replacement of many cofactors may be carried out utilizing FFP and should be utilized for extended therapies. Specific cofactors may need to be measured and replaced as needed. Many centers routinely measure IgG levels and replace accordingly. Careful monitoring of inflammatory mediators, coagulation profiles, protein, and immunoglobulins will trace improvement and depletion of cofactors.

It is important to calculate the plasma volume to exchange. One blood volume plasma exchange will replace 63% of the circulating blood volume or toxin. A two blood volume plasma exchange will remove 86%. Single volume exchanges are typically performed, better tolerated, and successful when repeated after a day or two time delay. TPE can be performed on an either daily or every other day profile depending on the indication. The typical total course for sepsis is four to ten treatments. Many centers will increase this to fourteen treatments for sepsis, although supporting data is not available. Unpublished data from Miami Children's Hospital (MCH) typically will provide five to seven treatments that successfully treat the rapid responders. We will institute a two day holiday before proceeding with additional treatments for slow responders, as all plasma and protein bound substances are readily removed during TPE and need to be reconstituted. The initial TPE calculation commonly recommends that a one and one half (1½) blood volume exchange is appropriate. Although many centers continue to perform single volume exchanges for consecutive treatment we perform 1½ volume exchanges throughout the TPE therapy for the sicker patients. It should be noted that the plasma volume calculated includes the plasma volume of the patient and the plasma volume of the extracorporeal ECMO circuit.

Sedation

The care for any patient receiving plasmapheresis depends on the patient's age, underlying condition, and cooperation. Conscious sedation is rarely required for a pheresis run.

It has been our experience that cooperation from the patient allows the pheresis operator the ability to concentrate more on the process rather than issues with the pheresis catheter and pheresis machine.

Uncooperative patients uncommonly may require conscious sedation to allow for an easier and, more importantly, complete pheresis run. We often use sedatives such as dexmedetomidine hydrochloride or chloride hydrate when sedation is necessary in our institution's PICU.

ECMO patients are traditionally sedated, which in turn allows the operator to concentrate more on the pheresis process.

Patients rarely experience pain during the process, other than catheter placement.

Psychosocial

Plasmapheresis is often well received by families and patients when the purpose and benefits are fully explained before the process. Practitioners should attempt to understand the patient's education, cultural, and religious background prior to discussing pheresis. It is imperative to explain the process to the family (and the patient), both before and during pheresis. At our institution, the ordering physician explains the processes in detail and obtains written consent prior to placing the apheresis catheter and placing the patient on the pheresis machine.

Furthermore, educational handouts, quantitative surveys, posters and child life specialists help both patients and parents become more comfortable with the pheresis process.

Cardiorespiratory considerations

Sudden decreases in preload, acute changes in peripheral vascular resistance, and alteration of right ventricular compliance may occur from both the exposure to the extracorporeal circuit and volume shifting. The initiation of any extracorporeal circuit must take into consideration the underlying right and left ventricular lusitropic and inotropic states, as well as the peripheral vascular resistance. Ventilated ECMO patients who are marginally preload-dependent may suffer a decrease in pulmonary blood flow and left ventricular pressure. Larger patients generally respond to flow adjustments and volume replacement with solutions containing protein, rarely requiring additional inotropic support. Warming of the replacement fluids can help prevent complications such as hypothermia and "sickling" in susceptible patients. There is no evidence of a primary change in pulmonary compliance or of alteration in gas exchange, but there may be a sudden change in peripheral vascular resistance from exposure to foreign surfaces, usually amenable to volume infusion. There may be an improvement in left ventricular function after therapy with the reduction of circulating mediators, seen more commonly in gram-negative sepsis.[65]

Metabolic

The most frequently encountered electrolyte disturbances and complications result from abnormalities in ionized calcium when citrate is used as an additional anticoagulant. Hypocalcaemia is most frequently seen in patients with severe liver dysfunction, those receiving FFP, or during procedures with a high citrate to whole blood ratio.[45,60] Children should also be observed for complications of hypokalemia as a result of citrate toxicity. Depletion of plasma proteins, especially coagulation factors, and immunologic factors may occur if repeated procedures are required. Prevention and management of hypocalcaemia includes administration of supplemental calcium (gluconate or chloride). Monitoring of pH, base excess, and metabolic alkalosis should be performed.

Hematologic

High blood flow rates may contribute to hemolysis if the circuit is twisted or kinked.

Significant hemolysis may precipitate DIC or mimic a transfusion reaction. Hemolysis may be detected by monitoring the plasma color or obtaining plasma hemoglobin levels. Monitoring of hemoglobin, hematocrit, platelets and coagulation factors such as PT/PTT, fibrinogen, and FDP are also essential for evaluation of hematologic status. There may changes in the ACTs as well. A decrease in circulating immunoglobulins or coagulation cofactors may be addressed by the infusion of FFP, IVIG, fibrinogen concentrates, or cryoprecipitate.

Complications

The Apheresis Program at Miami Children's Hospital began in 1994 and has provided care to over 340 patients with almost 1200 procedures.[29] Clinical events that required intervention occurred in 37% of our treatments, with one fatality. Decreased blood pressure was noted in 5.6%, increased blood pressure 3.5 %, and hypocalcaemia in 9%. Noninterventional events (nausea, vomiting, increased heart rate, tingling) occurred in 6.2% of patients. Other complications of vascular access included hematoma at the site of catheter insertion, pneumo/hemothorax, retroperitoneal bleed, infection, thrombosis, and air embolism.

Coagulation abnormalities are commonly twofold. First is a depletion of coagulation factors as they are removed during TPE. This can be compounded by the fact that an albumin solution, or any replacement fluid, that does not contain coagulation factors will dilute the patient's plasma. Recovery of coagulation factors is characterized by a rapid four hour increase and a slower rise in circulating cofactors during the next 24 hours after a single exchange. When multiple treatments are performed over a short period (three or more treatments per week), the depletion in clotting factors is more pronounced and may require several days for spontaneous recovery. By using FFP as a replacement fluid, the risks of iatrogenic hemodilution of circu-lating coagulation cofactors can be minimized. There is an increased risk of using human products that should always be considered. One of the other considerations in the use of FFP is the need to maintain antithrombin III levels for heparin effectiveness.

Transfusion reactions are an obvious risk if allogeneic products are required as replacement. Contributing factors include ABO mismatch (not following blood bank and hospital protocols) and multiple transfusions. Prevention includes administration of leuko-depleted blood products and pre-medication of sensitive patients. Patients that receive multiple treatments or transfusions may have a better response if an antihistamine is administered before treatment. When a transfusion reaction occurs, the procedure is discontinued and transfusion reaction protocols are followed. Maintain perfusion by giving crystalloids and osmotic diuretics. Check urine for hemolysis.[46] Thrombocytopenia can result from loss of platelets in the discarded plasma, during dilution, or via filter thrombosis. There is a greater loss of platelets using the centrifugal method than by membrane plasma separation. Wood and Jacobs have also shown decreases in the hematocrit by 10% after each plasmapheresis treatment in the absence of any extracorporeal losses or hemolysis.[53]

Hypothermia is another potential complication. Contributing factors are due to circuit exposure, the use of cold/cool replacement fluids, and patient size. Rapid loss of circulating volume may cause chills or shivering. Preventive measures include using warmed replacement fluids. Slowing down the inlet flow may improve hypothermia. It may help to also warm to the infusing replacement fluid via circuit warmer.

Medications Removed by Plasmapheresis

There are many drugs affected by plasmapheresis (Table 25-4). Certain drugs that are specifically circulating in the plasma compartment and specific antibodies circulating within the plasma are affected in plasmapheresis. For example, autoantibodies to cholinesterase will affect anticholinesterase drugs if these autoantibodies that are circulating within the plasma are removed during apheresis. Practitioners are encouraged to review patient medications and adjust them prior to starting plasmapheresis (in consultation with a pharmacist if needed). Owing to this ability, plasmapheresis can also be used therapeutically for pharmaceutical overdoses.

Agents with a low volume of distribution (Vd) and/or agents with higher tendency to be protein bound are most likely to be removed or decreased after plasmapheresis. Table 25-4 represents a general summary of about four decades of publications, mostly case reports on use of plasmapheresis in the setting of overdoses. If possible, practitioners should measure levels of agents after plasmapheresis and administer them after apheresis to assure therapeutic levels.

Table 25-4. Drugs affected by plasmapheresis

Drug/Agent	Theoretical Effect on Plasma Drug concentration after Plasmapheresis
Immunosupressants	
Corticosteroids	None/minimal Change
Cyclosporine	None/minimal Change
Tacrolimus	None/minimal Change
Basiliximab	None/minimal Change
Chemotherapeutic Agents	
Cisplatin	Decrease in levels
Vincristine	Decrease in levels
Cardiovascular Agents	
Digoxin	None/minimal Change
Calcium Channel Blockers	Decrease in levels
Homeostatic Agents	
Aspirin	Decrease in levels
Anti-viral	
Acyclovir	Minimal change
Antibiotics	
Ampicillin	Decrease in levels
Ceftiaxone	Decrease in levels
Chloramphenicol	Decrease in levels
Gentamicin	Decrease in levels
Vancomycin	Decrease in levels
Antieplieptics	
Phenytoin	Decrease in levels
Miscellaneous Agents	
Acetaminophen	Decrease in levels
Diclofenac	Decrease in levels
Quinine	Minimal change
Propoxyphene	Decrease in levels
Theophylline	Decrease in levels
Thyroxine	Decrease in levels
Amitriptyline	Decrease in levels

References

1. Szcepiorkowski ZM et al, Guidelines for the use of therapeutic apheresis in clinical preactise: evidence based from the Apheresis Applications Committee of the American Society for Apheresis, J. Clin Apher: Jun;22(3): 106-75, 2007.
2. Madore F. Plasmapheresis: technical aspects and indications. Crit Care Clin. 2002; 8:375-392.
3. McMaster P., Shann F; The use of Extracorporeal Techniques to remove humoral factors in sepsis, Pediatr Crit Care med. 2003;30,4(1):2-7.
4. Smith JW, Weinstein R, Hillyer KL, Therapeutic apheresis: A summary of current indication categories endorsed by the AARB and the American Society of Apheresis. Transfusion 43:820,2003.
5. Clark WF, Rock GA, Buskard N, et.al. Therapeutic plasma exchange: An update from the Canadian Apheresis Group. Ann Int Med. 1999; 131:453-462.
6. Nenov VD, Marinov P, Sabeva J. Current applications of plasmapheresis in clinical toxicology. Nephrol Dial Transp. 2003; 18 Suppl 5:56-58.
7. Adams WS, Bland WH, Bassetts H. A method of human Plasmapheresis. Proc Soc exp Biol Med 1952; 20:371-7.
8. Ni Maoshiing, The Yellow Emperor's Classic of Medicine, Shambhala Publications, Inc. 1995.
9. Grammaticos PC, Diamantis A., Useful known and inknown views of the father of modern medicine, Hippocrates and his teacher Democritus, Hell J Nucl Med, Jan-Apr; 11(1): 2-4, 2008.
10. Jones WHS, Hippocrates Collected Works I, Cambridge Harvard University Press, 1968
11. Kambic HE, Nose Y. Historical perspective on plasmapheresis. Therapeutic Apheresis, 1997. 1:83-108.
12. Shigehisa K, Interpreting the History of Bloodletting, Journal of the History of Medicine and Allied Sciences, 50 pg. 11-46, 1995.
13. Custis, George Washington Parke, Recollections of Washington (1860); " The Death of George Washington, 1799".
14. Vadakan MD, Vibul V, "A Physicians Looks At The Death of Washington", Early American Review, Early American Archiving.
15. Abel J. " Plasma Removal with return of corpuscles" in, Introduction to the article on Plasmaphersis, J. Pharmacol Exp, 5:625-641, 1941.
16. Co Tui, Bartter FC, Wright AM, Holt RD, Red Cell reinfusion and the frequency of donations, JAMA 124:331, 1944
17. Kambic HE, Nose Y. Historical perspective on plasmapheresis. Therapeutic Apheresis, 1997. 1:83-108.
18. Pool JG, Cryoprecipitated Factor VIII concentration, Bibleotheca Haematologica, 34:23, 1970.
19. Lockwood CM, Rees AJ, Pearson TA, Evans DJ, Peters DK, Wilson CB, Immunosuppression and plasma exchange in the treatment of Goodpasture's syndrome, Lancet ii;711-5, 1976.
20. Pinching AJ, Peters DK, Newsom, Davies J, Remission of myasthenia gravis following plasma exchange, Lancet ii; 1373-6, 1976
21. Brecher ME, Plasma Exchange: why we do what we do, J Clin Apher, 2002:17:204-211
22. Madore F. Plasmapheresis: technical aspects and indications. Crit Care Clin. 2002; 8:375-392.
23. Pisani E. Regulatory framework for plasmapheresis in the European Union: industry's viewpoint. Hematology & Cell Therapy, 1996, 38 Suppl 1:S35-38.
24. Rock G, Tittley P, McCombie N: Plasma collection using an automated membrane device, Transfusion 26:269, 1986.
25. Pisani E. Regulatory framework for plasmapheresis in the European Union: industry's

viewpoint. Hematology & Cell Therapy, 1996, 38 Suppl 1:S35-38.

26. Linenberger ML. Price TH. Use of cellular and plasma apheresis in the critically-ill patient: Part 1: technical and physiological considerations. J Int Care Med. 2005; 20:18-27.

27. DePalo T, Giordano M, Bellantuono, et al. Therapeutic apheresis in children, Int J Artif Org. 2000; 23:834-839.

28. Lindberger ML, Price , Use of cellular and plasma apheresis in the critically ill patient: Part I: Technical and Physiologic Considerations, J Intensive Care Med: 20, 18, 2005.

29. Sussmane J, Fifteen Years of Plasmapheresis Experience at Miami Children's Hospital, Int pediatrics, Vol 24., No. 3,116-119, 2009.

30. Kellum JA, Venkataraman R. Blood purification in sepsis: an idea whose time has come. Crit Care Med. 2002; 30:1387–1388.

31. Busund R, Koukline V, Utrobin U, et al. E Plasmapheresis in severe sepsis and septic shock: a prospective, randomised, controlled trial. Int Care Med. 2002; 28:1434-1439.

32. Stegmayr B.Plasmapheresis in severe sepsis or septic shock. Blood Purif. 1996;14:94101.

33. Busund R, Koukline V, Utrobin U, et al. E Plasmapheresis in severe sepsis and septic shock: a prospective, randomised, controlled trial. Int Care Med. 2002; 28:1434-1439.

34. Rock G, Buskard NA. Therapeutic plasmapheresis. Curr Opin Hematol. 1996; 3:504-510.

35. Ronco C., Tetta C, Mariano F. et. al., Interpreting the mechanism of continuous renal replacement therapy in sepsis: the peak concentration hypothesis, Artif Organs 27:792-801, 2003.

36. Watson RS, Caricillo JA, Scope and epidemiology of pediatric sepsis, Pediatr Crit care Med 6:S3-S5, 2005.

37. Malchesky PS. Sueoka. A. Matsubara S. et al. Membrane plasma separation. 1983. Therapeutic Apheresis. 2000; 4:47-53.

38. Pisani BA, Mullen GM, Malinowska K, et.al, Plasmapheresis with intravenous immunoglobulin G is effective in patients with elevated panel reactive antibody prior to cardiac transplantation. J Heart Lung Transplant. 1999; 18:701-706.

39. Gardlund B, Sjolin J, Nilsson A, et al. Plasma levels of cytokines in primary septic shock in humans: correlation with disease severity. J Inf Dis. 1995; 172:296–301.

40. McMaster P, Shann F. The use of extracorporeal techniques to remove humoral factors in sepsis. Ped Crit Care Med. 2003; 4:2-7.

41. Weinstein R, Basic principles of therapeutic blood exchange, Apheresis : Principles and Practice, 2nd Edition, Bethesda, Md., American Association of Blood Banks, 295-320, 2003.

42. Kaplan A, Therapeutic Plasma Exchange: Core Curriculum 2008,Am J of Kidney Disease, Vol. 52, Issue 6, 360, 2008

43. Reverberi R, Riverberi L., Removal kinetics of therapeutic apheresis, Blood Trans, July; 5(3):164-174,2007.

44. Nguyen TC, Stegmayr B, Busund R, et al. Plasma therapies in thrombotic syndromes. Int J Artif Organs. 2005; 28:459-465.

45. Baldini GM, Silvestri MG. Quality assurance in hemapheresis: quality of fresh frozen plasma. Int J Artif Organs. 1993; 16 Suppl 5:226-228.

46. Strauss RG. Apheresis donor safety--changes in humoral and cellular immunity. J Clin Apheresis. 1984; 2:68-80.

47. Kliman A, Carbone PP, Gaydos LA, et al. Effects of intensive plasmapheresis on normal blood donors. Blood.1964; 23:647-656.

48. Rock GA, Shumak KH, Buskard NA, et. al, Comparison of plasma exchange with plasma infusion in the treatment of throm-

botic thrombocytopenia purpura. NEJM, 1991; 325:393-397.

49. Madore F. Plasmapheresis. Technical aspects and indications. Crit Care Clinics. 2002; 18:375-392.

50. Weinstein R, Basic principles of therapeutic blood exchange, Apheresis : Principles and Practice, 2nd Edition, Bethesda, Md., American Association of Blood Banks, 295-320, 2003.

51. Yeh JH, Chen WH, Chiu HC. Complications of double-filtration plasmapheresis. Transfusion. 2004; 44:1621-1625.

52. Unger JK, Haltern C, Dohmen B, et al. Maximal flow rates and sieving coefficients in different plasmafilters: effects of increased membrane surfaces and effective length under standardized in vitro conditions. J Clin Apheresis. 2002; 17:190-198.

53. Wood L., Bond R., Jacobs P. Comparison of Filtration to continuous flow centrifugation for plasma exchange. J Clin Apheresis 2:155-162 1984.

54. Burgstaler EA, Current Instrumentation for apheresis. McLeod BC et al, Apheresis Principles and Practice. 2nd Edition Bethesda Md: American Assocation of Blood Banks; 95:-130, 2003.

55. Motohashi K, Yamane S. The effect of apheresis on adhesion molecules. Therapeutic Apheresis & Dialysis: Journal of the International Society for Apheresis, the Japanese Society for Apheresis, the Japanese Society for Dialysis Therapy. 2003; 7:425-430.

56. Gardlund B, Sjolin J, Nilsson A, et al. Plasma levels of cytokines in primary septic shock in humans: correlation with disease severity. J Inf Dis. 1995; 172:296–301.

57. Warren DS, Zachary AA, Sonnenday CJ,. et al. Successful renal transplantation across simultaneous ABO incompatible and positive crossmatch barriers. Am J Transp. 2004; 4:561-568.

58. Abraham KA, Brown C, Conlon PJ, et al. Plasmapheresis as rescue therapy in accelerated acute humoral rejection. J Clin Apheresis. 2003; 18:103-110.

59. Debray D, Furlan V, Baudoouin V, et. al, Therapy for acute rejection in pediatric organ transplant recipients. Pediatr Drugs. 2003; 5:81-93.

60. Berlot G, Tomasini A, Silvestri L, et al. Plasmapheresis in the critically-ill patient. Kidney International - Supplement. 1998; 66:S178-181.

61. Gorlin JB. Therapeutic plasma exchange and cytapheresis in pediatric patients. Transfus Sci. 1999; 21:21-39.

62. Urbaniak SJ. Therapeutic plasma and cellular apheresis. Clinics in Haematology. 1984; 13:217-251.

63. Grima KM. Therapeutic apheresis in hematological and oncological diseases. J Clin Apheresis. 2000; 15:28-52.

64. Kessinger A, Armitage JO, Landmark JD, et al. Reconstitution of human hematopoietic function with autologous cryopreserved circulating stem cells. Exp Hematol. 1986; 14:192-196.

65. Pahl E, Crawford SE, Cohn RA, et al. Reversal of severe late left ventricular failure after pediatric heart transplantation and possible role of Plasmapheresis. Am J Cardiol. 2000; 85:735-739.

26

Artificial Lung

William R. Lynch MD

Introduction

The concept of chronic implanted devices for pulmonary assistance is easy to imagine. The device would be continuously perfused by blood at flow rates high enough to exchange most or all of the oxygen and carbon dioxide requirements. Design considerations would include vascular access, thrombogenicity, durability, gas supply, infection, and patient mobility. Candidates for this technology would be patients with acute or chronic respiratory failure. The concept of applying membrane gas exchange as a pulmonary assist device has been suggested in the literature during the past fifty years. Laboratory success has been realized demonstrating durable partial and total support in large animal models. Recently, clinical application of extracorporeal pulmonary support has been realized. Why is this happening now?

The past thirty years has seen the maturation of temporary extracorporeal life support and lung transplantation into clinically successful strategies. Extracorporeal membrane oxygenation (ECMO) has become a reliable technology making prolonged support a reality. The application of ECMO allows support of patients in respiratory failure that, prior to this technology, had little chance for survival. ECMO provides a window of opportunity for recovery from respiratory insult. Early on, the practical application of ECMO for adults was only 30 days. However, with innovations in cannula design, pump technology, and membrane construction, adults are being supported successfully for longer and longer periods of time. That being said, associated complications continue to limit reliable and safe ECMO support. Lung transplantation has also become a clinical reality through advances in surgical technique and immunosuppression. This treatment can extend the lives of those suffering from endstage irreversible respiratory failure. The therapy is limited because of donor supply and many patients die waiting for a suitable organ. A device that would simplify ECMO technology and lengthen the therapeutic window would offer relief to patients dying from irreversible respiratory failure and provide a bridge to transplantation.

An implanted artificial lung could fulfill this role. The device would need to be compact, efficient in gas exchange, and durable. An artificial lung, like the artificial heart and the ventricular assist device, is unlikely to be a permanent organ replacement in the foreseeable future. Reliable performance for 1-6 months is feasible and such a device could support prolonged reversible acute respiratory failure or, bridge those in irreversible failure to transplantation. The stage is set for design, development, and testing of an artificial lung.

History of Artificial Lung Development

The technological advances making the development of an artificial lung possible provide an interesting review. Most significant has been the science and engineering of oxygenator technology. The development of CPB, ECMO, and the devices for ECMO are discussed in Chapters 1 and 8.

Design and Application of an Artificial Lung

Oxygenators and their membranes have been designed with cardiac surgery in mind. Some are used for prolonged support in ECMO. These devices are intended for short periods of use and with extensive heparinization. Most have very high resistance to blood flow, areas of stagnation, and little attention has been paid to mixing of blood. Condensation, which accumulates on the gas side of the membrane in a matter of hours, has drawn little attention. These characteristics make the existing oxygenators designed for cardiac surgery unsuitable as implantable devices. In the past decade, advances in membrane technologies have started to change this landscape, bringing the concept of a true "artificial lung" closer to clinical reality. These advances in membrane technology are allowing progress towards a clinically relevant artificial lung.

Design of an Artificial Lung

The first step is to define the qualities of an artificial lung. The device should have minimal resistance to blood flow while having high efficiency in gas exchange. Minimizing the thrombogenic potential will be necessary to extend membrane life and stagnant areas should be avoided. Taking advantage of secondary flows and blood mixing will help reduce thrombogenesis while improving gas exchange efficiency. These efforts should be made in concert with reducing or eliminating dependence on anticoagulation. Protecting the gas side of the membrane from plasma and water will also pose a design challenge necessary to extend membrane life. As each of these goals is accomplished, efficiency will increase, size will decrease, and durability will improve.

There are four practical design strategies for an artificial lung:

1. A gas exchange device within the vascular system. This intravascular oxygenator is referred to as the IVOX
2. A gas exchange device perfused by a systemic arteriovenous shunt. This is partial support, capable of clearing CO_2 but limited in oxygen delivery
3. A gas exchange device perfused by the right ventricle with the potential of total lung support
4. A gas exchange device and an extracorporeal pump. This combination would also provide total lung support.

Intravascular Oxygenator: The intravascular oxygenator (IVOX) is an intracorporeal bundle of hollow fiber membranes inserted into the vena cava, initially demonstrated by JD. Mortenson. The fiber bundles require surgical insertion. There is no need for extracorporeal blood circulation since the fibers are within the native circulation. Oxygen is pulled through the fibers with the assistance of vacuum. The inlet and outlet gas conduits are tunneled through a skin incision over the femoral vessels, passing into the femoral vein and into the device within the vena cava. With the gas exchange device in vivo, there is no extracorporeal circulation required. The capabilities of the device are less than full support. Early animal studies demonstrated approximately 40 cc/min of oxygen and carbon dioxide exchange which is 25-30% of a typical adults metabolic demands.[1,2] Engineering evolution of the IVOX concept investigated strategies to enhance mixing to improve gas exchange. Work continues on this concept of extracorporeal support as a means of partial support of the failing lung.[3]

Arteriovenous Shunt: Shunting blood via an arteriovenous connection has been used for years as access for renal dialysis. An arteriovenous shunt takes advantage of the pressure gradient that exists between the arterial and venous systems as a means of creating durable "pumpless" blood flow. The obvious disadvantage of the arteriovenous connection is diversion of oxygenated blood away from the arterial tree. Larger shunts can be easily created diverting up 25% of the cardiac output. This high pressure, high flow diversion of blood can be passed through a low resistance membrane oxygenator as a strategy of extracorporeal gas exchange. The advantages are the system is simple. A pair of cannulas, an oxygenator, and some anticoagulation are all that is needed. There is no need for an extracorporeal pump and it typically can be done without a heat exchanger. This strategy has two significant limitations. Blood flow can only be a fraction of the cardiac output and oxygen loading is minimal because of the relatively high oxygen content of arterial blood. These features are not limitations for carbon dioxide removal. In fact, because of membrane efficiency in CO_2 clearance, almost all the metabolic production of CO_2 can be removed.

Extracorporeal arteriovenous removal of CO_2 is abbreviated $AVCO_2R$. This can quite easily be done with the newer generation low resistance membrane oxygenators (Avecor, Quadrox-D, Novalung) and relatively small cannulas (12-14 Fr arterial, 16-21 Fr venous). This extracorporeal strategy is quite effective for hypercarbia from COPD exacerbations and status asthmaticus. It can only supplement oxygenation and is not adequate support for hypoxia. $AVCO_2R$ is considered partial respiratory support and is sometimes referred to as "pumpless extracorporeal lung assist", or PECLA.[4-7]

"Pumpless" Paracorporeal Artificial Lung: Total pulmonary support requires enough blood flow to exchange metabolically significant amounts of oxygen. For neonates, approximately 100 cc/kg/min are necessary; for adults, 60 cc/kg/min. If oxygen needs are met, carbon dioxide will be cleared. There are now membrane oxygenators that are considered low resistance at blood flow rates comparable to the cardiac output. Some devices have a pressure gradient of 10-20 mmHg at 3-4 liters per minute blood flow. The right ventricle is capable of overcoming this pressure gradient in many circumstances. In some chronic lung disease, the pulmonary vascular resistance slowly increases over time. This prepares the right ventricle in a way that it can tolerate the increased resistance of these low resistance oxygenators. Primary pulmonary hypertension is another condition that prepares the right ventricle. This strategy of support has been demonstrated to be practical for days in laboratory studies.[8-10] The right ventricle must be able to tolerate the "vascular" resistance of the membrane oxygenator. Laboratory work suggests when the membrane oxygenator is placed in series with the native pulmonary vasculature, the increased resistance to flow can result in right heart failure. When the oxygenator is placed in parallel with the native circulation, overall resistance is decreased. These parallel flow pathways (native pulmonary vasculature and the artificial lung) offer an opportunity to "decompress" the right ventricle. The right ventricular performance can be stabilized or even improved. Recently, this technique has been used clinically to support patients to lung transplantation.[11-14] The "in parallel" arrangement delivers the arterialized blood to the arterial circulation; typically the left atrium. The consequence of emboli would be end organ injury; most significant would be a stroke.

"Pump Assisted" Paracorporeal Artificial Lung: Integrating an extracorporeal pump with an oxygenator is the other strategy that can offer total support. Traditional adult ECMO could be considered a "pump assisted" paracorporeal artificial lung. However, adult ECMO commonly required femoral cannulation, a large collection of technology with complexity that demanded a bed side specialist. The new pumps and oxygenators have begun to change this landscape. The technology is now less cumbersome and more reliable. In addition, a dual lumen cannula is now available for adults. This bi-caval cannula allows single site cannulation, most typically in the right internal jugular. These new cannulas are capable of delivering enough flow for total support and since there is no longer a need to have cannulas in the groin, patients can get out of bed.[15-19] Laboratory work has demonstrated a pump assisted strategy is practical. Animals have been supported for days and weeks with an integrated pump/oxygenator paracorporeal artificial lung.[12] While these studies demonstrate proof of concept, most available pumps are either designed as ventricular assist pumps, cardiopulmonary bypass pumps, or ECMO pumps.[20] The pump technology is adequate for generating the necessary flow but these pumps are not uniquely designed with an artificial lung in mind.

Access to the blood stream offers choices and controversy. Different investigators are pursuing various approaches when configuring the artificial lung. One option, as previously described, is a configuration which is parallel to the native pulmonary circulation. To achieve this, venous blood is drained from the pulmonary artery (PA) and returned as arterialized blood to the left atrium (LA). A second option is to drain venous blood from the PA and return arterialized blood to the PA. This configuration is an "in series" arrangement with the pulmonary circulation. A third approach could be draining from the right atrium (RA) and returning to the LA. A final possibility would be a miniaturized form of traditional ECMO via a dual lumen cannula inserted in the vena cava. There are advantages and disadvantages with each vascular access approach. It is likely that some of these strategies will offer distinct advantages in specific patient populations.

Applications for an Artificial Lung

Acute Respiratory Failure: Currently, ECMO is the only mechanical support system for patients with acute respiratory failure who are failing on mechanical ventilation. Eighty five percent of neonates managed in this fashion recover and survive with normal lung function. With the exception of lung hypoplasia, neonatal respiratory failure is successfully treated by ECMO and there would be no application for an implantable device. However, older children and adults with severe acute respiratory failure have only a 50-70% survival with temporary ECMO support. The patients, who do not survive, usually die from multiple organ failure or from the effects of progressive irreversible pulmonary fibrosis. The ECMO survivors typically require 1-4 weeks of ECMO support. Many of these survivors require weeks in the hospital and extended care facilities prior to return home. The application of an artificial lung in this large patient group would be two fold. First, early use of an artificial lung for those requiring prolonged ECMO support, could simplify nursing care, reduce costs, and allow management outside of an ICU. Second, for the patients who progress to end-stage pulmonary fibrosis, return of pulmonary function is not expected. These patients usually have infections and many are suffering other organ system dysfunction. Because of the acute nature of their illness, these patients are not candidates for lung transplantation and go on to die. An artificial lung could support these patients through the acute illness, allowing recovery of other organ function and making transplantation a reasonable goal.

Graft failure in a recent lung transplant patient leaves few options. Whether acute respiratory failure, rejection, or bronchiolitis, the acute nature of the process precludes re-transplantation. Temporary support with an artificial lung would allow the transplant lung time to recover function or provide time for a second transplant. Use of the artificial lung in this situation could be used to rescue the graft or support patients until a replacement organ is found. The artificial lung, in this application, would be similar to reverting to hemodialysis in patients with failed transplanted kidneys.

Chronic Respiratory Failure: The largest group of patients to be candidates for an artificial lung is sufferers of chronic lung diseases of a destructive nature such as emphysema, cystic fibrosis, idiopathic fibrosis, or chronic rejection of a transplanted lung. Currently, these diseases are treated with supplemental oxygen and for a select few, lung transplantation. Some have worsening respiratory failure, requiring mechanical ventilation. For many centers, this is reason to remove a patient from the transplant list and these patients die on the ventilator. The use of an artificial lung could rescue these patients from the ventilator and provide a bridge to transplantation. When supported by the device, there would be an opportunity to improve nutrition, exercise tolerance, and clear infections while waiting for an appropriate donor. The time could also be used to facilitate treatment of the underlying disease, such as lung volume reduction surgery for bullous emphysema, or prolonged treatment of transplant rejection, or aggressive lavage of the infected lungs of a cystic fibrosis patient.

Patients with chronic respiratory failure might also benefit from application of partial, instead of total support. The device could potentially be implanted but more likely these artificial lungs would be paracorporeal. Perhaps the device could be perfused by an arteriovenous shunt designed to provide only enough flow to remove metabolically produced carbon dioxide while providing a supplemental amount of oxygen. The inability to clear CO_2 causes increased work of breathing that is debilitating to many of these patients. A strategy of partial support directed at relieving this aspect of the disease might be a simple and effective means of stabilizing the patient's condition, requiring no further treatment.

Chronic Right Ventricular Failure: There is a small group of patients that die from high pulmonary vascular resistance that is unresponsive to medical treatment. The etiology might be primary pulmonary hypertension or chronic obstructive pulmonary disease but death is from progressive right ventricular failure. Lung transplantation is the only treatment when right ventricular function is preserved. If the right ventricle is not salvageable, both heart and lung must be transplanted. The use of an implantable artificial lung perfused by the right ventricle would provide sufficient respiratory support while also reducing right ventricular work. The device would serve as a bridge to lung transplantation while rescuing the native right ventricle.

Theoretical and Speculative Applications: Treatment of patients with minimal or no native lung function might one day be possible. Consider infants with bilateral pulmonary hypoplasia, often associated with diaphragmatic hernias. Presently, these infants can be supported with ECMO but with minimal chance for recovery. Promising methods to induce lung growth exist, but these treatments would require time. An implantable or paracorporeal device could sustain life, providing time for lung maturation to occur. Even more speculative, would be using an artificial lung in conjunction with lung cancer therapy. Patients with primary or metastatic pulmonary disease could be supported with an artificial lung and their native lungs removed. Perhaps one or both lungs could be removed for treatment of the neoplasm while an implantable artificial lung supports the patient's respiratory function. The excised native lungs could be perfused with a chemotherapeutic regimen, too caustic for systemic exposure. Once the lungs were verified to be tumor free, they would be reimplanted into the patient for a cure.

Innovative applications would evolve as the device and technique improved with experience. Figure 26-1 represents treatment strategies in use today while Figure 26-2 suggests ways an artificial lung could impact treatment in the future.

**Treatment Algorithm
2011**

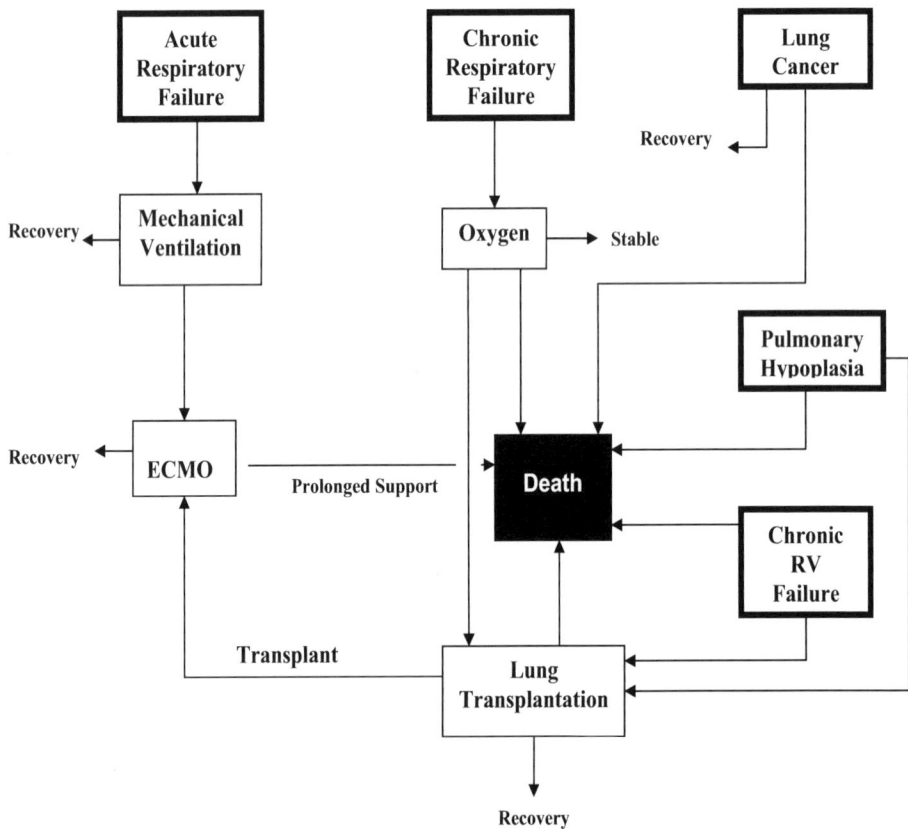

Figure 26-1. Treatment strategies currently in use.

**Treatment Algorithm
2020**

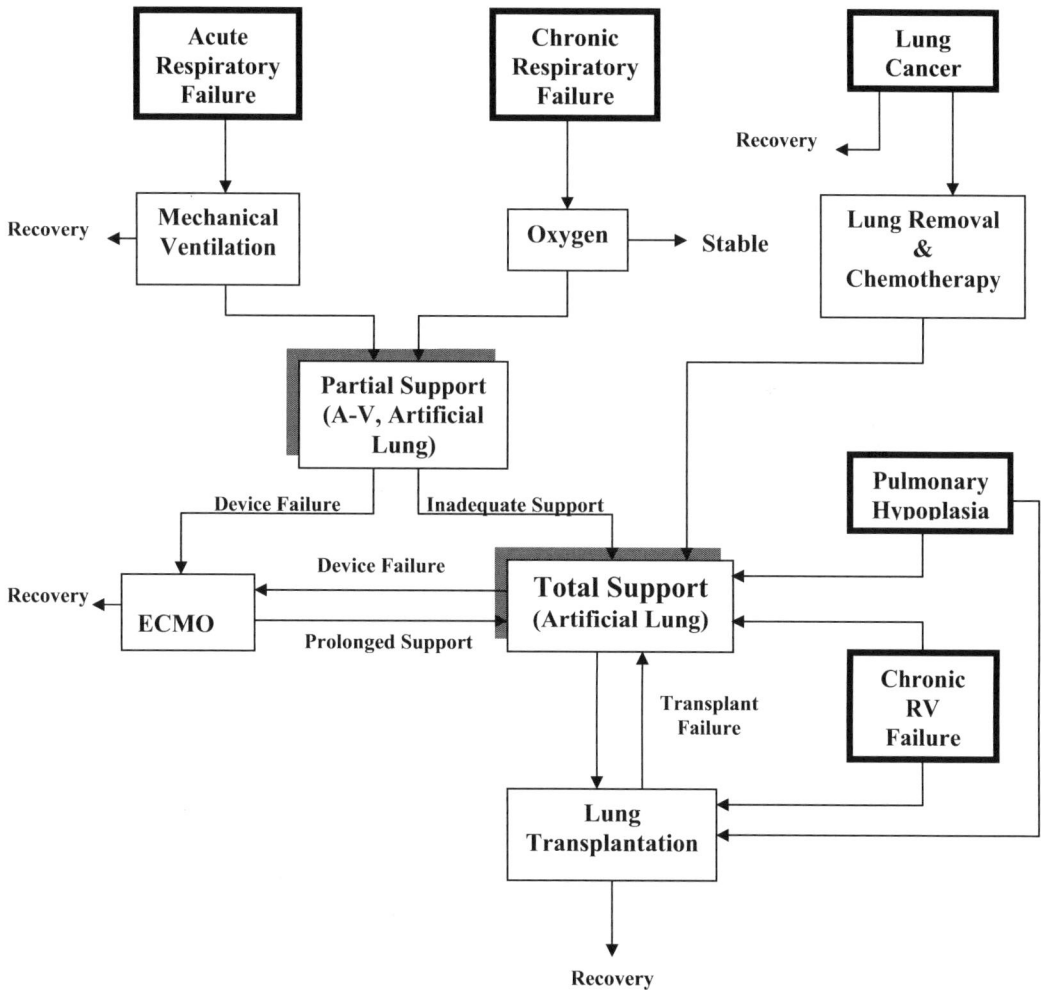

Figure 26-2. Artificial lung impact on future treatment treatment.

References

1. Cox CS, Zwischenberger JB, Graves DF. Intracorporeal CO_2 removal and permissive hypercapnia to reduce airway pressure in acute respiratory failure. The theoretical basis for permissive hypercapnia with IVOX. ASAIO j 1993;39(2):97-102.

2. Zwischenberger JB, Cox CS, Traber LD. Use of an intravascular oxygenator/carbon dioxide removal device in an ovine smoke inhalational injury model. ASAIO Trans 1991;37(3):M411-M413.

3. Polk AA, Maul TM, McKeel DT, Snyder TA, Lehocky CA, Pitt B, Stolz DB, Federspiel WJ, Wagner WR. A biohybrid artificial lung prototype with active mixing of endothelialized microporous hollow fibers. Biotech Bioengr 2010;106:490-500.

4. Conrad SA, Zwischenberger JB, Gier LR, Alpard SK, Bidani A. Total extracorporeal arteriovenous CO_2 removal in severe respiratory failure: a phase I clinical study. Intens Care Med 2001;27:1340-51.

5. Zwischenberger JA, Conrad SA, Alpard SK, Gier LR, Bidani A. Percutaneous extracorporeal arteriovenous CO_2 removal for severe respiratory failure. Ann Thorac Surg 199;68:181-7.

6. Flörchinger B, Philipp A, Klose A, Hilker M, Kobuch R, Rupprecht L, Keyser A, Pühler T, Hirt S, Wiebe K, Müller T, Langgartner J, Lehle K, Schmid C. Pumpless extracorporeal lung assist: a 10 year institutional experience. Ann Thorac Surg 2008;86:410-17.

7. Müller T, Lubnow M, Philipp A, Bein T, Jeron A, Luchner A, Rupprecht L, Reng M, Langgartner J, Wrede CE, Zimmermann M, Birnbaum L, Schmid C, Riegger GAJ, Pfeifer M. Extracorporeal pumpless interventional lung assist in clinical practice: determinants of efficacy. Eur Respir J 2009;33:551-8.

8. Sato H, Griffith GW, Hall CM, Toomasian JM, Hirschl RB, Bartlett RH, Cook KE. Seven-day artificial lung testing in an In-parallel configuration. Ann Thoracic Surg 2007;84:988-94.

9. Camboni D, Akay B, Sassalos P, Toomasian JM, Haft JW, Bartlett RH, Cook KE. Use of venovenous extracorporeal membrane oxygenation and an atria septostomy for pulmonary and right ventricular failure. Ann Thorac Surg 2011;91:144-9.

10. Wang D, Lick SD, Zhou X, Liu X, Benkowski RJ, Zwischenberger JB. Ambulatory oxygenator right ventricular assist device for total right heart and respiratory support. Ann Thorac Surg;84:1699-703.

11. Schmid C, Philipp A, Hilker M, Arlt M, Trabold B, Pfeiffer M, Schmid F. Bridge to lung transplantation through a pulmonary artery to left atrial oxygenator. Ann Thorac Surg 2008;85:1202-5.

12. Camboni D, Philipp A, Arlt M, Pfeiffer M, Hilker M, Schmid C. First experience with a paracorporeal artificial lung in humans. ASAIO 2009;55:304-307.

13. Haneya A, Philipp A, Mueller T, Lubnow M, Pfeiffer M, Zink W, Hilker M, Schmid C, Hirt S. Extracorporeal circulatory systems as a bridge to lung transplantation at remote transplant centers. Ann Thorac Surg 2011;91:250-6.

14. Wiebe K, Poeling J, Arlt M, PhilippA, Camboni D, Hofmann S, Schmid C. Thoracic surgical procedures supported by a pumpless interventional lung assist. Ann Thorac Surg 2010;89:1782-8.

15. Kaar JL, Heung-Il O, Russell AJ, Federspiel WJ. Towards improved artificial lungs through biocatalysis. Biomaterials 2007;28:3131-39.

16. Camboni D, Akay B, Pohlmann JR, Koch KL, Haft JW, Bartlett RH, Cook KE. Veno-venous extracorporeal membrane oxygenation with interatrial shunting: a novel approach to lung transplantation for

patients in right ventricular failure. J Thorac Cardiovasc Surg 2011;141:537-42.

17. Srivastava MC, Ramani GV, Garcia JP, Griffith BP, Uber PA, Park MH. Veno-venous extracorporeal membrane oxygenation bridging to pharmacotherapy in pulmonary arterial hypertensive crisis. J Heart Lung Transplant 2010;29:811-3.

18. Mangi AA, Mason DP, Yun JJ, Murthy SC, Pettersson GB. Bridge to lung transplantation using short-term ambulatory extracorporeal membrane oxygenation. J Thorac Cardiovasc Surg 2010;140:713-5.

19. Garcia JP, Iacono A, Kon ZN, Griffith BP. Ambulatory extracorporeal membrane oxygenation: A new approach for bridge-to-lung transplantation. J Thorac Cardiovasc Surg 2010;139:e137-9.

20. Matheis G. New technologies for respiratory assist. Perfusion 2003;18:245-51.

27

Extracorporeal Support Assisted Organ Donation

Alvaro Rojas-Pena MD, Robert H. Bartlett MD, Jeffrey D. Punch MD

Introduction

The ability of extracorporeal support (ECS) to provide normal tissue perfusion in the absence of cardiac activity has the potential to improve organ quality when initiated following cessation of circulation and declaration of death. This chapter will summarize the world experience with the use of ECS in organ donors in both clinical and laboratory settings.

In 2004, HSRA and the Greenwall Foundation asked the Institute of Medicine (IOM) to study issues relating to the shortage of viable organs, resulting in a 370 page report published in 2006 entitled Organ Donation; Opportunities for Action.[1] The recommendation to increase donated organs is focused on organ recovery from donors after cardiac death (DCD), building on similar recommendations from the IOM in 1997 and 2000. The report estimates that 22,000 additional donors could be candidates for DCD after unexpected cardiac arrest (uncontrolled DCD). The IOM report[1] recommends expansion of the population of potential donors via the implementation of initiatives to increase DCD donation, and research on organ quality and enhanced organ function.

There are at least three clinical scenarios where ECS can be applied to DCD organ donation (Table 27-1).

Table 27-1. Clinical Scenarios for Organ Donation After Cardiac Death (DCD)

Donor Type	Maastricht Category	Description
Unexpected DCD (Uncontrolled NHBD)	Maastricht Type I and II	Individuals that suffer cardiac arrest and are declared dead because the treating team determines that they cannot be resuscitated.
Expected DCD (Controlled NHBD)	Maastricht Type III	Deaths that occur following planned withdrawal of ventilatory and other support.
Brain Dead Donors	Maastricht Type IV	Brain dead donors that either suffer cardiac arrest prior to organ recovery or that manifest profound ventilator or hemodynamic dysfunction.

NHBD: non-heart beating donors. Maastricht Categories[2]

Rapid Recovery (RR, conventional) technique for procuring organs of Donors after Cardiac Death (DCD)

Rapid recovery (RR) instituted five minutes after cardiac death is the standard procedure for organ retrieval, but it accounts for only 4% of organ transplantation (and is almost exclusively to renal grafts donation). The reason is that the organs begin to sustain warm ischemic (WI) injury when the circulation stops. After declaration of death it is standard clinical practice to wait at least five minutes before beginning any organ procurement process. Therefore the WI period is at least five minutes. When RR is instituted after the five minute period the organs are typically retrieved within 30-45 minutes so the total WI time is prolonged in the RR-DCD procurement technique.

When the grafts are transplanted, reperfusion injury takes place in the recipient, affecting immediate graft function directly proportional to the WI times. Adequate graft function may not occur for days or weeks, perhaps not at all. For this reason DCD is largely limited to kidney donation because the recipient can be managed on other renal replacement therapies (dialysis) when the graft lacks function. This is a major limitation when liver grafts from DCD are used, especially if primary graft non-function occurs; however, common complications seen with hepatic grafts are stenosis of the biliary conducting system.

Because of the urgency of instituting RR within five minutes death declaration, all of this must be done in the operating room. The entire procedure is scheduled and elective for controlled (Maastricht 3) donors. Supportive care is stopped and the transplant team stands by until the heart stops (typically 20 minutes). The family says goodbye at the operating room door. If the heart does not stop within 90 minutes the procedure is abandoned because the organs are excessively damaged by poor perfusion during the agonal period.

In RR the abdomen is quickly opened after death and the peritoneum filled with iced solution, the aorta is flushed until the blood is removed, then the kidneys are removed, flushed, and stored until transplantation. Another technique of rapid recovery includes cannulation of the femoral artery for immediate cold perfusion of the body before opening the abdomen, while other centers maintain chest compressions during the RR organ procurement. Successful transplantation after RR has been reported for as long 45 minutes from asystole to organ procurement, although the longer procurement time the less successful the transplant.

Livers and kidneys from RR donors have been used with adequate long-term outcome, but their use has been limited due to higher risk of developing primary graft non-function (PGN). PGN is a catastrophic consequence seen more often in transplanted livers than kidneys from DCD due to warm ischemic injury. Also, 60% of these kidneys have delayed graft function (DGF) requiring renal support.

Between 2000 and 2005, some single center series of liver transplants with RR were reported with mixed results. D'Alessandro et al.[3] reported a series of 36 recipient allografts from DCD performed between 1993 and 2002, graft and patient survival were considerably worse at three years (56% graft and 68% patient) compared with those in recipients of BDD (80% graft and 84% patient). In a series of 15 patients with a mean follow up of 818 days, Abt and collaborators[4] reported graft and patient survival rates equivalent to those in a cohort of BDD grafts. One third of the recipients had a major biliary complication including intrahepatic strictures, resulting in the need for multiple interventional procedures, retransplantation, or death. The largest experience with RR-DCD is from Spain[5-10] and the Netherlands[11,12] where implied consent for organ donation after cardiac arrest is the norm. RR in these countries usually includes arterial cannulation and cold flushing within a few minutes after arrest. Ex vivo kidney perfusion may follow. The incidence of DGF reported was up to 47% in the Netherlands group and 13% in the Spanish group.

ECS assisted DCD technique

ECS-DCD involves placement of femoral arterial and venous cannulae either percutaneously or via cutdown. Depending on the clinical scenario and local practice, the cannulae may be placed prior to, or following declaration of death. The circuit consists of, at a minimum, a centrifugal pump, and an oxygenator. A heat exchanger may, or may not be included in the circuit. If included, circulation is normothermic (37°C). If not included, ECS occurs at ambient room temperature (~30°C). The entire system is about the size of a hemodialysis unit and can be transported on a wheeled cart. A proximal aortic occlusion balloon is inserted into the thoracic aorta to enable selective perfusion of the abdominal organs. This improves the efficiency of the ECS circuit by limiting the circulating volume, it avoids reanimation of the heart and it avoids violation of the dead donor rule in donors that are declared dead by circulatory criteria. Typically ECS target flow is >50mL/Kg/min (2-5 L/min).

ECS of Maastricht type III DCD

The process for Maastricht type III DCD must begin with the determination by the treating medical team that continued ventilatory support of the patient is futile. This circumstance is usually associated with a patient that has suffered a severe neurological injury without potential for meaningful survival, but in whom criteria for brain death cannot be satisfied. This decision must be made without consideration of the patient's potential as an organ donor. Once this decision to withdraw support has been made, the next step is for the medical team to inform the family of their recommendations. Depending on their state of mind, families may

immediate accept withdrawal of support as the appropriate thing to do, or they may resist for a time, and initially refuse to allow support to be withdrawn. The family may also be initially divided in their acceptance of withdrawal. It is appropriate to provide additional time to allow families to come to grips with the loss of their loved one. However, the vast majority of families do not want their loved one subjected to futile care that is viewed as undignified, and many individuals have stated in living wills or otherwise that they do not want to be kept alive if meaningful survival is not possible.

Once the team and the family agree to withdrawal of support, it is appropriate at that time to offer the family the option of organ donation when the patient expires. At the University of Michigan, ECS assist is then offered. It is explained that this technique may improve the likelihood of success for transplanted organs that are recovered, and that it involves placement of catheters into the groin prior to the withdrawal of support. A separate consent is signed. Objection to the ECS assist technique is only observed rarely. In general, families that have embraced the concept of organ donation want to do whatever they can to improve the odds that the organs will be functional in the recipient. During the consent process for donation after cardiac death, it is important to inform the family that death may not occur at the time of lifesupport withdrawal and if this happens, organ donation will not be possible.

Policy regarding intervention for ECS prior to withdrawal of care prior to death is hospital-specific. The UM protocol includes placement of cannulas and heparinization before withdrawal of care. Once consent for ECS assisted DCD is given, the ECS team is notified and femoral arterial and venous catheters are placed percutaneously. Local anesthesia is used in case the patient has sensation. The catheters are heparinized and clamped. The family is usually asked to step out of the room during this sterile procedure. An ECS circuit is primed with crystalloid and connected to the cannulae, but circulation is routed through a bridge catheter, rather than into the patient. The ECS team then leaves the room until death has been declared. The treating medical team then gives the orders for withdrawal of support, including discontinuation of intravenous infusions and mechanical ventilation. Palliative treatments such as narcotics and benzodiazipines should be given by the treating physician exactly as they would if organ donation is not occurring. As described below, the family may be present during the withdrawal. When circulation ceases and death is declared by the treating physician, the bridge on the ECS circuit is clamped while the cannulae are unclamped, and ECS begins. An aortic occlusion balloon is placed in the descending thoracic aorta through a side port of the arterial cannula. The family may then remain with the patient for a brief period of grieving if they desire.

Following the institution of ECS, the operating room team is activated and when everything is ready the patient is moved to the operating theater with the ECS system wheeling alongside the bed. In the operating room the body is prepped and draped as usual. All of these processes can happen at a comfortably normal pace, without any need to rush because the organs are well perfused by the ECS. A conventional organ recovery incision is made. When the blood supply to the abdominal organs has been dissected cold perfusate is connected to the arterial limb of the ECS circuit and perfused through arterial cannula. Topical ice is applied to the organs and the venous system is vented into the abdomen. Once the organs have been exsanguinated and cold perfused, they are removed surgically using conventional organ recovery technique.

In other centers cannulation and heparinization are done after declaration of death. An intermediate step is to place small intravascular catheters in the femoral vessels while the heart is still beating, and place perfusion cannulas

over a wire after death. In theory the treatment team is solely in control until death is declared and no organ salvage interventions are begun until 5 minutes after death. In practice the treatment team and the transplant team must work closely in DCD. The Michigan policy is based on the fact that the donating family wants every chance for success of the donated organs. All the details have been discussed with the family and consent is given.

EDCD compared to RR

There are several logistical and physiologic hurdles to the utilization of organs from Maastricht type III DCD. The chief physiologic barrier is warm ischemia. The ability to reestablish the flow of oxygenated blood after the declaration of death using ECS offers the ability to keep warm ischemia to the bare minimum.[13,14] During the time that it takes for the patient to be prepared for the recovery operation, fully warmed and oxygenated blood can be provided to the organs. The magnitude of this advantage over traditional rapid recovery DCD organ recovery techniques depends on the location where withdrawal of support occurs, the degree to which preparations for recovery such as skin prep and sterile draping have been made, and the time it takes to for vascular cannulation in order to begin cold perfusion. The latter time can be highly variable depending on the experience of the recovery surgeon, the body habitus of the donor, and the presence or absence of prior abdominal operations.

ECS assisted DCD also offers the advantage of allowing support to be withdrawn in the ICU, rather than in another setting, such as an anesthetic induction room or an operating room. The family can attend the death, without reducing the likelihood of successful transplantation of their loved one's organs. At the declaration of death, the ECS can be initiated, and the thoracic aortic balloon inflated, allowing the organs to be perfused and oxygenated while the family says their last goodbye. If death does not occur after 60-90 minutes after withdrawal of support, the patient does not have to be moved again back to a conventional hospital room.

Another significant advantage of ECS assisted DCD that has been observed is that it makes the practice of DCD easier to accept by hospital staff. In most ICUs withdrawal of ventilatory support is a common practice when further aggressive medical intervention is deemed by the treating team to be futile. The ICU nurses and staff are thus accustomed to having patients that are expected to expire following discontinuation of ventilation. They are more likely to have specific experience and training for supporting grieving families. The nurses are also comfortable with treating these patients with "comfort measures" including sedatives and narcotics, since these treatments are appropriately given to eliminate suffering in this setting. The setting of an ICU is also a much more palatable and peaceful setting for the family compared to either a holding room outside of an operating room, or to the operating room itself.

ECS assisted DCD also allows for greater efficiency of resources since an operating room and team do not need to be on standby, waiting for declaration of death with instruments opened and preparations complete. Rather the preparation for the recovery procedure can be initiated following declaration of death. If the patient does not expire, the operating room staff has not been inconvenienced and no expense has been undertaken. This can lead to greater acceptance of the DCD practice by hospitals, and a greater willingness on the part of clinicians to attempt DCD organ recovery, even when it is unclear whether expiration will occur soon after withdrawal of support or not.

Outcome of organs transplanted from ECS assisted DCD

Experience with ECS assisted DCD of Maastricht type III DCD has been reported by the University of Michigan, the National Taiwan University Hospital, and Wake Forest University.[15-18] The largest experience in the US is ours at the University of Michigan. We initially reported experience with 20 donors, resulting in 24 kidneys, 7 livers, and one pancreas transplant, all of which were very successful.[15] We have now used ECS-DCD for 50 patients. Organs were not taken from 11 because of prolonged agonal period (>90min), one donor with positive serologies, and one technical difficulty during perfusion. Organs from 37 donors were taken, resulting in the procurement of 73 kidneys, 21 livers, and two pancreata. From these organs 48 renal grafts, 13 livers, and one pancreas were successfully transplanted. All but one kidney had immediate and prolonged graft function, better than BDD donors over the same time period. In our institution an average of rate of 1.7 organs are transplanted per DCD. Graft survival for kidneys procured from ECS assisted Maastricht type III donors appears to be similar to that observed for kidney obtained from brain dead donors. The University of Michigan experience noted a reduced rate of delayed graft function in DCD supported by ECS compared to conventional DCD.[15] Liver grafts have also been utilized from ECS assisted DCD Maastricht type III donors, but the experience to date is limited and does not allow firm conclusions regarding outcomes.

ECS of Maastricht type I and II DCD

In Spain, cultural and legal barriers currently preclude organ donation following planned withdrawal of ventilatory support (Maastricht type III DCD). Instead, ECS has been applied to organ donors that suffer cardiac arrest outside of the hospital. Published reports from Madrid, La

Coruña and Barcelona describe the techniques used, which are similar at each location.[5-10] Spain possesses an excellent system for prompt emergency medical care. Emergency physicians are dispatched to the scene of cardiac arrest victims and institute manual cardiopulmonary resuscitation and advanced cardiac life support is initiated. Patients that fail resuscitation are considered candidates for DCD donation if they meet standardized criteria: time of cardiac arrest is known; cardiopulmonary resuscitation was begun with 10 minutes after arrest; age between 7 and 55; cause of death is known or supposed; non-bleeding injuries in thorax and abdomen; no evidence of risk factors for AIDS; and the time between arrest and organ recovery is limited to 2 hours.[10] Potential lung and liver donors have additional, more stringent, criteria. The patients are transferred to the hospital and declared dead when there is "unequivocal and irreversible absence of electrocardiographic activity and spontaneous breathing during a period of at least five minutes."

The transplant team is notified when potential DCD enters the hospital, but they remain uninvolved until death has been declared by the treating physicians. Once death is declared, the donor is given intravenous heparin, endotracheally intubated if this has not already been done, and an automatic external cardio-compression device is used while perfusion catheters are being inserted in the femoral artery and vein. When the cannulae are in place, cardiac massage is terminated and extracorporeal circulation is then begun using a heat exchanger in the circuit to maintain normothermia.

Evaluation of the donor begins simultaneously with the declaration of death by trained transplant coordinators that contact the next of kin to request consent. If consent is obtained, additional information regarding the donor's medical history is collected. If consent is declined, the extracorporeal pump is discontinued.

The Madrid experience in calendar year 2004, includes 74 potential donors, of which 62 were considered potential donors and 55 were actual donors. In comparison, during that year the program had only nine brain dead donors (BDD). The group reports that 105 kidneys, 22 lungs, 14 pancreata, and numerous tissues were recovered from the ECS supported DCD. Details of organ function are not clearly reported, except that kidney function is stated to be as good or better than those results obtained with kidneys from brain dead donors.[10] Jimenez-Galanes et al. have been using normothermic ECS for unexpected DCD since 2005. They recently reported experience with 20 livers recovered with ECS, and compared the results to 40 livers from conventional brain dead donors.[19] The incidence of primary non-function was 10% (2.5 for BDD), and cholangiopathy was 5% (0% BDD). The graft and patient survival at one year was not different from the DCD-ECS and BDD groups. Animal studies by Garcia-Valdecasas et al. using DCD-ECS in swine have demonstrated a significant advantage of normothermic ECS compared to continue CPR. They believe that the postmortem in situ ECS serves to resuscitate the liver following ischemia preconditioning. This group also studied modification of the reperfusion syndrome with selected amino acid additives. The DGF rate was only 12.5% in animals that received ECS support, much lower than in situ perfusion or total body cooling.[20,21]

In Barcelona, ECS assisted recovery of livers from 40 DCD over a four year period, has been reported.[9] Ten livers were transplanted at their program, and 30 were excluded for a variety of reasons including age, medical condition, poor perfusion, intra-abdominal sepsis, hepatic trauma, and others. One year patient survival was 70% with two patients requiring retransplantation due to primary non-function or hepatic artery thrombosis. A comparison with matched controls that had livers from brain dead individuals revealed no statistical difference in graft or patient survival. The Barcelona experience with the other organs transplanted from these donors has not yet been published.

The group at La Coruña has reported both renal[5] and liver[22] transplantation in uncontrolled cardiac death with different methods of resuscitating the organs. This group prefers external compression CPR while cooling and removing organs. They evaluated in situ cooling, cooling during CPR, and cardiopulmonary bypass (ECS) in some cases. The patient survival of liver recipients from CPR donors was only 42% at two years. The numbers of donors managed by normothermic ECS was small, and it is difficult to draw conclusions regarding the effectiveness of normothermic ECS from this report.

Similar DCD programs utilizing ECS assist for Maastricht type II DCD are in the planning stages in New York City, Ann Arbor, Michigan, and France.

ECS assist for brain dead donors

In addition to maintaining circulation after cardiac cessation in DCD, ECS can also be used to support brain dead donors that have severe cardiac or pulmonary dysfunction, including cardiopulmonary arrest that occurs before the team is assembled to recover organs.[23] While this is an unusual indication for ECS, it may allow organs to be recovered in a setting where otherwise recovery of viable organs would have been impossible. In this situation the aortic occlusion balloon can be omitted in order to expedite the process of placing the donor on ECS since there is no need to avoid blood flow to the coronary and carotid arteries.

Laboratory Experience

We have recently published that normothermic ECS restores renal function after 30 minutes of WI in our animal model.[24] An accompanying editorial in the American Journal of Transplantation asks[25] "Is Extracorporeal Support becoming the New Standard for the Preservation of DCD Grafts?" The top priority for innovation is to solve the shortage of donor organs. Although the use of ECS methodology to resuscitate organs in the donor is not new, prolongation of the warm ischemic time to 60 minutes could make donation in unexpected DCD routine, and that would be truly innovative.

In a relevant model we have studied many of the variables in ECS-DCD.[26-28] We have demonstrated and published that 90 minutes of normothermic ECS can resuscitate kidneys

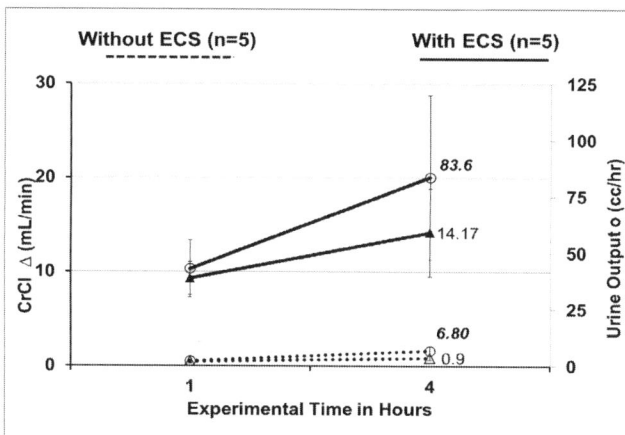

Figure 27-1. Immediate post-transplant function of DCD swine kidneys after 30 min WI with and without ECS assisted donation. Creatinine clearance (Δ-left axis), and urine output (O-right axis) at 1hr and 4hr post transplantation using renal grafts from DCD that sustained 30min of warm ischemia, with and without ECS for organ procurement. Renal function was restored only in grafts from the ECS-DCD (solid line) group.

to routinely successful transplantation after 30 minutes of warm ischemia. Rapid recovery technique at 30 minutes in the same model is never successful (Figure 27-1).[24] We now propose to extend the tolerable WI time to 60 minutes. In unpublished pilot studies we have similar success with 45 and 60 minutes of warm ischemia followed by 90 minutes of ECS, leading to normal renal function in the donor (without transplantation) (Figure 27-2).

We have demonstrated that lungs can be resuscitated with ECS in the animal model of DCD. Because there is no lung blood flow, the function of the lungs cannot be evaluated by gas exchange; however compliance in the normal range (50-100 cc/ cm H_2O) is a good surrogate marker of lung function.[29]

Future Directions

At the ECS lab of the University of Michigan five critical variables of ECS are currently being studied: duration, temperature, steroids,

pulsatility, and anticoagulation. We have previously studied temperature, and determined that room temperature perfusion is as effective as 37°C.[28] However, the details of the model were different than the current model. Published studies have been conducted with non-pulsatile flow. Since there is evidence that pulsatile flow may improve perfusion and outcome, it is important to determine if pulsatility adds benefit. The timing of anticoagulation is an important factor with potential ethical implications. Some consider it unacceptable to administer heparin prior to declaration of death. The Institute of Medicine concluded that whether to administer heparin should be a decision left up to the treating physician that is directing the withdrawal of support.[30] We have shown that heparin given five minutes after death is as effective as five minutes before in our porcine model.[31] Therefore, DCD-ECS could be simplified if anticoagulation is used only at the time of perfusion. Other preliminary studies in our ECS lab, have demonstrated that heparin can

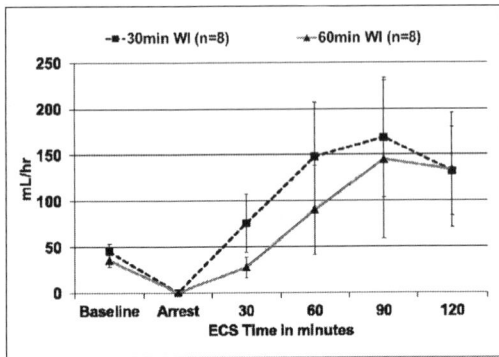

Figure 27-2. Swine DCD urine output during ECS assisted donation. Urine output was obtained after a prolonged time of warm ischemia (30 and 60min) in heparinized DCD swine during assisted ECS donation.

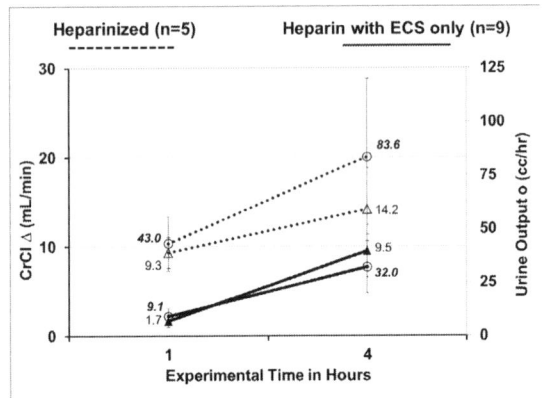

Figure 27-3. Immediate post-transplantation renal function after 30 min WI after ECS assisted donation in pre-heparinized and non-heparinized DCD Swine. Creatinine clearance (Δ-left axis), and urine output (O-right axis) at 1hr and 4hr post transplantation using renal grafts from pre-heparinized (controlled DCD) braked line, and non-heparinized DCD (uncontrolled DCD) that sustained 30min of warm ischemia and ECS for organ procurement. Renal function was restored in both type of DCD groups.

be given 30 minutes after death if followed by 180 minutes of ECS perfusion with satisfactory kidney function following transplantation of the recovered organs (Figure 27-3).

The VA ECS circuit animal model is represented in (Figure 27-4) and includes: a roller pump, an external heat exchanger, and a membrane oxygenator, and is then stepped up to 3/8" tubing to connect them to the oxygenator outlet. Pump flows are continuously monitored using a Transonic T208 monitor. The membrane oxygenator is primed with saline, 100 mEq of HCO_3, 12.5g mannitol, 125mg Methylpredinisolone and maintained at 38°C. After WI venoarterial perfusion will start and be maintained at 50 cc/kg/min for up to 3hrs, aiming to maintain SvO_2 at 75%, a CVP between 7–16 cmH_2O during ECS, avoiding cavitation or hemodilution (targeting hematocrit value >23%). The apparatus used for ECS in these experiments is standard in our lab, but any blood pump and membrane lung can be used.

Conclusion

Donation by ECS after cardiac death has many advantages over RR, most importantly better organ function after transplant. ECS assisted DCD is relatively easy to organize in controlled (Maastricht III) DCD. In uncontrolled DCD ECS must be immediately available and implemented by a combination of ER and transplant teams. Laboratory studies indicating that ECS can successfully resuscitate abdominal organs and lungs after a total arrest time up to 60 minutes will facilitate the use of ECS in uncontrolled DCD.

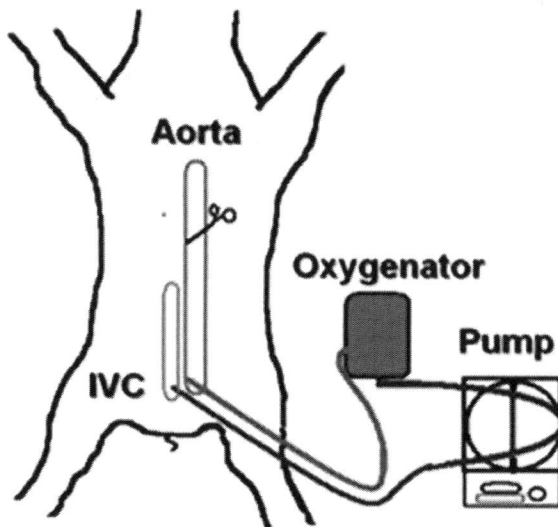

Figure 27-4. University of Michigan DCD-ECS assisted swine Model

References

1. (IOM) IOM. Organ Donation: Opportunities for Action. 2006 ed. Washington, D.C: The National Academies Press; 2006.
2. Kootstra G, Daemen JH, Oomen AP. Categories of non-heart-beating donors. Transplant Proc 1995;27:2893-4.
3. D'Alessandro AM, Fernandez LA, Chin LT, et al. Donation after cardiac death: the University of Wisconsin experience. Ann Transplant 2004;9:68-71.
4. Abt P, Crawford M, Desai N, Markmann J, Olthoff K, Shaked A. Liver transplantation from controlled non-heart-beating donors: an increased incidence of biliary complications. Transplantation 2003;75:1659-63.
5. Alonso A, Fernandez-Rivera C, Villaverde P, et al. Renal transplantation from non-heart-beating donors: a single-center 10-year experience. Transplant Proc 2005;37:3658-60.
6. Sanchez-Fructuoso AI, de Miguel Marques M, Prats D, Barrientos A. Non-heart-beating donors: experience from the Hospital Clinico of Madrid. J Nephrol 2003;16:387-92.
7. Sanchez-Fructuoso A, Prats Sanchez D, Marques Vidas M, Lopez De Novales E, Barrientos Guzman A. Non-heart beating donors. Nephrol Dial Transplant 2004;19 Suppl 3:iii26-31.
8. Sanchez-Fructuoso AI. Kidney transplantation from non-heart-beating donors. Transplant Proc 2007;39:2065-7.
9. Fondevila C, Hessheimer AJ, Ruiz A, et al. Liver transplant using donors after unexpected cardiac death: novel preservation protocol and acceptance criteria. Am J Transplant 2007;7:1849-55.
10. Nunez JR, Del Rio F, Lopez E, Moreno MA, Soria A, Parra D. Non-heart-beating donors: an excellent choice to increase the donor pool. Transplant Proc 2005;37:3651-4.
11. Kievit JK, Oomen AP, de Vries B, Heineman E, Kootstra G. Update on the results of non-heart-beating donor kidney transplants. Transplant Proc 1997;29:2989-91.
12. Keizer KM, de Fijter JW, Haase-Kromwijk BJ, Weimar W. Non-heart-beating donor kidneys in the Netherlands: allocation and outcome of transplantation. Transplantation 2005;79:1195-9.
13. Rudich SM, Kaplan B, Magee JC, et al. Renal transplantations performed using non-heart-beating organ donors: going back to the future? Transplantation 2002;74:1715-20.
14. Rudich SM, Arenas JD, Magee JC, et al. Extracorporeal support of the non-heart-beating organ donor. Transplantation 2002;73:158-9.
15. Magliocca JF, Magee JC, Rowe SA, et al. Extracorporeal support for organ donation after cardiac death effectively expands the donor pool. J Trauma 2005;58:1095-101; discussion 101-2.
16. Gravel MT, Arenas JD, Chenault R, 2nd, et al. Kidney transplantation from organ donors following cardiopulmonary death using extracorporeal membrane oxygenation support. Ann Transplant 2004;9:57-8.
17. Lee CY, Tsai MK, Ko WJ, et al. Expanding the donor pool: use of renal transplants from non-heart-beating donors supported with extracorporeal membrane oxygenation. Clin Transplant 2005;19:383-90.
18. Farney AC, Singh RP, Hines MH, et al. Experience in renal and extrarenal transplantation with donation after cardiac death donors with selective use of extracorporeal support. J Am Coll Surg 2008;206:1028-37; discussion 37.
19. Jimenez-Galanes S, Meneu-Diaz MJ, Elola-Olaso AM, et al. Liver transplantation using uncontrolled non-heart-beating donors under normothermic extracorporeal membrane oxygenation. Liver Transpl 2009;15:1110-8.
20. Garcia-Valdecasas JC, Tabet J, Valero R, et al. Liver conditioning after cardiac arrest:

the use of normothermic recirculation in an experimental animal model. Transpl Int 1998;11:424-32.

21. Valero R, Garcia-Valdecasas JC, Tabet J, et al. Hepatic blood flow and oxygen extraction ratio during normothermic recirculation and total body cooling as viability predictors in non-heart-beating donor pigs. Transplantation 1998;66:170-6.

22. Otero A, Gomez-Gutierrez M, Suarez F, et al. Liver transplantation from maastricht category 2 non-heart-beating donors: a source to increase the donor pool? Transplant Proc 2004;36:747-50.

23. Englesbe MJ, Woodrum D, Debroy M, et al. Salvage of an unstable brain dead donor with prompt extracorporeal support. Transplantation 2005;79:378.

24. Rojas-Pena A, Reoma JL, Krause E, et al. Extracorporeal support: improves donor renal graft function after cardiac death. Am J Transplant 2010;10:1365-74.

25. Fondevila C. Is extracorporeal support becoming the new standard for the preservation of DCD grafts? Am J Transplant 2010;10:1341-2.

26. Obeid NR, Rojas A, Reoma JL, et al. Organ donation after cardiac determination of death (DCD): a swine model. ASAIO J 2009;55:562-8.

27. Rojas A, Chen L, Bartlett RH, Arenas JD. Assessment of liver function during extracorporeal membrane oxygenation in the non-heart beating donor swine. Transplant Proc 2004;36:1268-70.

28. Rojas A LN, Arenas J.D, Bartlett R.H, Punch J.D. Normothermic .vs. Hypothermic extracorporeal membrane oxygenation (ECMO) support during procurement of abdominal organs from donors after cardiac death (DCD) in swine. . American Journal of Transplantation and Transplantation 2006;Supplement for WTC 2006:629.

29. Reoma JL, Rojas A, Krause EM, et al. Lung physiology during ECS resuscitation of DCD donors followed by In Situ assessment of lung function. ASAIO J 2009;55:388-94.

30. Abouna GM. Ethical issues in organ and tissue transplantation. Exp Clin Transplant 2003;1:125-38.

31. Rojas A GG, Cook K.E, Bartlett R.H, Punch J.D, Arenas J.D. . Role and Timing of Heparin During Procurement of Organs with Extracorporeal Life Support (ECLS). In: 8th Congress of the International Society for Organ Donation and Procurement (ISODP) 2005; Gramado, Brasil. December 4-7, 2005; 2005.

28

Sepsis and ECMO

Graeme MacLaren MBBS FCICM FCCM, Warwick Butt MBBS FCICM

Introduction

Sepsis is defined as the systemic inflammatory response to infection. A systemic inflammatory response consists of two or more of the following:

- Fever or hypothermia
- Tachycardia (or bradycardia in infants)
- Tachypnea or hypocapnia
- Leucocytosis, leucopenia, or >10% immature neutrophils

The exact values that define many of these parameters vary with age and can be found in the consensus statements of various Societies.[1-3] Severe sepsis occurs when organ dysfunction, hypoperfusion, or hypotension are present. Septic shock is defined as severe sepsis with hypotension and hypoperfusion which persist despite adequate fluid replacement. The definition of refractory septic shock varies[4] but the most comprehensive and apposite is that of the American College of Critical Care Medicine (ACCM): shock that persists despite goal-directed use of inotropes, vasopressors, vasodilators, and maintenance of metabolic and hormonal homeostasis.[5]

Sepsis is one of the leading causes of mortality and morbidity worldwide. Although case fatality rates appear to be falling in some countries, population-based mortality rates and hospitalization rates with severe sepsis are increasing.[6,7] In high income countries, adult patients admitted to the intensive care unit (ICU) with a diagnosis of severe sepsis have hospital mortality rates of between 27.6 – 32.1%.[7-10] In the United States, children hospitalized with severe sepsis have mortality rates of up to 10.3%.[10,11] The most important determinant of the likelihood of death is the development of shock.[12,13]

Sepsis was historically regarded as a contraindication to ECMO. In the 1990s, however, a number of studies demonstrated that it could be lifesaving in neonatal and pediatric septic shock,[14-17] a view strengthened by recent reports involving larger numbers of patients.[18-20] ECMO for refractory septic shock in neonates is now regarded as a standard indication for extracorporeal support, with survival rates of approximately 75-80%.[5,19,21] However, universal acceptance of ECMO for septic shock in older patients has been limited by the retrospective uncontrolled studies on the subject, historically poor outcomes in some centers, lack of comparative evaluation of cannulation strategies, and perhaps by an under-appreciation of the pathophysiological and hemodynamic responses to infection with changes in age. The ACCM recommend that ECMO be considered for refractory septic shock in children, but they anticipate survival rates no higher than 50%.[5] Whether better survival can be achieved with newer and safer types of ECMO technology is a question awaiting multicenter evaluation.

Sepsis is predominantly associated with only one pulmonary pathophysiological response (i.e., acute respiratory distress syndrome; ARDS) but a multitude of hemodynamic responses, including dilation and failure of one or both ventricles, an increase in pulmonary vascular resistance, and a fall in systemic vascular resistance, all of which may exist in relative isolation or in combination.[4,5] ECMO can be used to support patients with severe sepsis and any combination of:

- ARDS,
- Right heart failure,
- Left heart failure, and/or
- Combined cardiogenic and distributive shock.

This chapter will outline the indications and contraindications for ECMO in sepsis, review the hemodynamic responses to infection in patients of all ages and the consequent effects upon cannulation strategies, discuss circuit management in sepsis, and briefly summarize outcomes. The chapter will primarily focus on the use of ECMO as circulatory support in refractory septic shock, which requires more detailed consideration than isolated respiratory failure from sepsis.

Indications

It was suspected for many years that septic patients being placed on ECMO for respiratory support of sepsis-induced ARDS or bacterial pneumonia had worse outcomes than similar patients without sepsis. This has been shown not to be the case and neither sepsis nor bacteremia at the initiation of ECMO are predictors of poor outcome[22,23] (although, not surprisingly, the acquisition of new, nosocomial infection during an ECMO run can be detrimental[24-27]). Pneumonia or sepsis-induced ARDS often present without

significant circulatory dysfunction, in which case the indications and cannulation strategies for ECMO are similar as for other causes of hypoxic respiratory failure (see Chapter 4). Some of these patients may have hypotension, caused by many factors including severe hypoxia, hypercapnia, pulmonary hypertension, or right heart dysfunction. However, these secondary cardiovascular effects usually improve substantially with adequate venovenous (VV) ECMO, with its attendant effects on oxygenation, acid-base balance, carbon dioxide, temperature, and intrathoracic pressure.

In septic shock, the indication for ECMO is straightforward only in principle: it has been regarded as the therapy of last resort, when shock is refractory and continues to progress despite all attempts at ventilation, fluid, pharmacological, and disease-modifying therapy, or when cardiac arrest has ensued. However, the exact criteria when ECMO should be instituted have not been the subject of prospective study and clinicians must rely on clinical experience and judgment. The ACCM have summarized one approach in a consensus statement on the hemodynamic management of pediatric septic shock.[5] The rapidity of shock progression and physiological decline is more important than the absolute amount of inotropic support, but in general ECMO should be considered if a child:

- is receiving doses of >1 mcg/kg/min of epinephrine or its equivalent (i.e., an inotrope score[28] > 100),
- has already had aggressive fluid replacement and other pharmacological strategies described by the ACCM consensus statement,[5]
- is continuing to deteriorate with worsening hypotension, rising lactates, or rapidly progressive multiorgan dysfunction.

The speed at which ECMO can be initiated is very institution-dependent and this must be borne in mind by clinicians seeking to try every possible, less invasive strategy in children with rapidly progressive shock. Although several children have been successfully resuscitated from cardiac arrest caused by progressive septic shock and yet made complete recoveries,[18] it is clearly more desirable to intervene before arrest occurs. The timing of this will depend on how quickly an institution can mobilize an emergency ECMO team. Parallels can be drawn to fulminant myocarditis, where the exact timing of mechanical support is based on clinical experience and institutional resources, rather than by prospectively studied, specific criteria.

ECMO has been used in adult septic shock as well[29-32] but this is very rare and generally only seen in younger adults, for reasons that will be discussed under the section on cannulation.

Contraindications

The standard relative contraindications apply in septic patients being considered for ECMO, such as preexisting severe neurological dysfunction or advanced malignancy.[33] An additional consideration in sepsis is the septic oncology patient. Oncology patients have been regarded as poor ECMO candidates, but this view is anachronistic and outcomes can be reasonably good in many instances.[34] One exception to this is allogeneic bone marrow transplant recipients, who have dismal outcomes.[35] Septic shock with neutropenia may also be regarded as a relative contraindication, although ECMO has been successfully employed in a small number of select cases.[36]

The type of infecting organism should not be regarded as a major determinant of the appropriateness of ECMO, although some organisms, most notably *Bordetella pertussis* and herpes simplex in infants, are associated with poorer outcomes than others.[37,38] In the absence of other contraindications, the infecting microbe usually has minimal bearing on whether ECMO is offered or not (and is often not known at the time). Some known microbiological causes of septic shock in patients successfully supported with venoarterial (VA) ECMO are listed in Table 28-1.

Table 28-1. Reported microbiological causes of septic shock in patients successfully treated with venoarterial ECMO. Sourced from personal and published experience[14,15,18,20,37-42]

Gram-Negative Bacteria	Gram-Positive Bacteria	Other Bacteria	Viruses	Fungi
Neisseria meningitidis	*Staphylococcus aureus*	*Mycoplasma*	Influenza	*Candida* spp.
Neisseria gonorrhoea	Coagulase-negative	*Leptospira*	Parainfluenza	*Aspergillus* spp.
Klebsiella pneumoniae	*Staphylococcus*		Respiratory syncytial	
Enterobacter spp.	Group A *Streptococcus*		Herpes simplex	
Escherichia coli	Group B *Streptococcus*		Hanta	
Campylobacter jejuni	*Streptococcus pneumoniae*			
Salmonella spp	*Enterococcus* spp.			
Pseudomonas aeruginosa	*Listeria monocytogenes*			
Burkholderia cepacia				
Bordetella pertussis				
Haemophilus influenza				

Cannulation

The type of cannulation is one of the most important management issues in ECMO for sepsis and must be individually tailored to the patient's circulatory and respiratory status. An understanding of the pathophysiology of septic shock coupled with adequate hemodynamic information is vital in planning an appropriate cannulation strategy.

For sepsis-induced isolated respiratory failure requiring ECMO, VV cannulation is preferred as extracorporeal life support may be required for six weeks or more. VV ECMO avoids the complications of VA ECMO such as systemic embolization, arterial trauma, and increased left ventricular afterload, while preserving pulmonary blood flow, pulsatile systemic flow, and oxygenation of blood in the left ventricle and thus the coronary arteries.[43,44] VV ECMO is also preferred in those patients with ARDS that persists after resolution of shock, when the patient is ready to be weaned off mechanical circulatory support but not ready to cease extracorporeal gas exchange because of ongoing respiratory failure. In these instances, consideration should be given to changing to VV cannulation if it is anticipated that lung recovery will require more than 1-2 days of further ECMO.

If ECMO is being considered primarily as circulatory support for refractory septic shock, then the patient's hemodynamic response to sepsis must first be established. Septic shock has three principle hemodynamic manifestations based on the most compromised part of the circulation: right heart failure, left heart failure with poor systemic oxygen delivery, or distributive shock with poor oxygen extraction.[5] In advanced cases a mixture of these may occur, e.g., adult patients who present with distributive shock but later develop progressive ventricular failure, or children with a combination of cardiogenic and distributive shock.[18,20,29,31,32]

Right heart failure associated with persistent pulmonary hypertension of the newborn is the most frequent manifestation of septic shock in neonates. A component of right heart failure from a combination of sepsis-induced ventricular dysfunction and high positive pressure ventilation can also be seen in older patients. After the neonatal period, septic children suffer from left ventricular failure with preserved vasomotor tone and impaired oxygen delivery. The age at which a child will alter their hemodynamic response from left heart failure ('cold' shock) to distributive shock ('warm' shock) is highly variable and cannot be reliably predicted from the child's age. However, by late adolescence and into adulthood, the near universal hemodynamic response to sepsis is distributive shock. This is characterized by a reduction in ventricular function and an increase in heart rate, a reduction in vasomotor tone, and often by a reduction in oxygen extraction at a mitochondrial level. The categorization of shock requires a combination of clinical assessment, blood tests (e.g., venous oximetry, lactate), and echocardiography, with or without measurement of cardiac output, and is best done by an experienced intensivist.[5]

Possible ECMO cannulation strategies become apparent once the hemodynamic pattern of shock has been identified (Table 28-2). Those with right heart failure and concomitant respiratory failure can be supported with VV ECMO if the shock is not particularly advanced, as the consequent reduction in intrathoracic pressure and optimization of oxygenation and carbon dioxide clearance may be sufficient to improve myocardial performance and peripheral circulation, especially in small children. Otherwise, peripheral VA ECMO or central ECMO can be used.

In left heart failure, peripheral or high flow central ECMO is appropriate. Serial echocardiograms must be performed to monitor left heart distension. If this is severe or worsening, then steps should be taken to alleviate it before left atrial distension and hypertension lead to pulmonary edema or pulmonary hemorrhage. Increasing circuit flow may limit atrial distension; if unsuccessful then percutaneous atrial septostomy can be performed on peripheral ECMO, or a left atrial vent cannula can be inserted on central ECMO i.e., biatrial drainage. If the femoral artery is used in older children or adults then some centers advocate the routine use of an anterograde perfusion cannula to supply oxygenated blood to the affected leg to prevent limb ischemia. An additional consideration in patients on peripheral VA ECMO is that coronary and cerebral arterial blood may be supplied by the left ventricle and not the ECMO circuit. It is thus of considerable importance that an appropriate amount of oxygen is provided by the ventilator depending on the severity of respiratory failure, and that a surrogate marker of coronary oxygenation (e.g., right radial artery blood) is used to monitor for possible complications.[43,44] If there is decreased oxygen saturation in the right arm, then increasing peripheral VA

Table 28-2. ECMO cannulation strategies in septic shock

Hemodynamic Pattern	Usual Patient	Cannulation Options	Advantages	Caveats	Ref
Right heart failure	neonate	VV	- Avoids risk of systemic embolization - Avoids maldistribution of oxygenated blood - Fast cannulation - Can use 1 cannula	- Cannot provide complete circulatory support - Inappropriate for very advanced shock	45
		Peripheral VA (carotid)	- Can provide complete circulatory support - Fast cannulation	- Limited flows - May cause maldistribution of oxygenated blood	14,15,18
		Central VA	- Allows the highest flow rates - Avoids maldistribution of oxygenated blood	- Requires cardiac surgeon to cannulate - Theoretically higher bleeding or infection risk	18
Left heart failure	Young child	Peripheral VA (carotid or femoral)	- As above	- As above - Femoral cannulation may require an anterograde perfusion cannula to avoid limb ischemia	16-18
		Central VA	- May be associated with better outcomes	- As above	18,20
Distributive	Older child or adult	Central VA	- Only strategy likely to achieve sufficiently high circuit flows	- ECMO unnecessary / inappropriate unless pre-arrest physiology	18,20
Mixed shock (cardiogenic and distributive)	Any age	Central VA	- May be associated with better outcomes	- As above	18,20

VV: venovenous
VA: venoarterial
Peripheral: Drains deoxygenated blood via jugular vein, femoral vein, or both. Returns oxygenated blood to carotid artery (young children) or femoral artery (older children or adults)
Central: Drains deoxygenated blood directly from right atrium ± left atrium. Returns oxygenated blood to ascending aorta.

flow (if possible) and thus decreasing flow through the pulmonary circulation may be sufficient to allow for adequate coronary and cerebral oxygenation; if not, then an additional venous drainage cannula may provide sufficient flow to avoid cerebral injury.

Further explanation is necessary regarding distributive shock and any possible role of ECMO. Adults with fatal septic shock die as a consequence of one of three mechanisms: multiorgan failure (by far the most common), progressive ventricular dilatation and cardiogenic shock (rare), or early refractory vasodilation (rare).[46] Although distributive shock is associated with high cardiac output and vasoplegia, the left ventricular ejection fraction is usually depressed. In fact, preservation of ejection fraction and failure of the left ventricle to dilate in response to infection is associated with higher mortality,[47] perhaps as a result of preexisting diastolic dysfunction and poor ventricular compliance. Unlike in children,[48] deaths from multiorgan failure in adults are late in the course of illness and there is no evidence that ECMO would be useful in these patients. However, ECMO may have a role to play in those with progressive ventricular dilatation who maintain a high cardiac output initially, but later decline and suffer cardiovascular collapse. This scenario has been described in adults with bacterial septic shock, but is uncommon.[29,30,32] Distributive shock with early refractory vasodilation may also eventually lead to periods of cardiac arrest. In these rare patients, central ECMO has been used in adolescent patients to achieve flows of up to 10 L/min with good outcomes.[20,31]

Central cannulation

Central cannulation is commonly used in most major pediatric and adult cardiac transplantation centers. With this technique, analogous to cardiopulmonary bypass, a cardiac surgeon performs a sternotomy and cannulates the right atrium directly. Venous blood is pumped through the circuit and returned through a cannula placed in the ascending aorta. The largest available cannulae should be placed so as to maximize laminar flow and minimize excessive negative pressures, which might otherwise promote turbulent flow leading to shear-stress on blood components and hemolysis.[49] Many ECMO programs use the roller pump with gravity drainage into a bladder, but more recently the safety and portability of Mendler-designed centrifugal pumps have seen them increasingly used. These pumps generate negative pressure which draws blood out of the patient and through the circuit. The intensity of this pressure requires monitoring, as hypovolemia or cannula obstruction will limit inflow and create an increase in suction, with resultant turbulent flow and potential red cell hemolysis. In small children and newborn infants in whom constrained vortex pumps are being used, the pump inlet pressure should be measured at the connection between the atrial cannula and the inlet tubing, and should be maintained between -20 mmHg and zero. If the pressure is consistently more negative than -20 mmHg, then it should be assumed that the pump revolutions have been set too high, the patient is hypovolemic, or the cannulae are kinked, obstructed, or too small. Suggested cannula sizes and estimated flow ranges are listed in Table 28-3. In older children being cared for in dedicated pediatric hospitals and requiring higher flows, either a second drainage cannula can be inserted, or larger sized cannulae may have to be sourced from amongst cardiopulmonary bypass cannulae in nearby adult institutions. If possible, the skin should be sutured around the cannulae to minimize bleeding, and the defect

Table 28-3. Suggested cannula sizes for central ECMO

Patient Weight (kg)	Atrial Cannula (Fr)	Aortic Cannula (Fr)	Anticipated Flows (L/min)
<10	14-28	10-16	1-2
10-20	20-36	14-20	3-4
21-40	24-46	18-21	4-6
41-60	28-50	20-24	6-8
>60	36-52	22-24	8-10

between the sternal edges closed over with a Silastic membrane sutured into place.

Possible benefits of this technique include:[18,20,31,49]

- Achieving very high flow rates, which may lead to faster resolution of shock
- Avoiding maldistribution of oxygenated blood (as all blood is introduced into the ascending aorta)
- Complete cardiac and pulmonary support

Possible disadvantages include:

- Requires specialty cardiac surgical services
- Risk of mediastinitis (increases substantially after 5-7 days)
- Risk of local hemorrhage is greater than percutaneous techniques

There is some evidence that high flow, central ECMO is associated with improved survival in pediatric septic shock. In one study of 45 children with refractory septic shock, 73% of patients who received central ECMO survived compared to 38% who received peripheral ECMO (p=0.05).[5] However, this was an uncontrolled, retrospective study with limited numbers and there were a number of other possible reasons for these results, such as improved circuit technology and better intensive care provision in the more recent, high flow, central ECMO group. Nonetheless, the study highlighted that central ECMO is a valid technique in septic shock. At the Royal Children's Hospital, Melbourne, Australia, 25 children suffering from refractory septic shock have been supported with central ECMO over the last 10 years. Eighteen (72%) of these children have survived to hospital discharge. Many of these patients have received long-term followup. There have been no survivors with severe disability and the majority of survivors made a complete recovery.[18,50]

Management on ECMO

For patients with circulatory failure on VA ECMO, the goals of ECMO are the same as for other indications: restore organ blood flow and adequate tissue oxygenation while awaiting recovery, without causing damage to the lungs or circulation. The ECMO pump now becomes analogous to the heart. Instead of adjusting inotropes to enhance cardiac output, circuit flows 'replace' the cardiac output and thus must be titrated to provide adequate oxygen delivery. A term that is frequently used when referring to ECMO circuit flows is 'full flow.' However, this term is misleading and should be abandoned. Analogous to the concept that no given cardiac output can ever be considered 'normal,'[51] there is no circuit flow that can be regarded as 'full-flow.' The term fails to take oxygen consumption into consideration and falsely implies that there is a universally applicable level above which no benefit would be seen from further increases in flow. Instead, circuit flows should be goal-directed, targeting rapid normalization of lactate, improvement in $SvO_2 > 70\%$, and restoration of age-appropriate mean arterial pressures. In sepsis, this often requires very high flows (e.g., >150-200 ml/kg/min). Although the ACCM has recommended that flows be kept <110 ml/kg/min to minimize the risk of hemolysis,[5] this should be reconsidered in view of more recent information.[49] Instead, the target should be whatever flow is needed to promptly reverse shock and restore tissue oxygenation. In order to do this safely, appropriate monitoring of pump inlet pressures (see above) and regular measurement of plasma free hemoglobin should be used to detect excessive pump revolutions or cannula misplacement.[18] These goals are more easily executed with central ECMO than with other cannulation strategies. Appropriate flows that minimize hemolysis are often less than 110 ml/kg/min, but flows for adequate tissue oxygen delivery in sepsis are most often in excess of this figure, frequently 150-200 ml/kg/min.[18,20,49]

Therefore, other circuit considerations, such as maximizing cannula size and minimizing the presence of low flow zones (e.g., circuit bridges and the number of taps and access points), become very important to address in order to minimize the risk of hemolysis.[49]

Inotropes can usually be weaned off or to minimal doses within a few hours of achieving goal directed circuit flows. Vasoconstrictors may be necessary to maintain age appropriate mean arterial pressures but it is not unusual to see hypertension ensue around this time, particularly with the high flows of central ECMO, in which case short acting vasodilators (e.g., sodium nitroprusside or phentolamine) should be started to improve centrifugal pump flow and improve peripheral circulation. Ventilation settings should be reduced to lung-protective settings (e.g., rate 5-10, peak inspiratory pressure <25 cmH$_2$O, PEEP 5-12, FiO$_2$ <0.5) unless on peripheral VA ECMO, in which case FiO$_2$ must still be set high enough to maintain coronary oxygenation[43,44] (and, as the heart recovers, cerebral oxygenation).

The coagulation cascade is intricately involved in the process of inflammation and septic patients frequently have disseminated intravascular coagulation (DIC). Thrombus may form in parts of the ECMO circuit or patient's blood vessels while there is profuse hemorrhage from other areas. DIC should be aggressively treated with blood products while heparin is titrated to activated clotting times (ACT) and thromboelastography, if the latter is available. In sepsis, the target ACT is generally two times normal unless bleeding is profuse, in which case the target may be temporarily lowered to 1.5 times normal until the bleeding slows or stops. Aggressive blood product support with fresh frozen plasma (aiming INR<1.3-1.5), cryoprecipitate (aiming fibrinogen > 2.5 g/L), and platelets (aiming >100 x 10^9/L) is routine. Coagulopathy should never be allowed to replace controlled pharmacological anticoagulation in circuit management. A minimum of 10 U heparin/kg/hr should continue because of circulating procoagulants triggered by the septic process. Occasionally very large doses of heparin may be required (e.g., >30 U/kg/hr). In these patients, antithrombin-III levels may be low, in which case there may be a role for administering intravenous antithrombin-III concentrate, aiming for 100-120% of the reference value. In particularly difficult cases of DIC and hemorrhage, thromboelastography can be useful in identifying the most important elements of coagulopathy which can then be targeted for treatment.

Other measures such as effective empiric antibiotics and immediate treatment of any septic foci are vital. The pharmacokinetics of antibiotics for patients receiving extracorporeal life support have been inadequately studied. As failure to provide adequate and timely empiric antibiotics have been associated with substantial increases in mortality,[52,53] initial antibiotics should be given as early as possible, cover all likely pathogens, and be at the maximum dose recommended by standard formularies, especially those with a wide therapeutic index such as β-lactam antibiotics.[54]

The role of other extracorporeal life support modalities in sepsis to remove inflammatory mediators or modulate the immune response is controversial. These techniques, classified as Extracorporeal Blood Purification (EBP), include continuous renal replacement therapy (CRRT), plasmapheresis, plasma exchange, and hemoadsorption.[55,56] CRRT is frequently required in septic patients on ECMO to compensate for sepsis-induced acute kidney injury and provide adequate solute clearance, as well as to prevent severe volume overload from blood product, nutrient, and drug administration. Although some investigators have seen hemodynamic benefits in children receiving high-flux CRRT,[5] CRRT should not been regarded as standard management for septic patients on ECMO unless severe renal injury or diuretic-resistant fluid overload are present.[56-58] Plasma exchange and plasmapheresis have shown some promise in small trials but again cannot be considered standard therapy and await proper evaluation in large prospective multicenter studies.[48,59,60] Many other forms of EBP are undergoing phase II or III trials. One prospective, randomized, controlled trial of intraabdominal sepsis and shock showed decreased mortality with the use of polymyxin B hemoperfusion.[61] Although this finding was a secondary endpoint and just achieved statistical significance, the study demonstrated that EBP may well have an important role to play in the management of septic shock and further trials need to be conducted urgently.

Most patients on ECMO for septic shock recover quickly and do not require ECMO for more than 3-4 days. Failure of the heart to recover after seven days should trigger a search for additional pathologies such as myocardial infarction or bacterial myocarditis, and is usually a poor prognostic indicator. Occasionally, patients suffer from persistent ARDS, necessitating conversion to VV ECMO when the circulatory component of their illness resolves. This scenario is seen particularly with disseminated *Staphylococcus aureus* and can be challenging to deal with, as necrotizing staphylococcal pneumonia can cause substantial lung parenchymal destruction. After a trial of prolonged VV ECMO in some patients with this condition, the only option other than withdrawal of support may be to perform lung transplantation directly from ECMO. However, this scenario is uncommon and some patients can still be successfully weaned.

Outcomes

ECMO for neonatal sepsis is associated with survival rates of about 75%.[21] This age group is unique in having sufficient data to comment on pathogen-specific outcomes. In one survey sent to 16 ICUs worldwide, 117 septic patients were identified, 107 of whom were neonates.[39] Survival in patients with gram-positive, gram-negative, or viral sepsis was 77%, 60%, and 40% respectively, although the study was published over a decade ago and it is likely that outcomes are better now. One study of neonates on ECMO with herpes simplex virus showed survival to hospital discharge was only 25%.[37]

Data from the ELSO Registry reveal that survival in children after the neonatal period with isolated respiratory failure from bacterial or viral pneumonia are 57% and 63%, respectively.[21] The corresponding figures for adult patients are 56% and 64%. 55% of children and 49% of adults with ARDS have survived, but this includes all causes of ARDS and is not specific to sepsis. However, as noted above, there is no reason to believe that outcomes are different in septic patients.[22,23]

In septic shock, historical experience suggests that the use of ECMO in children is associated with survival to hospital discharge of 50% at best.[5,18] However, the use of high flow, central ECMO with modern circuitry and intensive care is associated with survival rates approaching 75%.[18,20] Hopefully, further assessment will support these more recent, improved survival figures, which are comparable to survival in neonatal sepsis.

The infrequent use of ECMO for adult septic shock has only been described in isolated case reports, so outcome data are not available.

Conclusions

Our understanding of ECMO for septic shock has progressed considerably in the last 20 years, through being regarded by many practitioners in the early 1990s as a complete contraindication, to modern published case series demonstrating up to 75% survival. However, many questions remain unanswered, particularly those concerning the optimal timing for commencement of ECMO, the optimal circuit flow and cannula configuration. Whether higher blood flows, and central cannulation are unequivocally associated with better survival and, if so, whether they should become a universal standard of care are issues currently in need of further evaluation.

ECMO is generally required very early in the course of sepsis, usually before antibiotics have taken effect.[20] The beneficial effects it exerts on reversing shock and halting the evolution of multiorgan failure are usually very apparent, particularly with central cannulation. As the technological advancements in ECMO circuitry have made extracorporeal support safer than ever before, it is interesting to speculate whether in time ECMO will move higher up the algorithm of septic shock management. Instead of being the therapy of last resort, it may become a more widely accepted treatment for septic shock, instituted earlier in the course of illness to prevent the establishment of multiorgan failure.

Septic shock remains a rare indication for ECMO in experienced centers yet up to 10% of children hospitalized with sepsis die.[10,11] While not all of these deaths can be prevented, some of these patients probably could be rescued with ECMO. With wider acceptance of sepsis as an indication for ECMO and greater engagement of institutions to refer to ECMO-capable centers, we believe this unacceptably high figure will fall. Extracorporeal therapy, whether it is ECMO, EBP, or both, holds the promise of significantly improving outcomes in septic shock.

References

1. Bone RC, Balk RA, Cerra FB, et al. Definitions for sepsis and organ failure and guidelines for the use of innovative therapies in sepsis. The ACCP/SCCM consensus conference committee. American College of Chest Physicians/Society of Critical Care Medicine. Chest 1992;101:1644-1655.

2. Levy MM, Fink MP, Marshall JC, et al. 2001 SCCM/ESICM/ACCP/ATS/SIS International sepsis definitions conference. Crit Care Med 2003;31:1250-1256.

3. Goldstein B, Giroir B, Randolph A, et al. International pediatric sepsis consensus conference: definitions for sepsis and organ dysfunction in pediatrics. Pediatr Crit Care Med 2005;6:2-8.

4. Annane D, Bellisant E, Cavaillon JM. Septic shock. Lancet 2005;365:63-78.

5. Brierley J, Carcillo JA, Choong K, et al. Clinical practice parameters for hemodynamic support of pediatric and neonatal septic shock: 2007 update from the American College of Critical Care Medicine. Crit Care Med 2009;37:666-688.

6. Dombrovskiy VY, Martin AA, Sunderram J, Paz HL. Rapid increase in hospitalization and mortality rates for severe sepsis in the United States: a trend analysis from 1993 to 2003. Crit Care Med 2007;35:1244-1250.

7. Australasian Resuscitation in Sepsis Evaluation (ARISE) Investigators and the Australian and New Zealand Intensive Care Society (ANZICS) Adult Patient Database (APD) Management Committee. The outcome of patients with sepsis and septic shock presenting to emergency departments in Australia and New Zealand. Crit Care Resusc 2007;9:8-18.

8. Barnato AE, Alexander SL, Linde-Zwirble WT, Angus DC. Racial variation in the incidence, care, and outcomes of severe sepsis: analysis of population, patient, and hospital characteristics. Am J Respir Crit Care Med 2008;177:279-284.

9. Levy MM, Dellinger RP, Townsend SR, et al. The surviving sepsis campaign: results of an international guideline-based performance improvement program targeting severe sepsis. Crit Care Med 2010;38:367-374.

10. Angus DC, Linde-Zwirble WT, Lidicker J, et al. Epidemiology of severe sepsis in the United States: analysis of incidence, outcome, and associated costs of care. Crit Care Med 2001;29:1303-1310.

11. Watson RS, Carcillo JA, Linde-Zwirble WT, et al. The epidemiology of severe sepsis in children in the United States. Am J Respir Crit Care Med 2003;167:695-701.

12. Watson RS, Carcillo JA. Scope and epidemiology of pediatric sepsis. Pediatr Crit Care Med 2005;6:S3-S5

13. Leclerc F, Leteurtre S, Duhamel A, et al. Cumulative influence of organ dysfunctions and septic state on mortality of critically ill children. Am J Resp Crit Care Med 2005;171:348-353.

14. McCune S, Short BL, Miller MK, Lotze A, Anderson KD. Extracorporeal membrane oxygenation therapy in neonates with septic shock. J Pediatr Surg 1990;25:479-482

15. Hocker JR, Simpson PM, Rabalais GP, Stewart DL, Cook LN. Extracorporeal membrane oxygenation and early-onset group B streptococcal sepsis. Pediatrics 1992;89:1-4

16. Beca J, Butt W. Extracorporeal membrane oxygenation for refractory septic shock in children. Pediatrics 1994;93:726-729.

17. Goldman AP, Kerr SJ, Butt W, et al. Extracorporeal support for intractable cardiorespiratory failure due to meningococcal disease. Lancet 1997;349:466-469.

18. MacLaren G, Butt W, Best D, Donath S, Taylor A. Extracorporeal membrane oxygenation for refractory septic shock

in children: one institution's experience. Pediatr Crit Care Med 2007;8:447-451.

19. Bartlett RH. Extracorporeal support for septic shock. Pediatr Crit Care Med 2007;8:498-499.

20. MacLaren G, Butt W, Best D, Donath S. Central extracorporeal membrane oxygenation for refractory pediatric septic shock. Pediatr Crit Care Med 2011; 12:133-136.

21. Extracorporeal Life Support Organization (ELSO). ECLS registry report, International Summary. January 2011.

22. Meyer DM, Jessen ME. Results of extracorporeal membrane oxygenation in children with sepsis. The Extracorporeal Life Support Organization. Ann Thor Surg 1997;63:756-761.

23. Rich PB, Younger JG, Soldes OS, Awad SS, Bartlett RH. Use of extracorporeal life support for adult patients with respiratory failure and sepsis. ASAIO J 1998;44:263-266.

24. Montgomery VL, Strotman JM, Ross MP. Impact of multiple organ dysfunction and nosocomial infections on survival of children treated with extracorporeal membrane oxygenation after heart surgery. Crit Care Med 2000;28:526-531.

25. Burket JS, Bartlett RH, Vander Hyde K, Chenoweth CE. Nosocomial infections in adult patients undergoing extracorporeal membrane oxygenation. Clin Infect Dis 1999;28:828-833.

26. O'Neill JM, Schutze GE, Heulitt MJ, Simpson PM, Taylor BJ. Nosocomial infections during extracorporeal membrane oxygenation. Intensive Care Med 2001;27:1247-1253.

27. Hsu MS, Chiu KM, Huang YT, et al. Risk factors for nosocomial infection during extracorporeal membrane oxygenation. J Hosp Infection 2009;73:210-216.

28. Wernovsky G, Wypij D, Jonas RA, et al. Postoperative course and hemodynamic profile after the arterial switch op-

eration in neonates and infants. Circulation 1995;92:2226-2235.

29. MacLaren G, Pellegrino V, Butt W, Preovolos A, Salamonsen R. Successful use of ECMO in adults with life-threatening infections. Anaesth Intensive Care 2004;32:707-710.

30. Vohra HA, Adamson L, Weeden DF, Haw MP. Use of extracorporeal membrane oxygenation in the management of septic shock with severe cardiac dysfunction after Ravitch procedure. Ann Thorac Surg 2009;87:e4-5.

31. MacLaren G, Cove M, Kofidis T. Central extracorporeal membrane oxygenation for septic shock in an adult with H1N1 influenza. Ann Thorac Surg 2010; 90:e34-35.

32. Firstenberg MS, Abel E, Blais D, et al. The use of extracorporeal membrane oxygenation in severe necrotizing soft tissue infections complicated by septic shock. Am Surg 2010; 76:1287-1289.

33. Extracorporeal Life Support Organization. ELSO general guidelines. Available at: http://www.elso.med.umich.edu/Guidelines.html. Accessed April 13, 2010

34. Gow KW, Heiss KF, Wulkan ML, et al. Extracorporeal life support of children with malignancy and respiratory or cardiac failure: The extracorporeal life support experience. Crit Care Med 2009;37:1308-1316.

35. Gupta M, Shanley TP, Moler FW. Extracorporeal life support for severe respiratory failure in children with immune compromised conditions. Pediatr Crit Care Med 2008;9:380-385.

36. Best D, MacLaren G, Butt W. Extracorporeal membrane oxygenation and oncological disease: one institution's experience. Presented at the 6th World Congress on Pediatric Critical Care, Sydney, Australia, March 2011.

37. Prodhan P, Wilkes R, Ross A, et al. Neonatal herpes virus infection and extracor-

poreal life support. Pediatr Crit Care Med 2010;11:599-602.

38. Pooboni S, Roberts N, Westrope C, et al. Extracorporeal life support in pertussis. Pediatr Pulmonol 2003;36:310-315.

39. Stewart DL, Dela Cruz TV, Ziegler C, Goldsmith LJ. The use of extracorporeal membrane oxygenation in patients with gram-negative or viral sepsis. Perfusion 1997;12:3-8.

40. Kahn JM, Muller HM, Kulier A, Keusch-Preininger A, Tscheliessnigg KH. Veno-arterial extracorporeal membrane oxygenation in acute respiratory distress syndrome caused by leptospire sepsis. Anesth Analg 2006;102:1597-1598.

41. Minette MS, Ibsen LM. Survival of candida sepsis in extracorporeal membrane oxygenation. Pediatr Crit Care Med 2005;6:709-711.

42. Crowley MR, Katz RW, Kessler R, et al. Successful treatment of adults with severe Hantavirus pulmonary syndrome with extracorporeal membrane oxygenation. Crit Care Med 1998;26:409-414.

43. Keckler SJ, Laituri CA, Ostlie DJ, St Peter SD. A review of venovenous and venoarterial extracorporeal membrane oxygenation in neonates and children. Eur J Pediatr Surg 2010;20:1-4.

44. Kinsella JP, Gerstmann DR, Rosenberg AA. The effect of extracorporeal membrane oxygenation on coronary perfusion and regional flow distribution. Pediatr Res 1992;31:80-84.

45. Roberts N, Westrope C, Pooboni SK, et al. Venovenous extracorporeal membrane oxygenation for respiratory failure in inotrope dependent neonates. ASAIO J 2003;49:568-571.

46. Court O, Kumar A, Parrillo JE, Kumar A. Clinical review: myocardial depression in sepsis and septic shock. Crit Care 2002;6:500-508.

47. Parker MM, Shelhamer JH, Bacharach SL, et al. Profound but reversible myocardial depression in patients with septic shock. Ann Intern Med 1984;100:483-490.

48. Carcillo JA. Multiple organ system extracorporeal support in critically ill children. Pediatr Clin North Am 2008;55:617-646.

49. MacLaren G, Butt W, Best D. Pediatric septic shock guidelines and extracorporeal membrane oxygenation management. Crit Care Med 2009;37:2143-2144.

50. Taylor A, Cousins R, Butt WW. The long-term outcome of children managed with extracorporeal life support: an institutional experience. Crit Care Resusc 2007;9:172-177.

51. Pinsky MR. Hemodynamic evaluation and monitoring in the ICU. Chest 2007;132:2020-2029.

52. Kumar A, Roberts D, Wood KE, et al. Duration of hypotension before initiation of effective antimicrobial therapy is the critical determinant of survival in human septic shock. Crit Care Med 2006;34:1589-1596.

53. Kumar A, Ellis P, Arabi Y, et al. Initiation of inappropriate antimicrobial therapy results in fivefold reduction of survival in human septic shock. Chest 2009;136:1237-48.

54. Lipman J, Boots R. A new paradigm for treating infections: "go hard and go home". Crit Care Resusc 2009;11:276-281.

55. House AA, Ronco C. Extracorporeal blood purification in sepsis and sepsis-related kidney injury. Blood Purif 2008;26:30-35.

56. Rimmele T, Kellum JA. Clinical review: Blood purification for sepsis. Crit Care 2011; 15:205.

57. MacLaren G, Butt W. Controversies in paediatric continuous renal replacement therapy. Intensive Care Med 2009;35:596-602.

58. Ronco C, Kellum JA, Bellomo R, House AA. Potential interventions in sepsis-related acute kidney injury. Clin J Am Soc Nephrol 2008;3:531-544.

59. Busund R, Koukline V, Utrobin U, et al. Plasmapheresis in severe sepsis and septic shock: a prospective, randomized, controlled trial. Intensive Care Med 2002;28:1434-1439.

60. Stegmayr BG, Banga R, Berggren L, et al. Plasma exchange as rescue therapy in multiple organ failure including acute renal failure. Crit Care Med 2003;31:1730-1736.

61. Cruz DN, Antonelli M, Fumagalli R, et al. Early use of polymyxin B hemoperfusion in abdominal septic shock: the EU-PHAS randomized controlled trial. JAMA 2009;301:2445-2552.

29

Extracorporeal Life Support Pre and Post Lung Transplantation

Shaf Keshavjee MD MSc FRCSC FACS, Marcelo Cypel MD MSc

Abstract

Patients who are otherwise excellent candidates for lung transplantation often die on the waiting list because they are too sick to survive until an organ becomes available. Improvements in lung transplant outcomes, patient selection, and improvements in artificial lung device technologies have made it possible to bridge these very sick patients to successful life saving transplantation. Extracorporeal life support (ECLS) can be tailored to minimize morbidity and provide the appropriate mode and level of cardiopulmonary support for each specific patient's physiologic requirements. Novel device refinements and simplification of ECLS will help to maintain these patients in improved condition until transplantation. In the recent years, improved outcomes have been also achieved with use of ECLS as a bridge to recovery after primary graft dysfunction after lung transplantation.

Introduction

Lung transplantation (LTx) is effective life saving therapy for patients with endstage lung disease.[1] However, patients who are otherwise excellent candidates for LTx often die on the waiting list because they are too sick to survive until an organ becomes available. Traditionally, these patients are supported by maximal mechanical ventilation in the ICU, but this further aggravates the lung injury[2] and often leads to remote organ dysfunction with subsequent high mortality prior to or after LTx.[3] For most of these patients, refractory hypercapnia, and/or hypoxia will develop despite maximal ventilatory support and therefore extracorporeal life support (ECLS) is their only chance to survive until a compatible donor lung becomes available. Initial attempts at utilizing ECLS as a bridge to LTx were hindered by a high rate of complications and poor outcomes.[4] In fact, the very initial attempts of lung transplantation were frequently in patients on ECLS. In 1975, the first case of extracorporeal membrane oxygenation (ECMO) as a bridge to lung transplant was performed for posttraumatic respiratory failure. The patient was successfully weaned from ECMO after the transplant; however, he died 10 days posttransplant from a combination of sepsis and bronchial dehiscence.[5] Subsequently in 1982 in Toronto, a further case of ECMO as a bridge to lung transplant was attempted in a patient with severe paraquat poisoning, but the patient died 92 days after the procedure with a tracheal-innominate artery fistula.[6] ECMO, and subsequently mechanical ventilation, were viewed as contraindications to lung transplantation as it was believed that both compromised bronchial healing – a major obstacle to LTx success in the early days.[4] Around the same time, a negative NIH randomized controlled trial was published in which survival after venoarterial (VA) ECMO was only 10% in patients with severe acute respiratory failure.[7] This combination of factors resulted in the concept of using ECMO as a bridge to lung transplant being largely discouraged.

However, in the last decade, improvements in lung transplant outcomes and patient selection, a better understanding of ventilator-associated lung injury, and improvements in artificial lung device technologies have made it possible to successfully bridge selected extremely sick patients to LTx.[8-12] In addition, recent studies have shown more promising results using ECLS for adults with ARDS with survival rates ranging from 50 to 80%. This includes the experience from Michigan in 100 patients,[13] the UK CESAR trial,[14] and H1N1/ARDS reports.[15,16] Significant improvements in survival for patients requiring ECLS as bridge to recovery from primary lung graft dysfunction (PGD) have also been achieved.

ECLS Pre-Lung Transplantation

Indications

The main indications for ECLS as a bridge to lung transplant include patients with irreversible endstage lung diseases presenting with rapid deterioration of respiratory status as reflected by refractory hypercapnic and/or hypoxic respiratory failure (usually $pCO_2 > 80$ mmHg and P/F < 80 mmHg). Another important indication for ECLS in the pretransplant setting is in patients with severe pulmonary hypertension and hemodynamic collapse due to severe dysfunction of the right ventricle.[11,17] Given the level of resource utilization and the scarcity of donor organs, careful patient selection is clearly needed. No specific criteria for this group of patients can yet be suggested due to the small

number of reported cases, but in general, young age, absence of multiple-organ dysfunction, and good prospects for rehabilitation after LTx should be considered. Usually, these patients have already been assessed by the LTx team and listed for LTx; however, in exceptional instances, urgent assessments and listing can be performed. With increased experience, there is also a trend towards implementing ECLS earlier in the course of the respiratory failure in order to avoid the need for prolonged high pressure mechanical ventilation leading to a systemic inflammatory response and secondary organ dysfunction.[2,3] Furthermore, recent reports have shown the feasibility of ECLS as bridge to LTx in awake and nonintubated patients allowing them to ambulate and potentially be in better physical condition by the time of the transplant.[9,18]

Contraindications

Contraindications for the use of ECLS in this population are: septic shock, multiorgan dysfunction, severe arterial occlusive disease, and heparin-induced thrombocytopenia type II. Unfavourable prognostic factors include: acute renal failure, high vasopressor requirements, a long preceding duration of mechanical ventilation, advanced age, and obesity.[19] Another contraindication is a patient with poor prospect for effective rehabilitation after transplantation.

Modes of ECLS–Configuration of Device

In addition to the technical advances, device configuration can be individualized and tailored for specific patient ventilatory and hemodynamic requirements. The configuration and mode of ECLS will depend on the specific clinical scenario (Figure 29-1).

Hypercapnic Respiratory Failure

Refractory hypercapnic respiratory failure and acidosis is a common scenario in patients with cystic fibrosis (CF) waiting for lung transplantation. Noninvasive ventilation (NIV) has become an important option as a treatment modality in acute respiratory failure in CF, avoiding endotracheal intubation with its attendant complications.[20] If a suitable organ does not become available in time, respiratory failure progresses and mechanical ventilation becomes necessary. At that stage, management becomes increasingly difficult as high pressure ventilation is required and alveolar hypoventilation and hypercapnia often persists despite it. The large amounts of bronchopulmonary secretions in these patients make ventilation even more difficult. Traditionally, patients with hypercapnia and respiratory acidosis required ECLS with the use of a pump. However, with the advent of an interventional lung assist device (iLA, Novalung,® Germany), the Hannover group demonstrated the feasibility of bridging these patients with the iLA in a ***pumpless*** arteriovenous (AV) mode.[8] This low resistance (11mmHg) hollow fiber polymethylpentene membrane is attached to the systemic circulation (usually femoral artery) and receives only part of the cardiac output (15 to 20%) for extracorporeal gas exchange. This allows prompt and effective CO_2 removal and correction of respiratory acidosis. CO_2 removal rates

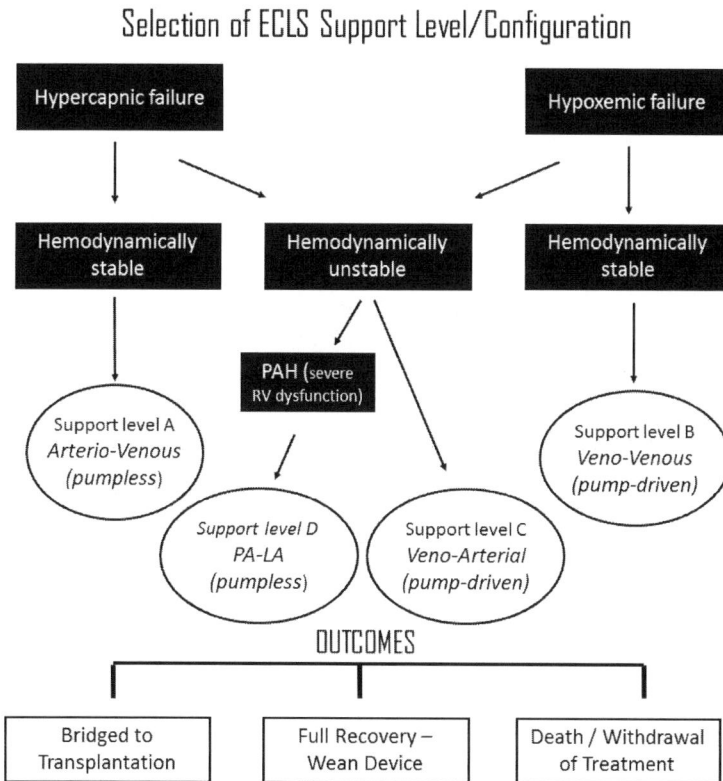

Figure 29-1. Algorithm for selection of ECLS support mode. Support Level A: AV pumpless ECLS mode-for patients with hypercapneic respiratory failure; Support Level B: VV ECLS mode-for patients with hypoxic respiratory failure; Support Level C: VA ECLS mode-for patients with hypoxic respiratory failure with hemodynamic compromise; and Support Level D: PA-LA pumpless ECLS mode-for patients with pulmonary hypertension causing RV failure.

can be controlled by varying the sweep of gas flow up to 15 L/min. The usual recommended rate of CO_2 clearance is 20 mmHg/hour. In order to use the pumpless device, the patient must have an adequate mean arterial blood pressure to be able to sustain good flows through the device (mean arterial pressure > 80 mmHg). Since only about one fifth of the cardiac output can be oxygenated via this AV mode of ECLS, it is not recommended for patients with severe hypoxia (PaO_2/FiO_2 < 80 mmHg).[8] Cannulation is usually achieved percutaneously using a Seldinger technique (or an open modified Seldinger technique) in the femoral artery (13-15Fr) and femoral vein (17 Fr). Insertion of long ECMO cannulas on the venous side provide too much resistance to flow when AV mode is being applied and therefore should be avoided. Since a centrifugal pump is not required and the circuit is fully heparin coated, anticoagulation levels can be similar to those used in pump assisted ECLS (traditional venovenous [VV] or VA ECMO). When measured using activated clotting times (ACT), a typical range of 160-200 seconds is used. If there is a concern about bleeding, an ACT of 150-180 seconds is acceptable.

In the initial publication from Fischer et al. 12 patients were bridged to transplantation using the iLA. The underlying diseases were bronchiolitis obliterans in three patients who were listed for redo LTx, idiopathic pulmonary fibrosis in four patients, cystic fibrosis in two patients, emphysema in one patient, inhalation trauma in one patient, and lymphangioleiomyomatosis in another patient. The mean duration of iLA support in the 12 patients was 15±8 days (4-32 days). Efficient CO_2 removal was rapidly achieved in all patients. Four patients died of multiorgan failure, two before LTx and two on days 16 and 30 after LTx. Thus, 10 of the 12 patients were successfully bridged to LTx, and 8 of the 10 were alive one year posttransplantation.[8]

Ricci attempted the use of CO_2 removal devices in 12 patients as bridge to LTx.[21] Causes of respiratory failure that led to implantation of iLA were cystic fibrosis (n=6), pulmonary emphysema (n=5), and chronic rejection of a previous double lung transplant (n=1). Mean time on extracorporeal support was 13.5±14.2 days. However, 8 of the 12 patients died on the device prior to transplantation despite efficient CO_2 removal.

In Toronto, four patients underwent femoral iLA applied in the AV mode as bridge to LTx and all of them were successfully transplanted.[12] Another four patients were initiated in the pumpless AV mode, and were successfully transplanted, but had to be converted to pump assisted VV or VA ECLS.

Hypoxemic Respiratory Failure

Some patients will progress to hypoxemic respiratory failure and a different level of support is required. Whereas CO_2 removal can be achieved with low membrane flows (0.5-1 L/min),[22] substantial oxygenation requires more physiologic flows over the membrane (3-5 L/min). In order to achieve this, VV or VA pump-driven ECLS support is required. VV mode is the preferred choice if the patient is hypoxic, but hemodynamically stable. The advantages of the VV mode in comparison to VA mode are the decreased rates of bleeding, arterial thrombosis, and neurologic complications. Generally, a 22Fr canula is inserted into a femoral vein for drainage and a 17Fr single-stage cannula inserted into an internal jugular vein percutaneously for patient inflow. More recently, a dual lumen single cannula system has been developed for VV ECLS that has the advantage of simplicity, and importantly, allows for patient mobilization.[18] Usual ACTs should range from 160-200 seconds.

Fischer et al. demonstrated the use of iLA Novalung in VV mode in two patients successfully bridged to transplantation.[23] In a recent report from Scandinavia, seven patients were supported with VV ECLS for a mean of 17±19 days (median 12, range 1–59) before LTx. Two patients had to be converted to VA ECLS. One patient was weaned from ECLS before LTx; in all the other patients, ECLS was continued until the LTx was performed. None of the patients needed ECLS postoperatively. By intention-to-treat, the success for bridging was 81% and one year survival was 75%.[24]

Hypoxemic Respiratory Failure and Hemodynamic Compromise

For patients with respiratory failure and hemodynamic compromise, VA ECLS is the recommended option since it provides both cardiac and pulmonary support. In fact, the initial experience with ECLS in LTx was using this mode.[6] Usually a femoral vein is cannulated for drainage and a femoral artery cannulated for blood return. Some authors also propose the use of the axillary artery with an interposition graft.[25-27] Although vascular access is a bit more difficult, the advantages of the axillary artery in this setting are the possibility of better patient mobilization and the low incidence of atherosclerosis in this vessel. Improved upper body oxygenated perfusion is also an important advantage. Another option to improve central oxygenation is to insert an additional cannula into the internal jugular vein and convert the circuit to a hybrid VAV (V: femoral vein - VA: jugular vein and femoral artery) ECLS. This configuration of VAV ECMO can also be used to provide partial cardiac support when cardiac function is depressed and does not improve with improved oxygenation on VV support alone.[28-30]

A recent report demonstrates the application of VA ECLS as bridge to LTx in awake and spontaneously breathing patients, avoiding the drawbacks and complications associated with intubation and prolonged mechanical ventilation. All five patients described in this series presented with cardiopulmonary failure due to pulmonary hypertension with or without concomitant lung disease. ECLS application

was performed under local anaesthesia without sedation and resulted in immediate stabilization of hemodynamics and gas exchange as well as recovery from secondary organ dysfunction. Two patients later required endotracheal intubation because of bleeding complications and both of them eventually died. The other three patients remained awake on ECMO support for 18–35 days until the time of transplantation after which full recovery was achieved.[9]

Pulmonary Hypertension and Right Ventricular Failure

A novel mode of ECLS that we recently described is pulmonary artery to left atrium (PA to LA) ECLS configuration.[11,31] Although progress has been made for isolated lung failure, no truly effective solution existed for patients with primary pulmonary arterial hypertension (PAH). Compared to patients with lung failure due to isolated lung parenchymal disorders, patients with endstage PAH develop severe right heart failure. VV ECLS does not effectively unload the right ventricle (RV). An atrial septostomy is sometimes performed to create a right to left shunt, thereby unloading and protecting the RV from failing. The consequence of right to left shunt will also be desaturated blood reaching the left sided circulation. This can result in an unacceptable hypoxia. In this patient with PAH, we have demonstrated that the connection of a low resistance gas exchange device (Novalung[R]) between the main trunk of the pulmonary artery and the left atrium (PA-LA) in a pumpless mode effectively creates an *oxygenating* shunt that pressure unloads the right ventricle much like an atrial septostomy (Figure 29-2). However, the important advantage in this case, is that the membrane oxygenates the blood and thus the central hypoxia seen with a simple septostomy is avoided. In our experience, patients improve dramatically as soon as flow across the Novalung[R] is instituted.[11] The elevated pressure in the pulmonary arteries serves as the driving force for the device and obviates the need for a pump. From a technical standpoint, patients are often so unstable they usually require femoral–femoral VA ECLS support just prior to anesthetic induction. This is followed by median sternotomy and cannulation of the right superior pulmonary vein with a 17-23 Fr Pacifico canula (Bard Inc.). The PA is then cannulated with a 21-24 Fr canula (Medtronic arterial canula). The femoral ECLS support is then discontinued. Extubation, physiotherapy, and ambulation are achievable while a patient is on pumpless PA-LA ECLS awaiting a compatible donor lung (Figure 29-3). Eight successful cases have been reported using this technique to bridge PAH patients for LTx.[11,12,31] In our experience, these patients become remarkably stable during PA-LA ECLS and three of these patients stayed on the device for more than 30 days without significant complications. Of note, in most cases, heart-lung transplantation is not required since the unloaded right ventricle recovers on the Novalung[R] and bilateral LTx provides ongoing remodelling and recovery of the right heart.[11]

Another innovative ECLS approach to bridge patients with severe PAH to lung transplantation is VV ECLS with added atrial septostomy. In two studies using adult sheep, right to left atrial shunting of oxygenated blood with VV ECMO was capable of maintaining normal systemic hemodynamics and normal arterial blood gases during high right ventricular afterload dysfunction.[32,33] The theoretical advantage in comparison to PA-LA mode is the avoidance of sternotomy and central cannulation, however, the use of a pump is required.

Patient Management

Patients receiving ECLS as a bridge to LTx require clinical management comparable to an ECLS patient being supported secondary to ARDS. Once ECLS is initiated, the ventilator should be adjusted to "resting" lung settings. The ECLS flow should be maintained to sustain a venous blood saturation of 80-85% and an arterial saturation of 80-95%. Diuretics are given as required, to maintain adequate urine output and remove excess fluid. If negative

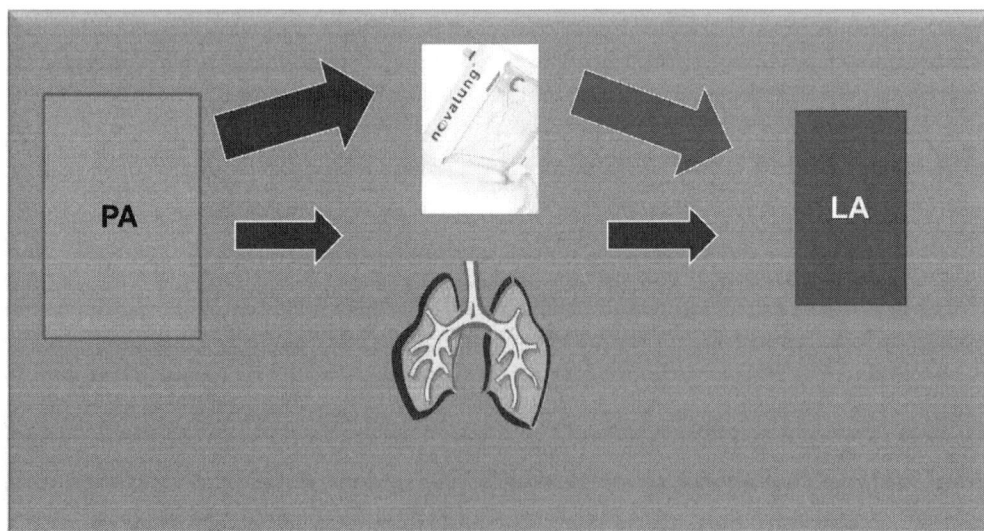

Figure 29-2. Pumpless pulmonary artery (PA) to left atrium (LA) ECLS support for patients with pulmonary hypertension. An oxygenating shunt is created providing both right ventricular decompression and oxygenation.

fluid balance cannot be achieved with diuretics, hemofiltration should be initiated early. Neurologic status is frequently checked and any deterioration should prompt further investigations. Cannulation sites and limb perfusion status are also frequently checked for bleeding and distal perfusion respectively. Prophylactic antibiotics are given prior to insertion of cannulas. General target guidelines used by the Toronto General Hospital ECLS/Lung Transplant Program are listed in Table 29-1.

Outcomes

The outcomes of patients bridged to LTx using mechanical support have been improving and are satisfactory considering the severity of their diseases and the overall survival of LTx recipients. A recent review from the UNOS experience totalling 51 patients bridged to LTx with ECLS from 1987 to 2008, showed a 1, 6, 12, and 24 month survival of 72%, 53%, 50%, and 45% respectively; compared to 93%, 85%, 79%, and 70% for unsupported patients, respectively.[34] Most recent reports from experienced centers in both LTx and ECLS have shown that 80% or more of patients can be successfully bridged to LTx and outcomes after LTx in these selected patients can approach that of conventional lung transplants.[8,9,11,12,21,24,35,36] These results demonstrate that outcomes in this patient population are better than the results of ECLS use to bridge patients to recovery from severe primary graft dysfunction after LTx,[19] (which is usually a tougher salvage situation); although improved results have been recently obtained in this latter group as well.[37,38] Table 29-2 demonstrates reported series of cases in which more than four patients were included.[8,9,11,12,21,24,35,36]

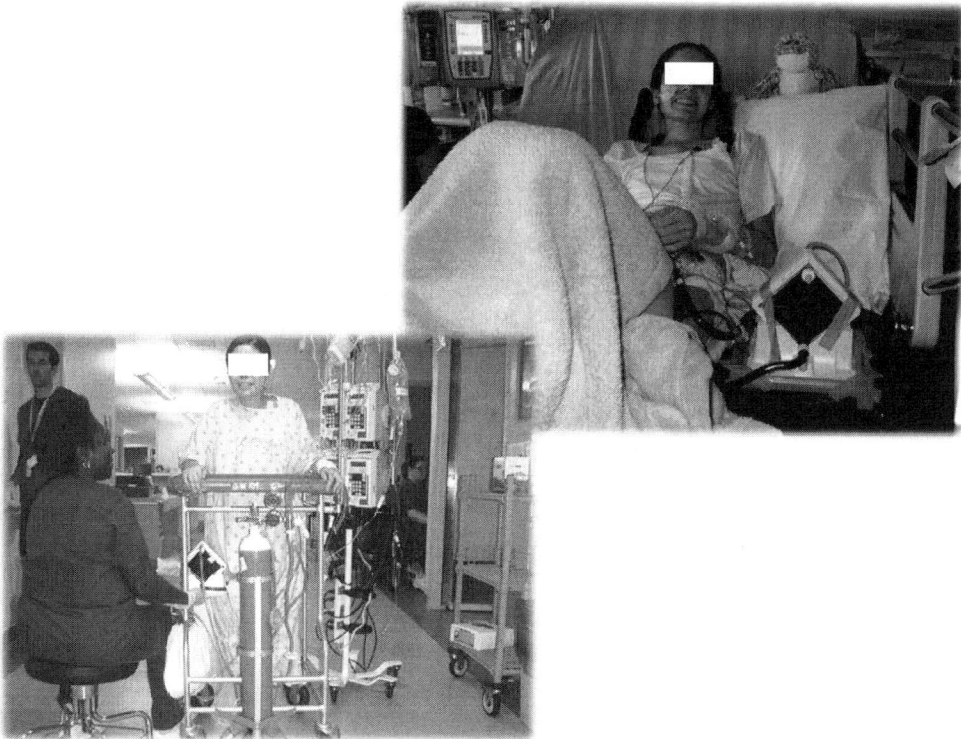

Figure 29-3. Extubated, rehabilitating and ambulatory patients with PA-LA ECLS (Novalung®) waiting for lung transplantation.

Perioperative ECLS

The group from Vienna has the largest experience with the use of VA ECMO instead of central cardiopulmonary bypass (CPB) for intraoperative and perioperative support during the transplantation procedure.[10] The theoretical advantages of VA ECMO in that setting are the avoidance of heparinization as indicated for cardiopulmonary bypass (300 U/kg heparin with target ACT > 400 sec) and the potential to prolong the support beyond the operation. ECMO was used in 147 patients in total. Two patients were bridged to transplantation. A total of 130 patients received intraoperative ECMO support. In 51 of these patients ECMO was prolonged into the perioperative period. A total of 149 patients without relevant risk factors were transplanted without any intraoperative extracorporeal support. Six of these patients required ECMO support in the postoperative period for treatment of primary graft dysfunction. The 3, 12, and 36 month survival rates were 85.4%, 74.2%, and 67.6% in the intraoperative ECMO group; 93.5%, 91.9%, and 86.5% in the no support group and 74.0%, 65.9%, and 57.7% in the CPB group. Select patients, who may be at a higher risk for developing PGD posttransplant, may benefit from prophylactic institution of ECMO at the beginning of the surgery, with continuous ECMO-assisted respiratory and hemodynamic support during surgery, enabling optimally controlled ventilation, and graft reperfusion methods as well as controlled early posttransplant management. However, most lung transplant centers still use CPB during LTx if temporary support is required.

ECLS Post Lung Transplantation

Primary graft dysfunction (PGD) affects 15-50% of lung transplant recipients and remains a significant cause of early morbidity and mortality after lung transplantation (30-day mortality of 42% in severe PGD compared to 6% in PGD-free patients).[39,40] In most cases of post-LTx PGD, optimization of conventional mechanical ventilator support allows for recovery of the injured lung; however, mechanical ventilation alone cannot achieve sufficient gas exchange in some patients with severe PGD and pushing mechanical ventilation to the limits risks adding further injury to the already injured lung. In such cases, therapeutic interventions such as the administration of inhaled nitric oxide,[41] intravenous prostacyclins,[42] or surfactant[43,44] have all been tried with variable results in the setting of severe PGD. If these agents are ineffective, then the only life-prolonging option is extracorporeal gas exchange using ECLS. This

Table 29-1. Target guidelines for a patient on ECLS.

Target guidelines for a patient on ECLS	
Temperature	*35.5 – 37.0 °C*
pH	*7.35 – 7.45*
pCO$_2$	*35 – 45 mmHg*
pO$_2$	*> 100 mmHg*
Hemoglobin Saturation	*> 85%*
Hemoglobin	*80-100g/L*
INR	*<1.8*
	<1.5 if bleeding
Platelets	*> 80,000/mm^3*
	> 100,000/mm^3 if bleeding
Fibrinogen	*> 1.5 - 4.0 g/l*
Factor X Concentration	*0.4 - 0.6 u/ml*
Anticoagulation Time (ACT)	*160 – 200 sec.*
Pump Flow	*Aim for 60cc/kg/min*

theoretically will also give the injured lung graft a chance to recover.

The international experience (ELSO Registry) for the use of ECLS for PGD after LTx was recently reviewed by Fischer et al.[19] Out of 31,340 ECLS cases, 151 were post-LTx patients with PGD. The mean age was 35 ± 18 years. Indications for LTx were acute respiratory distress syndrome (15%), cystic fibrosis (15%), idiopathic pulmonary fibrosis (8%), primary pulmonary hypertension (10%), emphysema (15%), acute lung failure (11%), other (23%), and unknown (3%). ECMO run time was 140 ± 212 hours. VV ECMO was used in 25, VA in 89, and other modes in 15 patients. In total 63 (42%) patients survived the hospital stay.

ECLS after LTx is predominantly instituted for pulmonary support, which is generally achievable in the VV mode. However, in the ELSO Registry review, a high proportion of adult patients received VA support, which is well known to have more side effects than the VV mode. In the pediatric setting, VA support was used in 60% of cases. Investigators may consider VA ECMO to be a safer approach because many patients develop hemodynamic instability in addition to poor gas exchange. It is frequently the case, however, that this instability can resolve when adequate gas exchange is achieved with VV ECMO. Some groups also have preferred VA ECMO due to a more efficient unloading of the pulmonary circulation[10,45]

Hartwig et al. reported superior outcomes after VV ECMO vs. VA ECMO for post-LTx PGD. They reported a 30-day survival of 88% in the VV group vs. no 30-day survival in the VA cohort.[37] In contrast, Ailwady et al. demonstrated that using VA ECMO, the mortality of patients with reperfusion injury requiring ECMO has significantly improved in the recent era (25% vs. 80% in the previous era).[45] Bermudez et al. reported their experience with 58 patients (7.6% of LTx) requiring early (0 to 7 days after transplant, VV [n=32] or VA [n=26]) ECMO support for PGD.[38] Mean duration of support was 5.5 days. Thirty-day, 1-year, and 5-year survivals were 56%, 40%, and 25%, respectively. Survival at 30 days and at one and five years was similar for the patients supported in VA or VV ECMO modes.

One important predictor of patient outcome has been the timing of ECLS initiation after transplantation. In the report by Wigfield, 30-day, 1-year and 3-year survival of LTx recipients with ECMO support postoperatively were 74.6%, 54%, and 36%, respectively. Late institution of ECMO (>24h) was associated with 100% mortality in their experience.[46] Meyers et al. reviewed their experience with 12 patients (2.7% of LTx).[47] Seven patients (58.4%) survived, including one of two patients who underwent retransplantation while being supported by ECMO. All survivors had ECMO instituted either perioperatively or during the first postop-

Table 29-2. Experience with ECLS as a bridge to lung transplant (series with more than 4 cases).

Author	# Cases	Days on Device (mean)	Mode ECLS	Bridged to Tx (%)	30 Day Survival after LTx (%)	1 Yr Survival (%)
Fischer 2006	12	15	AV pumpless	83	80	80
Strueber 2009	4	17	PA-LA pumpless	100	100	75
Cypel 2010	12	10	VA (3), VV (1), AV (4), PA-LA (4)	100	100	83
Yun 2010	7	7	VV (5) VA (2)	86	83	NA
Ricci 2010	12	13.5	AV pumpless	25	NA	NA
Nosoti 2010	4	9	VV	100	75	NA
Hämmäinen 2010	16	17	VV (7) VA(6)	81	100	92

erative day--again underscoring the importance of early institution of support. Glassman et al. compared patients with early (up to seven days posttransplant) ECMO institution (10 patients, 7 long term survivors) to those with late (>7 days) ECMO placement (6 patients, no survivors).[48] Nguyen et al. reported their experience in 14 patients (5.5% of LTx) that received posttransplant ECMO support. Seven of nine patients that had early (≤24 hours) graft failure survived in comparison to 0/5 for late (>7 days) graft failure.[49] In summary, reported outcomes are uniformly dismal if ECMO is initiated later than seven days posttransplant because in most of these cases the occurring problem is not related to recoverable PGD, but more likely due to other complicating factors such as irreversible lung injury, rejection, or infection.

Conclusions

Although experience is still limited, ECLS clearly can be an effective tool to bridge critically ill patients to a lifesaving lung transplant. Technological advances have permitted safer, less complicated application of ECLS for longer periods of time. Support can be tailored to minimize morbidity and provide the appropriate ECLS mode and level of cardiopulmonary support for each specific patient's physiologic requirements. Novel device refinements and further development of ECLS in an ambulatory and simplified manner will help to maintain these patients in better condition until transplantation. Further experience is required to ultimately define the optimal timing and criteria for initiation of ECLS in patients requiring bridging to lung transplantation. After LTx, ECLS is a potentially lifesaving treatment option for patients with severe primary graft dysfunction, who are not improving with conventional supportive therapy. It is expected that 2 to 8% of patients after LTx will require some form of ECLS. Each individual patient should be carefully considered with regard to other comorbidities to determine the overall likelihood of success. Currently, available data indicate that early (< 24 hour) institution offers a significant survival benefit. Expected survival to hospital discharge in these patients have ranged from 40 to 80% in different series; however, outcomes have significantly improved in more recent reports.

References

1. Christie JD, Edwards LB, Aurora P, et al. The Registry of the International Society for Heart and Lung Transplantation: Twenty-sixth Official Adult Lung and Heart-Lung Transplantation Report-2009. J Heart Lung Transplant 2009;28:1031-49.

2. Slutsky AS, Imai Y. Ventilator-induced lung injury, cytokines, PEEP, and mortality: implications for practice and for clinical trials. Intensive Care Med 2003;29:1218-21.

3. Imai Y, Parodo J, Kajikawa O, et al. Injurious mechanical ventilation and end-organ epithelial cell apoptosis and organ dysfunction in an experimental model of acute respiratory distress syndrome. JAMA 2003;289:2104-12.

4. Jurmann MJ, Haverich A, Demertzis S, Schaefers HJ, Wagner TO, Borst HG. Extracorporeal membrane oxygenation as a bridge to lung transplantation. Eur J Cardiothorac Surg 1991;5:94-7; discussion 8.

5. Nelems JM, Duffin J, Glynn FX, Brebner J, Scott AA, Cooper JD. Extracorporeal membrane oxygenator support for human lung transplantation. J Thorac Cardiovasc Surg 1978;76:28-32.

6. Sequential bilateral lung transplantation for paraquat poisoning. A case report. The Toronto Lung Transplant group. J Thorac Cardiovasc Surg 1985;89:734-42.

7. Zapol WM, Snider MT, Hill JD, et al. Extracorporeal membrane oxygenation in severe acute respiratory failure. A randomized prospective study. JAMA 1979;242:2193-6.

8. Fischer S, Simon AR, Welte T, et al. Bridge to lung transplantation with the novel pumpless interventional lung assist device NovaLung. J Thorac Cardiovasc Surg 2006;131:719-23.

9. Olsson KM, Simon A, Strueber M, et al. Extracorporeal Membrane Oxygenation in Nonintubated Patients as Bridge to Lung Transplantation. Am J Transplant 2010.

10. Aigner C, Wisser W, Taghavi S, et al. Institutional experience with extracorporeal membrane oxygenation in lung transplantation. Eur J Cardiothorac Surg 2007;31:468-73; discussion 73-4.

11. Strueber M, Hoeper MM, Fischer S, et al. Bridge to thoracic organ transplantation in patients with pulmonary arterial hypertension using a pumpless lung assist device. Am J Transplant 2009;9:853-7.

12. M. Cypel, T.K. Waddell, M. de Perrot, et al. Safety and Efficacy of the Novalung Interventional Lung Assist (iLA) Device as a Bridge to Lung Transplantation J Heart Lung Transplant 2010;February 2010 (Vol. 29, Issue 2, Supplement, Page S88.

13. Kolla S, Awad SS, Rich PB, Schreiner RJ, Hirschl RB, Bartlett RH. Extracorporeal life support for 100 adult patients with severe respiratory failure. Ann Surg 1997;226:544-64; discussion 65-6.

14. Peek GJ, Mugford M, Tiruvoipati R, et al. Efficacy and economic assessment of conventional ventilatory support versus extracorporeal membrane oxygenation for severe adult respiratory failure (CESAR): a multicentre randomised controlled trial. Lancet 2009;374:1351-63.

15. Freed DH, Henzler D, White CW, et al. Extracorporeal lung support for patients who had severe respiratory failure secondary to influenza A (H1N1) 2009 infection in Canada. Can J Anaesth 2010;57:240-7.

16. Davies A, Jones D, Bailey M, et al. Extracorporeal Membrane Oxygenation for 2009 Influenza A(H1N1) Acute Respiratory Distress Syndrome. JAMA 2009;302:1888-95.

17. Puehler T, Philipp A, Schmid C. Paracorporeal artificial lung circuit as a possibility for bridge to lung transplantation. Ann Thorac Surg 2009;88:352; author reply -3.

18. Garcia JP, Iacono A, Kon ZN, Griffith BP. Ambulatory extracorporeal membrane oxygenation: a new approach for bridge-to-lung

transplantation. J Thorac Cardiovasc Surg 2010;139:e137-9.

19. Fischer S, Bohn D, Rycus P, et al. Extracorporeal membrane oxygenation for primary graft dysfunction after lung transplantation: analysis of the Extracorporeal Life Support Organization (ELSO) registry. J Heart Lung Transplant 2007;26:472-7.

20. Noone PG. Non-invasive ventilation for the treatment of hypercapnic respiratory failure in cystic fibrosis. Thorax 2008;63:5-7.

21. Ricci D, Boffini M, Del Sorbo L, et al. The use of CO2 removal devices in patients awaiting lung transplantation: an initial experience. Transplant Proc 2010;42:1255-8.

22. Zwischenberger BA, Clemson LA, Zwischenberger JB. Artificial lung: progress and prototypes. Expert Rev Med Devices 2006;3:485-97.

23. Fischer S, Hoeper MM, Tomaszek S, et al. Bridge to lung transplantation with the extracorporeal membrane ventilator Novalung in the veno-venous mode: the initial Hannover experience. ASAIO J 2007;53:168-70.

24. Hammainen P, Schersten H, Lemstrom K, et al. Usefulness of extracorporeal membrane oxygenation as a bridge to lung transplantation: A descriptive study. J Heart Lung Transplant 2010.

25. Iglesias M, Jungebluth P, Sibila O, et al. Experimental safety and efficacy evaluation of an extracorporeal pumpless artificial lung in providing respiratory support through the axillary vessels. J Thorac Cardiovasc Surg 2007;133:339-45.

26. Yokota K, Fujii T, Kimura K, Toriumi T, Sari A. Life-threatening hypoxemic respiratory failure after repair of acute type a aortic dissection: successful treatment with veno-arterial extracorporeal life support using a prosthetic graft attached to the right axillary artery. Anesth Analg 2001;92:872-6.

27. Mangi AA, Mason DP, Yun JJ, Murthy SC, Pettersson GB. Bridge to lung transplantation using short-term ambulatory extracorporeal membrane oxygenation. J Thorac Cardiovasc Surg 2010.

28. Chou NK, Chen YS, Ko WJ, et al. Application of extracorporeal membrane oxygenation in adult burn patients. Artif Organs 2001;25:622-6.

29. Madershahian N, Wittwer T, Strauch J, et al. Application of ECMO in multitrauma patients with ARDS as rescue therapy. J Card Surg 2007;22:180-4.

30. Stohr F, Emmert MY, Lachat ML, et al. Extracorporeal membrane oxygenation for acute respiratory distress syndrome: is the configuration mode an important predictor for the outcome? Interact Cardiovasc Thorac Surg 2011.

31. Camboni D, Philipp A, Arlt M, Pfeiffer M, Hilker M, Schmid C. First experience with a paracorporeal artificial lung in humans. ASAIO J 2009;55:304-6.

32. Camboni D, Akay B, Pohlmann JR, et al. Veno-venous extracorporeal membrane oxygenation with interatrial shunting: a novel approach to lung transplantation for patients in right ventricular failure. J Thorac Cardiovasc Surg 2011;141:537-42, 42 e1.

33. Camboni D, Akay B, Sassalos P, et al. Use of venovenous extracorporeal membrane oxygenation and an atrial septostomy for pulmonary and right ventricular failure. Ann Thorac Surg 2011;91:144-9.

34. Mason DP, Thuita L, Nowicki ER, Murthy SC, Pettersson GB, Blackstone EH. Should lung transplantation be performed for patients on mechanical respiratory support? The US experience. J Thorac Cardiovasc Surg 2010;139:765-73 e1.

35. J.J. Yun, A.A. Mangi, L.C. Benjamin, et al. ECMO as a Bridge to Lung Transplantation: The Cleveland Clinic Experience J Heart Lung Transplant 2010;February 2010 (Vol. 29, Issue 2, Supplement, Page S31).

36. Nosotti M, Rosso L, Palleschi A, et al. Bridge to lung transplantation by venove-

nous extracorporeal membrane oxygenation: a lesson learned on the first four cases. Transplant Proc 2010;42:1259-61.

37. Hartwig MG, Appel JZ, 3rd, Cantu E, 3rd, et al. Improved results treating lung allograft failure with venovenous extracorporeal membrane oxygenation. Ann Thorac Surg 2005;80:1872-9; discussion 9-80.

38. Bermudez CA, Adusumilli PS, McCurry KR, et al. Extracorporeal membrane oxygenation for primary graft dysfunction after lung transplantation: long-term survival. Ann Thorac Surg 2009;87:854-60.

39. Lee JC, Christie JD, Keshavjee S. Primary graft dysfunction: definition, risk factors, short- and long-term outcomes. Semin Respir Crit Care Med 2010;31:161-71.

40. Christie JD, Sager JS, Kimmel SE, et al. Impact of primary graft failure on outcomes following lung transplantation. Chest 2005;127:161-5.

41. Pasero D, Martin EL, Davi A, Mascia L, Rinaldi M, Ranieri VM. The effects of inhaled nitric oxide after lung transplantation. Minerva Anestesiol 2010;76:353-61.

42. Khan TA, Schnickel G, Ross D, et al. A prospective, randomized, crossover pilot study of inhaled nitric oxide versus inhaled prostacyclin in heart transplant and lung transplant recipients. J Thorac Cardiovasc Surg 2009;138:1417-24.

43. Amital A, Shitrit D, Raviv Y, et al. Surfactant as salvage therapy in life threatening primary graft dysfunction in lung transplantation. Eur J Cardiothorac Surg 2009;35:299-303.

44. Amital A, Shitrit D, Raviv Y, et al. The use of surfactant in lung transplantation. Transplantation 2008;86:1554-9.

45. Ailawadi G, Lau CL, Smith PW, et al. Does reperfusion injury still cause significant mortality after lung transplantation? J Thorac Cardiovasc Surg 2009;137:688-94.

46. Wigfield CH, Lindsey JD, Steffens TG, Edwards NM, Love RB. Early institution of extracorporeal membrane oxygenation for primary graft dysfunction after lung transplantation improves outcome. J Heart Lung Transplant 2007;26:331-8.

47. Meyers BF, Sundt TM, 3rd, Henry S, et al. Selective use of extracorporeal membrane oxygenation is warranted after lung transplantation. J Thorac Cardiovasc Surg 2000;120:20-6.

48. Glassman LR, Keenan RJ, Fabrizio MC, et al. Extracorporeal membrane oxygenation as an adjunct treatment for primary graft failure in adult lung transplant recipients. J Thorac Cardiovasc Surg 1995;110:723-6; discussion 6-7.

49. Nguyen DQ, Kulick DM, Bolman RM, 3rd, Dunitz JM, Hertz MI, Park SJ. Temporary ECMO support following lung and heart-lung transplantation. J Heart Lung Transplant 2000;19:313-6.

30

Cardiac Catheterization Procedures for ECMO Patients

Ravi R. Thiagarajan MBBS MPH, Joshua W. Salvin MD MPH

Introduction

The use of cardiac catheterization to provide diagnostic information for patients on Extracorporeal Membrane Oxygenation (ECMO) has increased with the increasing utilization of ECMO to support children with cardiac disease.[1] Similarly, the advances in cardiac catheterization techniques have allowed the application of a number of interventional catheterization-based therapeutic interventions to improve myocardial function and outcomes in patients supported with ECMO. Approximately 23–28% of children with cardiac disease supported with ECMO undergo cardiac catheterization for either diagnostic information or therapeutic intervention during ECMO support, although this may vary with center experience.[1,2] The utilization of cardiac catheterization in adults supported with ECMO is much harder to estimate. In this chapter we will review indications for the use of cardiac catheterization in ECMO patients, management of patients on ECMO in the cardiac catheterization laboratory, some technical aspects of left ventricular decompression in the cardiac catheterization laboratory, and the use of ECMO as prophylactic or rescue therapy in children and adults for hemodynamic instability in the cardiac catheterization laboratory.

Indications for the use of Cardiac Catheterization in ECMO patients

Cardiac catheterization plays an important role in the diagnosis and management of children and adults with critical heart disease.[1-4] For critically ill children and adults requiring ECMO due to myocardial dysfunction from underlying cardiac disease, diagnostic, and physiological information obtained from cardiac catheterization may be invaluable in patient management, determining prognosis, and assessing candidacy for cardiac transplantation. Because surgical correction of the cause of underlying myocardial dysfunction carries a high risk for mortality in some patients, the risk of surgical mortality can be mitigated by undertaking catheter-based interventional therapies while on ECMO, as this may temporarily restore cardiac output, improve end-organ perfusion, and may help decrease the risk of mortality until a more definitive surgical procedure can be attempted at a later time.

In critically ill patients, the risk of dangerous hemodynamic perturbation from manipulation of catheters placed in the heart during the catheterization procedure to gather hemodynamic data or perform interventions may worsen the hemodynamic state or lead to cardiac arrest. Here, ECMO deployed electively prior to the procedure can maintain adequate cardiac output and tissue perfusion and improve the safety of the procedure.[5-11] Furthermore, ECMO can also be used to rescue patients in whom hemodynamic perturbation during cardiac catheterization may lead to cardiac arrest when cardiopulmonary resuscitation fails to establish an adequate circulation.[7] Here, ECMO can aid in the resuscitation efforts by providing cardiac output during cardiopulmonary resuscitation. Finally, in patients requiring ECMO for myocardial failure, decompression of the left heart to decrease myocardial wall stress and promote myocardial recovery can be achieved safely and effectively in the catheterization laboratory.[12-17]

Booth et al. from Children's Hospital Boston reported on indications for cardiac catheterization in a series of 54 patients with heart disease supported with ECMO.[1] The most common reason for cardiac catheterization in these children included assessment of adequacy of operative repair of congenital heart disease (35%) and to provide left heart decompression (20%). In a more recent series of consecutive patients from Children's Hospital Boston requiring catheterization in the early postoperative period, 30 of 226 (13%) were catheterized while supported with ECMO.[18] The utility of these procedures was high, with the majority yielding anatomic or hemodynamic information leading to re-operation (47%) or catheter-based intervention (20%). Early postoperative catheterization on ECMO was performed safely, with a low serious adverse event rate. Thus, cardiac catheterization should not be delayed for patients requiring ECMO following cardiac surgery.

Although indications for the use of cardiac catheterization in adult ECMO patients have not been comprehensively reported, based on the many case reports available, the most common indication in adults is evaluation and high risk intervention of coronary artery disease in patients presenting with cardiogenic shock following acute myocardial infarction.[9-11]

Left Heart Decompression on ECMO

Left heart distension requiring decompression may be seen in patients with severe cardiac failure supported with venoarterial (VA) ECMO, especially in those where ECMO results in a further decrease or loss of left ventricular ejection.[12-17,19] The physiology of left ventricular distension is detailed in other chapters of this textbook (see Chapters 2,3). Briefly, left heart distension is caused by severe myocardial dysfunction resulting in impaired left ventricular contractility, continued filling of the left ventricle from return of blood from the bronchial circulation to the left atrium, and from the increased afterload posed by the arterial cannula. Left heart distension results in high left ventricular end-diastolic pressure and severe left atrial (LA) hypertension. The increased left ventricular end-diastolic pressure results in increased wall stress, increased myocardial oxygen consumption, and sub-endocardial ischemia. Left heart distension may thus impair myocardial recovery or even cause further myocardial injury. Clinical manifestations of left heart distension are due to left atrial hypertension, and include severe pulmonary edema, hemoptysis due to pulmonary hemorrhage, and "whiteout" on chest radiographs causing respiratory failure. Left heart decompression should be undertaken expeditiously in these patients as it may promote myocardial recovery and prevent lung injury and pulmonary hemorrhage. Left heart decompression can be achieved through either surgical or transcatheter-based techniques. In patients who have undergone a recent cardiac surgical procedure through a sternotomy, surgical placement of a venting cannula in the left atrium through the right pulmonary veins is used to decompress the heart.[20] The venting cannula is then attached to the venous limb of the ECMO circuit. In some patients who have undergone cardiac surgery and in many noncardiac surgical patients, left heart decompression is usually accomplished by catheter-based interventional procedures to drain the left atrium.[12-17]

Several techniques to provide left atrial decompression in the cardiac catheterization laboratory have been described (Figure 30-1).[21] Detailed descriptions of the transseptal atrial puncture procedure can be found in most textbooks on cardiac catheterization.[21] For most patients access to the left atrium is through the femoral vein, inferior vena cava, right atrium, then via a transseptal puncture of the atrial septum or through a preexisting atrial communication such as a patent foramen ovale. The method of choice for creating the atrial communication depends on the age and size of the patient, and may vary with institutional experience. In the neonatal age group, a communication between the atrium is created by tearing the atrial septum using a balloon catheter.[12,13] The atrial septum in neonates is usually pliable and an adequate atrial septal communication can usually be created.[21]

In children beyond a month of age the atrial septum is less pliable and usually not amenable to tearing with a balloon catheter.[21] These patients usually require the atrial communication to be created using a blade atrial septostomy catheter.[13,14] The atrial communication can then be further enlarged by static balloon dilation (balloon atrial septoplasty). Occasionally, an intravascular stent is required to maintain the

Left Sided Decompression During VA ECMO

A. Balloon Atrial Septostomy

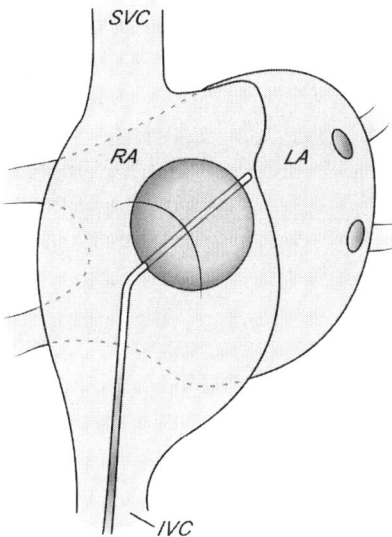

B. Percutaneously Placed ECMO Cannula in Left Atrium (LA Vent)

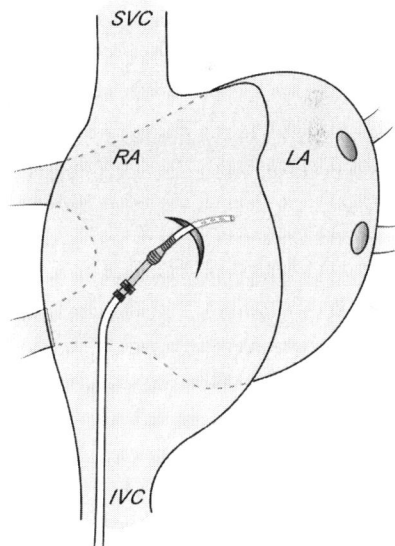

Figure 30-1. Trans-catheter procedures for creating and enlarging atrial septal defects: A). Balloon atrial septostomy; B). Percutaneous left atrial vent. SVC: superior vena cava, RA: right atrium, LA: left atrium, IVC: inferior vena cava.

atrial communication.[14] Occasionally, balloon atrial septoplasty can be used to enlarge a preexisting natural atrial communication. Alternative approaches to left atrial decompression include placing a transseptal catheter in the left atrium or in the left ventricle after transseptal puncture to access the left atrium[15-17,19] The types of transseptal catheters used for left atrial drainage may include a transseptal sheath or even ECMO cannulae. The transseptal catheter drains blood from the left atrium into the venous limb of the ECMO circuit. Transseptal catheters should be withdrawn into the right atrium or removed to allow filling of the left atrium prior to weaning ECMO. Many centers use transseptal catheters to decompress the left heart for ECMO patients but it is unclear whether this approach is better than the atrial septostomy or septoplasty procedures.[22] The size of the transseptal catheter used depends on patient size, but the goal should be to use the largest possible cannula to provide adequate decompression. Aiyangari et al. suggested an 8 Fr sheath in infants and toddlers, 10 -12 Fr sheath in larger children, and 15 Fr sheath in adult-sized patients.[17] Balloon atrial septostomy and, rarely, placement of a transseptal catheter can be undertaken at the bedside in ECMO patients too unstable to move to the cardiac catheterization laboratory using transthoracic or transesophageal echocardiographic guidance.[23]

Regardless of the method used, it is imperative to provide good left atrial decompression for ECMO patients for relief of left heart distension, as this may improve the chances of myocardial recovery and survival. Aiyangari et al. reported a trend towards improved survival in children with adequate left atrial decompression compared to those whose left sided decompression was thought to be inadequate[17] In the catheterization laboratory, adequacy of left atrial decompression can be confirmed by a decrease in left atrial pressures immediately following left sided decompression. At the bedside, the adequacy of left atrial decompression can be

confirmed by resolution of pulmonary edema on chest radiographs, resolution of pulmonary hemorrhage, and improvement in respiratory mechanics and gas exchange. The size and flow across the defect can also be monitored periodically using echocardiography. Recently, Falkshammer et al. demonstrated resolution of elevated serum brain natriuretic peptide (BNP) following left atrial decompression in an ECMO patient who developed left heart distension, and suggested that it may be a useful marker of the adequacy of left atrial decompression.[24]

Complications following percutaneous decompression of the left atrium in the catheterization laboratory include bleeding from the vascular access site and retroperitoneal hemorrhage, rupture of the left atrium, inadequate left atrial decompression, and arrhythmia during manipulation of catheters in the heart. Although many created atrial communications may close spontaneously in the future, the natural history of atrial communications created in the setting of ECMO is unknown and may merit followup, due to the potential risk of thromboembolic stroke. Clinical followup and consideration for closure of these defects when the patient is fully recovered from ECMO could be considered. Finally, Vlasselaers et al. described the use of a novel miniature axial flow pump (Impella, Abiomed INC, Danvers MA) to decompress the left ventricle in an ECMO patient who developed left ventricular distension during VA ECMO support.[25] In this report, the intravascular pump was placed in the left ventricle via the femoral artery, advanced through the aorta and provided adequate decompression of the left ventricle by pumping blood out of the left ventricle into the aorta.

ECMO to Support High Risk Cardiac Catheterization Procedures

Advances in the procedural, technical aspects, and development of devices has made diagnostic and interventional cardiac catheterization an important aspect of management of patients with heart disease.[26] Critically ill patients with heart disease and severe hemodynamic instability become candidates for transcatheter based intervention because the risk of undertaking a surgical procedure in such patients may be prohibitively high. Catheter manipulation within the heart during interventional therapies in these patients may result in further hemodynamic deterioration and cardiac arrest. Elective ECMO deployment in these patients may provide hemodynamic stability for the safe conduct of cardiac catheterization.[5-11]

There are several published case reports of the elective use of ECMO to support interventional cardiac catheterization procedures in children and adults. Butler et al. described the use of prophylactic VA ECMO prior to aortic balloon valvuloplasty in a hemodynamically unstable neonate with critical aortic stenosis.[8] ECMO was deployed in this patient to provide cardiac output in anticipation of severe hemodynamic instability during balloon aortic valvuloplasty. Ward et al. describe the use of ECMO to provide oxygenation in a 4 year old with pulmonary atresia and ventricular septal defect during dilation of right pulmonary artery (RPA) stenosis.[5] This patient was extremely cyanotic at baseline and had an absent left pulmonary artery and was thus dependent on the right pulmonary artery as the only source of pulmonary blood flow. ECMO was deployed in anticipation of extreme hypoxemia that would result from complete occlusion of the RPA during balloon dilation. In another report, Carmichael et al. described the use of VA ECMO to provide circulatory support in a patient with severe Ebstein's anomaly undergoing ablation for supraventricular tachycardia (SVT).[6] Prophylactic ECMO was used in anticipation of the severe hemodynamic perturbation anticipated from induction of SVT for purposes of identification of the pathway for ablation. Finally, Allan et al. reported on the use of prophylactic ECMO in three patients. Anticipation of severe hemodynamic instability during

myocardial biopsy, assessment of hypoxemia in a patient with a Blalock-Taussig shunt, and arrhythmia ablation prompted the use of ECMO to provide hemodynamic stability during these procedures.[7] In the same report, Allan et al. described 19 patients for whom ECMO was initiated during resuscitation of cardiac arrest during a high risk cardiac catheterization procedure. The need for preprocedure ECMO support was not anticipated in these patients. Only 15 (78%) of the 19 patients requiring CPR during the high risk procedure survived to hospital discharge and 9 (47%) had clinical evidence of neurological injury. All three patients in whom ECMO was initiated in anticipation of hemodynamic compromise survived with intact neurological function. Because of better outcomes for patients who received anticipatory ECMO for hemodynamic support prior to catheterization, the authors suggest consideration of ECMO for hemodynamic support for those patients in whom their severity of illness is associated with a high risk of cardiac arrest during procedures in the catheterization laboratory.

Similar to the use of ECMO to support high risk catheterization procedures in children, many reports of the use of ECMO to support high risk cardiac catheterization procedures in adults exist. In these reports ECMO has been most commonly used in the setting of cardiogenic shock complicating myocardial infarction. ECMO has also been shown to be useful in patients with myocardial infarction with left ventricular function with ejection fraction of <25%-35%, and for those in whom the vessel considered for angioplasty supplied >50% of the viable myocardium.[9] Shawl et al. reported on eight patients with cardiogenic shock following myocardial infarction supported with a cardiopulmonary support system consisting of a centrifugal pump without an oxygenator.[10] Seven of these patients underwent angioplasties and survived to hospital discharge. In another report, von Segesser et al. described 11 patients supported with the cardiopulmonary support

(CPS) circuit during angioplasties for cardiogenic shock following myocardial infarction. Nine patients survived to hospital discharge.[27] In a 1994 report by Sivanathan et al. 13 patients underwent angioplasty procedures with CPS support and 11 patients survived to hospital discharge.[9]

Anticipation of the need for hemodynamic support and coordination of experts for patients electively supported with ECMO for procedures is critical to obtaining a successful outcome. The benefits of ECMO in these situations should always be weighed against the risk of ECMO complications. Discussion of ECMO cannulation sites, conduct of ECMO during the diagnostic aspects of the case where ECMO flows may need to be reduced for pressure measurements or angiography, management of anticoagulation during catheterization, transport of the patient on ECMO, anticipated duration of ECMO use, and a weaning strategy should be discussed among the healthcare team and a plan of action should be made prior to the procedure. In addition, the risk and benefits of the use of ECMO and decision making regarding the use of ECMO should be clearly explained to the patient's family and their consent should be obtained prior to the procedure.

Preparation and Patient Management during Cardiac Catheterization

The decision to embark on cardiac catheterization for ECMO patients should be made jointly between the interventional cardiologist, cardiac surgeon, intensive care physician, bedside nursing staff, and ECMO specialist caring for the patient. Safe transport of the ECMO patient to the catheterization laboratory requires adequate preparation, multidisciplinary collaboration, and available personnel to help move ECMO equipment to the catheterization laboratory.[26] In general, ECMO transports for the purposes of imaging or operative procedures are safe when conducted by well trained and coordinated teams. Once the patient arrives in the catheterization laboratory, the patient should be properly positioned on the operating table, with the ECMO equipment situated in such a manner that it allows for movement of the patient on the operating table for fluoroscopy and does not interfere with the camera and other catheterization equipment. Given that most catheterization laboratories use both lateral and anteroposterior cameras (biplane), the space available for ECMO equipment may be minimal. Adequate communication regarding planning and positioning to allow easy access to ECMO equipment is essential for the smooth conduct of cardiac catheterization.[26] Depending on the type of ECMO pump used, it is important to allow adequate lengths of ECMO tubing (especially in circuits with roller pumps) to allow for movement of the patients for imaging during cardiac catheterization. Some centrifugal pump systems can be placed on or attached to the operating table, allowing it to move with the patient, and may not require additional length of ECMO circuit tubing. Patient monitoring during the procedure should include hemodynamic and respiratory monitoring and should be checked and confirmed to be in good working order prior to the start of the procedure.

Vascular access for cardiac catheterization depends on the type of procedure performed and sites available for use. Preexisting indwelling vascular access could be exchanged for a venous or arterial sheath to provide vascular access for cardiac catheterization.[4] Since most patients are already anticoagulated with intravenous heparin for ECMO, a discussion between the physician caring for the patient, interventional cardiologist, and ECMO specialist should occur regarding administration of additional heparin during cardiac catheterization. Interpretation of hemodynamic data is often inaccurate during full ECMO support and ECMO flows may need to be reduced to gather useful diagnostic information in terms of physiological measurements and angiography. Reducing ECMO flows to obtain hemodynamic data will depend on the patient's circulation and should be conducted after discussion among the care team. The patient's vasoactive and ventilatory support may need to be increased when ECMO support is reduced to maintain organ perfusion. Generally, the lowest flow tolerated by the patient that allows collection of adequate hemodynamic and angiographic data to facilitate clinical decision making should be used. Following cardiac catheterization, vascular access sheaths may be left in place if the risk of bleeding from their removal is high. Complications including vessel injury, bleeding, arrhythmia, cardiac perforation, device embolization, and cerebrovascular accidents should be anticipated and managed appropriately.[28] Finally, the safe conduct of cardiac catheterization in patients supported on ECMO depends on good communication and collaboration among all the members of the care team.

Summary

Cardiac catheterization both for diagnostic and therapeutic purposes can be an invaluable adjunct to the management of patients supported with ECMO for cardiac failure. Similarly, the anticipatory use of ECMO in select patients with severe hemodynamic instability may allow safe conduct of lifesaving interventional cardiac catheterization procedures.

References

1. Booth KL, Roth SJ, Perry SB, del Nido PJ, Wessel DL, Laussen PC. Cardiac catheterization of patients supported by extracorporeal membrane oxygenation. J Am Coll Cardiol. 2002;40(9):1681-1686.

2. Zahn EM, Dobrolet NC, Nykanen DG, Ojito J, Hannan RL, Burke RP. Interventional catheterization performed in the early postoperative period after congenital heart surgery in children. J Am Coll Cardiol. 2004;43(7):1264-1269.

3. desJardins SE, Crowley DC, Beekman RH, Lloyd TR. Utility of cardiac catheterization in pediatric cardiac patients on ECMO. Catheter Cardiovasc Interv. 1999;46(1):62-67.

4. Ettedgui J, Fricker FJ, Park SC, Fischer DR, Siewers RD, Del Nido PJ. Cardiac catheterization in children on extracorporeal membrane oxygenation. Cardiol Young. 1996;6:59 -61.

5. Ward CJ, Mullins CE, Barron LJ, Grifka RG, Gomez MR, Cuellar-Gomez MR. Use of extracorporeal membrane oxygenation to maintain oxygenation during pediatric interventional cardiac catheterization. Am Heart J. 1995;130(3 Pt 1):619-620.

6. Carmichael TB, Walsh EP, Roth SJ. Anticipatory use of venoarterial extracorporeal membrane oxygenation for a high-risk interventional cardiac procedure. Respir Care. 2002;47(9):1002-1006.

7. Allan CK, Thiagarajan RR, Armsby LR, del Nido PJ, Laussen PC. Emergent use of extracorporeal membrane oxygenation during pediatric cardiac catheterization. Pediatr Crit Care Med. 2006;7(3):212-219.

8. Butler TJ, Yoder BA, Seib P, Lally KP, Smith VC. ECMO for left ventricular assist in a newborn with critical aortic stenosis. Pediatr Cardiol. 1994;15(1):38-40.

9. Sivananthan MU, Rees MR, Browne TF, Verma SP, Hick DG, Whittaker S, Davies GA, Tan LB. Coronary angioplasty in high risk patients with percutaneous cardiopulmonary support. Eur Heart J. 1994;15(8):1057-1062.

10. Shawl FA, Domanski MJ, Hernandez TJ, Punja S. Emergency percutaneous cardiopulmonary bypass support in cardiogenic shock from acute myocardial infarction. Am J Cardiol. 1989;64(16):967-970.

11. Teirstein PS, Vogel RA, Dorros G, Stertzer SH, Vandormael MG, Smith SC, Jr., Overlie PA, O'Neill WW. Prophylactic versus standby cardiopulmonary support for high risk percutaneous transluminal coronary angioplasty. J Am Coll Cardiol. 1993;21(3):590-596.

12. Koenig PR, Ralston MA, Kimball TR, Meyer RA, Daniels SR, Schwartz DC. Balloon atrial septostomy for left ventricular decompression in patients receiving extracorporeal membrane oxygenation for myocardial failure. J Pediatr. 1993;122(6):S95-99.

13. Seib PM, Faulkner SC, Erickson CC, Van Devanter SH, Harrell JE, Fasules JW, Frazier EA, Morrow WR. Blade and balloon atrial septostomy for left heart decompression in patients with severe ventricular dysfunction on extracorporeal membrane oxygenation. Catheter Cardiovasc Interv. 1999;46(2):179-186.

14. Haynes S, Kerber RE, Johnson FL, Lynch WR, Divekar A. Left heart decompression by atrial stenting during extracorporeal membrane oxygenation. Int J Artif Organs. 2009;32(4):240-242.

15. Cheung MM, Goldman AP, Shekerdemian LS, Brown KL, Cohen GA, Redington AN. Percutaneous left ventricular "vent" insertion for left heart decompression during extracorporeal membrane oxygenation. Pediatr Crit Care Med. 2003;4(4):447-449.

16. Hlavacek AM, Atz AM, Bradley SM, Bandisode VM. Left atrial decompression by percutaneous cannula placement while on extracorporeal membrane oxygenation. J

Thorac Cardiovasc Surg. 2005;130(2):595-596.

17. Aiyagari RM, Rocchini AP, Remenapp RT, Graziano JN. Decompression of the left atrium during extracorporeal membrane oxygenation using a transseptal cannula incorporated into the circuit. Crit Care Med. 2006;34(10):2603-2606.

18. Salvin JW, Bergeresen L, Laussen PC, Teele SA, Marshall AC, Mayer JE, McElhinney DB. Early cardiac catheterization following congenital heart surgery is not associated with increased risk of serious adverse events. Journal of the American College of Cardiology. 2010;55(10):A:45, E437.

19. Ward KE, Tuggle DW, Gessouroun MR, Overholt ED, Mantor PC. Transseptal decompression of the left heart during ECMO for severe myocarditis. Ann Thorac Surg. 1995;59(3):749-751.

20. Duncan BW. Extracorporeal Membrane Oxygenation for Children with Cardiac Disease. In: Duncan BW, ed. Mechanical Support for Cardiac and Respiratory Failure in Pediatric Patients. First ed. New York, NY: Marcel Dekker Inc; 2001:1 - 20.

21. Lang P. Other Catheterization Laboratory Techniques And Interventions: Atrial Septal Defect Creation, Transseptal Pericardial Drainage, Foreign Body Retrieval, Exercise and Drug Testing. In: Lock JE, Keane JF, Perry SB, eds. Diagnostic and Interventional Catheterization in Congenital Heart Disease. Second ed. Norwell, MA: Kluwer Academic Press; 2000:245 - 268.

22. Hanna BD. Left atrial decompression: Is there a standard during extracorporeal support of the failing heart? Crit Care Med. 2006;34(10):2688-2689.

23. Johnston TA, Jaggers J, McGovern JJ, O'Laughlin MP. Bedside transseptal balloon dilation atrial septostomy for decompression of the left heart during extracorporeal membrane oxygenation. Catheter Cardiovasc Interv. 1999;46(2):197-199.

24. Falkensammer CB, Heinle JS, Chang AC. Serial plasma BNP levels in assessing inadequate left ventricular decompression on ECMO. Pediatr Cardiol. 2008;29(4):808-811.

25. Vlasselaers D, Desmet M, Desmet L, Meyns B, Dens J. Ventricular unloading with a miniature axial flow pump in combination with extracorporeal membrane oxygenation. Intensive Care Med. 2006;32(2):329-333.

26. Laussen P, Nugent A. Diagnostic and Therapeutic Cardiac Catheterization. In: Fuhrman BP, Zimmerman JJ, eds. Pediatric Critical Care. Third ed. Philadelphia: Mosby Elsevier; 2006:285 - 297.

27. von Segesser LK. Cardiopulmonary support and extracorporeal membrane oxygenation for cardiac assist. Ann Thorac Surg. 1999;68(2):672-677.

28. Vitiello R, McCrindle BW, Nykanen D, Freedom RM, Benson LN. Complications associated with pediatric cardiac catheterization. J Am Coll Cardiol. 1998;32(5):1433-1440.

31

The Future of Extracorporeal Life Support

Robert H. Bartlett MD, Graeme MacLaren MBBS FCICM FCCM,
Gail M. Annich MD MS FRCP(C)

Since our last speculation on the future of ECLS in the 2005 edition of the Red Book, several important things have happened.

Most important is ECMO II, the second generation of ECMO devices, which makes ECMO much safer, simpler, and less expensive.

The new technology facilitated the widespread use of ECMO during the worldwide H1N1 influenza epidemic of 2009. ECMO was remarkably successful for moribund patients and awoke the attention of skeptical adult intensivists throughout the world.

The prospective randomized trial (CESAR) in acute respiratory distress syndrome (ARDS) and the matched pairs study in H1N1 patients proved the value of ECMO in adult respiratory failure.[1,2] In addition, these studies demonstrated the superiority of the matched pairs approach to study interventions in acute fatal illness. Skeptics with no ECMO experience criticized these studies with the courage of the noncombatant. They now seem as out of touch as the skeptical neonatologists did 30 years ago.

The advantage of managing ECMO patients awake and breathing, demonstrated long ago by the Karolinska group, is now widely recognized. Hard to learn, to be sure, but widely recognized. This led to ambulatory ECMO in many experienced centers, both in ARDS and also as a bridge to lung transplantation. The availability of a practical double lumen catheter for those patients facilitates this process.

The simplicity and safety of ECMO II devices has prompted us to reexamine the role of the ECMO specialist. With specialized training, ICU nurses can learn to manage the circuit and the patient. This leads to two categories of ECMO specialists: 1) the core team responsible for managing the entire program, triaging patients, initiating and troubleshooting ECMO, and education; and 2) the ICU nurse ECMO specialist responsible for hour to hour care of both patient and circuit with support and education from the core team. The important results of this expanded specialist role makes the number of simultaneous patients in any hospital almost unlimited and significantly lowers the cost compared to ECMO I.

In 2008, ELSO published guidelines for the management of patients in all categories, helping standardize the practice worldwide. The guidelines are updated regularly and provide a starting point for new centers and a reference for new personnel in established centers.

What will be the seminal events when we discuss the future in the 5th edition of the Red Book several years from now?

The ECMO Circuit

ECMO III will be based on pumps which have the advantages, but none of the disadvantages, of both roller and centrifugal pumps. Systemic anticoagulation will be used only for patient (not circuit) indications, such as poor cardiac function with the possibility of intracardiac clot. Circuits will be small and easily portable. They will be totally automatic, servo regulated based on the patient's physiology. Circuits will include integrated plugin modules for liver support, renal replacement therapy, plasmapheresis, and extracorporeal blood purification.

New Applications

The major growth will be in ECPR in emergency rooms. Half of these resuscitations will result in successful return of stable circulation, which will result in a new problem: patients on full ECMO support being admitted to unprepared ICUs.

Some transplant centers will use ECMO to resuscitate abdominal organs for transplantation in controlled and uncontrolled cardiac death.

Modified ECMO systems will be used in the management of very premature infants as an alternative to intubation and mechanical ventilation. Transportation of ECMO patients will be routine and largely managed by emergency room teams.

Extracorporeal gas exchange technology, with or without noninvasive ventilation, will lead to a new paradigm which obviates endotracheal intubation in severe respiratory failure.

Global applications

ECMO will be widely adopted in medium to high income countries across the globe. In patients with advanced circulatory or respiratory failure, ECMO will be used routinely everywhere, analogous to the widespread application of continuous renal replacement therapy in acute kidney injury.

Clinical Research

A protocol for instituting ECMO early in progressive ARDS will evolve (Pplat>25, P/F<200, pCO_2>50 at 24 hrs after intubation, for example). This protocol will be studied compared to conventional care in a matched pairs trial. The result will be 80% vs. 50% survival.

Implantable artificial lungs perfused by the right ventricle will be used for acute lung disease which is not improving after seven days on ECMO, and for chronic lung disease as a bridge to transplantation, or destination for endstage lung disease. Experience has taught us to predict not the limitations but rather the possibilities.

ECMO is no longer a salvage therapy to be used in the most extreme cases when all else fails. It is an important tool in the toolbox of critical care medicine alongside high frequency oscillatory ventilation, inhaled nitric oxide, and continuous renal replacement therapy. It is organ support therapy upon which the future of critical care medicine will be built.

References

1. Peek GJ, Mugford M, Tiruvoipati R, et al. Efficacy and economic assessment of conventional ventilatory support versus extracorporeal membrane oxygenation for severe adult respiratory failure (CESAR): a multicentre randomised controlled trial. *Lancet* 2009;374:1351-1363.
2. Noah MA, Peek GJ, Finney SJ, et a. Referral to an extracorporeal membrane oxygenation center and mortality among patients with severe 2009 influenza A(H1N1). *JAMA*. 2011;306:1659-1668.

32

Regionalization and Triage

John Beca FCICM FRACP

Which centers should provide ECMO?

Extracorporeal Life Support Organization (ELSO) guidelines outline the ideal institutional requirements for an ECMO center in terms of organizational structure, staffing, physical facilities, equipment, staff training, continuing education, and ongoing program evaluation. These guidelines recommend that ECMO centers should be located in tertiary hospitals receiving referrals from geographic areas that can support a *minimum* of six ECMO patients per year.[1] This is because treating fewer patients than this will very likely be associated with loss or lack of clinical expertise and reduced cost effectiveness. While there are many case series reporting outcomes from ECMO centers of varying sizes, there are no published studies assessing the influence of ECMO center size on patient outcomes. However, there is a considerable body of evidence supporting that greater patient volumes improve patient outcomes, especially for low volume complex conditions and procedures, which provides strong indirect support for the ELSO recommendation. For conditions in which there is a strong volume-outcome relationship, there will be benefits to establishing a regionalized system of care.

The benefits of regionalization

Regionalization may improve patient outcomes in two ways. First, outcomes will be better in high volume specialized centers. Second, outcomes will also be better where regionalization is associated with improved coordination between centers within a geographical area.[2]

Volume-outcome benefits

The pioneering work in this area was published by Luft in 1979, who showed that mortality rates from higher risk surgical procedures (e.g., vascular surgery) were 25-41% lower in hospitals that performed >200 procedures per year compared to those who performed <200 procedures per year. However, for lower risk procedures (e.g., total hip replacement), mortality plateaued at much lower volumes.[3] Subsequent publications have shown that "this relationship between high volume and better outcomes is strong and persistent, with approximately 300 studies on the subject having been reported in the English-language literature."[4] Two systematic reviews found that approximately 70% of studies reported associations between higher volume (both hospital and physician volume) and better outcomes and that no studies showed poorer outcomes.[5,6] It has been estimated that referral of appropriate patients to high volume centers in California could reduce overall hospital mortality in the State by approximately 600 deaths per year.[7]

There are two important further themes to this literature. First, the strength of the association between volume and outcome varies considerably between conditions, and tends to be strongest for low volume higher risk procedures and diagnoses. It is very strong for surgical procedures such as pancreatic resection, esophagectomy and pneumonectomy, moderately strong for gastrectomy, cystectomy, non-ruptured abdominal aneurysm, and replacement of either the aortic or mitral valve, and weak for coronary artery bypass surgery, colectomy, lobectomy, nephrectomy, and lower extremity bypass.[8] Second, there are volume thresholds above which the volume-outcome effect is attenuated or lost. For example, hospital volume is associated with reduced mortality for three common medical conditions: acute myocardial infarction, heart failure, and pneumonia, but there are thresholds above which this effect is no longer significant. These thresholds are 610 patients (95% CI: 539-679) for myocardial infarction, 500 patients (95%CI: 433-566) for heart failure, and 210 patients (95%CI: 142-284) for pneumonia.[9] Further examples where mortality rates were lower above a certain threshold are liver transplantation (more than 20 per year), congenital diaphragmatic hernia (more than 6 per year), and insertion of ventricular assist devices in children (more than 5 per year).[10-13]

The benefit of high volume specialized centers is not restricted to lower death rates. Complication rates, hospital length of stay and hospital costs have all been found to be reduced in a range of conditions and services, including pediatric intensive care,[14-16] lung cancer surgery,[17] radical prostatectomy,[18] and percutaneous coronary interventions.[19] Decentralized services will be more expensive for two reasons. First, length of stay and complication rates will be increased. Second, there will be duplication of staff and equipment.

The relationship between volume and outcome has been studied in three areas of importance to any ECMO program: pediatric intensive care, adult intensive care, and pediatric cardiac surgery.

Volume-outcome in pediatric intensive care

Pearson et al. published a landmark study specifically addressing the effect of regionalization and specialization in pediatric intensive care in 1997.[14] The authors compared severity-adjusted pediatric intensive care unit (ICU) mortality between Victoria in Australia (where care is highly centralized to a single pediatric ICU) and Trent in the United Kingdom (where care was not centralized). The population and admission rates were very similar between regions. The odds ratio for the risk of death was 2.1 (95% CI: 1.4-3.2) and the mean ICU length of stay was over a day longer in Trent compared to Victoria. The authors estimated that the excess death rate was equivalent to 11% of all childhood deaths in the region. In a subsequent before and after study assessing the consequences of regionalization in a different area of the United Kingdom, the proportion of children admitted to a specialist pediatric ICU rose from 60% to 90%, length of stay fell by over a day, and the overall child mortality rate fell in the region.[20]

Further studies in pediatric intensive care have shown that admission to specialist tertiary units was associated with similar or greater mortality reductions as those described by Pearson. Increased admissions have also been associated with better outcomes. In three separate studies, mortality fell by 10% with an extra 31, 120, and 200 admissions per year.[15,16,21] The optimal number of admissions was >840 per year in one study[15] and 992-1491 per year in another.[21] The latter study suggested that the relationship between volumes and mortality might be U-shaped, with increased mortality if a pediatric ICU becomes too big. Increasing volumes were consistently associated with reduced length of stay in all reports.

Volume-outcome in adult intensive care

There are at least six studies that have specifically examined volume-outcome relationships in different patient populations of adult ICU patients and shown consistent beneficial effects with increased patient volumes.[22] Of particular relevance to ECMO are two studies in adults requiring mechanical ventilation. In a study of 20,241 non-surgical patients requiring ventilation, admission to a hospital in the highest volume quartile (>400 per year) had a 37% reduction in the adjusted odds of death in the ICU compared to admission to hospitals in the lowest quartile (<150 per year).[23] A study in all of the acute care hospitals in Pennsylvania of a similar population found an absolute risk reduction of 3.4% in 30-day mortality at high volume hospitals (≥ 300 per year) compared to low volume hospitals (<300 per year).[24]

Volume-outcome in congenital heart surgery

An early paper from 1995 assessing volume-outcome in congenital heart surgery in California and Massachusetts found that the risk of dying in hospital was much lower in programs performing >300 operations per year.[25] More recent work shows that this relationship is complex and is related to case complexity. There was no volume effect for low difficulty operations, but for difficult operations (as defined by the Aristotle technical difficulty score) the mortality decreased by approximately 50% from small centers to very large (≥ 350 cases per year) centers.[26]

Understanding the volume-outcome relationship

There are multiple mechanisms postulated for the better results observed in busier hospitals.

These include increased clinical experience ("practice makes perfect"), selective referral (hospitals with good results are referred more patients), increased individual physician workload, the benefits of greater specialization, and the system improvements that can occur in bigger, busier hospitals. While the relative importance of each of these has been debated, all have consistently been shown to be important.

Increasing hospital volumes over time improves outcomes. These effects are best seen in longitudinal studies, showing greater effects of volume on outcome than cross-sectional studies.[27,28] Equally, selective referral has been shown to play a larger role in some conditions (e.g., coronary artery bypass grafting). Both surgeon volume and specialization improve outcome, independent of hospital volume and of each other.[4,5,27]

Mortality rates for some complex operations are not only inversely related to hospital volumes of that procedure but also to the hospital volumes of other procedures i.e., it is not specific to the procedure being studied.[29] This suggests that systems and support services present in busier hospitals also contribute to the outcome improvements. For example, organizational characteristics of intensive care units are related to outcome. "Closed" or intensivist-run ICUs, daily ward rounds by an intensivist, and nursing ratios of 1:2 or better are associated with reduced mortality and complications, shorter length of stay, and reduced cost.[30] Evidence-based care guidelines, standardization, nursing staff ratios, education, a culture of teamwork and communication, multidisciplinary rounds, and the presence of a clinical pharmacist are all thought to contribute to improved outcome and these are more likely to occur in large busy hospitals.[22] Understanding this aspect of the volume-outcome relationship is especially important because it may have implications for health policy beyond simply transferring patients with certain conditions to high volume hospitals. Larger hospitals without such systems may perform worse than their smaller counterparts with such systems. Quality improvement programs targeted to hospitals that do not have these systems may also improve outcomes.

Limitations of the volume-outcome literature

There are methodological limitations compromising interpretation of the volume-outcome literature. Most studies are retrospective and used either clinical or administrative databases of varying detail and reliability. Retrospective studies report a greater association between volume and outcome compared with prospective studies.[5] The degree of risk adjustment has also varied widely. Thresholds are commonly arbitrary and variable, making metaanalysis of data difficult. Volume is easy to measure but is a poor surrogate for quality. Understanding what it is about volume that improves outcome is not purely academic and is critical to making appropriate recommendations.

Regionalized systems of care

Regionalization may also improve outcomes when systems are established that increase coordination of care and knowledge transfer between centralized, specialized hospitals and non-specialty hospitals. This has been demonstrated for the establishment of trauma systems with integration between pre-hospital and hospital care. Population-based evidence shows that implementation of a trauma system improves survival 15%-20% among seriously injured patients.[31] Similarly, a large centralized pediatric ICU with a coordinated network of referring hospitals and a retrieval team is associated with a mortality rate 57% of that where there was no regionalized system.[14]

Recommendation

There is strong and consistent evidence that outcomes are improved in high volume programs and hospitals and this effect is strongest for low volume, higher risk conditions and procedures. Regionalized high volume programs have better outcomes in pediatric and adult intensive care and pediatric cardiac surgery. While there are no studies specifically assessing volume in relation to outcome for ECMO, patients requiring ECMO are those with severe cardiorespiratory failure in ICU. ECMO is therefore a relatively low volume procedure performed in high risk patients. We might anticipate that such patients would be optimally managed in a high volume specialist unit, with ECMO available if required. In addition, outcomes are also likely to be improved if ECMO units are part of a regionalized integrated network sharing similar systems and processes for patient management.

There are two further corollaries to providing a centralized ECMO service. First, there is a requirement for the ECMO service to provide an ECMO retrieval team for the transfer of patients who are too sick to safely transfer using standard therapies. Second, since there is no guarantee that centralized services will have better outcomes, all programs should routinely measure and publically report their outcomes.

The ELSO recommendation of a minimum of six patients per year in order to maintain expertise provides guidance as to the size of program required. Local solutions can also be found to maximize experience and expertise. This will depend on the size of individual ICUs and the geographical configuration within campuses and regions. For example, the Auckland program at Starship Children's Hospital and Auckland City Hospital is the national program for New Zealand (population 4.4 million). Within the hospital campus there are four ICUs – NICU, PICU (general and cardiac), adult general ICU, and adult cardiothoracic ICU – all of which have patients that may need ECMO. In order to maximize ECMO team experience and expertise, ECMO is provided by a single team of ECMO nurse specialists who work in either PICU or the adult cardiothoracic ICU. All pediatric and neonatal ECMO is performed in the PICU and all adult ECMO is performed in the adult cardiovascular ICU. This means that the ECMO specialists care for 25-30 patients per year and the medical staff in each unit care for approximately 12-15 patients per year. An ECMO specialist roster of approximately 20 accredited nurses can be maintained and has managed up to 5 patients simultaneously.

Triage of patients for ECMO

ECMO is indicated when the risk of the patient dying from respiratory and/or cardiac failure is 80% or greater, and there are no contraindications to ECMO. Both indices that predict mortality and contraindications will differ according to the nature of cardiorespiratory failure, patient age and institution. Indices may also vary over time, typically over-predicting mortality as treatments and systems improve; they require periodic revalidation. Contraindications may also change as technology improves. All ECMO centers must therefore establish their own inclusion and exclusion criteria and review these regularly.

General oxygenation indices for respiratory failure have been reasonably robust over time. In neonatal respiratory failure, the oxygenation index (OI, which is 100 x [mean airway pressure x FiO_2] / PaO_2) is used. An OI $\geq$ 40 predicts a mortality of at least 80%. For ARDS in adults and children, a PaO_2/FiO_2 < 80 mmHg and a Murray score of 3-4 predict an 80% risk of mortality.[32] Indices for cardiac support are less specific and relate to the presence of signs of shock despite maximal medical therapy.

Wherever possible, ECMO should be considered early for all patients in intensive care with severe respiratory and/or cardiac failure. In some patients undergoing planned surgical procedures, especially high risk cardiac operations, this decision may be made before surgery. ELSO recommends consideration of ECMO

when the probability of dying is approximately 50%. In neonatal respiratory failure this is an OI $\geq$ 20, and in adult ARDS it is PaO_2/FiO_2 < 150 mmHg and a Murray score of 2-3.[32] In many other conditions it will be judged on the basis of the underlying etiology, level of therapy, and a consensus of the multidisciplinary team caring for the patient.

When a patient has severe respiratory and/or cardiac failure and has an approximately 50% or greater risk of dying with no obvious absolute contraindications, there should be discussion with the relevant ECMO service. Early discussion with the ECMO service allows for two possible outcomes. The patient may have definite contraindications to ECMO, in which case this can be clarified, documented, and standard therapy continued. If, however, the patient is a potential ECMO candidate, management depends on whether the patient is in an ECMO center. If in an ECMO center, the ECMO team can ensure that staff and equipment are prepared and be involved in regular review of the patient and decision making about the optimal timing of ECMO should it be required. If the patient is not in an ECMO center, triage decision making must take account of the nature of the ICU and hospital where the patient is at the time, the ability to safely transfer the patient using standard therapies, the availability of an ECMO retrieval service, and resource constraints in the ECMO center.

Ideally, patients who may need ECMO should be treated in a high volume intensive care unit because of the better outcomes associated with this. Where the patient can be transferred safely, one approach would be to transfer to an ECMO center early, once approximately 50% mortality criteria are met. The alternative, following early notification, is regular review of the patient's progress by both the referring and ECMO teams. If ECMO criteria are subsequently met, then retrieval on ECMO can be instigated. There is now considerable experience with retrieval on ECMO in many areas of the world showing that it can be performed safely.[33-37] Where referral is from a smaller secondary ICU, early transfer on standard therapy may be appropriate. Where referral is from a larger tertiary unit and/or there are limited beds available at the ECMO center, regular review followed by ECMO retrieval may be more appropriate. Unusual circumstances with high demand for intensive care beds, such as the 2009 pH1N1 influenza virus pandemic, may modify these triage decisions. For example, patients with pH1N1 influenza in 2009 occupied up to 25% of intensive care beds in New Zealand. Most ICUs were operating near to maximum capacity. A decision was therefore made to only transfer patients to the national ECMO center once ECMO was required and then retrieval on ECMO was performed. There were no patient-related complications with this approach.

Triage of patients during events requiring mass critical care

An outbreak of pandemic influenza or other infectious diseases, or natural or man-made disasters may result in patient numbers that overwhelm the healthcare system. Such events require systems and processes both to increase capacity beyond normal ("surge capacity") and then, if surge capacity is also overwhelmed, to prioritize and allocate limited resources ("triage"). Management of such events requires preparation and planning at hospital, regional, and national levels. Essential components are planning for surge capacity levels, coordination within the hospital and between healthcare facilities, manpower requirements, education, essential equipment and supplies, patient and staff protection, and triage protocols. Most mass casualty events, especially infectious pandemics, are likely to result from agents or events of which we have little experience. Therefore it will be unknown early in the course of a new pandemic what proportion of patients will be hospitalized, require intensive care, or require

ECMO. For example, the severe acute respiratory syndrome (SARS) caused severe illness in adults but very few children were seriously affected.[38] The 2009 pH1N1 influenza pandemic required a fraction of the ICU capacity compared to what was initially predicted.

A full discussion of all aspects of this topic is beyond the scope of this chapter but several comprehensive reviews have been published.[39,40] Most aspects are generic to hospital, ICU, and ECMO service planning (e.g., infrastructure, communication, education). However, planning for surge capacity and triage protocols are aspects that may require specific preparation and involvement by ECMO services.

Surge capacity planning

Surge capacity planning is a stepwise approach to an increase in intensive care capacity above normal. One task force recommends that ICUs should be able to expand to 300% of usual capacity and maintain this for 10 days without external assistance.[41] While this may not be possible for many facilities, clear targets must be set along with plans showing how this will be achieved. Most centers should plan to at least double capacity. There are three phases to expansion:[42]

1. Conventional. This involves using spaces usually used for intensive care. Many ICUs are not resourced in terms of staff and equipment for full physical occupancy. Conventional expansion maximizes ICU occupancy by increased staffing (e.g., overtime, cancelling leave, etc), using adjacent step-down and high dependency (HDU) areas, and ensuring that there is sufficient equipment to support this.
2. Contingency. This involves using spaces similar to ICU spaces, such as post-anesthesia care units (PACU), emergency department spaces, operat-

ing rooms, and procedure areas. Hospitals need to define the number of spaces potentially available in each area and then prioritize in terms of suitability for this purpose. It may involve the use of equipment not usually used routinely in intensive care, such as transport ventilators and anesthetic machine ventilators. Usually the most critically ill patients will be cared for within the ICU and less critically ill in other areas. Staff contingency planning may involve changing the scope of practice and responsibilities of some staff and/or altered models of care, along with legal protection for staff involved in these changes.

3. Crisis. This is the provision of intensive care either in areas not designed for high intensity care (e.g., hospital ward bed spaces) and/or by staff who are not trained in intensive care but are supported by trained intensive care staff. When demand exceeds capacity of either critical care equipment (e.g., mechanical ventilators, ECMO equipment) or staff, triage protocols should be invoked.

With respect to the ECMO service, conventional expansion includes planning to fully use all of the available ECMO equipment. This requires being explicit about how many pumps, heat exchangers, and essential monitors are available along with the maximum staffing capacity. Contingency expansion planning includes defining processes for sourcing additional equipment, such as from other cardiac surgical programs, equipment companies, and other ECMO programs (if not affected by the same event). ECMO specialist models of care may also need to be altered. The accepted standard is one nurse and one ECMO specialist per patient in many current programs. Contingency planning may require reduction of these ratios;

for example, an ECMO specialist looking after the patient and circuit or else an ECMO specialist looking after multiple circuits. A clear plan needs to establish how many additional patients contingency expansion will allow both in terms of ECMO staff, including using reduced staffing models, and also equipment. Crisis levels of planning are unlikely to be relevant for ECMO since an event requiring expansion of intensive care to low intensity areas of the hospital will be of such magnitude as to preclude the widespread use of ECMO because it is so labor and resource intensive.

During 2009 in Australia and New Zealand (total population approximately 25 million), patients with pH1N1 influenza occupied 7.4 (95%CI: 6.3-8.5) ICU beds per million inhabitants. This accounted for 5.2% of ICU bed-days and a peak percentage of 8.9-19% of ICU beds over a three month period. Approximately 12% of mechanically ventilated patients received ECMO. This corresponded to 2.6 patients per million people requiring ECMO. ECMO was provided in 15 units and, at the peak of the pandemic, 23 concurrent patients required ECMO (see Figure 32-1). This was performed using conventional expansion alone.

Triage protocols

Triage protocols should only be implemented when all efforts to increase capacity have been exhausted. Limitations should also be proportional to the actual shortfall and are likely to need modification as data about the characteristics of the event become clearer. Other principles of rationing are that it occur uniformly and be transparent and that it apply equally to withholding and withdrawing life support, since these are ethically equivalent. Patients not eligible for intensive care should continue to receive supportive and/or palliative care.[43]

There are four main components to a triage protocol, defined in 2006 by Christian et al.[44,45] These are:

1. Inclusion criteria. This identifies patients who require and are likely to benefit from intensive care and principally focuses on ventilatory support, but may also include some hemodynamic support.

2. Exclusion criteria. These include patients (a) with a poor prognosis despite ICU care, (b) those who may benefit but require intensive use of resources and prolonged care that cannot be justified during a pandemic, and (c) those with severe comorbidities that have a poor prognosis.

3. "Minimum qualifications for survival." These are a ceiling on the amount of resources that can reasonably be expended on any one person. It requires reassessment of patients admitted at fixed intervals (e.g., 2 and 5 days) to identify patients who are not improving, in whom life support may be withdrawn.

4. A prioritization tool. Commonly this involves categorization and allocation of a color according to category, together with an ICU priority ranking and general plan of treatment if not admitted.

Triage protocols require individuals with training in the triage process and a central triage committee made up of experts with broad regional situational awareness, and the capability to assess data and outcomes and modify protocols as required. All staff need to understand that decisions made during a mass casualty event are made in the best interests of the population as opposed to the individual. Each institution should determine its own triage criteria. The most widely proposed prioritization tool is the Sequential Organ Failure Assessment (SOFA) score (see Table 32-1).[43,45] This is because it is easy to collect using simple laboratory tests, can be performed daily, and has been validated in a diverse range of intensive care conditions. A predicted mortality of >80% has been suggested as a basis for exclusion from intensive care and this is predicted with a SOFA score of ≥15 at any time and a score of ≥5 for at least 5 days that is either flat or rising. Others have suggested a SOFA score of >11 be the basis for exclusion. However the SOFA score was not designed for triage and there is conflicting opinion as to its validity for this purpose.

Decisions about ECMO will depend on the scale of the event. ECMO may not be appropriate at all if hospitals and ICUs are overwhelmed. However, in a lesser event where intensive care capacity is being maintained but conventional ECMO surge capacity is exceeded, "ECMO-specific" triage criteria may be required. These will also need to be institution-specific and based on local data and resources. However, appropriate approaches might, for example, limit ECMO to patients with single organ failure or limit ECMO duration to 10-12 days, since this is the average time for recovery to occur.

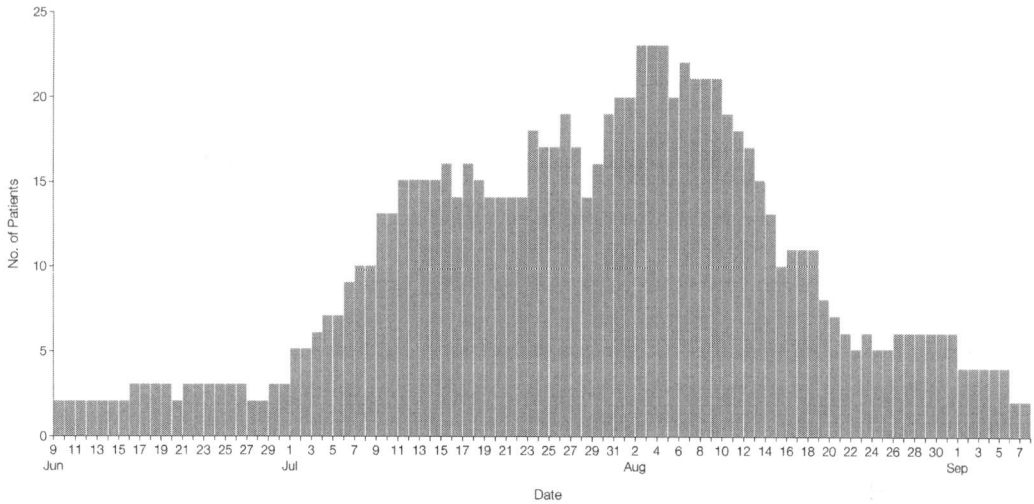

Figure 32-1. Histogram of the number of concurrent patients across Australia and New Zealand receiving ECMO during the pH1N1 influenza pandemic in 2009.[47]

Table 32-1. Sequential Organ Failure Assessment (SOFA) Score[46]

Score	0	1	2	3	4
PaO$_2$/FiO$_2$ mmHg	>400	400	300	200	100
Platelets	>150	150	100	50	20
Bilirubin mg/dl (μmol/l)	<1.2 (<20)	1.2-1.9 (20-32)	2.0-5.9 (33-100)	6.0-11.9 (101-203)	>12 (>203)
Hypotension	None	MABP<70 mmHg	Dop=5	Dop>5, Epi=0.1, Norepi=0.1	Dop>15, Epi>0.1, Norepi>0.1
Glasgow Coma Score	15	13-14	10-12	6-9	<6
Creatinine mg/dl (μmol/l)	<1.2 (<106)	13-14 (106-168)	2.0-3.4 (169-300)	3.5-4.9 (301-433)	>5 (>434)

References

1. ELSO Guidelines for ECMO Centers. Extracorporeal Life Support Organization. 2010;Version 1.7.

2. Lorch SA, Myers S, Carr B. The regionalization of pediatric health care. Pediatrics. Dec 2010;126(6):1182-1190.

3. Luft HS, Bunker JP, Enthoven AC. Should operations be regionalized? The empirical relation between surgical volume and mortality. N Engl J Med. Dec 20 1979;301(25):1364-1369.

4. Kizer KW. The volume-outcome conundrum. N Engl J Med. Nov 27 2003;349(22):2159-2161.

5. Chowdhury MM, Dagash H, Pierro A. A systematic review of the impact of volume of surgery and specialization on patient outcome. Br J Surg. Feb 2007;94(2):145-161.

6. Halm EA, Lee C, Chassin MR. Is volume related to outcome in health care? A systematic review and methodologic critique of the literature. Ann Intern Med. Sep 17 2002;137(6):511-520.

7. Dudley RA, Johansen KL, Brand R, Rennie DJ, Milstein A. Selective referral to high-volume hospitals: estimating potentially avoidable deaths. JAMA. Mar 1 2000;283(9):1159-1166.

8. Birkmeyer JD, Siewers AE, Finlayson EV, et al. Hospital volume and surgical mortality in the United States. N Engl J Med. Apr 11 2002;346(15):1128-1137.

9. Ross JS, Normand SL, Wang Y, et al. Hospital volume and 30-day mortality for three common medical conditions. N Engl J Med. Mar 25 2010;362(12):1110-1118.

10. Bucher BT, Guth RM, Saito JM, Najaf T, Warner BW. Impact of hospital volume on in-hospital mortality of infants undergoing repair of congenital diaphragmatic hernia. Ann Surg. Oct 2010;252(4):635-642.

11. Edwards EB, Roberts JP, McBride MA, Schulak JA, Hunsicker LG. The effect of the volume of procedures at transplantation centers on mortality after liver transplantation. N Engl J Med. Dec 30 1999;341(27):2049-2053.

12. Grushka JR, Laberge JM, Puligandla P, Skarsgard ED. Effect of hospital case volume on outcome in congenital diaphragmatic hernia: the experience of the Canadian Pediatric Surgery Network. J Pediatr Surg. May 2009;44(5):873-876.

13. Morales DL, Zafar F, Rossano JW, et al. Use of ventricular assist devices in children across the United States: analysis of 7.5 million pediatric hospitalizations. Ann Thorac Surg. Oct 2010;90(4):1313-1318; discussion 1318-1319.

14. Pearson G, Shann F, Barry P, et al. Should paediatric intensive care be centralised? Trent versus Victoria. Lancet. Apr 26 1997;349(9060):1213-1217.

15. Ruttimann UE, Patel KM, Pollack MM. Relevance of diagnostic diversity and patient volumes for quality and length of stay in pediatric intensive care units. Pediatr Crit Care Med. Oct 2000;1(2):133-139.

16. Tilford JM, Simpson PM, Green JW, Lensing S, Fiser DH. Volume-outcome relationships in pediatric intensive care units. Pediatrics. Aug 2000;106(2 Pt 1):289-294.

17. Bach PB, Cramer LD, Schrag D, Downey RJ, Gelfand SE, Begg CB. The influence of hospital volume on survival after resection for lung cancer. N Engl J Med. Jul 19 2001;345(3):181-188.

18. Begg CB, Riedel ER, Bach PB, et al. Variations in morbidity after radical prostatectomy. N Engl J Med. Apr 11 2002;346(15):1138-1144.

19. Shook TL, Sun GW, Burstein S, Eisenhauer AC, Matthews RV. Comparison of percutaneous transluminal coronary angioplasty outcome and hospital costs for low-volume and high-volume operators. Am J Cardiol. Feb 15 1996;77(5):331-336.

20. Pearson G, Barry P, Timmins C, Stickley J, Hocking M. Changes in the profile of paediatric intensive care associated with centralisation. Intensive Care Med. Oct 2001;27(10):1670-1673.

21. Marcin JP, Song J, Leigh JP. The impact of pediatric intensive care unit volume on mortality: a hierarchical instrumental variable analysis. Pediatr Crit Care Med. Mar 2005;6(2):136-141.

22. Kahn JM. Volume, outcome, and the organization of intensive care. Crit Care. 2007;11(3):129.

23. Kahn JM, Goss CH, Heagerty PJ, Kramer AA, O'Brien CR, Rubenfeld GD. Hospital volume and the outcomes of mechanical ventilation. N Engl J Med. Jul 6 2006;355(1):41-50.

24. Kahn JM, Ten Have TR, Iwashyna TJ. The relationship between hospital volume and mortality in mechanical ventilation: an instrumental variable analysis. Health Serv Res. Jun 2009;44(3):862-879.

25. Jenkins KJ, Newburger JW, Lock JE, Davis RB, Coffman GA, Iezzoni LI. In-hospital mortality for surgical repair of congenital heart defects: preliminary observations of variation by hospital caseload. Pediatrics. Mar 1995;95(3):323-330.

26. Welke KF, O'Brien SM, Peterson ED, Ungerleider RM, Jacobs ML, Jacobs JP. The complex relationship between pediatric cardiac surgical case volumes and mortality rates in a national clinical database. J Thorac Cardiovasc Surg. May 2009;137(5):1133-1140.

27. Farley DE, Ozminkowski RJ. Volume-outcome relationships and in-hospital mortality: the effect of changes in volume over time. Med Care. Jan 1992;30(1):77-94.

28. Finks JF, Osborne NH, Birkmeyer JD. Trends in hospital volume and operative mortality for high-risk surgery. N Engl J Med. Jun 2 2011;364(22):2128-2137.

29. Urbach DR, Baxter NN. Does it matter what a hospital is "high volume" for? Specificity of hospital volume-outcome associations for surgical procedures: analysis of administrative data. BMJ. Mar 27 2004;328(7442):737-740.

30. Pronovost PJ, Jenckes MW, Dorman T, et al. Organizational characteristics of intensive care units related to outcomes of abdominal aortic surgery. JAMA. Apr 14 1999;281(14):1310-1317.

31. Mullins RJ, Mann NC. Population-based research assessing the effectiveness of trauma systems. J Trauma. Sep 1999;47(3 Suppl):S59-66.

32. ELSO Patient Specific Supplements to the ELSO General Guidelines. Extracorporeal Life Support Organization. 2009;Version 1.1.

33. Cabrera AG, Prodhan P, Cleves MA, et al. Interhospital transport of children requiring extracorporeal membrane oxygenation support for cardiac dysfunction. Congenit Heart Dis. May 2011;6(3):202-208.

34. Ciapetti M, Cianchi G, Zagli G, et al. Feasibility of inter-hospital transportation using extra-corporeal membrane oxygenation (ECMO) support of patients affected by severe swine-flu(H1N1)-related ARDS. Scand J Trauma Resusc Emerg Med. 2011;19:32.

35. Forrest P, Ratchford J, Burns B, et al. Retrieval of critically ill adults using extracorporeal membrane oxygenation: an Australian experience. Intensive Care Med. May 2011;37(5):824-830.

36. Javidfar J, Brodie D, Takayama H, et al. Safe transport of critically ill adult patients on extracorporeal membrane oxygenation support to a regional extracorporeal membrane oxygenation center. ASAIO J. Sep-Oct 2011;57(5):421-425.

37. Knapik P, Przybylski R, Borkowski J, et al. Interhospital transport of patients requiring extracorporeal membrane oxygenation

ECMO. Anestezjol Intens Ter. Jul-Sep 2011;43(3):142-145.

38. Kissoon N, Bohn D. Use of extracorporeal technology during pandemics: ethical and staffing considerations. Pediatr Crit Care Med. Nov 2010;11(6):757-758.

39. Sprung CL, Cohen R, Adini B. Chapter 1. Introduction. Recommendations and standard operating procedures for intensive care unit and hospital preparations for an influenza epidemic or mass disaster. Intensive Care Med. Apr 2010;36 Suppl 1:S4-10.

40. Devereaux A, Christian MD, Dichter JR, Geiling JA, Rubinson L. Summary of suggestions from the Task Force for Mass Critical Care summit, January 26-27, 2007. Chest. May 2008;133(5 Suppl):1S-7S.

41. Rubinson L, Hick JL, Hanfling DG, et al. Definitive care for the critically ill during a disaster: a framework for optimizing critical care surge capacity: from a Task Force for Mass Critical Care summit meeting, January 26-27, 2007, Chicago, IL. Chest. May 2008;133(5 Suppl):18S-31S.

42. Hick JL, Christian MD, Sprung CL. Chapter 2. Surge capacity and infrastructure considerations for mass critical care. Recommendations and standard operating procedures for intensive care unit and hospital preparations for an influenza epidemic or mass disaster. Intensive Care Med. Apr 2010;36 Suppl 1:S11-20.

43. Devereaux AV, Dichter JR, Christian MD, et al. Definitive care for the critically ill during a disaster: a framework for allocation of scarce resources in mass critical care: from a Task Force for Mass Critical Care summit meeting, January 26-27, 2007, Chicago, IL. Chest. May 2008;133(5 Suppl):51S-66S.

44. Christian MD, Hawryluck L, Wax RS, et al. Development of a triage protocol for critical care during an influenza pandemic. CMAJ. Nov 21 2006;175(11):1377-1381.

45. Christian MD, Joynt GM, Hick JL, Colvin J, Danis M, Sprung CL. Chapter 7. Critical care triage. Recommendations and standard operating procedures for intensive care unit and hospital preparations for an influenza epidemic or mass disaster. Intensive Care Med. Apr 2010;36 Suppl 1:S55-64.

46. Ferreira FL, Bota DP, Bross A, Melot C, Vincent JL. Serial evaluation of the SOFA score to predict outcome in critically ill patients. JAMA. Oct 10 2001;286(14):1754-1758.

47. Davies A, Jones D, Bailey M, et al. Extracorporeal Membrane Oxygenation for 2009 Influenza A(H1N1) Acute Respiratory Distress Syndrome. JAMA. Nov 4 2009;302(17):1888-1895.

33

Transport of the ECMO Patient: From Concept to Implementation

Jeremy W. Cannon MD SM, Patrick F. Allan MD, Eric C. Osborn MD, Alois Phillip, Matthias Arlt MD, Melissa M. Tyree MD

Introduction

Matching patients who require ECLS for cardiopulmonary or respiratory failure with centers that offer these services sometimes requires inter-hospital transfer. Because these patients are highly unstable, the resources required to affect such a transfer are substantial, and few teams have the expertise to perform these transports safely. At the same time, broader indications for ECLS[1] and improved patient outcomes at specialty centers[2] may lead to increased demand for such transport services in the coming years. Intra-hospital ECMO transport also continues to be required for certain diagnostic and therapeutic interventions. Increasing awareness and training for both forms of transport will serve to enhance the capability of entire ECMO community in the art of transport medicine.

Medical teams who perform ECLS transports have significant experience in rescue resuscitation techniques using a number of different advanced technologies. As a result, the transport configuration can take many forms. By the strictest definition, ECLS transport between hospitals represents movement of a patient who is on either VV or VA ECMO by ground or air ambulance, sometimes termed mobile ECMO. In some cases, ECMO teams who respond to a transport request may find that following rescue maneuvers, the patient can be safely transported

without ECMO. For example, an ECMO-capable team may elect to use advanced ventilator modes, adjuncts such as inhaled nitric oxide (iNO), or pumpless extracorporeal lung assist (PECLA) to stabilize the patient. However, the discussion that follows presumes that the safest approach to moving potential ECMO candidates is by a team capable of implementing mobile ECMO if these maneuvers have previously failed or prove ineffective.

This chapter reviews the modern approach to movement of these ultra-tenuous patients by examining several key topics. The history of mobile ECMO is briefly reviewed to underscore the role of ECMO-capable transport teams as an extension of the ECMO center. The process of ECMO referral is described to provide intensivists who recognize the potential need for ECMO the resources to initiate such a transfer. For those considering adding mobile ECMO to their existing transport team, the particulars of the ECMO transport process is discussed in detail from team preparation to mission completion. Considerations for the Transport Medical Director including team training, equipment selection, and in-transport emergencies are also reviewed. The collaborative effort between the US military Acute Lung Injury Rescue Team (ALIRT, also known as the "Lung Team") and the ECMO center at University Hospital Regensburg, Germany, which has enabled the use of extracorporeal support in combat casualty care is described. Results from several transport teams are updated from previous reports[3] to illustrate the current state of inter-hospital ECMO transport in the US and across the world. Finally, the elements unique to intra-hospital transport (IHT) are highlighted, and the risks versus the diagnostic and therapeutic benefits of IHT are assessed.

History of inter-hospital ECMO transport

With the recent descriptions of Critical Care Air Transport Teams (CCATT),[4] long-range military subspecialty transport teams,[5,6] and a ground-based mobile Intensive Care Unit,[7] an entire field of so-called "transit care medicine" has emerged.[8] Guidelines for safely transporting critically ill adults[9] and children[10] have been published with improved outcomes in patients transported by these specialized teams well-documented.[11] Of course the ECMO community has a rich history of transporting the sickest of patients and would do well to lend this expertise to future guidelines which should include the role of ECMO and other advanced technologies in stabilizing patients for inter-hospital transport. This section reviews the origins of transport ECMO which developed as a hedge against the so-called "hidden mortality" of ECMO referral.

The hidden mortality of ECMO referral

The history of inter-hospital ECMO transport parallels that of ECMO development. Bartlett and colleagues reported two ECMO transports in their original series of 28 ECMO patients.[12] One of their five survivors in this series was a 17 year-old female with pulmonary hemorrhage from Goodpasture's Syndrome. After initiating VA ECMO and stabilizing the patient with four Landé-Edwards oxygenators, the ECMO team moved her from Albuquerque, NM, to Orange County Medical Center on a US Air Force C-130. The team hand cranked the

pump to and from the airfield in the back of a bread truck that was acquisitioned for ground transport on either end.[13]

As the benefits of ECMO became apparent, referrals of tenuous ICU patients at outlying hospitals for possible ECMO increased. However, transporting these critically ill patients to ECMO centers carried significant risk and seemed to uncover a "hidden" mortality associated with ECMO referral. In 1986, Cornish and colleagues alluded to this phenomenon among military dependents who were identified as ECMO candidates in geographically remote medical centers but expired either prior to or during transport.[14] This issue was first reported by Boedy and colleagues who found that 18 of 158 (11%) neonates referred to their center for ECMO died either before, during, or shortly after conventional ground transport.[15] Similarly, University of Michigan Medical Center (UMMC) found that of 107 referrals for ECMO in two years, 11 (10.3%) expired either during transport or at the referring center because they were denied transport due to cardiopulmonary instability.[16] Arkansas Children's Hospital (ACH) described three in-transport deaths in cases where ECMO was not available. This represented a 12% mortality in their non-ECMO transport group.[17] Wilson et al. noted at least six deaths in neonates referred for ECMO over a three-year period where the patient could not be converted from high frequency oscillatory ventilation to conventional ventilation for transport after referral to an ECMO center.[18] These observations directly motivated the development of portable ECMO equipment and transport teams who could place a patient on ECMO prior to transport.[14]

More recently, the CESAR investigators reported three deaths prior to transport and two in-transport deaths of 90 patients randomized for transport to the ECMO center.[2] In this study, mobile ECMO was not used; however, the ECMO team performed all inter-facility transports. These cases demonstrate that a "hidden" risk of mortality in patients referred for ECMO still exists. However, as transport equipment becomes more compact and the physiologic derangements associated with ECMO lessen, recognition of these potentially avoidable deaths may compel more ECMO centers with transport teams to incorporate mobile ECMO into their armamentarium.

Currently, ECMO-capable transport teams in the US routinely performing ECMO transport include WHMC, UMMC, ACH, and the Hanuola ECMO Program of Hawaii. In addition, multiple international centers have reported a growing experience of inter-hospital ECMO transport. Results reported by these US and international teams suggest their expertise and ability to use advanced therapies in transport have greatly reduced mortalities in ECMO candidates following referral to an ECMO center.[16,19,20]

In addition to the transport services provided by these academic centers, a company called ECMO Advantage now offers commercial ECMO transport in partnership with AirMed International.[21] Although this group has significant ECMO expertise, given the complexity of this endeavor, ECMO Advantage and transport agencies who offer mobile ECMO in the future should espouse the ELSO guidelines, report results to the ELSO Registry, and share lessons learned with others in the field.

Transport ECMO equipment

Outfitting an ECMO-capable transport team involves specialized equipment, and over time, this equipment has evolved. Transport teams have described a number of different transport carts which hold the pumps, monitors, gas tanks, and the patient and have used custom vehicles ranging from specialized ambulances to specially configured fixed wing aircraft. In every case, the transport setup must have sufficient capacity and power for the ECMO equipment

and a mechanism for loading the patient and circuit into the vehicle.[16,20,22,23]

The first custom transport ECMO cart used by Cornish, et al, was a modified Rubbermaid® cart which could only hold neonates.[14] Subsequent versions of this cart were incredibly heavy at 740 lb (336 kg) but could accommodate both pediatric and adult patients.[20] This cart and its various components have been subjected to rigorous air worthiness testing which allow it to be used worldwide on US Air Force transport aircraft.[3] This testing ensures that aircraft and medical device electromagnetic interaction is minimized, that aircraft power and gas stores can sustain device function, and that the equipment can be securely anchored to the aircraft cabin. An updated version of this cart recently passed these rigorous tests and is presently in use by the WHMC Neonatal & Pediatric ECMO transport team (Figure 33-1). However, given the size and weight of this cart and its components, a specialized ambulance with a

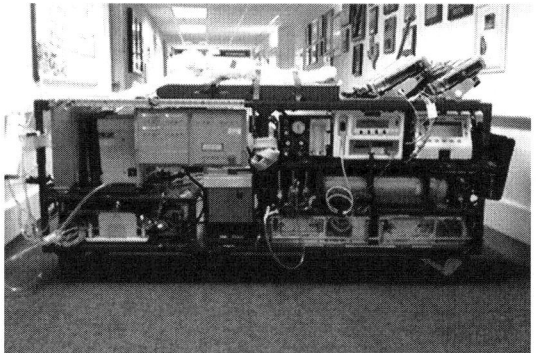

Figure 33-1. The 2005 WHMC ECMO transport cart. This cart can support neonates, children, and adults and is certified for both ground and air transport with US Air Force safe-to-fly designation for the C 17 and C-130 aircrafts. The system is based on the Stockert SIII Roller Pump Console servoregulated system (Cobe Cardiovascular, Arvada, CO). The component shelves slide out for accessibility and lock in place for stability. The cart is self-contained with its own gas (air, O2, carbogen Q tanks) and power source (2 Energy Technologies ETI0001-1240 UPS units) which can provide up to 3 hours of independent emergency function. Photo courtesy Kreangkai Tyree, MD, Wilford Hall Medical Center, San Antonio, TX.

hydraulic lift or access to a loading dock is required for each mission. UMMC also continues to use a cumbersome roller pump-based transport stretcher for infant ground transport (Figure 33-2).

With the increased use of centrifugal pump-based systems which permit short circuit lengths and with the miniaturization of many of the required monitors, ECMO transport carts have shrunk dramatically in recent years. The Hanuola and ACH teams have partnered with aeromedical companies (Elliott Aviation, Moline, IL, and JetMed, Little Rock, AR, respectively) to design relatively streamlined sleds which can fit on small fixed wing aircraft (Figure 33-3). UMMC employs a compact overbed tray module and console for its pediatric and adult transport setup (Figure 33-4). Similarly, a new hand-held mini-ECMO device developed by Arlt and colleagues (ELS-System, Maquet Cardiopulmonary, Hechingen, Germany) can be placed directly on a platform over a conventional stretcher[24] or suspended from the siderail (Figure 33-5).[19,25,26] An enclosed self-contained system based on a centrifugal pump termed the Lifebridge B2T (Lifebridge Medizintechnik AG, Ampfing, Germany) has recently been described for inpatient use,[27,28] and given its convenient packaging and compact size, it has some potential for use as a transport system. Other similar transport-specific systems are currently in development. As these and future systems complete clinical evaluation and FDA review, they should rapidly enter the FAA and US Air Force air worthiness testing process[3] so that US ECMO centers considering the establishment of transport programs will have this equipment available for use at their discretion.

A complete extra or backup ECMO circuit should be part of the ECMO team's equipment list, including extra cannulas, tubing, and an oxygenator. Although some groups advocate packing lightly, this must be balanced against

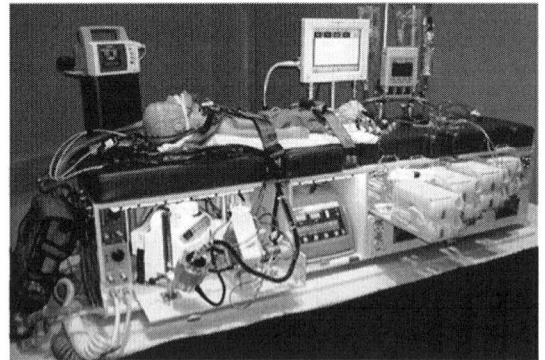

Figure 33-3. The Hanuola ECMO program of Hawaii ECMO transport sled. The modular sled can support infants, children, and adults. It is shown with the Levitronix CentriMag centrifugal pump (Levitronix LLC, Waltham, MA), Quadrox D gas exchange membrane (Maquet, Inc. Bridgewater, NJ), B Braun infusion pumps (B Braun, Bethlehem, PA) and Spectrum M3 monitor, (Spectrum Medical, Fort Mill, SC) with slide-out trays for easy access. Components can be interchanged to accommodate all pump and membrane models. The total sled weight as shown is 250lbs. It requires 10 amp power support. The sled's base includes a Lifeport Clipdeck mounting bracket which secures it to the Stryker Power Pro IT hydraulic ambulance gurney (International Biomed, Austin,TX). Photograph courtesy Kristen Costales, CCP, Hanuola ECMO Program, Honolulu, HI.

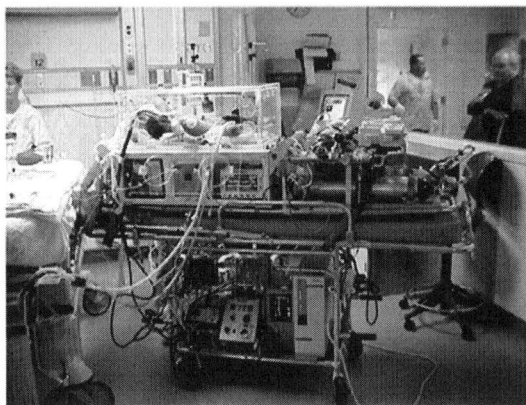

Figure 33-2. University of Michigan Medical Center infant ground roller pump transport stretcher. Photograph courtesy William Copenhaver, RN, BSN, University of Michigan Medical Center, Ann Arbor, MI.

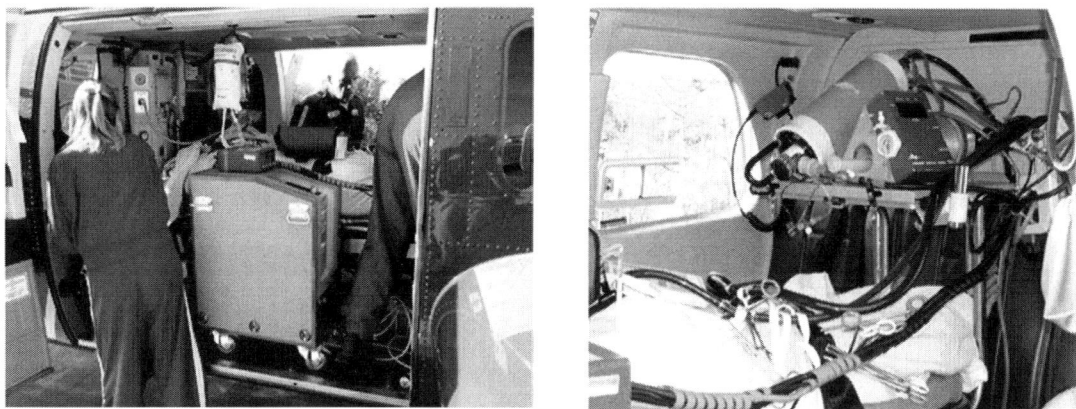

Figure 33-4. A.) University of Michigan pediatric and adult centrifugal pump transport system. The Heli-Dyne console box (Heli-Dyne Systems, Inc, Hurst, TX) houses the centrifugal pump control module, Hemochron 401 (International Technidyne Corp., Edison, NJ), and CSZ Microtemp water heater (Cincinnati Sub Zero, Cincinnati, OH) and is secured to the aircraft via 6 quick connect tie downs. B.) The overbed table slides into the litter frame and supports the pump motor, oxygenator, and DLP monitor. A tether consisting of the drive motor cable, flow probe cable, and water heater lines (shown crossing from picture bottom left to the right side of the overbed table) connects to the Heli-Dyne console box. Photographs courtesy William Copenhaver, RN, BSN, University of Michigan Medical Center, Ann Arbor, MI.

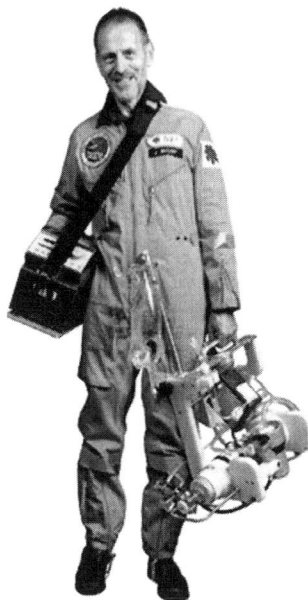

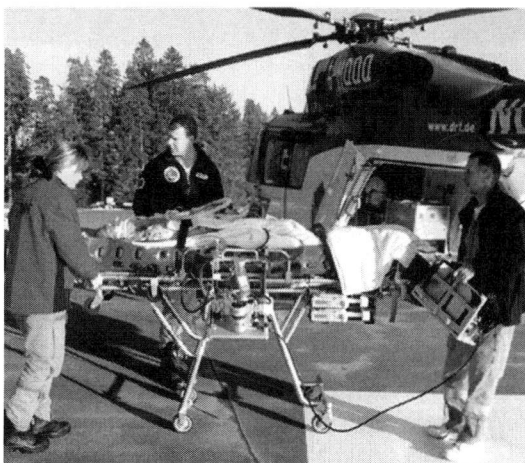

Figure 33-5. A.) New hand-held mini-ECMO system (ELS-System, MAQUET Cardiopulmonary AG, Hechingen, Germany) which consists of a custom frame housing the pump head, gas exchange membrane, and an oxygen tank. This compact, lightweight system can be carried by a member of the ECMO transport team. B.) Inter-hospital transfer using the mini-ECMO system. The custom frame is mounted to the siderail of the stretcher while the pump controller is carried by a member of the transport team. Photographs courtesy Matthias Arlt, MD, University Hospital Regensburg, Germany.

preparation for unforeseen mechanical problems in order to perform ECMO transport safely. For brief helicopter flights and ambulance drives, many transport teams will not take the extra equipment. This is not unreasonable, but advance planning and packing allows for the presence of extra contingency equipment and enhances patient safety. For example, the water heater can be disconnected for short ambulance ground transports and helicopter rides, but a water heater is necessary for longer helicopter and fixed wing transports.

In addition to specific ECMO equipment, materials and medicines to augment support enroute should be present, especially on longer trips. A portable ultrasound can help with bedside interventions including line placement and final cannula positioning. A portable fiberoptic bronchoscope can be used for airway clearance and delivery of medications if necessary. For adults, specialty medications including inhaled prostacyclin and intravenous tromethamine, for example, should be available along with the other medications used during long-range critical care transport.

Logistics of inter-hospital transport

Over time, transport medicine has evolved from emergency technicians performing hand bag ventilation to in-flight trauma surgeons and intensivists equipped with advanced capabilities including high frequency ventilation and extracorporeal life support.[5,6,8] In this paradigm, medical transport does not suspend but rather facilitates patient care. However, the logistics of this transport process can be quite complex. Transporting a patient on ECMO requires out-of-hospital management of a patient in the midst of advanced cardiopulmonary life support in which the transport team must become a self-contained, self-sufficient entity. The transport then involves a complex interplay between the referring facility, the transport team, and the receiving ECMO center with the Transport

Medical Director responsible for planning the mission, preparing and assembling the transport team, and ultimately safely delivering the patient to the accepting facility. This section reviews in detail the many considerations involved in these transports.

Referring center preparation

Patients considered for ECMO transport include those who have potential indications for ECMO initiation outside an ECMO center, those who have already been placed on ECMO at a center unable to support long-term ECMO management, and those who have been placed on ECMO as a potential bridge to transplant in a non-transplant center. Once the candidate patient with potentially reversibly respiratory and/or cardiac failure has been identified using the ELSO guidelines and selection criteria detailed in this book, the referring hospital should contact a potential accepting center. A newly developed ECMO center map on the ELSO web site allows referring physicians to quickly identify nearby ECMO centers and the categories of patients these centers can accommodate (Figure 33-6).[29]

Upon receiving a potential referral, the ECMO center should elicit the patient's history, current physiologic state, and the reason for consultation. Referring and accepting centers are encouraged to have specific acceptance criteria in place as described by existing ECMO transport programs.[16,20,23] In general, early referral is preferred so that the ECMO center team can apply rescue therapies that may not have been considered or implemented before committing to ECMO.

Once the receiving center accepts the referral, the transport modality should then be decided by the referring and receiving centers. Options for transport include conventional emergency medical transport, transport by a specialty team from the ECMO center without ECMO backup, or transport by an ECMO-capable team. As described above, we firmly believe that ECMO candidates should be transported by an ECMO-capable team to avoid unnecessary deaths in transport if at all possible. Accordingly, contact information for the most experienced US and international transport teams is provided in Table 33-1.

Prior to the transport team's arrival, the referring center can begin to prepare the patient for transport by attending to several details as described in the ELSO General Guidelines. For local or regional transports (< 150 miles and 150-1,000 miles, respectively), the transport team usually arrives within 2 to 4 hours of the referral request. If the transport logistics are complicated or long-range military transport is required (>1,000 miles), there may be as much as a 72 hour interval between referral and arrival of the transport team. During this time, the transport team will often fax ahead a list of required equipment, preferred patient positioning (e.g., in the largest ICU room available with the ventilator on the patient's left), any required personnel from the referring center, blood bank requests, and a consent packet for review. For legal purposes, the UMMC transport team has developed an "umbrella" policy in which the referring physician signs orders which transfer care of the patient to the transport team upon their arrival.[16]

Transport team preparation

Preparation for ECMO transports involves significant advanced planning on the part of the Transport Medical Director. Ultimately, the Medical Director is responsible for the safe and efficient movement of the patient by a team of highly trained personnel. With this in mind, the principal roles and the many responsibilities of the Medical Director are summarized in Table 33-2. For team sustainment, the Transport Medical Director is responsible for training the transport team, identifying proficient team members for future missions, and keeping transport equipment and supplies current and serviceable (Tables 33-3 and 33-4). Then, when a transport request is received, the Medical Director or a designated Mission Commander makes the logistical arrangements for transport of the team and the equipment to the referring facility, assesses the capabilities of the referring facility's blood bank, determines the optimal transport mode for the patient (ground vs. rotary wing vs. fixed wing), and identifies medical center waypoints for emergency intervention if the patient deteriorates in transport.

For transport between two hospitals that do not include the transport team's home facility

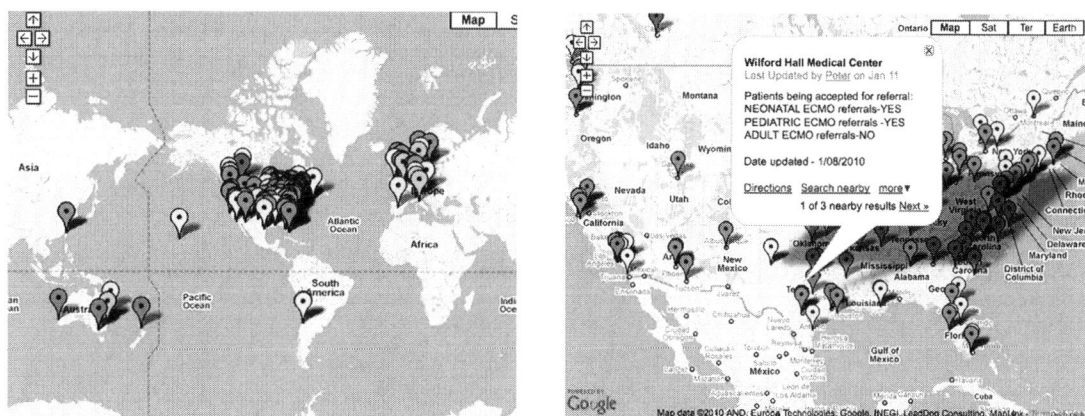

Figure 33-6. A.) ECMO center bed status map which can be accessed on the ELSO web site (http://www.elso.med.umich.edu/Maps.html). B.) Contributing centers can update current availability for accepting ECMO patients in transfer. Each center is color coded according to their designation in the ELSO registry.

Table 33-1. Contact information for ECMO transport services.

	Patient Type	Point of Contact	Contact Information
Arkansas Children's Hospital	Neonatal Pediatric	Richard Fiser	800-372-2229 (Central Dispatch)
Hanuola ECMO Program	Neonatal Pediatric Adult[#]	Melissa Tyree	808-983-6555 (Transport Hotline) 210-787-9685 (cell) mtyree@usuhs.mil 808-294-2275
		Melody Kilcommons	
University of Michigan Medical Center	Neonatal Pediatric Adult	Jonathan Haft	734-936-6626, pager 9766 734-216-5763 734-763-9919 (ECMO office)
San Antonio Military Medical Center	Neonatal Pediatric	Susan Dotzler	210-292-7850 (NICU) 210-292-2442 (MD workroom)
	Adult	Jeremy Cannon	210-222-2876 (ICU) 210-594-2742 (pager) 210-289-7672 (cell) jcannon@massmed.org jeremy.w.cannon@us.army.mil
Karolinska University Hospital Stockholm, Sweden	Neonatal Pediatric Adult	Kenneth Palmer Bjorn Frenckner	+46 8 517 70000 +46 8 517 78000
Landstuhl Regional Medical Center, Ramstein Air Base, Germany	Adult (Combat Casualties)	David Zonies	Military only
National Taiwan University Hospital, Taipei, Taiwan	Neonatal Pediatric Adult	Yih-Sharng Chen	0972651433 (cell) yschen1234@gmail.com
Oslo Universitetshospital-Rikshospitalet, Oslo, Norway	Neonatal Pediatric Adult	Kari Wagner	+47 23070000 kari.wagner@oslo-universitetshospital.no
University Hospital Regensburg, Germany	Adult	Matthias Arlt	+49 941-944-0 matthias.arlt@klinik.uni-regensburg.de
Royal Children's Hospital, Melbourne, Australia	Neonatal Pediatric	Warwick Butt	+613 93455522

[#]only for transport to/from Hawaii.

Table 33-2. Responsibilities of the Transport Medical Director.

	Specific Tasks
Transport Team Training	- Mannequin drills - Use in-hospital moves as an opportunity to train - Train to recognize and resolve in-flight emergencies such as power failure, tubing rupture, pneumothorax, endotracheal tube dislodgement
Team Assembly; Selection of Proficient Members	- Pre-determine team structure - Bring additional trainees on transports - Have a recall roster and keep vacation schedules current - Maintain an active transport team roster updated weekly
Transport Equipment & Supplies	- Service transport equipment regularly - Maintain equipment bags containing cannulae, insertion supplies, surgical instruments, chest tubes, endotracheal tubes, and surgical airway supplies - Work with pharmacy to develop an allowance standard for transport medications - For team activations, bring backup equipment and hand-crank pump heads; bring advanced adjuncts including iNO and high frequency ventilator as indicated
Team travel to referral center	- Use commercial transport for personnel - The circuit can travel separately from the team
Assess blood bank capability	- If patient needs are likely to outstrip in-house blood product availability, bring products from the transport team's home facility
Referral center tasks	- Locate the loading dock in the hospital for use by the transport team if ambulance not equipped with hydraulic lift and the team is using a transport sled - Arrange for transport team police escort from referral center back to flightline - Prepare working space for ECMO team (clear out adjacent areas for equipment in the ICU, place ventilator on patient's left for neck cannulation, code cart and medications at the bedside) - Surgical equipment (cautery, headlamp, instrument table) at bedside and surgical scrub tech available
Mode of patient transportation	- Local (<150 miles)=typically use ground transport - Regional (150-1,000 miles)=helicopter vs. fixed wing - Long-distance (>1,000 miles)=jet transport (this is likely to be an "aircraft of opportunity;" so the specific model will not be known until it arrives)
Check Transport Vehicle	- Door dimensions to ensure sled or stretcher will fit - Determine electrical power capacity of the ambulance - Check ambulance inverter for functionality - Locate the ambulance breaker box
Travel route	- Discuss the route of travel with the ambulance driver or pilot to identify waypoints where the team can stop to perform advanced medical interventions or to address equipment problems

Table 33-3. Representative ECMO cart characteristics.

	Wilford Hall Medical Center	University of Michigan Medical Center	Arkansas Children's Hospital	Hanuola ECMO Program	University Hospital Regensburg, Germany
ECMO Cart	2005 Custom Cart Military Aircraft Approved	<10Kg, Ground: Custom Stretcher >10kg Air: Custom Stretcher: Harrington Board Heli-Dyne Console Box	Ground: Custom Stretcher Fixed wing: Custom Sled	2010 Custom Sled Stryker Power Pro IT Ambulance Cot Lifeport Clipdeck	Standard Adult Stretcher (Stryker or Ferno)
Pump	Stockert Roller Pump	<10Kg Baxter Century Roller Pump >10kg Medtronic Biomedicus 550 Centrifugal	Stockert-Sorin Roller Pump; Maquet Rotaflow; Levitronix Centrimag	Maquet Rotaflow; Levitronix Centrimag	Maquet Rotaflow ELS or Cardiohelp HLS*
Oxygenator	Medtronic or Quadrox D	Medtronic silicone	Avecor, Medtronic; After 2008 Quadrox D	Quadrox D	Quadrox PLS or Integrated Cardiohelp HLS*
Water heater	Cincinnati Subzero ECMO-Heater	Cinncinati Subzero Microtemp	Gaymar Allegiance K-MOD107	Cinncinati Subzero Microtemp	None
SVO2	Terumo CDI 100	< 10kg Oximetrix 3 >10Kg Gish Biomedical Stat-Sat	None	Spectrum M3 Monitor	Integrated Cardiohelp HLS*
Pressure Monitor	DLP Medtronic Stockert S3 System	DLP Medtronic	DLP Medtronic	DLP Medtronic	Integrated Cardiohelp HLS*
Cardio - respiratory monitor	Propaq	<10kg Welch-Allen >10kg Lifepak	GE Dash 3000	Phillips Intellivue MP2 Monitor	Dräger Oxylog 3000
UPS/ Battery	2 Energy Technologies ETI0001-1240	<10kg Cleary On Guard >10Kg none	ATC Smart UPS 1000 or Tripp Lite BC Pro	1 Geo Data System (Part of Back up pack)	None
Ultrasonic Flow Probe	Transonic HT109	Biomedicus 550 system	None	Spectrum M3 Monitor	Integrated Cardiohelp HLS*
IV Pumps	Baxter AS 50 and IVAC Medsystem III DLE	Medfusion 3500	Medfusion 3500; Sigma	B Braun Syringe Pump and IVAC Medsystem III DLE	B Braun Perfusor compact
Ventilator	MVP-10	Carefusion LTV	LTV 1000	LTV 1200	Oxylog 3000
Blender	Custom Air/ O2 Flowmeters	None	None	Terumo Sechrist	None
Air Tank	Q Tank	None	None	E Tank	None
Oxygen Tank	Q Tank	D tank	E Tank	E Tank	O Tank
ACT device	i-Stat 1 Analyzer	Hemochron 401	Hemochron Jr	i-Stat 1 Analyzer	None

*Cardiohelp HLS only available in Europe.

Table 33-4. Representative ECMO transport team characteristics.

	Wilford Hall Medical Center	University of Michigan Medical Center	Arkansas Children's Hospital	Hanuola ECMO Program	University Hospital Regensburg, Germany
Regional	Yes	Yes	Yes	Yes	Yes
Global	Yes	No	No	No	No
Extra-institutional "Taxi Runs"	Yes (26%)	No	Yes (7%) (not routine)	No	No
Ground	38% Custom: Generator, 1200 lb lift	70% Custom: Generator, 800lb lift, 250 gallon fuel tank	12.50%	Yes	Yes Specialized ICU Ambulance
Helicopter	No	20% Bell 230, Bell 430	75% Sikorsky S-76	No	Yes BK-117
Fixed Wing	62% Military Aicraft C-17, C-130	10% Lear Citation 5 jet Cessna Citation Encore	12.5% JetMed Lear Jet	100% Hawker Falcon 50 Gulfstream 3	No
Typical Team Size:	10-15	5-6	4	4-5	3-4
Physician	1 ECMO MD 1 Patient MD	1 ICU Fellow	1 ICU MD	1 ICU MD	1 Anesthesiologist
Nurse	1 ECMO Coordinator 1-2 Patient RN's 1-2 Circuit RN's	2 Flight nurses 2 ECMO Specialists	1 ECMO Coordinator	1	1
Perfusionist	No	No	No	1	1
Respiratory Therapist	1-2	2 ECMO Specialists	No	1	No
Surgeon	1	1-2	1 CT Surgeon 1 Surgical assistant	1	1
Cardiologist	1	No	No	No	No
Other	NICU/PICU Fellow	NA	NA	NA	NA
VA	99%	50%	100%	67%	50%
VV	1%	50%	0	33%	50%
Other	Additional back up of all equipment Total weight 2000 lbs	Use 2 helicopters or jets for extra personnel	NA	Back Up Pack: Geo Data System UPS Rotaflow Hand Crank Levitronix console Battery packs to Braun, LTV, Phillips	NA

(so-called "Taxi Runs"), the Medical Director or Mission Commander must take extra care to speak with the principal physicians at both the referring and receiving facility to ensure that all involved have the most up to date information on the patient's status throughout the entire planning process. In particular, any consideration of circuit changes should include an analysis of the condition of the patient's current circuit, the circuit requirements of the transport system and the anticipated circuit requirements of the receiving facility to ensure that the patient does not needlessly undergo the inherent risks of 2 to 3 circuit changes in a 24 to 48 hour period solely due to unforeseen system incompatibilities or institutional preferences. Furthermore, the Medical Director should ensure that candidacy criteria for the anticipated intervention such as Ventricular Assist Device (VAD) placement or cardiac transplant have been fully discussed and that all efforts to identify potential exclusionary findings (e.g., intracranial hemorrhage) have been completed to avoid a futile transport.

ECMO transport teams range in size from 3 to 15 depending on the length of the transport and the complexity of the transport equipment (Table 33-4).[19,20] The essential members include an ECMO-trained physician experienced in cardiopulmonary resuscitation, a critical care nurse with ECMO experience, and an ECMO specialist to manage the circuit. For vascular access, many teams include a surgeon if the lead ECMO physician is not a surgeon. Most teams perform regional transports for which 3 to 6 person teams supported by helicopter or fixed wing transport suffice. However, long-range transports require larger teams so that personnel can work in shifts to avoid fatigue-related errors.

At the referring center

Once the ECMO transport team assembles, the candidate patient should be evaluated comprehensively to include a thorough bed-side evaluation and review of laboratory and radiographic studies. The referring team should describe any interval changes in the patient's cardiopulmonary function. Based on both the current physiologic status of the patient and the recent trend in these parameters, the ECMO team must decide upon a course of treatment. If advanced maneuvers have not been performed and the patient is not rapidly deteriorating, these can be instituted and the patient observed.

If rescue maneuvers have failed or if the patient is rapidly declining and otherwise meets criteria for initiation of ECMO, the patient should be cannulated without delay. Likewise, the transport ECMO mindset requires recognition that some critically ill patients who would have undergone further observation prior to cannulation in an ECMO center, may need to be placed on ECMO at an earlier time-point in their clinical course as the only means of safe transport to definitive care. Once a decision has been made, the transport team should meet the patient's family to describe the transport plan and to obtain informed consent for transport and for the initiation of ECMO, as required.

If the patient meets criteria for ECMO, the transport team must decide the mode of ECMO. Historically, the WHMC team preferentially performed VA ECMO for all transports given the difficulty in converting a patient from VV to VA support during transport.[3,20] However, other teams report placing patients on the mode they would normally have selected based on the patient's underlying physiologic derangement if the patient were in their home ECMO center.[19,30,31]

Some teams have also described the use of PECLA as an alternative to ECMO for transport.[5,32-34] Based on an AV shunt through a gas exchange membrane, PECLA is both conceptually and logistically straightforward. It has no moving parts and no power requirement. However, it does require arterial cannulation, the patient must have sufficient cardiac output to perfuse the membrane, and it affords only modest improvements in oxygenation due to the relatively low flow rates through the membrane. However, because of the membrane's efficient CO_2 handling properties, the ideal patient candidate for PECLA is the head injured patient with intractable hypercarbia.[35] Given these considerations, we believe PECLA has an important role in transport but that it is best used by ECMO-capable teams.

Once the ECMO transport team performs an advanced rescue maneuver or initiates ECMO, the patient should be observed for a period of time to ensure stability prior to transport. During this time, the patient's ventilator can be adjusted to transport settings, vasopressor and medication infusions converted to the transport pumps, and the patient moved to the transport stretcher or sled. If the patient has any intracavitary air such as a pneumothorax, or the transport plan should be revised (e.g., use ground transport for a patient with intraocular air). The transport team should evaluate all tubes, lines, and drains for proper placement, functionality, and security. Deep sedation is strongly recommended, and chemical paralysis with adequate analgesia and anxiolysis should be considered. The team should refill its supply of oxygen, ensure full battery charge on all equipment, and reload all medication infusions for transport. The Medical Director or Mission Commander has the final authority over the final transport plan (ground vs. helicopter vs. fixed wing) based on patient factors and transport vehicle availability. Prior to departure, this individual should update the receiving ECMO center of the patient's status and potential need for additional diagnostic studies or interventions on arrival.

In transport

The most important considerations for the actual transport include patient movement to and from the transport vehicle, the effects of altitude on membrane gas exchange for air transports, and the recognition and management of in-transport emergencies. Mishaps during patient movement represent the most obvious additional risk attending medical transportation. The military transport community has successfully minimized transport-related complications such as tube dislodgment, patient falls, or equipment failure through the attentiveness of an experienced support staff which rehearses patient transfers. For the average litter-borne, mechanically ventilated patient there are typically 4 to 6 non-medical staff that physically haul the patient to and from the aircraft cabin or ambulance and 2 to 3 aeromedical support crew who watch for obstacles or possible gear and tubing hang-ups. Meanwhile the 3-person CCATT continues to monitor the patient's status.[36] Other teams have minimized these patient transfers during air transport missions by simply driving the transport ground vehicle onto the transport aircraft.[31,37] Another vulnerable time in transport is the power and gas source transfer from the transport vehicle to the mobile sled, transport platform, or stretcher. Because this transfer must be perfectly synchronized, we strongly recommend a team "time-out" with verbal rehearsal to ensure that everyone is clear on their role prior to the transfer. This practice prevents any interruption in oxygen supply and blood flow support to the patient.

Effects of altitude on membrane gas exchange

Because the gas exchange capacity of the membrane declines with the reduction in atmospheric pressure, transport teams initially restricted cabin altitude to "field level."[38] This adds a significant logistical burden to the mission and is no longer felt to be required given the high efficiency of modern gas exchange membranes. At an altitude of 6900 ft (2300 m) an oxygenator supplied with an FiO_2 of 1 has the same capacity as with an FiO_2 of 0.8 at sea level. When using an unpressurized helicopter below 5000 ft, the reduced atmospheric pressure typically leads to a saturation drop of 3-4% on pulse oximetry.[19] For fixed-wing air transports, the WHMC neonatal and pediatric team uses a 5000 ft (1524 m) cabin altitude restriction.[20] For adult VV ECMO transport, the standard cabin altitude of 8000 ft has been used more recently without complication. During air transport, acceleration and deceleration forces do not typically substantially alter venous return or cause other problems with the circuit during takeoff and landing. However, the circuit and patient must be well secured to the aircraft and watched carefully during takeoff and landing to avoid any inadvertent shift in cannula position or kinking of the circuit.

Recognition and management of in-transport emergencies

The most common in-transport emergencies result from tube dislodgement (endotracheal tube or tube thoracostomy) or equipment malfunction. Although reports of these events are rare during ECMO transport,[16,37] their occurrence can be catastrophic. Early recognition of these mechanical problems or troubleshooting the etiology of a sudden change in the patient's status can be especially challenging in the transport environment given the low lighting, significant noise, and limited access to the patient. Team training around common emergency scenarios and a systematic approach to troubleshooting physiologic problems can greatly reduce the rate of major and minor complications.[25] The most widely recognized in-transport complications are summarized in Table 33-5 with recommendations for both prevention and resolution of each. For patients on ECMO, each intervention to resolve a complication can escalate the morbidity to the patient significantly. Pericardiocentesis, tube thoracostomy placement, or even reintubation can result in life-threatening hemorrhage; so when considering an intervention, transport teams should take an extra measure of caution

to ensure the solution is not more risky than the original problem.

At the ECMO center

Upon arrival of the transport team to the receiving ECMO center, the ECMO transport team meets with the ICU team and reviews the patient's history, in-flight events, and current condition. Transport equipment is disassembled, and the ECMO circuit evaluated for compatibility. If the transport team originated from the receiving center, compatibility should not be a problem. However, in the case of a Taxi Run by the transport team, this consideration becomes much more important. If a complete circuit switch out is required, both the Transport Medical Director and the receiving ECMO physician should be present to minimize the time "off-pump" as much as possible. Once again a "time-out" protocol is advised including a recap of each person's role and a physical practice walk-through of the circuit transfer maneuver in advance. In our experience this practice facilitates a smooth transfer particularly in the setting of unfamiliar circuit layouts and alternate circuit components used by other facilities. The transport team typically hands over responsibility of the patient to the receiving team once the patient has been reestablished on ECMO and stabilized.

Military ECMO transport and lessons from combat casualty care

The US Air Force has offered transport ECMO to military beneficiaries and civilian neonates since November 1985 through its program at WHMC.[3,14,20,38] In 1993, the program was expanded to also include pediatric patients, and to date, our team has performed a total of 76 transports over distances of up to 7,500 miles. WHMC is the only program capable of global ECMO transport due to its utilization of US Air Force aircraft such as the C-17 and C-130 which can refuel in-flight. Due to the extensive

Table 33-5. Widely recognized in-transport emergencies and the recommended prevention or resolution.

Complication	Prevention/Resolution
Airway	
Endotracheal Tube Kinking/Dislodgement	Prevention: Re-secure airway prior to transport; assign a team member to monitor airway position. Resolution: Continue ECMO; controlled re-intubation; if the patient remains well oxygenated with little air hunger, consider leaving extubated vs. surgical airway if initial attempts fail
Breathing	
Delayed pneumothorax	Prevention: Carefully review pre-flight radiographs. Resolution: Tube thoracostomy insertion (Note: for the hypoxic/hypotensive patient on ECMO during transport, first perform a complete circuit check, increase flow and sweep gas rate, and observe before considering needle decompression or chest tube placement.)
Chest tube dislodgement	Prevention: Check tube position and anchor prior to departure; assign a team member to monitor tubes during movement. Resolution: Replace chest tube
Ventilator malfunction	Resolution: Backup ventilator; increase ECMO flow
Oxygen supply exhaustion	Prevention: Assign this pre-transport check to multiple team members and put on a pre-launch checklist. Resolution: Rapidly proceed to the nearest waypoint to re-supply.
Circulation	
ECMO tubing rupture	Preparation: Have tubing rupture kit available Resolution: Clamp and replace the tubing section; re-initiate ECMO
Partial cannula dislodgment	Prevention: Use multiple anchoring sutures; Transparent dressing; Medical Director hold the cannula during movement Resolution: If the side holes are out of the vessel, remove and rapidly proceed to the nearest waypoint to re-initiate ECMO.
Pericardial tamponade	Prevention: For single site R IJ cannula insertion, consider fluoroscopic wire positioning and using a Rosen wire (relatively stiff with a J-tip) Resolution: Diagnose with FAST; pericardiocentesis and proceed to the nearest waypoint. (Note: for the hypotensive patient on ECMO during transport, first perform a complete circuit check, increase flow and sweep gas rate, and observe before considering pericardiocentesis)
Battery failure	Prevention: Ensure maximal charge on all components prior to departure; assign this pre-transport check to multiple team members and put on a pre-launch checklist or "time out." Consider bringing additional battery packs or a backup power source. Resolution: Rapidly proceed to the nearest waypoint to re-supply.

range of its travel, the WHMC program is also currently the only program routinely capable of Taxi Runs. These missions have typically been used to move patients to specialty centers for placement of a VAD or organ transplantation although this capability could also be employed during times of national crisis to match patients in need of ECMO with centers who have available ECMO beds.

In recent years, another role for a military ECMO-capable team has been recognized: the transport of combat casualties with severe respiratory insufficiency.[39] A recent review of the combat casualty registry from Operations Iraqi and Enduring Freedom found that up to 6.6% of deaths among intubated combat casualties are in patients with ARDS and that ARDS is an independent predictor of mortality in this population.[40] This section describes the development of the military ALIRT which transports combat casualties with severe ARDS and the expansion of this team's capabilities to include ECMO is also being added to the WHMC team.

From AE to ALIRT

The basic aeromedical evacuation (AE) team is comprised of a nurse and a medical technician support staff. Each AE team can safely convey more than 20 stable patients per flight. If one or more critically ill patient(s) is assigned to a scheduled flight the AE team then configures the aircraft for an additional three person CCATT which consists of a critical care-experienced physician, a critical care nurse, and a respiratory therapist.[6,36,41] The CCATT is stocked with critical care medications (typically a three day supply), 2-4 Univent 754 ventilators (Impact Instrumentation, Inc., West Caldwell, NJ), and multiple intravenous infusion and suction pumps which allow them to care for up to 4 mechanically ventilated patients. Since their implementation in 1994, these teams have continued the care of critically ill combat casualties in their evacuation from overflowing

combat support hospitals to the next echelon in the military evacuation chain.[4]

This concept has flourished during the conflicts in Iraq and Afghanistan with a trend now towards moving not only the "stable" but also the "stabilizing" casualty. CCATT became adept at continuing the care of patients with extensive burns, elevated intracranial pressure, acute respiratory distress syndrome (ARDS), sepsis, cardiac failure, and post-combat trauma hemorrhagic shock. This was accomplished by the widespread adoption of the Acute Respiratory Distress Syndrome Network (ARDSnet) ventilator algorithm, US Army Institute of Surgical Research (USAISR) burn and blood product ratio protocols, and standardized intracranial pressure management algorithms. CCATT has, in essence, become an extension of the ICU resuscitation phase of combat casualty care.

In some cases, a CCATT's ability to safely transport patients has been constrained by the capabilities of their flight-approved ventilator. For instance, the Univent 754 ventilator has a 60 liter per minute (Lpm) flow capacity which is insufficient in the young, healthy male who typically demands flows in excess of 80 Lpm. In these cases, dys-syncrhoncy can develop leading to precipitous hypoxia and increased doses of sedative-analgesic agents which can exacerbate hemodynamic instability. Similarly, many portable ventilators have a very limited I:E ratio inversion range and lack the servo-controlled expiratory valves required for modes such as airway pressure release ventilation. In some cases, the ventilator needs of patients with severe ARDS precluded their evacuation from burdened or embattled combat support hospitals. In response, in 2005, after returning from their respective deployments several trauma surgeons, intensivists, and CCATT members created an aeromedical team specifically suited to care for these patients: the Acute Lung Injury Response Team (ALIRT).[5,42,43] As of February 2011, this team has successfully transported

29 patients whose critical care support requirements exceeded regular CCATT capabilities.

Adding adult ECMO to military transport teams

Over time, formal criteria were adopted and published to inform all deployed medical services of the indications, manning, and capabilities of the ALIRT service. Each ALIRT consists of a pulmonary-critical physician, a trauma surgeon, two critical care nurses, and two respiratory therapists from the LRMC staff who augment the basic AE + CCATT transport teams when activated. ARDS-specialized clinician experience combined with high frequency percussive ventilation, nebulized prostacyclin, intra-tracheal calfactant, standardized albumin-furosemide infusions, prone positioning, PECLA, and VV ECMO used individually or in combination expanded the gamut of ARDS severity which could be safely evacuated from the combat theater.

Use of high frequency percussive ventilation (HFPV) via the flight approved VDR4 (Percussionaire Corporation, Sandpoint, Idaho) allows for a higher level of respiratory support than other transport and even conventional ventilators.[44] The incidence of ARDS in military trauma casualties approaches 25%, due to the ARDS inducing pentad of blast, contusion, aspiration, massive transfusion, and polytrauma. HFPV is effective in the majority of cases, but the higher pressures and volumes necessary do not help the underlying lung injury. Additionally, proper use of HFPV in transport is arguably more complex and difficult than use of VV ECMO. Extensive experience with HFPV in flight exists among only a few individuals of the ISR's Burn Team and the ALIRT. Respiratory failure refractory even to HFPV and the desire to deliver the highest level of lung protective therapy demonstrated the need for extracorporeal therapies.

Subsequently, this need to augment therapy for respiratory failure using pump-driven extracorporeal support and LRMC's geographic proximity to one of the leaders in ECMO transport, the University Hospital at Regensburg, led to a close collaboration between the two centers. At the time, Regensburg's team had successfully transported over 60 patients on VV or VA ECMO as well as PECLA-dependent combat casualties transported from the theater of operations.[19,34,45] With ECMO training and mentorship provided by the Regensburg team and the acquisition of state of the art equipment, the ALIRT has now added ECMO to its armamentarium.

As of February 2011, the ALIRT has successfully transported patients long distances using PECLA and VV ECMO.[46] Similar to the experience of the team from Karolinska University in Sweden, the US military experience illustrates that adults can be transported safely over great distances. Evacuation of a young soldier on VV ECMO from Kandahar, Afghanistan, to Germany was completed successfully in October 2010. A member from the Lung Team in Germany now stationed at Tripler Army Medical Center in Hawaii collaborated with the Hanuola ECMO program in Hawaii to complete the longest recorded adult VV ECMO transport in November of 2010. A Gulf Stream III equipped for medical transport was able to fly directly from Honolulu to an ECMO center of excellence at the University of Iowa, a distance of 4,052 miles or 6,519 km. The patient was transferred without incident to Iowa City after six days of VV ECMO in Hawaii when it became evident that a longer course of ECMO treatment was necessary at a more experienced center. Advances in technology and critical care medicine have allowed ECMO to develop as a successful therapy in selected adults. As more evidence accumulates about the benefits of ECMO in adults and more ECMO centers arise, safe transportation over short and long distances to centers of excellence will become increasingly important.

The WHMC team simultaneously recognized the need to provide ECMO transport for combat casualties on ECMO at LRMC who need to return to the US and for civilian adults who are identified as ECMO candidates outside the relatively few adult ECMO centers across the US. We have been able to leverage our significant historic transport ECMO experience and rich research collaborations with the University of Michigan and clinical collaboration with Maryland Shock Trauma to develop the adult Critical-care Resuscitation And Support (CRASh) team at the new San Antonio Military Medical Center (SAMMC). This team has robust multidisciplinary support and sufficient funding for initial equipment and training expenses to permit a formal launch shortly after the publication of this book.

Results of inter-hospital transport

Although WHMC, UMMC, and ACH remain the major ECMO transport centers in the US, as many as 23 ECMO centers worldwide have had inter-facility ECMO experience on a limited basis in recent years.[47] Among these centers, the survival to discharge rate ranges from 56% to 66% which is comparable to age and disease-matched non-transport ECMO cases for each facility and the ELSO Registry (Table 33-6).[16,20,48] As is the case with in-house ECMO, cardiac cases tend to have a lower survival to discharge (35% -46%) than respiratory cases (60-80%).

Initially ACH reported a low survival of their extra-institutional Taxi Runs and no longer routinely performs them; however, the Taxi Runs performed by WHMC provide an interesting insight into the changing demographics of transport ECMO. A growing subset of transport ECMO cases are patients on ECMO at ECMO centers as a bridge to cardiac repair, VAD, or heart transplant. Since 2006 77% of extra-

institutional ECMO cases performed by WHMC have been for pediatric cardiac cases with an 87% survival to discharge. Of the eight pediatric cardiac extra-institutional transports, all three that used ECMO as a bridge to congenital heart disease repair underwent successful repair for Tetrology of Fallot, Total AV Canal and Transposition of the Great Vessels, respectively. Of the remaining five pediatric cardiac extra-institutional transports three had spontaneous recovery from myocarditis including a seven year-old ECPR case who underwent over 60 minutes of CPR, one underwent successful VAD and transplant for myocarditis, and one died following a failed valve replacement attempt after MI secondary to Anomolous Left Coronary from the Pulmonary Artery (ALCAPA).[49]

As described above, ECMO transport team dispatches do not always result in ECMO cannulation. In some cases, the patient's condition improves prior to arrival of the transport team while in others, advanced rescue maneuvers by the transport team stabilize the patient and permit transport without ECMO. Since 2006, 4 of 21 (19%) dispatches of the WHMC ECMO transport team did not require ECMO. Two patients (10%) improved after pulmonary management by the ECMO team on site at the referral center and were transported using high-frequency ventilation (Bronchotron, Percussionaire Corp., Sandpoint, Idaho) and iNO. Both patients subsequently recovered completely without ever requiring ECMO. The other two patients improved at the referral facility following a management strategy developed in consultation with the ECMO Transport Medical Director while the ECMO transport team was en route.[49] Similar cases have been reported by UMMC and ACH where 7% and 6% of their respective dispatches did not result in ECMO transport.[47,48] Both centers also report that although they have not had any in-transport deaths, 5% of ECMO patients for which a transport team was dispatched expired prior to arrival of the transport team or during

Table 33-6. Cumulative ECMO transport experience.

ECMO Center	Year Founded	Patient Category	n	Survival to Discharge (%)
Wilford Hall Medical Center	1985	Neonatal Respiratory	41	66
		Pediatric Respiratory	10	60
		Cardiac *	5	40
		Taxi Runs ^	20	75
		Total	**76**	**66**
Arkansas Children's Hospital	1990	Neonatal Respiratory	35	80
		Pediatric Respiratory #	21	62
		Cardiac #	48	42
		Taxi Runs†	8	14
		Total	**112**	**56**
University of Michigan	1990	Neonatal Respiratory	4	100
		Pediatric Respiratory	51	80
		Cardiac	31	35
		Adult Respiratory	117	64
		Total	**203**	**65**

*Pediatric cases only; #pediatric and adult cases; ^3 neonatal respiratory, 2 pediatric respiratory, 15 cardiac; †1 lost to follow-up

Table 33-7. International ECMO transport reports.

ECMO Center	ECMO Transport Reports	Patient Category	n	Survival to Discharge (%)
Oslo Universitetshospital-Rikshospitalet, Oslo, Norway	1992-2008			
		Neonatal Respiratory	8	
		Pediatric Respiratory	3	
		Pediatric Cardiac	1	
		Adult Respiratory	8	
		Adult Cardiac	3	
		Total	**23**	**67**
The Karolinska University Hospital, Stockholm, Sweden*	1996-2009			
		Neonatal Respiratory	91	91
		Pediatric Respiratory	41	76
		Adult Respiratory	104	67
		Total	**236**	**78**
National Taiwan University Hospital, Taipei,Taiwan	1998-2004			
		Adult Cardiac	31	32
		Total	**31**	**32**
University Hospital Regensburg, Regensburg, Germany	2000-2009	Adult Respiratory (Interventional Lung Assist)	20	45
		Adult Respiratory	9	44
		Adult Cardiac	9	56
		Total	**38**	**47**
Royal Children's Hospital, Melbourne, Australia	2003-2007#			
		Neonatal Respiratory	2	100
		Pediatric Respiratory	3	0
		Neonatal Cardiac	1	100
		Pediatric Cardiac	2	100
		Total	**8**	**63**

*An additional 36 patients were transported to other centers.
#As of 2012 doing an average of 3-5 per year usually several hundred kilometers at a time

assessment of the patient by the team. This represents a residual although greatly improved "hidden mortality" associated with ECMO referral Furthermore, many of these patients had already been placed on ECMO by the referring center. Thus as transport ECMO has become more prevalent, the mortality associated with ECMO referral has become less a consequence of ECMO non-availability and inherent delays, and more a result of the disease process itself.

A number of international centers have reported transport ECMO experience as well (Table 33-7). The largest reported experiences to date include 33 ECMO transports over 9 years by the team from Regensburg, Germany;[19] 31 ECMO transports over 6 ½ years by the team from National Taiwan University Hospital, Taipei, Taiwan;[50] 23 ECMO transports over 16 years by the team from Oslo Universitetshospital-Rikshospitalet, Norway;[31] and the largest series of 272 ECMO transports from 1996-2009 by the team from the Karolinska University Hopital, Stockholm, Sweden, which is greatly expanded from their original report of 30 transports as of 2001.[37,51] Smaller series and case reports have been published by the team from Berlin, Germany;[22] Melbourne, Australia;[30,52] and Glenfield Hospital, Leicester, United Kingdom.[53] All centers report that ECMO transport is safe and feasible, with survival of ECLS and survival to discharge rates comparable to those of non-transport ECMO cases.

Intra-hospital transport

Patients on ECMO may require transport within the hospital for diagnostic or therapeutic procedures. Depending on the patient population, the need for one or more such transports varies significantly from 8% of ECMO patients in a pediatric cardiac ICU to 48% in a mixed ECMO population.[54,55] These patient moves impose a significant risk which must be weighed against the potential benefits of the planned study or intervention. The previously

discussed principles required for safe, effective inter-hospital transport are also essential to intra-hospital transport. In general, a significant degree of provider preparation and experience is required to be proficient in the recognition and management of mechanical complications or patient emergencies during these excursions. Consequently, these moves should be performed by an expert multidisciplinary team which has rehearsed the transport sequence and the intended route. A checklist can facilitate preparation by prompting the assignment of specific tasks to team members and by spelling out the required supplies such as emergency "jump bags," pharmacy kits, and blood products. The following section describes these steps in further detail along with the published experience of centers that use this type of approach to safely transport ECMO patients throughout the hospital.

ACH has published an in-depth review of 57 intra-hospital transport procedures performed over a 10 year period for children on ECMO in their institution.[54] The authors sub-divide these transports into three phases: preparatory, transfer, and post-transport stabilization. During the preparatory phase, the timeline of the procedure should be outlined, with the recommendation to build in a minimum of 30 minutes for transport equipment and supply acquisition, up to 30 minutes of travel time en route to the destination, anticipated procedure time, and return travel time. In this review, median travel times away from the ICU for interventional catheterizations (most commonly blade and balloon atrial septostomy), diagnostic catheterizations, and head CT were 158, 119, and 40 minutes, respectively.

During the preparatory phase, an institutional specific checklist should be used to ensure sedation, muscle relaxation, transport cardiorespiratory monitors, ACT or blood gas device, backup battery, gas supply, blood products, blankets for thermoregulation, the patient's chart, emergency drug code box, and resuscitation cart are available and packaged to be mobilized with the transport team

Figure 33-8. Hanuola ECMO Program of Hawaii checklist for intra-hospital transport.

Hanuola Intra-Hospital Transport Checklist

TRANSPORT PREPARATION

ECMO Physician
- Confirm need for ECMO transport with 2 ECMO physicians
- Notify ECMO Medical Director and ECMO Coordinator
- Notify parents of transport
- Call radiology to arrange time for study -- aim for low volume time of day
- Order appropriate sedation, vasopressors, blood products
- Discontinue non-essential infusions

ECMO Coordinator
- Assign ECMO transport team: ECMO coordinator; ECMO attending physician; bedside ICU nurse (RN); perfusionists (CCP) x2; respiratory therapists (RT) x2
- Assign en route roles (see table) and review transport schematic with team
- Have RN, RT, CCP acquire and inventory specialty specific ECMO Jump bags
- Notify blood bank, and ensure bedside blood product cooler is adequately re-stocked
- Call security to cordon off back hallway and secure back service elevator during transport
- Call housekeeping to clean service elevator before and after transport
- Ensure back up battery (UPS) is available
- Ensure power supply extension cords are available at destination
- Ensure code card/defibrillator available at destination site
- Place imaging approved transport board under patient if >10kg

RN
- Transfer patient cardiorespiratory cables to transport monitor
- Assess and secure all tubes and lines
- Secure all ancillary devices (Pleur-evac, foley) to ICU bed
- Place chest tube to water seal or portable suction.
- Discontinue non-essential infusions (e.g. lipids) per physician orders
- Ensure vasopressor(s) spiked and hung for emergency access
- Consolidate all IV pumps onto one mobile IV pole
- Identify and isolate a dedicated IV lumen to push code medications or volume to patient if needed for possible circuit emergency. Add extenders to ensure adequate IV tubing length is available to reach site while in CT
- Place patient chart and flowsheets for charting
- Bring blankets for thermoregulation
- RN Jump Bag: 30 mL pre-filled syringes (1 unit PRBC, 1 unit FFP, saline); sedation & muscle relaxant (x3 doses); epinephrine, CaCl, NaHCO3 (x3 doses); empty syringes, alcohol pads, flush solutions

RT
- Place full E-cylinder of O_2 in the HL-20 tank holder or bring a tank roller with full E-cylinders of air and O_2
- Add length of high pressure gas tubing to reach the wall source at the destination
- Place full E-cylinder of O_2 on the patient bed
- Ensure ETT secured
- Set up manual ventilation source (anesthesia bag, self-inflating bag, or Neopuff)
- Set up ventilator at destination site and have settings adjusted (leave in Standby mode)
- RT Jump Bag: flow meters and quick connect styles for universal compatibility

CCP
- Turn water heater off but leave in place on HL-20 cart
- Disconnect bubble detector from circuit if needed to free up circuit tubing length. Reposition support clamp
- Pre-position Rotaflow handcrank to maintain optimal access while in transit and in elevator configuration
- Bring ECMO flowsheets for charting
- CCP Jump Bag: mini circuit rupture kit (6 circuit clamps, 1 sterile scissors, sterile gloves, 2 60 mL syringes for de-airing, 2 60 mL syringes with sterile saline for volume, 2 stopcocks, 2 (1/4 x ¼ or 3/8 x3/8) circuit connectors, 6 ChloraPrep® swabs); i-STAT® module; 6 i-STAT® ACT cartridges; 6 3 mL syringes; 6 needle-less injection tips; 6 ChloraPrep® swabs

AT RADIOLOGY OR CT SUITE

- Enter room head first (circuit on patient's right)
- Drop CT scanner stretcher to match inpatient bed height
- ECMO MD coordinates verbal time out for lateral pull from inpatient bed to scanner stretcher.
- Move empty patient bed to hall
- Plug all equipment into wall AC power (HL-20 base, water heater, transonic, monitor)
- Connect to wall gas and oxygen source, turn off tanks and recheck PSI
- Connect patient to ventilator.
- Turn on water heater
- Reassess temperature
- Do slow walk through of full range of motion through scanner to ensure circuit length / HL-20 position is appropriate before imaging starts.
- CCP and ECMO MD wear led aprons and remain in room with patient during testing to monitor pump and circuit
- Continue ACT's per usual protocol

AFTER RETURN TO UNIT

- Plug all equipment into wall AC power (HL-20 base, water heater, transonic)
- Connect to wall gas and oxygen source
- Connect patient to ventilator.
- Turn on water heater
- Confirm bubble detector is connected and turned on
- Reassess temperature.
- Obtain CXR for ETT and cannula position if clinically indicated
- Get CBC, Coags, ACT, Circuit and patient ABG if clinically indicated

(Table 33-8). The Hanuola ECMO Program of Hawaii has found it helpful during the preparatory phase to prepackage perfusion, respiratory therapist, and nursing related "jump bags" and streamline all auxiliary support devices. During this phase, team member assignments and circuit preparation are completed. The makeup of the transport team will be based on institutional experience and protocol. Larger volume ECMO centers such as ACH with a higher frequency of IHT performed on a regular basis recommend a minimum 4 person team (ECMO specialist, ECMO coordinator, bedside ICU nurse, and attending physician). On the other hand, centers with only a few IHT procedures annually such as the Hanuola ECMO program of Hawaii have found benefit from a slightly larger team for additional backup (two perfusionists, bedside ICU nurse, ECMO coordinator, two respiratory

therapists, and an ECMO attending physician).[54] The team member task assignments are detailed in Table 33-9.

Circuit preparation is then completed. Although some centers transfer the patient to a dedicated transport cart, many centers simply streamline the existing circuit as much as possible to minimize the risk of mechanical problems (e.g., fracturing the water heater connections off of the membrane). The Hanuola program transports the patient remaining on their original ICU bed or infant warmer along with the ECMO circuit (Rotaflow pump, Quadrox D oxygenator) mounted on the Maquet HL-20 PerfusionSystem (Maquet, Wayne, NJ). The water heater is turned off due to lack of internal battery power but is left in place to be restarted at the IHT destination site. The Rotaflow remains servo regulated through the HL20 system

Table 33-9. Hanuola ECMO Program of Hawaii intra-hospital transport team roles and responsibilities.

Transport Team Member	Intra-hospital Transport Responsibilities
ECMO Physician	Manage the patient and circuit during transport; perform "time out" and call out movement commands for transfer of patient off and back on hospital bed
ECMO Coordinator	Assign ECMO transport team, review transport roles and en-route positioning schematic; notify blood bank; place imaging approved transport board under patient (if > 10kg); clear transport hallways and place elevators on standby; monitor power and gas supply transitions
Bedside Nurse	Eliminate unnecessary infusions with MD direction; consolidate remaining infusions to a single IV pole prior to transport; prepare all transport medications including ACLS/PALS medications, muscle relaxants, and sedatives; ensure blood products available; administer medications as necessary; push infusion pump IV pole
Respiratory Therapist 1	Ensure circuit and patient E tanks are full; bring additional pressurized gas tubing and all quick connects/flow meter styles; travel with patient to secure the airway and gently hand ventilate the patient
Respiratory Therapist 2	Pre-positioned at destination with a ventilator on standby
Perfusionist 1	Prepare the circuit for transport; monitor circuit function during transport; carry circuit rupture kit
Perfusionist 2	Serve as "bridge" between the patient and circuit during transport by manually holding the tubing near the patient and regulating tension on the tubing (alternatively done by ECMO coordinator); assist Perfusionist 1 with circuit emergencies

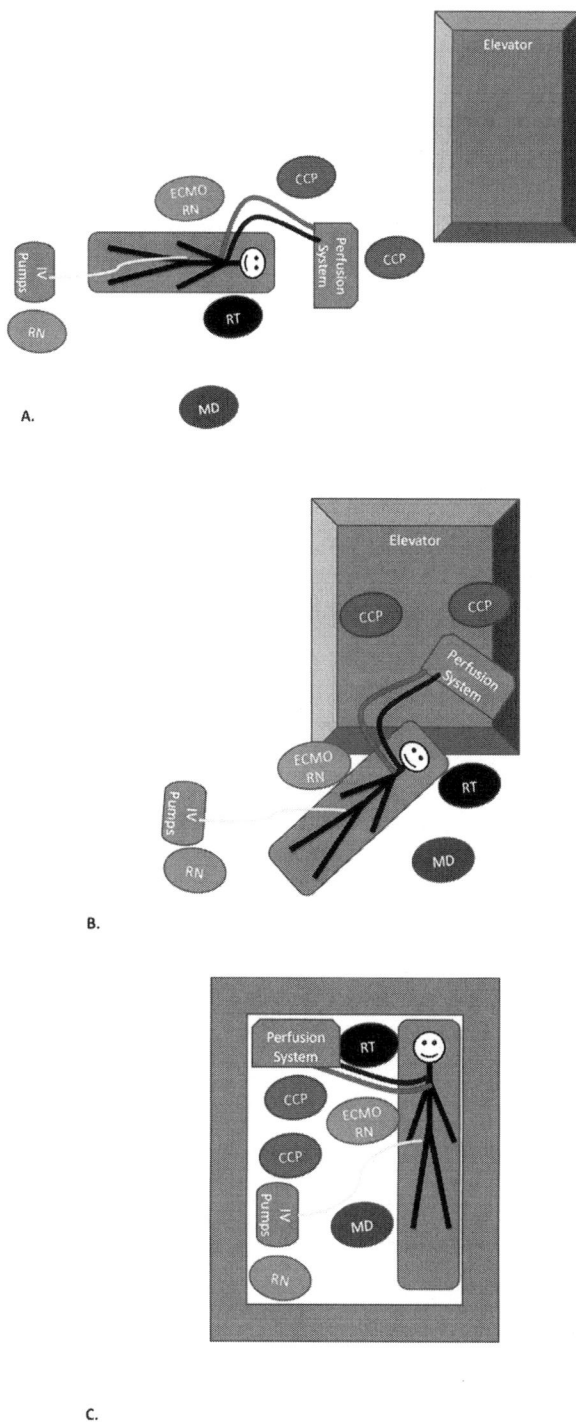

Figure 33-7. Hanuola ECMO Program of Hawaii schematic for intra-hospital transport. A.) Configuration for hallway travel. B.) Configuration of elevator entry. C). Configuration inside elevator.

which remains powered by its internal battery. If necessary, the bubble detector is disconnected to minimize the perfusion system footprint and to allow additional slack in the ECMO circuit to attain the greatest range of patient mobility. The Hanuola circuit tubing is 75 inches long from the venous cannula connection site to the first immobile site at the pump inflow, and 70 inches long from the arterial cannula connection site to the first immobile site at the membrane. These dimensions have allowed adequate mobility to transfer neonates up to large adult sized patients from the hospital bed to the CT scanner stretcher without circuit disruption. In addition to circuit preparation, the transport team also prepares the patient by discontinuing all non-essential infusions and then consolidating all the remaining infusions such as sedation and vasopressors onto one IV pole.

Once the ECMO coordinator ensures the planned route is cleared and the elevators secured, the team proceeds to the destination. Hanuola has found that it has been helpful to create a schematic to illustrate the required positioning of all personnel and equipment for optimal medical management and logistical maneuvering both while in motion and in the elevator or CT suite with minimal space (Figure 33-7). At the destination, power to the water heater and pump as well as institutional gas supply to the oxygenator are immediately reestablished to avoid complications of inadvertent battery and equipment failure. During the post-transport stabilization phase, the transport is completed in reverse to ensure a safe return to the ICU. In addition, a new baseline should be established with a complete circuit check, verification of cannula position with x-ray or ultrasound, and a new set of labs to include blood gas analysis, CBC, electrolytes, ACT, coagulation profile.

Multiple centers report that with such a systematic approach, these transports can be performed safely with the diagnostic studies and therapeutic interventions practice significantly altering the course of clinical care for the patient. The Karolinska team has reported successful intra-hospital transport in 63 of 131 ECMO patients (48%) for a total of 118 chest and abdominal CT scans.[55] A mobile ECMO system was used with 100 cm of additional tubing length. Of the 118 studies, 30 (25%) revealed significant complications that prompted 26 interventions. Total time out of the ICU was typically less than 60 minutes. In another study, ACH reported that intra-hospital transport for diagnostic catheterization resulted in a management change in 70% of the patients.[54] Diagnostic capability of bedside echocardiography was limited in 59% of these patients, particularly in patients with branch pulmonary artery and systemic-to-pulmonary artery shunt abnormalities. All patients who underwent transport for interventional catheterization received the intervention indicated by the findings on diagnostic catheterization including blade and balloon atrial septostomy, cardiac biopsy, radiofrequency ablation, and aortic valvotomy. Of the patients who underwent transport for a head CT because of a significant change in neurologic status, 88% had significant intracranial pathology which frequently resulted in withdrawal of life support. Thus IHT like inter-hospital transport has proven to be safe and feasible in the hands of experienced and highly trained personnel with diagnostic and therapeutic benefits in targeted clinical scenarios that outweigh the inherent risks of transport.

Conclusions

Originally developed to limit mortality in patients referred for ECMO and to transport military dependents with severe cardiopulmonary failure, transport ECMO teams and their equipment have evolved significantly over the past 25 years. Outcomes from the three principal US transport teams and a growing number of international teams demonstrate that transport ECMO can be safely and effectively applied in a variety of healthcare settings and that the hidden mortality of ECMO has been greatly reduced. These results stem from the careful attention to a number of details ranging from team training to the power capacity of the transport ambulance by a handful of Transport Medical Directors and their cadre of dedicated staff. As the demand for ECMO increases, existing ECMO transport teams should lend their expertise to the growing field of transit care medicine and work to train new teams as recently demonstrated by the collaboration between the transport team from University Hospital Regensburg and the US military ALIRT.

Disclaimer

The opinions contained in this chapter are solely the authors' private ones and are not to be construed as official or reflecting the views of the United States Air Force, the United States Army, or the Department of Defense. The authors received no financial support for this work.

Acknowledgment

The authors would like to thank the members of the Wilford Hall Medical Center transport team for their help in conducting transport cases from 2006-present including LtCol Dan Dirnberger, MD, ECMO Co-Director, Ms. Cheryl Collicott, ECMO Coordinator, RN, and Capt Terry Bailey, RN, ECMO Coordinator; staff from Arkansas Children's Hospital including Katherine C. Clement, MD and Richard Fiser, MD, ECMO Medical Director, for sharing their pre-publication and transport data; and the staff from University of Michigan Medical Center for their mentorship in expanding the Wilford Hall Medical Center transport capabilities to include adult patients and William Copenhaver, RN, BSN, ECMO Specialist, and Paula Baldridge, RN, ECMO Program Manager, for sharing their personal observations on ECMO transport and their transport team data.

References

1. Arlt M, Philipp A, Voelkel S, et al. Extracorporeal membrane oxygenation in severe trauma patients with bleeding shock. Resuscitation. 2010; 81:804-809.
2. Peek GJ, Mugford M, Tiruvoipati R, et al. Efficacy and economic assessment of conventional ventilatory support versus extracorporeal membrane oxygenation for severe adult respiratory failure (CESAR): a multicentre randomised controlled trial. Lancet. 2009;374:1351-1363.
3. DiGeronimo RJ, Henderson CL, Grubb PH. Referral and transport of ECMO patients. In: Van Meurs K, Lally KP, Peek G, Zwischenberger JB, eds. ECMO: Extracorporeal cardiopulmonary support in critical care. 3rd ed. Ann Arbor, MI: Extracorporeal Life Support Organization; 2005:157-172.
4. Grissom TE, Farmer JC. The provision of sophisticated critical care beyond the hospital: lessons from physiology and military experiences that apply to civil disaster medical response. Crit Care Med. 2005;33:S13-21.
5. Dorlac GR, Fang R, Pruitt VM, et al. Air transport of patients with severe lung injury: development and utilization of the Acute Lung Rescue Team. J Trauma. 2009;66:S164-171.
6. Renz EM, Cancio LC, Barillo DJ, et al. Long range transport of war-related burn casualties. J Trauma. 2008;64:S136-144; discussion S144-135.
7. Gebremichael M, Borg U, Habashi NM, et al. Interhospital transport of the extremely ill patient: the mobile intensive care unit. Crit Care Med. 2000;28:79-85.
8. Nagappan R. Transit care medicine--a critical link. Crit Care Med. 2004;32:305-306.
9. Warren J, Fromm RE, Jr., Orr RA, Rotello LC, Horst HM. Guidelines for the inter- and intrahospital transport of critically ill patients. Crit Care Med. 2004;32:256-262.
10. Ajizian SJ, Nakagawa TA. Interfacility transport of the critically ill pediatric patient. Chest. 2007;132:1361-1367.
11. Orr RA, Felmet KA, Han Y, et al. Pediatric specialized transport teams are associated with improved outcomes. Pediatrics. 2009;124:40-48.
12. Bartlett RH, Gazzaniga AB, Fong SW, Jefferies MR, Roohk HV, Haiduc N. Extracorporeal membrane oxygenator support for cardiopulmonary failure. Experience in 28 cases. J Thorac Cardiovasc Surg. 1977;73:375-386.
13. Bartlett RH, University of Michigan, personal communication, 2010.
14. Cornish JD, Gerstmann DR, Begnaud MJ, Null DM, Jr., Ackerman NB. Inflight use of extracorporeal membrane oxygenation for severe neonatal respiratory failure. Perfusion. 1986;1:281-287.
15. Boedy RF, Howell CG, Kanto WP, Jr. Hidden mortality rate associated with extracorporeal membrane oxygenation. J Pediatr. 1990;117:462-464.
16. Foley DS, Pranikoff T, Younger JG, et al. A review of 100 patients transported on extracorporeal life support. ASAIO J. 2002;48:612-619.
17. Heulitt MJ, Taylor BJ, Faulkner SC, et al. Inter-hospital transport of neonatal patients on extracorporeal membrane oxygenation: mobile-ECMO. Pediatrics. 1995;95:562-566.
18. Wilson JM, Bower LK, Thompson JE, Fauza DO, Fackler JC. ECMO in evolution: the impact of changing patient demographics and alternative therapies on ECMO. J Pediatr Surg. 1996;31:1116-1122; discussion 1122-1113.
19. Arlt M, Philipp A, Zimmermann M, et al. Emergency use of extracorporeal membrane oxygenation in cardiopulmonary failure. Artif Organs. 2009;33:696-703.
20. Coppola CP, Tyree M, Larry K, DiGeronimo R. A 22-year experience in global

transport extracorporeal membrane oxygenation. J Pediatr Surg. 2008;43:46-52; discussion 52.

21. First Airmed–ECMO Advantage transport a success. Available at: http://www. waypointmagazine.com/content/first-airmed%E2%80%93ecmo-advantage-transport-success. Accessed May 23, 2010.

22. Rossaint R, Pappert D, Gerlach H, Lewandowski K, Keh D, Falke K. Extracorporeal membrane oxygenation for transport of hypoxaemic patients with severe ARDS. Br J Anaesth. 1997;78:241-246.

23. Wilson BJ, Jr., Heiman HS, Butler TJ, Negaard KA, DiGeronimo R. A 16-year neonatal/pediatric extracorporeal membrane oxygenation transport experience. Pediatrics. 2002;109:189-193.

24. Impact Instrumentation Inc.: SMEEDTM. Available at: http://www.impactinstrumentation.com/SMEED.html. Accessed May 26, 2010.

25. Arlt M, Philipp A, Zimmermann M, et al. First experiences with a new miniaturised life support system for mobile percutaneous cardiopulmonary bypass. Resuscitation. 2008;77:345-350.

26. Arlt M, Philipp A, Iesalnieks I, Kobuch R, Graf BM. Successful use of a new hand-held ECMO system in cardiopulmonary failure and bleeding shock after thrombolysis in massive post-partal pulmonary embolism. Perfusion. 2009;24:49-50.

27. Krane M, Mazzitelli D, Schreiber U, et al. LIFEBRIDGE B2T--a new portable cardiopulmonary bypass system. ASAIO J. 2010;56:52-56.

28. Mehlhorn U, Brieske M, Fischer UM, et al. LIFEBRIDGE: a portable, modular, rapidly available "plug-and-play" mechanical circulatory support system. Ann Thorac Surg. 2005;80:1887-1892.

29. ECMO center bed status map. Available at: http://www.elso.med.umich.edu/Maps. html. Accessed May 23, 2010.

30. Perez A, Butt WW, Millar KJ, et al. Long-distance transport of critically ill children on extracorporeal life support in Australia. Crit Care Resusc. 2008;10:34.

31. Wagner K, Sangolt GK, Risnes I, et al. Transportation of critically ill patients on extracorporeal membrane oxygenation. Perfusion. 2008;23:101-106.

32. Kjaergaard B, Christensen T, Neumann PB, Nurnberg B. Aero-medical evacuation with interventional lung assist in lung failure patients. Resuscitation. 2007;72:280-285.

33. Zimmermann M, Bein T, Philipp A, et al. Interhospital transportation of patients with severe lung failure on pumpless extracorporeal lung assist. Br J Anaesth. 2006;96:63-66.

34. Zimmermann M, Philipp A, Schmid FX, Dorlac W, Arlt M, Bein T. From Baghdad to Germany: use of a new pumpless extracorporeal lung assist system in two severely injured US soldiers. ASAIO J. 2007;53:e4-6.

35. Bein T, Scherer MN, Philipp A, Weber F, Woertgen C. Pumpless extracorporeal lung assist (pECLA) in patients with acute respiratory distress syndrome and severe brain injury. J Trauma. 2005;58:1294-1297.

36. Beninati W, Meyer MT, Carter TE. The critical care air transport program. Crit Care Med. 2008;36:S370-376.

37. Linden V, Palmer K, Reinhard J, et al. Inter-hospital transportation of patients with severe acute respiratory failure on extracorporeal membrane oxygenation--national and international experience. Intensive Care Med. 2001;27:1643-1648.

38. Cornish JD, Carter JM, Gerstmann DR, Null DM, Jr. Extracorporeal membrane oxygenation as a means of stabilizing and transporting high risk neonates. ASAIO Trans. 1991;37:564-568.

39. Midla GS. Extracorporeal circulatory systems and their role in military medicine: a

clinical review. Mil Med. 2007;172:523-526.

40. Park PK, Cannon JW, Wen Y, et al. Incidence and mortality of ARDS in combat casualty care. Presented at the American Association for the Surgery of Trauma. Pittsburgh, PA; 2009.

41. Bridges E, Evers K. Wartime critical care air transport. Mil Med. 2009;174:370-375.

42. Allan PF, Codispoti CA, Womble SG, et al. Inhaled prostacyclin in combination with high-frequency percussive ventilation. J Burn Care Res. 2010;31:347-352.

43. Fang R, Pruitt VM, Dorlac GR, et al. Critical care at Landstuhl Regional Medical Center. Crit Care Med. 2008;36:S383-387.

44. Allan PF, Osborn EC, Chung KK, Wanek SM. High-frequency percussive ventilation revisited. J Burn Care Res. 2010;31:510-520.

45. Arlt M, Regensburg University Hospital, Germany. 2010; unpublished data.

46. Bein T, Osborn E, Hofmann HS, et al. Successful treatment of a severely injured soldier from Afghanistan with pumpless extracorporeal lung assist and neurally adjusted ventilatory support. Int J Emerg Med. 2010;3:177-179.

47. Copenhaver W, University of Michigan, personal communication, 2010.

48. Clement KC, Fiser RT, Fiser WP, et al. Single-institution experience with inter-hospital extracorporeal membrane oxygenation transport: A descriptive study. Pediatric Critical Care Medicine. 2010;11:In press.

49. Tyree M, Wilford Hall Medical Center. 2010; unpublished data.

50. Huang SC, Chen YS, Chi NH, et al. Out-of-center extracorporeal membrane oxygenation for adult cardiogenic shock patients. Artif Organs. 2006;30:24-28.

51. Holzgraefe B, Kalzen H, Broome M, Frenckner B, Palmer K. Inter-hospital transportation on extracorporeal membrane oxygenation (ECMO). The experience of the ECMO Centre Karolinska, Sweden. Presented at the European Society for Intensive Care Medicine. Barcelona, Spain; October 2010.

52. Rosengarten A, Elmore P, Epstein J. Long distance road transport of a patient with Wegener's Granulomatosis and respiratory failure using extracorporeal membrane oxygenation. Emerg Med (Fremantle). 2002;14:181-187.

53. Machin D, Scott R, Hurst A. Ground transportation of a pediatric patient on ECMO support. J Extra Corpor Technol. 2007;39:99-102.

54. Prodhan P, Fiser RT, Cenac S, et al. Intra-hospital transport of children on extracorporeal membrane oxygenation: indications, process, interventions, and effectiveness. Pediatr Crit Care Med. 2010;11:227-233.

55. Lidegran MK, Ringertz HG, Frenckner BP, Linden VB. Chest and abdominal CT during extracorporeal membrane oxygenation: Clinical benefits in diagnosis and treatment. Acad Radiol. 2005;12:276-285.

34

ECMO Administrative and Training Issues, and Sustaining Quality

Mark T. Ogino MD, John Chuo MD, Billie Lou Short MD

Introduction

ECMO procedures are technically complex, high risk, resource dependent, and unpredictable in terms of volume and timing. Safe, economical, and effective use of ECMO requires unique institutional resources and effective strategies to maintain optimal quality in the delivery of ECMO care.

The Extracorporeal Life Support Organization (ELSO) has developed "ELSO Guidelines for ECMO Centers" which outline institutional requirements for effective ECMO use.[1] The "ELSO Guidelines for Training and Continuing Education of ECMO Specialists" specifies the educational requirements of clinicians responsible for monitoring and maintaining ECLS support to the patient.[2] ELSO recognizes that differences in regional and institutional regulations impact each ECMO center, and these variations may result in deviation from these guidelines. Nevertheless, these guidelines establish standards for assessing current and future ECMO centers. All ELSO guidelines are reviewed and revised every three years, and are available on the ELSO website (www.elso.med.umich.edu).

In ELSO's commitment to promote patient safety and quality initiatives at each of its member institutions, the "ELSO Award of Excellence" has been established to recognize ECMO centers that have met or surpassed the ELSO guideline recommendations for hospital administrative support, facility and equipment requirements, and ECMO team administrative organization.[3] In addition to the administrative aspects of a program, the Award recognizes programs that have met or exceeded the recommendations that highlight clinical excellence with quality initiatives, clinical process evaluations and optimization, and support programs for family members. The subject matter discussed in this chapter is to encourage all ECMO centers to achieve the designation as an ELSO Center of Excellence.

Essential Hospital Support Components

Tertiary care centers providing ECMO services must provide institutional support systems to maintain the essential environment for safe delivery of comprehensive ECMO services. Although it is difficult to determine the actual minimum case load required to maintain clinical competency, at least six ECMO patients per center per year is the recommended standard. ELSO membership and active participation in the organization's activities, including involvement with the ELSO Registry, is recommended to enhance a program's quality review process through the availability of benchmark data.

Physical Facilities

ECMO centers are preferably located in tertiary care medical facilities with intensive care units able to care for a specific ECMO patient population: adult ICU, cardiac ICU, Level 3C neonatal ICU, and/or pediatric ICU. ECMO may be provided in a centralized intensive care location, in multiple intensive care unit settings, or in a space allotted for ECMO patients. If the location is located outside an intensive care setting, it is recommended that the critical care medical and support services to be in close proximity to the ECMO unit and a formal communication channel established with the critical care unit for summoning immediate additional staff support for emergency situations.

Equipment

The basic components of an ECMO system consists of tubing, blood pump, oxygenator, heat exchanger, and heating unit. Each center will determine the addition of supplemental circuit components to match the needs of the patient population and experience level of the program. Chapter 8 is devoted to a detailed review of the ECMO circuit and available components. Backup components of the ECMO system and the circuit must be available for potential emergencies. Additional equipment recommended to support bedside surgical procedures in the intensive care unit include: additional lighting, instrument sets, personal protective wear, and traffic barriers. Each center will need to establish an effective ordering and inventory system to ensure availability of essential supplies. Equipment maintenance and cleaning processes must be in place to ensure that the manufacturer's suggested periodic maintenance is performed and records documenting ECMO equipment maintenance are maintained per The Joint Commission (TJC) regulations. This process will be unique to the individual center and may require the involvement of the biomedical engineering department, cardiopulmonary perfusion services, and/or ECMO team members.

Support Personnel

Permanent hospital support personnel, available 24 hours a day seven days a week, include: population specific specialists in general surgery, cardiovascular surgery, anesthesiology, cardiology, neurosurgery, radiology, cardiovascular perfusion, biomedical engineering, and respiratory care (in applicable countries). Most ECMO centers also provide consultant services to assist with complex ECMO management including: population specific specialists in neurology, nephrology, infectious disease and genetics. Rehabilitation specialists, including occupational, physical, speech and language therapies, and specifically for the neonatal and pediatric populations, a developmental specialist, are essential to the meet the multidisciplinary needs of the ECMO patient. Support facilities with around the clock staff availability are required in the blood bank, radiology (cranial ultrasound and CAT scan included), and clinical laboratories for blood gas, chemistry, and hematological testing. Availability of cardiovascular operating room facilities with cardiopulmonary bypass capabilities located within the hospital campus is necessary 24 hours a day.

Policy and Procedures

The ECMO center is responsible for developing institutional selection criteria for ECLS support in patients with acute cardiac and/or respiratory failure and for outlining the indications and contraindications for ECMO. Formal policy and procedures are required for ECMO patient and circuit management, maintenance of equipment, termination of ECMO therapy, and ECMO patient followup. The policy and procedures should be easily accessed by all team members and regularly reviewed and updated, as determined by the ECMO center's institutional policy.

Transport of the ECMO patient within an ECMO center is a common requirement in clinical situations where the cardiac catheterization lab, diagnostic imaging facilities, or the operating room are necessary. Each center is responsible for developing policies and procedures for inter-hospital transport to ensure safe uninterrupted ECLS support. This requires an inventory of essential transport equipment, such as portable battery pack and emergency ECLS supplies. Staff training for safely transporting ECMO patients is a subject matter to be considered in a center's educational curriculum. If advanced medical or surgical services for ECMO patients are not available at an ECMO center, relationships with other referral ECMO centers will need to be established. The development of intra-hospital transport protocols and guidelines for transfer is also recommended. Transport of the ECMO patient to another ECMO center by ground and air is extremely complex and requires extensive coordination between the discharging and receiving hospitals, transport team, and carrier. Chapter 33 discusses inter and intra hospital ECMO transfers in detail.

For the discharged ECMO patient, a follow-up program with appropriate subspecialty support is necessary to address the long term medical, surgical, and psychosocial issues which may have developed during the ECMO course. For neonatal patients, a neurodevelopmental followup program is highly recommended.

ECMO Team Organization

Program Director

The overall operation of the center's ECMO program is the responsibility of a single ECMO physician designated as the program director. While there may be several associate directors with specific interests or focus in limited areas

of ECMO care, the primary program director is responsible for assuring appropriate specialist training and performance, directing quality improvement meetings and projects, validating proper and valid data submission to ELSO. The program director is also responsible for the credentialing of physicians who care for ECMO patients and/or who manage the ECMO circuit. The program director's qualifications include board-certification in one of the following specialties: critical care, neonatology, surgery (pediatric, cardiovascular, trauma, or thoracic), or any board-certified specialist with specific training and experience with ECMO support.

ECMO Physician

The clinical management of a patient on ECMO will be provided by an ECMO-trained physician. The physician may include neonatologists, pediatric or adult critical care specialists, neonatal or critical care fellows, or other physicians who have completed at least three years of post-graduate pediatric, surgical, or adult medical training and have had specific ECMO training. All ECMO trained physicians must meet the requirements of their subspecialty training as set forth by their specific governing board (e.g., the American Board of Surgery or American Board of Pediatrics) in addition to their institution's ECMO training requirements. Currently, ELSO does not have guidelines to define the competencies required of a physician responsible for a patient on ECMO. Each center's program director is responsible for defining the qualifications of a physician receiving privileges in ECMO management. Consideration for different levels of responsibility may be necessary depending on the experience of the medical and surgical staff.

ECMO Coordinator/Manager

The ECMO coordinator or manager's responsibilities include the non-physician management of the ECMO program. The ECMO coordinator may be an experienced (minimum of one year ICU experience) neonatal, pediatric, cardiac, adult intensive care registered nurse, registered respiratory therapist, or certified clinical perfusionist. The responsibilities of coordinators vary among centers, but typically they are responsible for the supervision, training and continuing education of the technical staff, maintenance of equipment, and collection of patient data. In addition, the ECMO coordinator acts as a clinical resource for all team members.

The ECMO program director and ECMO coordinator establish the leadership team to enhance their effectiveness to oversee all elements of a multidisciplinary care team. They work collaboratively to develop standard medical and nursing order sets, as well as formal policies and procedures regarding all aspects of ECMO.

ECMO Specialist

The ECMO specialist is defined in the ELSO guidelines as "the technical specialist trained to manage the ECMO system and the clinical needs of the patient on ECMO under the direction and supervision of an ECMO-trained physician," and the ECMO specialist provides 1:1 or 1:2 care throughout the course of ECMO. ECMO specialists are registered nurses, registered respiratory therapists, certified perfusionists, or physicians who have a strong intensive care background and have at least one year of neonatal, pediatric, cardiac, or adult intensive care experience. Specialists provide care to the patient on ECMO with primary responsibility for maintaining appropriate extracorporeal support, troubleshooting equipment, assessing the circuit, and managing circuit emergencies until additional assistance is available. In addition to the ECMO specialist, an intensive care nurse provides patient care throughout the ECMO course. In some centers, both the bedside nurse and the clinical personnel managing the ECMO system are trained ECMO specialists. This

allows the roles to be fluid and provides an immediate resource for troubleshooting, problem-solving, emergencies, and scheduling of breaks.

The strength of an ECMO team is fundamentally dependent on the ECMO specialists and the cohesiveness established between each member. It is important that the ECMO specialists are aware of all job expectations including training requirements, continuing education, alternate shift work, and on-call hours. In most ECMO programs, specialists are given a significant amount of responsibility and are required to work in stressful conditions. Common characteristics of successful ECMO specialists include: ability to think critically, support a team model of care, demonstrate effective communication skills, develop technical skillfulness, function in stressful situations, and demonstrate flexibility with work schedules. Training requirement recommendations differ based upon the specialist's clinical background. See Table 34-1 for recommended qualifications.

With advancements in equipment and simplification of circuits, the "Single Care Giver" bedside model has been adapted in some high volume ECMO centers. In this clinical setting, a single intensive care nurse provides patient care and monitors ECLS equipment. The intensive care nurse is specifically trained in ECMO patient and circuit management, and participation in this role requires approval by the ECMO program director. A separate ECMO specialist team is responsible for managing equipment and supplies, circuit preparation, and troubleshooting.

Primer

Most centers identify a team of personnel who are responsible for priming the ECMO circuit, that is, to prepare the circuit for patient use. A clinician assigned to set up the ECMO circuit will need additional training, practice, and skill assessments. The composition of the priming team varies from center to center. In some centers all of the ECMO specialists are primers; whereas in other centers, ECMO physicians, perfusionists, or a small group of specialists are responsible for the priming procedure. Prior to allowing individuals to prime alone, a priming trainee will need to demonstrate the procedure accurately and within a preestablished time frame. Repeated "practice" of the technique is necessary to maintain the accuracy and speed. For low volume centers, a defined maximum interval between performing either a practice or actual prime will help to maintain skill levels. Some centers have ECMO primers in-house around the clock, while others have established an on-call system. In many centers, members of the priming team also provide assistance for troubleshooting and component replacement. A comprehensive discussion on priming is covered in Chapter 8.

Educational Process

ECMO education is a challenge due to the different skill sets that an ECMO physician or specialist must achieve before they can be considered qualified to deliver ECLS care. Most centers have created a training program that involves writing a training manual and developing a didactic course. Since learning does not automatically occur with the transfer of information from an instructor to learner, the majority of ECMO centers will supplement their traditional didactic courses with additional "hands on" training to address the technical and behavioral skills (team interaction, communication, leadership skills) that are essential at the ECMO patient's bedside. Adult Educational Theory supports the use of an active learning environment and the use of an educational environment similar to the real working environment to optimize skill acquisitions and maintenance.[5] Effective learning can be further enhanced by applying new information to a learner's previous clinical experience.[6]

The framework for clinical education and assessment was eloquently described by Miller. The essay figuratively describes the ascent to attaining knowledge using a four tiered triangle as the assessment model; hence the learning process is known as "Miller's Triangle."[9] The base of the triangle begins with the learner who "knows" the knowledge, and advances to the second stage where the learner "knows how" to apply the knowledge. The third stage is when the learner "shows how" to use the knowledge and this can be related to performance in a test-

Table 34-1. ECMO Specialist Qualifications.

Specialist	Qualifications
Nurse	• Completion of an approved school of nursing
	• Passing score on state's Board of Nursing written examination
Respiratory Therapist	• Completion of an accredited school of respiratory therapy
	• Passing score on registry examinations for advanced level practitioners
	• Registered Respiratory Therapist with the National Board of Respiratory Care
Perfusionist	• Completion of an accredited school of perfusion
	• Certification by the American Board of Cardiovascular Perfusion
Physician	• Licensed by state's Medical Board
	• Completion of institutional training requirements for ECMO privileges
Other Medical Personnel	• Refer to "ELSO Guidelines for ECMO Centers" February 2010. Organization, Section B-6.

ing environment, such as, an ECMO training lab. Stage two and three combined describe the degree of competency achievable in ECMO training courses. The apex of the triangle is when the learner "does." This is the action phase of the clinical assessment process in which the learner applies the knowledge in the clinical environment. This cannot be tested in an artificial environment since unpredictable elements of an actual clinical setting cannot be replicated. The "does" is the decisive test of knowledge mastery. It is ELSO's recommendation that each center develop training programs that accomplish the first three steps of Miller's Triangle's framework, to allow the successful implementation of the "does" phase for each learner.

Defining training objectives designed for the specific needs of each center must be clearly distinguished and incorporated into an ECMO center's training outline. This will ensure the successful conveyance of essential concepts during the didactic course. In developing a course, principles of adult learning to consider include:[10]

- Involve the learner in the planning and evaluation of their instruction
- Experience, positive and negative, provides the basis for learning activities
- Generate motivation by having the learner participate in activities with immediate relevance to their job or personal life
- Recognize and incorporate previous experiences of the learner

Establishing ECMO Competency

The ECMO program director and ECMO coordinator are responsible for the training of the ECMO team, including assuring their ongoing competency, and also assuring that established guidelines and standards are clearly defined in each institution's policies and procedures. The Joint Commission defines competency as the knowledge, skills, ability,

and behaviors that a person possesses in order to perform tasks correctly and skillfully.[7] TJC standard HR 01.02.01 states, "The hospital defines staff qualifications" and HR 01.06.01 requires the hospital to ensure that "Staff are competent to perform their responsibilities."[8] The ECMO coordinator/manager and ECMO program director roles in competency assessment are to determine physician and specialist staff qualifications and job responsibilities, determine competencies required for each job, identify staff development needs, implement a system competency verification, and develop an individual development plan for employees who do not meet the defined standards.

With the diversity in ECMO program organization, it is recommended each center develop its own training program based on their patient population, equipment, and assigned responsibilities of team members. Since the educational backgrounds of ECMO specialists differ, each center will need to adjust its training program based on their staff's specific needs. For example, respiratory therapists will need more time to learn about transfusion procedures, IV pumps, and medications, whereas nurses may need more education in gas physics and circuit component physiology. Perfusionists will need to learn more about the effects of long-term bypass and patient care assessment. In addition, the bedside nursing staff will need additional training on caring for an ECMO patient along with a basic understanding of ECMO. The multidisciplinary composition of the ECMO team utilizes the strengths of each discipline to address the multisystem challenges in the care of an ECMO patient.

It is helpful to include representatives from other patient care services who are involved with the ECMO program in some portions of the training. This may include representatives from blood bank (hospital and regional), radiology, catheterization lab, operating room, laboratory medicine, and biomedical engineering. Multidisciplinary exposure to the ECMO patient will help improve communication among hospital services and will allow other services to understand and anticipate the needs of the ECMO patient.

Good team communication is an essential skill for the ECMO team to maintain and the training process should include team-building activities across all disciplines. Optimal care of ECMO patients requires specialized knowledge from the multiple disciplines to be integrated. Integration is best accomplished through frequent, respectful interaction, and competent communication. In today's healthcare system, working collaboratively with others is as important to successful ECMO care as expert clinical skills are to the individual practitioners. According to data from The Joint Commission (TJC), a breakdown in team communication is a top contributor to sentinel events.[4] Chapter 36 on safety includes more information on this topic.

ECMO Training Program

ELSO has developed "ELSO Guidelines for Training and Continuing Education of ECMO Specialists" and "Guidelines for ECMO Centers" which can be used as a reference for both current and future ECMO centers. Other ELSO training resources include the ECMO Red Book and ECMO Specialist Training Manual. Educational conferences are also offered by ELSO to assist new centers with training.

These guidelines recommend that a new ECMO program offer a didactic course lasting 24-36 hours, followed by water drills (described later in this chapter), and/or animal sessions. Although high fidelity simulation is not listed in the guidelines, simulation is a very effective educational tool for teaching, maintaining, and assessing ECMO skills.[11] The ELSO Guidelines recommended hours for the animal lab may be applied to time in a water drill or simulation lab. The advantage of animal laboratory training is real-time coagulation management and blood gas management which are difficult to simu-

late in either water drills or ECMO simulation laboratory settings, although these simulation techniques are becoming quite refined. Four to eight hours are recommended for review of ECLS equipment and basic procedures; four to eight hours for emergency procedures training; and minimum of 12 hours additional time with an instructor reviewing ECMO bedside skills. Most programs will require additional time with an instructor or a bedside preceptor until the specialist-in-training has gained a solid understanding of the management principles of ECLS and are fully competent managing ECMO emergencies.

Experienced center recommendations are the same, except that animal labs are not required. In most experienced centers, new specialists work with an experienced specialist at the bedside for a predetermined time.

Didactic Course

There are many topics to include in a didactic course and a sample outline is provided in Table 34-2. Most centers begin their course with an "Introduction to ECMO" which includes a discussion of the history of ECMO. An understanding of past successes and failures will lead to a better understanding of the basis for current practice. Other introductory discussions may include: different forms of ECMO support, general indications for ECMO, the risks and benefits for specific populations, as well as recent clinical research trials that outline the current status of ECLS therapy and define clinical outcomes.

Other topics recommended for specialist education include pathophysiology of diseases and current medical therapies in patients with severe respiratory failure. Institutions using ECMO for cardiac support may also include education on the anatomy, circulation and repairs of congenital heart disease patients, pathophysiology of cardiomyopathy and myocarditis, and principles of transplantation medicine.

Table 34-2. ECMO Didactic Topics.

Introduction to ECMO
- History
- Current status
- Risks and benefits
- Membrane gas exchange physics and physiology
- Oxygen content, delivery and consumption
- Shunt physiology
- Types of ECMO
- Future applications
- Research

Physiology of the diseases treated with ECMO
- Neonatal respiratory failure
- Pneumonia
- Aspiration pneumonia
- ARDS
- Pulmonary embolism
- Sepsis
- Postoperative congenital heart disease
- Heart transplantation
- Cardiomyopathy and myocarditis

Pre ECMO procedures
- Notification of the ECMO Team
- Cannulation procedure
  - open
  - percutaneous
- Initiation of bypass
- Responsibility of team members

Criteria for ECMO
- Patient selection
- Selection criteria
- Pre-ECMO evaluation
- Contraindications
- Selection of ECLS support (VA, VV, VA-V)

Blood products and coagulation
- Blood products and interactions
- Blood product management of the bleeding patient

- Coagulation cascade
- Blood surface interactions
- Heparin pharmacology
- Activated clotting times (ACT)
- Other laboratory anticoagulation monitoring studies
- Amicar, Protamine and other drugs
- Recombinant clotting factors
- Disseminated intravascular coagulation

ECMO equipment
- ECMO circuit design
- ECMO circuit components (cannula, compliance chamber, pump, venous return monitor, in-line saturation monitor, pressure monitor, heater, hemofilter, bubble detector)
- Oxygenator function and blood gas control
- ECMO supply cart

Physiology of venoarterial and venovenous ECMO
- Indications
- Vessel cannulation
- Physiology
- Advantages and disadvantages

Cannulation and initiation of ECMO support
- Circuit priming
- Preparing the patient
- Initiating ECLS support

Daily patient management on ECMO
- Bedside care of the ECMO patient
- Fluid, electrolytes and nutrition
- Respiratory
- Neurologic
- Infection control
- Sedation and pain control
- Hematology
- Cardiac
- Psychosocial
- Pharmacologic issues

Table 34-2. ECMO Didactic Topics.

- Lab schedule
- Documentation and orders

Daily circuit management on ECMO
- Aseptic technique
- Pump and gas flow
- Pressure monitoring
- Blood product infusion techniques
- Circuit infusions
- Management of anticoagulation
- Circuit checks
- Hemofiltrations setup

Medical emergencies and complications during ECMO
- Intracranial and other hemorrhage
- Pneumothorax and pneumopericardium
- Cardiac arrest
- Arrythmias
- Hypotension and hypovolemia
- Hypertension
- Severe coagulopathy
- Seizures
- Hemothorax and hemopericardium
- Uncontrolled bleeding
- Electrolyte imbalance
- Renal failure

Mechanical emergencies and complications during ECMO
- Circuit disruption
- Raceway rupture
- Cavitation
- System or component alarm and failure (pump, compliance chamber, venous return monitor, oxygenator, heater, flow sensor)
- Air embolus
- Inadvertent decannulation
- Clots

Management of complex ECMO cases
- Surgery on ECMO
  - post-operative bleeding
- Transport on ECMO
  - inter-hospital
  - intra-hospital

Weaning from ECMO
- Techniques and complications
- Clinical indications of pulmonary and cardiac recovery
- Pump and gas flow weaning techniques
- ACT changes during weaning
- Ventilator changes during weaning
- Trial off
- Decannulation from low flow

Decannulation
- Personnel needed
- Medications required
- Potential complications
- Vessel ligation
- Vessel reconstruction
- Percutaneous approach

Post ECMO complications
- Platelet and electrolyte alterations

Short and long-term developmental outcome of ECMO patients
- Institutional follow-up protocol
- Literature review

Ethical and social issues
- Consent process
- Parental and family support
- Withdrawal of ECMO support

Topics that review the pre-ECMO setting are also recommended. These include: pre-ECMO orders, informed consent for ECMO and blood transfusions, pre-ECMO laboratory sampling tests along with blood product type and cross match, neuro-imaging studies, and echocardiograms. Room setup, circuit priming, ECMO initiation, and necessary documentation tools are also important topics to be reviewed.

It is essential that each ECMO specialist gains a comprehensive understanding of blood gas interpretation and gas exchange. This includes knowledge of the principles involved with oxygen content, delivery, and consumption, and carbon dioxide production and elimination in normal physiologic and extracorporeal support conditions. It is recommended that all team members demonstrate an understanding of the impact ECMO pump and sweep flow changes upon gas exchange. Ventilator and airway management may be included in this session. A thorough demonstration of ECMO physiology and oxygen physics knowledge by the specialist is highly recommended at the end of a training course.

Table 34-3. ECMO Technical Skills.

Subject	Topics

Equipment Component check Function check	• "Circuit check"
	   o Tubing
	   o Sampling ports
	   o Pump head
	   o Pump controls and alarms
	   o Pressure monitoring
	   o Servo regulation panel
	   o Oxygenator
	   o Sweep gas monitoring
	   o Heat exchanger
	   o Water heater
	   o Other (bridge, compliance chamber, flow sensor, arterial filter, bubble detector, etc)

Basic procedures	• Blood sampling • Bedside ACT checks • Pigtail and stopcock changes • Blood product administration • IV infusion and medication administration • ECLS documentation • ECMO order set review • Other (roller pump head occlusion checks)
Emergency procedures	• Clamping off ECMO • Massive blood loss from circuit • Tubing replacement • Oxygenator failure • Air in circuit and de-airing circuit • Loss of venous return • Inadvertent decannulation • Pump head failure and hand cranking • Power failure • Circuit and/or component change

Each center will focus the majority of its training on the ECMO techniques that are site-specific; however, a discussion regarding different types of support in use at other centers will assist with inter-hospital communication and exchange of ideas. Blood product administration, coagulation management, medications commonly used in the blood prime and during ECMO, ECMO weaning, and decannulation procedures are other essential topics to be reviewed. In addition, a basic understanding of intra-hospital and inter-hospital ECMO transport requirements is recommended.

It is critical that all specialists gain a thorough understanding of ECMO equipment and circuit used in their institution, and receive training in discussing mechanical complications and preventative measures. Institutional guidelines will need to define the essential equipment and emergency skills each specialist must maintain. These skills may include: how to set alarm parameters, recognition of factors that cause alarm conditions, initiating appropriate response to the alarm conditions, and response to mechanical emergencies.

Patient and circuit management lectures cover a broad range of subjects which include the fundamentals of day to day management of a patient on ECMO, and recognition of medical emergencies that may occur during ECMO. Specialists in training will also benefit from lectures in ethical and social issues.

Training Labs

Technical skills and behavioral skills necessary for effective ECMO Team training can be accomplished using different "hands on" training methods. These training methods offer a unique opportunity to create, test, refine, and streamline ECLS processes without disrupting patient care or endangering patients. Water drills have been utilized to demonstrate functionality of ECMO components. Animal labs allow ECMO physiology to be demonstrated

in an in vivo model. The introduction of high fidelity simulation into ECMO training sessions enables the learner to experience a real-time situation with realistic sensory cues that mimic the critical care setting with an ECMO patient. For the purpose of this discussion, these "hands on" training sessions will be categorized as "training labs."

Training lab sessions are recommended to allow additional discussion and demonstration of ECMO and support equipment, instruction for the management of ECMO emergencies, and observation of ECMO specialist's bedside care performance. Table 34-3 outlines the recommended list of topics for training lab sessions.

The recommended basic session topics include a discussion and demonstration of all equipment including an explanation of the circuit configuration and function, alarm functions, and a routine circuit assessment, "circuit check." Basic and emergency procedures drills can also be developed based upon a center's equipment selection and practiced in the training labs. Standard emergency drills include managing power failures, clamping off ECMO, manually hand cranking the pump, de-airing a circuit, and managing accidental decannulations. Each program will need to define their specialist's role and the level of competency of each trainee. This will determine if advanced skills such as priming, replacing a circuit, oxygenator and/or individual components will be practiced. The goals of these training labs are to prepare each specialist to promptly identify any mechanical circuit problems and to initiate the appropriate problem solving response. The clinical specialist responsible for correcting the problem will depend on the defined responsibilities of a center's ECMO team members.

Water Drills

ECMO circuits can be assembled, filled with fluid, and run in non-clinical settings. This allows for opportunities to mimic many of the situations that occur during an actual ECMO run and is commonly referred to as a "water drill." To optimize hands on experience by each participant it is recommended that the number of water drills participants is limited.

Animal Lab Sessions

Animal labs are performed in accordance with institutional animal care guidelines. Because of the need for blood products to prime the ECMO circuit and transfuse during the training session, the newborn lamb (1-7 days of age) model has been used successfully. Several units of blood can be obtained from an adult sheep without complications to that animal, and sheep do not have major blood incompatibilities as do piglets, etc. If a 24 hour animal facility is available to a new ECMO center, the recommended time period for animal lab sessions is 24-72 hours with each trainee participating in a 4-8 hour session. This will simulate the around-the-clock management requirements of the ECMO patient and also decrease the number of animals needed. During these sessions, participants can practice tasks such as blood product administration, intravenous solution and medication administration, and blood sampling. The physiologic impact of the pump, sweep gas regulation, and heparin infusion adjustments can be demonstrated in an in vivo model. Many centers have difficulty accessing vivariums for training causing a decrease use of animals for ECMO training. Animal labs have become increasingly difficult to perform due to cost, availability of approved facilities, and rigorous institutional animal care guidelines; hence, alternative "hands on" training methods have been developed.

High Fidelity Simulation

High fidelity simulation has become a widely accepted educational tool for anesthesiology, surgery, obstetrics, neonatology, and critical care training programs. For decades, simulation has been used in the military, airline, and nuclear power industries to train their personnel for skill acquisition in routine and extraordinary emergency situations.[12] High fidelity simulation enhances learning through multiple factors such as: providing immediate feedback, allowing repetitive practice, increasing level of difficulty with attainment of skills, addressing multiple forms of learner strategies, and permitting clinical variation in learner reponses.[13] Simulation also addresses the traditional educational method deficiencies of technical and behavioral skill development by immersing the trainee in realistic environments populated with working equipment (including a functional circuit), a patient simulator capable of generating authentic physiologic cues, and living human beings who respond in a realistic manner to the events of the scenario. By creating a highly realistic environment where trainees must respond to problems with both the circuit and the patient, a more realistic and valuable learning opportunity is created. Halamek et al. from the Center for Advanced Pediatric and Perinatal Education at Packard Children's Hospital at Stanford published two articles describing the use of high fidelity simulation in ECMO training. The first article described ECMO simulation as a valid training tool, and the second demonstrated ECMO simulation's superiority in training technical and behavioral skills essential for ECMO specialists.[11, 14] This group has subsequently made several modifications to this system to allow an even more realistic simulation of circuit performance and patient physiology.[15]

High fidelity ECMO simulation offers an advantage over wet drills and animal labs because it adds "the patient's" physiologic parameters incorporated into the training session. This new educational tool has been introduced in many ECMO centers as an alternative training tool for new, as well as experienced specialists and physicians. ELSO has also instituted high fidelity ECMO simulation in its educational programs. If high fidelity simulation is available at an ECMO center, it is recommended that the ECMO Team should actively collaborate with the simulation center staff to develop and implement training and competency assessment programs.

Maintaining Competency Standards

Verifying ECMO Competency

ECMO competency can be verified by observation in actual clinical settings or in simulated settings. There are three skills to consider when assessing competency – cognitive (critical thinking), technical, and behavioral. Verification is the objective process of assuring that a staff member can perform the competency based on specific performance criteria used to ensure accurate and safe practice. Performance criteria must be outlined in a policy, procedure, standard, guideline, or reference. Institutional certification of ECMO specialists is achieved when performance criteria for clinical competency is fulfilled. The ELSO guidelines recommend that all specialists take an annual oral and/or written exam.

Table 34-4. Essential Behavioral Skills in ECMO.[11]

Behavioral Skills
• Familiar with ECMO equipment and bedside environment
• Anticipates and plans for crisis
• Assumes a leadership role
• Communicates effectively
• Distributes workload optimally
• Allocates attention wisely
• Utilizes all available resources
• Calls for help early
• Maintains professional behavior

A written test can be used to assess knowledge. Critical thinking skills include decision-making, prioritizing, troubleshooting, and responding to actual or potential events. Specific ECMO problems and the knowledge of how to handle problems can be simulated in a training lab session and an instructor can observe the ECMO specialist's response and assess critical thinking skills.

Technical skills include psychomotor activities that are part of every job. Training labs provide a simulated surrounding to determine by observation if a specialist is competent in performing the technical skills necessary for the care of an ECMO patient in routine and emergent situations. The instructor can observe the specialist performing the procedure. Simulation is the closest assessment of an individual's ability to apply their "know how" competency. True competency, the apex of Miller's Triangle, defined as "does," can only be verified by observation in actual patient situations, under real-life, stressful situations. It is here that the specialist's ability level can be most accurately determined.[9] Advanced Cardiac Life Support training skills begin to decay after six months.[16] It is therefore essential to have specialists practice infrequently used skills on a regular basis."

Behavioral skills reflect the ability to communicate effectively with individuals and groups. Professional communication skills include written, spoken, and non-verbal skills. Co-workers can identify ECMO specialists who lack the appropriate interpersonal skills. The difficulty lies in objectively identifying those skills. Some of the communication behavioral indicators include demonstrating courtesy, being respectful, and practicing good listening and feedback skills. Table 34-4 outlines the behavioral skills measured by the Stanford CAPE group in their original study measuring the effectiveness of high fidelity simulation in ECMO training.[11]

Maintaining ECMO Competency

Since ECMO is a high risk, low volume procedure, ECMO centers will need a process to ensure that all team members obtain the appropriate education and experience to retain their skills. Each center will need to determine their own timeline for competency evaluation based on their specific needs and specialist exposure to ECMO care. The ELSO guidelines recommend that training lab sessions be held at a minimum of every six months. It is also recommended that an annual examination be used to verify the knowledge and skills of all specialists. Each program will need to determine each team member's minimum number of pump hours in an established time period to maintain institutional certification. If the number of hours is not met, then a policy outlining a retraining program is recommended.

Most ECMO centers schedule specialist team meetings on a regular basis to discuss clinical and operational issues, quality assurance review findings, and any other topics pertinent to the team. Team meetings also provide an opportunity to offer continuing education sessions. Frequencies of these meetings are determined based on the size of the team and the volume of ECMO patients treated. It is recommended that the attendance of team members at these meetings is monitored and criteria for minimal attendance defined for specialists to ensure maintenance of institutional certification. Information on patient followup could be included here allowing specialists to be familiar with patient outcomes in order to appreciate the risks and benefits associated with ECMO.

Institutional Certification of the ECMO Specialist

Each institution is responsible for evaluating and certifying its own team members, and maintaining a written evaluation of each specialist's training history. Most centers include documentation of course attendance, successful performance at water drills or animal sessions or simulations, and completion of all required skills lists and competencies in the evaluations. In addition, each specialist must obtain a passing grade on a written and/or oral exam.

Table 34-5. ECMO Specialist Certification Examples.

Certification Requirements	
Institutional certification	• Minimum of 1 year critical care experience prior to training
	• Attendance at all didactic sessions
	• Attendance at all training lab sessions
	• Participation in ECLS emergency drills
	• Completion of pump time with a preceptor
	• Completion of technical skills list and/or competencies
	• Successful completion of written/oral exam with passing score
Institutional recertification	• Attendance at required team meetings
	• Participation in bi-annual ECLS training lab drills
	• Passing score on annual written or oral examination
	• Verification of ECLS competency
	• Performance of required number of pump hours per time period

Institutional certification can be granted after successfully completing the training course requirements and passing the exam. Sample institutional certification requirements are shown in Table 34-5.

Periodic review of the ECMO specialist's knowledge and skill level is essential. The frequency and the skills to be assessed are center-specific and based upon the center's specific requirements for recertification. All training expectations need to be established as well as criteria indicating success (e.g., a passing score on a test and a minimum number of pump hours). In addition, yearly requirements for attendance and participation in team meetings will need to be fulfilled. Sample recertification requirements are listed in Table 34-5.

Policy, Procedures, and Competency Revisions

Initial ECMO policy and procedures, and competencies may be completed in a set time frame and will need to be reviewed and updated on a regular basis. In general, ongoing or new competencies can be developed with review of the following questions:

1. Are there new procedures, polices, equipment, or initiatives? An example would be a new inline gas monitoring system or new ECMO pump.
2. Are there changes or revisions in procedures, policies, equipment, or initiatives? An example would be a change in anticoagulation management procedures.
3. What are the non-routine practices, procedures, equipment, or skills needed? An example would be the occasional use of hemofiltration.
4. What are the problem-prone aspects of ECMO? These can be identified through quality improvement data, incident reports, staff surveys, and other forms of evaluation.

5. What are the high risk aspects of this job? High risk is anything that would lead to harm, death, or legal action. Unfortunately, this about covers everything to do with ECMO.

A review of the ECMO center's most recent ELSO Registry report is recommended during a program's internal quality review. Twice annually, each ELSO member institution receives collective International Summary reports as well as Center-specific reports. The ELSO Registry report highlights the common problems reported by participating centers and their incidence, and also the rate of occurrence at the individual center. The Center-specific reports provide an ECMO program with a benchmark for comparison to the international ECMO community. There are potential limitations to interpreting and comparing outcomes due to inconsistencies in the diagnostic and monitoring parameters' definitions; however, the Registry report provides invaluable information to monitor a center's outcomes. More details about the ELSO Registry are included in Chapter 6.

Ensuring Quality

Promoting and maintaining quality in an ECLS program is essential. Continuous quality improvement is required by accrediting agencies; moreover, ECMO programs have a responsibility to their patients to monitor outcomes and continually seek opportunities for improvement. Membership in ELSO is of paramount importance. ELSO supports many quality improvement tools for centers to utilize such as national meetings that facilitate important collaboration, publications, research studies, and the Registry.

Sustaining the quality of an ECLS program requires a flexible operation that integrates people, processes, and tools to deliver care that is: effective, efficient, safe, timely, and equitable (Institute of Medicine indicators of quality healthcare).[17] Even the best thought out programs must seek opportunities for improvement once it goes 'live;" hence, methods for making real time improvements play an important role in sustaining excellence. Improvement areas can be divided into four areas: data acquisition, workflow processes, staff configuration, and communication. In some cases, established guidelines are determined by the institution, such as those for point of care testing, while in other cases, the guidelines originate locally. Regardless of who determined the guidelines, what is recommended practice and how practice is actually done must be the same. Tracking the proper process metrics and holding practitioners accountable for their practices will minimize this practice gap. Effective communication will ensure that staff understands the reasons for the recommendations and need for compliance.

Two key components of improvement operations to consider are: high reliability principles that describe the cultural strategy, and improvement methods which are the implementation strategy. As described by Weick and Sutcliffe, high reliability means constantly 1) learning from even the smallest failures and near misses, 2) avoiding simplification and understanding the complexities of context and problems, 3) relying on expertise regardless of organizational hierarchy, 4) attention to operations, and 5) building resilience.[18] These five principles, once embedded into an ECMO program, support the ability to detect weak signals of potential trouble early, identify problems within complex processes, leverage existing expertise within an organization to make improvements, and build capacity to absorb future strains and preserve function when unexpected adverse events occur. Applying these principles to an ECMO program would necessitate: 1) clearly identifying and recording all clinical and administrative processes that are involved in the ECMO program and understand their dependencies, 2) standardizing whenever possible, 3) identifying a process owner and specifying their responsibilities, 4)

seeking out subject matter experts, and 5) establishing a transparent system to detect, analyze, and react to failures.

While many excellent improvement methods are available, the process developed by Institute for Healthcare Improvement is one of the most widely used.[19-21] It begins with a charter that states three critical questions 1) What will you improve, by how much, by when? 2) How will you know that an improvement has been made? and, 3) How will you measure improvement? For instance, a plausible charter for an ECMO program may state an aim as "to reduce reporting time of antithrombin 3 (AT3) results to 30 minutes in 90 days." Key process "drivers" that will enable the successful achievement of reducing reporting time are determined by subject matter experts from within or outside of the organization; although frontline staff can often provide insight that outside experts cannot. In this example, two drivers could be 1) rapid processing of AT3 samples in the laboratory, and 2) communicating AT3 results quickly to the bedside ECMO specialist. Based on these drivers, the team could work on interventions that 1) ensure ECMO specimens are processed first in the laboratory, and 2) send results directly to the pagers of ECMO specialists. To monitor the progress of their efforts, the team will track the primary outcome (i.e., number of AT3 tests reported within 30 minutes / number of AT3 tests sent), and also the reliability of the interventions (i.e., number of AT3 tests processed first / number of AT3 tests sent). By monitoring outcome and process metrics simultaneously, the team can determine whether failure to reach the goal was because the interventions were poorly executed or because the interventions were the wrong ones.

Run and control charts are used to monitor how quality metrics (i.e., time it takes to get AT3 results) vary over time (i.e., month). These line plots have operating rules that will help users identify time points when the metric has unusual value, called a special cause signal, and prompt the user to investigate for possible reasons for this change. For instance, the chart may show the ECMO coordinator that the AT3 reporting time has significantly risen over the past month; upon investigating, the coordinator discovers that laboratory is currently short staffed, but new staff will receive special training on a better AT3 machine. In this improvement project, the charts will monitor whether the interventions (new staff, better machine) can shorten the AT3 result reporting time as Figure 34-1 illustrates.

Institutions will vary between the number and experience of the ECMO staff, the processes that are in place to run the program, and the tools used by staff to perform the processes. These three factors are co-dependent and each factor influences overall quality. Where tools fall short, better processes and more people will be needed. When staffing is inadequate, more efficient processes and better tools must be available. When processes are streamlined and have little waste, less staff is required. The "triple balance" of staff, process and tools is often challenged by unexpected events (i.e., equipment break down, specialist calls in sick). ECMO programs that can anticipate and can quickly maintain a balance of these factors to maintain quality have developed a highly reliable organizational structure that contain problems so that patients continue to experience seamless optimal clinical care

ECMO Program Evaluation

It is the responsibility of each center to ensure that ongoing quality improvement occurs. It is recommended that a multi-disciplinary ECMO team including all key ECMO team members be organized to assist the program director provide administrative oversight for the program. New centers may also wish to consider inviting subject matter experts from the established ELSO centers to participate in institution's formal program reviews during the initial years of program development. ELSO recommends that formal multi-disciplinary team meetings be held on a regular basis and the agenda include review of clinical cases, equipment, administrative and educational needs, and other pertinent issues. Written meeting minutes should be made available to all ECMO team members. The multidisciplinary ECMO team is responsible to have quality assurance review procedures in place for annual internal ECMO evaluation. It is expected that all team members have the responsibility to promote and maintain a quality program.

A prompt review of any major complication or death is recommended with ECMO team members and with the responsible hospital morbidity and mortality committee. These reviews are conducted under the relevant quality assurance laws for the state where the center is located. Formal clinical-pathological case reviews with a multidisciplinary approach are also suggested as regularly conducted meetings.

Summary

Although providing ECMO to critically ill patients is complex and uses many healthcare resources, it can be very rewarding to the institution, staff, and, especially, the infants, children, adolescents, adults, and families served. Meticulous attention to the areas of essential support systems, physical facilities and equipment, team and personnel issues, and quality assurance are the foundations of a successful ECMO program. Ongoing assessment of the program's outcome, not only mortality but review of complications using standard QI methodologies, is essential for a successful program. Continued education and assessment of clinical competency should be an integral part of the program, including competencies of ECMO specialist, ECMO physicians, and ECMO surgeons.

Acknowledgement: We thank Dr. Louis P Halamek, MD, FAAP for his critical review of this chapter.

References

1. ELSO Guidelines for ECMO Centers. Retrieved February 2010, from http://www.elso.med.umich.edu/guide.html.
2. ELSO Guidelines for Training and Continuing Education of ECMO Specialists. Retrieved February 2010, from http://www.elso.med.umich.edu/guide.html.
3. ELSO Award for Excellence in Life Support. Retrieved March 2011, from http://www.elso.med.umich.edu/award.html.
4. Joint commission on accreditation of healthcare organizations. Root causes of sentinel events 1995-2003. Retrieved May 25, 2005 from http://www.jcaho.com/accredited+organizations/ambulatory+care/sentinel+events/root+causes+of+sentinel+event.htm.
5. Misch DA. Andragogy and medical education: are medical students internally motivated to learn? Adv Health Sci Educ Theory Pract 2002;7(2):153-160.
6. Knowles MS, Holton E, Swanson R. The Adult Learner. Houston: Gulf Publishing Company, 1998.
7. Joint Commission on Accreditation of Healthcare Organizations. Building the Foundations. Oakbrook Terrace: Joint Commission Resources, 2002.
8. The Joint Commission. The Joint Commission E-dition: Accreditation. Oak Brook: Joint Commission Resources, July 1, 2011. Retrieved 21 September 2011, from https://e-dition.jrcinc.com/frame.aspx.
9. Miller GE. The Assessment of Clinical Skills, Competence, Performance. Acad Med 1990; 65:S63-7.
10. Conlan, J., Grabowski, S., & Smith, K.. (2003). Adult Learning. In M. Orey (Ed.), Emerging perspectives on learning, teaching, and technology. Retrieved 13 September 2011, from http://projects.coe.uga.edu/epltt/
11. Anderson J, Boyle K, Murphy A, Yaeger K, LeFlore J, Halamek L. Simulating Extracorporeal Membrane Oxygenation emergencies to improve human performance. Part II: Assessment of technical and behavioral skills. Simul Healthcare. 2006; 1(4):228-232.
12. Helmreich RL, Merritt AC, Wilhelm JA. The evolution of Crew Resource Management training in commercial aviation. Int J Aviat Psychol 1999; 9:19–32.
13. Issenberg S B, McGaghie W C, Petrusa E R, Gordon D L and Scalese R J. What are the features and uses of high-fidelity medical simulations that lead to most effective learning? BEME Guide No 4. Medical Teacher 2005; 27:10-28.
14. Anderson J, Boyle K, Murphy A, Yaeger K, LeFlore J, Halamek L. Simulating Extracorporeal Membrane Oxygenation emergencies to improve human performance. Part I: Methodologic and technologic innovations. Simul Healthcare 2006; 1(4):220-227.
15. Personal correspondence, Halamek, L to Ogino, M. September 30, 2011.
16. Chamberlain D, Smith A, Woollard M, et al. Trials of teaching methods in basic life support (3): Comparison of simulated CPR performance after first training and at 6 months, with a note on the value of retraining. Resuscitation 2002; 53:179–187.
17. Berwick DM. A User's Manual for the IOM's 'Quality Chasm' Report. Health Affairs 2002, 21(3): 80-90
18. Weick, Karl E.; Sutcliffe, Kathleen M. Managing the unexpected: Assuring high performance in an age of complexity. University of Michigan business school management series. San Francisco, CA, US: Jossey-Bass. (2001). xvi, 200 pp.
19. Institute of Healthcare Improvement. Retrieved May 2011, from http://www.ihi.org/ihi/topics.

20. Berwick DM. A primer on leading the improvement of systems. BMJ 1996; 312(7031):619-622.
21. Weeks, William B.; Mills, Peter D.; Dittus, Robert S.; Aron, David C.; Batalden, Paul B. Using an Improvement Model to Reduce Adverse Drug Events in VA Facilities. Joint Commission Journal on Quality and Patient Safety 2001; 27(5):243-254.

35

Economics of ECLS

Robert H. Bartlett MD, Robin A. Chapman RN

Introduction

Anyone walking into a modern ICU in any country is first impressed with the intense, professional, and highly technological atmosphere, and second with what must be an enormous expense. Any health care professional who spends a month in any modern ICU perceives that most patients recover, but some suffer expensively only to die or to be discharged to permanently nonproductive lives. Daily the question arises: Is it worth it? ECLS is an obvious example of the dilemma: how much time, effort, and money can we afford to spend on a single individual? ECLS is not very costly as compared with other high-tech therapies. It is less expensive than organ transplant, cancer chemotherapy, or the cost of maintenance hemodialysis for one year. The cost accrues over a short time in very accountable categories; however, the patient is often a small child, and the outcome is uncertain. Recently in a study by Angus et al. the high cost of nitric oxide (NO) was examined and they concluded that although the initial costs were high with NO treatment, the cost effectiveness profile was favorable.[1] This demonstrates that therapies with high initial costs can become cost effective if the therapy is successful and leads to many productive years of life. This aspect of ECMO was recently studied in a 4 year followup to the UK collaborative ECMO trial.[2] The study

concluded that ECMO was cost effective when compared to conventional treatment at 4 years.

As the indications for ECMO broaden, patient selection becomes a factor in ECMO's cost effectiveness, as was recently highlighted in a study by Van Litsenberg et al.[3] Therefore, the question, "Is this worth it?" is epitomized at the ECMO bedside. The answer to this question requires various facts which we will enumerate in this chapter. It also includes some intangible variables which must be addressed. The implications of the costs and benefits to a single patient, workers, payers, and to society have been addressed in several retrospective and prospective studies which we will examine, all in an effort to address this challenging question.

The first formal reports regarding the costs and benefits of ECLS were based on neonatal patients. Walsh-Sukys[4] compared resource utilization and outcome at 20 months of age in 43 neonates treated with ECLS to 26 infants with respiratory failure who did not receive ECLS. The hospital charges were similar (about $60,000 in 1994). Schumacher et al.[5] conducted a prospective, randomized study comparing the costs and outcome in neonates treated with ECLS at 50% mortality risk to neonates treated with ECLS at 80% mortality risk. The hospital charges were similar (about $51,000 in 1995). However, the ICU stay was shorter and the neurological complications less in the

50% mortality risk group, which was the early ECLS group.

ECLS for cardiac support has led to a dramatic improvement in the survival of children with congenital heart defects. The survival rate for cardiac ECMO is ~40%, leading some to question the utility of an expensive therapy such as ECLS in this patient population. Mahle et al. utilized an accepted cost-efficacy of <$50,000 per quality-adjusted life-year saved; the authors concluded that salvage ECMO in the cardiac population resulted in a $24,386 per quality-adjusted life-year saved and that ECMO was an economically viable treatment option in this high risk population.[6]

Using statewide databases, the number of neonatal cases considered for ECLS can be estimated, and the impact on neonatal mortality per dollar can be calculated.[7,8] The cost effectiveness of ECLS compared to other treatment can be analyzed using information from the ELSO Registry and some assumptions. Schumacher et al.[9] used this approach to estimate the number and costs of additional survivors with ECLS and included the added costs of caring for survivors with chronic pulmonary or neurological conditions.

Cost effectiveness in fatal illness is usually measured in expense required to produce surviving patients compared to the cost of treating all patients. This method was used in the studies of neonatal and adult ECMO in the UK.

The definitive United Kingdom neonatal trial published in 1996[10] proved that the survival rate in severe respiratory failure in neonates with ECMO was 29% better than conventional therapy, but also addressed the cost of ECMO in detail. This is particularly important in the United Kingdom because there is a single payer system and the government has to decide whether to pay for specific expensive programs, how many programs there should be in a given region and what the return on investment is to the society. In that study the conclusions were

that neonatal ECMO improves survival at a modest cost.

The CESAR trial of respiratory failure in adults was conducted in the UK using the same methodology, with the same goals.[11] The results were quite similar with 20% better 28 day survival in severe ARDS in an expert center that used ECMO when indicated compared to conventional treatment. The thorough financial analysis of that study showed that management of severe ARDS in the ECMO center was cost effective.[11]

Cost effectiveness is also measured by the number of "quality life years" after the treatment (QALYs). An acceptable cost per QALY depends on the society, but 50,000 USD is considered reasonable for treatment of cancer and organ transplantation. This requires standardized measure of quality of life by questionnaire. These measurements have not been widely done for ECMO survivors, but the quality of life is generally reported to be good for most patients. Assuming that the average cost of an ECLS hospitalization is $100,000, and life expectancy is 70 years, the cost per quality life year is 1,500 for neonates, 2,000 for children, and 5,000 for a 50 year old adult. By this measure, ECLS is economically sound.

The financial and intangible costs of maintaining an ECLS program are similar worldwide. The reimbursement system varies considerably between countries, as do the budgets for health care. In the U.S., any care which extends a healthy productive life is considered legitimate regardless of cost. In life threatening situations such as those requiring ECLS, care is given by doctors and hospitals regardless of the individual's ability to pay. An elaborate system of identifying costs and charges exists in the U.S., and the insurance carriers and tax supported agencies pay enough to cover the "bad debt" incurred by doctors and hospitals. In other countries, the reimbursement system ranges from a fee-for-service approach resembling that of the U.S. to a fixed annual rate for physicians and hospitals regardless of the amount or type of care rendered. Obviously, any decision by an individual physician, a hospital, a health care payor, or a society will depend on the variables of the reimbursement system for that group or individual. Therefore, the answer to the value question for any technology will be different for each person involved and for each societal group. In this chapter we will focus on the U.S. system for costs, charges, and reimbursement. Those existing within other systems can then modify this information to apply to their own health care finance systems. The cost, charges, and reimbursement numbers in this chapter are general approximations and serve only as examples for discussion.

Costs

The costs of maintaining ECLS capability are fairly easily enumerated: equipment, supplies, personnel, and some additional costs. In this section we will identify the specific costs associated with a hypothetical ECMO program with the capability for treating one patient at a time and a history of treating 20 patients per year with average time on ECLS 10 days. The costs are analyzed per day of ECLS and per case. The permanent hardware required for each case is listed in Table 35-1. This list assumes that a fully stocked and equipped ICU is the venue for the procedure. It is not necessary to have a separate room or location identified for ECLS, it is not necessary to use the OR for cannulation (although a scrub team from the OR is helpful), and it is not necessary to use additional space or nursing personnel than that usually allotted to a critically ill patient with cardiac or respiratory failure. In fact, the need for ICU nursing time is usually decreased when patients are on ECLS because the patients are very stable. The essential equipment is the blood pump, a servo regulation system for the pump, a flow meter (usually integral to the pump), a method to monitor pressures and saturation in the extra-

corporeal circuit, a device for measuring whole blood activated clotting time (ACT), an oxygen flow regulator and pressure popoff valve, a circulating waterbath to maintain the temperature in the heat exchanger, an emergency battery, and a small cart to carry this equipment. All of this equipment can be purchased prepackaged at a cost of ~$105,000 or individual components which costs about $42,000. The equipment cost is identified as a single item in this analysis but should be amortized over about seven years.

The pump can be a roller pump or a centrifugal pump. The characteristics of each pump are listed in Chapter 8. Roller pumps are less expensive but require more intensive monitoring. The pump hardware includes the drive motor, controller based in a console, battery, and systems for bubble detection, flow measurement and various built in monitors. A roller pump requires a servo-regulation system (mechanical or electronic) to prevent excessive suction on the inlet side. The disposables for a centrifugal pump may also include a shock absorbing bladder on the inlet side.

The disposables for a roller pump are tubing and a collapsable bladder for measuring and controlling inlet suction. The cost is $100-$200. The disposable for a centrifugal pump is the pump head. The cost for centrifugal pump heads designed for ECLS ranges from $400 for the Rotoflow or Sorin pump to $9,000 for the Levitronix Centrimag pump. Centrifugal pumps which are used for cardiac surgery such as the Biomedicus cost less but are not suited for prolonged use.

In addition to the equipment necessary to manage a single patient, at least one backup component should be available for each part of the system. This may require having a duplicate, unused, complete system available at all times, or may be simply a list of equipment which can be located in the OR, laboratory, or ICU storage area when needed. However, the backup equipment may be needed emergently on any night or weekend, so the backup equipment must be truly immediately available. With all these considerations, the cost of equipment for an ECMO program might range from $42,000 to $105,000 (Table 35-1). A safe and reasonable approach is to buy a new equipment component system and use old, recently serviced equipment as a backup, all of which will cost ~$40,000

Disposable supplies

Disposable supplies must be provided for each case, and must be custom designed for patient size and type of vascular access. Enough supplies must be kept on hand to respond to any type of patient and to replace disposable components as necessary. The supplies needed for the hypothetical ECMO center are listed in Table 35-2. The annual supply costs for a typical ECMO center are about $114,000. We have estimated conservatively, for safety, that two oxygenators and two circuits will be needed for each patient, but this is an overestimate and will result in some surplus stock. The supplies needed specifically for the ECMO system are oxygenators, access cannulas, various sizes of conduit tubing, connectors, Luer locks, pigtail adapters and stop cocks, a small venous bladder for servo regulation, disposable components needed for pressure monitoring and venous saturation monitoring, a heat exchanger, and tubes and syringes for blood sampling and ACT

measurements. The entire extracorporeal circuit, with the exception of the oxygenator and access cannulas, can be purchased as custom made tubing packs that include all the supplies, plus extra components necessary for priming and cannulation. Although commercially assembled tubing packs are convenient and safe, it is certainly possible to assemble the circuit components ahead of time, sterilize the entire system with gas sterilization, and achieve considerable cost savings. If an institution assembles its own tubing packs onsite, it is important to allow appropriate time for sterilization and full degassing. It is particularly important to have connectors and tubing in all appropriate sizes, and other components individually wrapped and sterilized in order to deal with any circuit emergency. The only ECMO-specific drug requirement is heparin, although there will be increased requests to the pharmacy for antibiotics, sedatives, and narcotics, as well as extra demands on the blood bank.

Personnel

Personnel costs described here relate to non-physician hospital based personnel only. Personnel costs unique to the ECMO program begin with a full time coordinator and include five full time ECMO technical specialists which comprise the core ECMO team. The team may

Table 35-1. Equipment for ECLS.

	New Components	Integrated System
Pump	$10,000	$50,000
Pump servo-regulation "Bladder Box" for roller pump	3,000	
Pressure sensors	1,000	
Saturation monitor	ICU Equipment	
Water bath	3,000	
Battery	1,000	
Cart	1,500	
Gas flow meter	ICU Equipment	
Gas valve	50	
Other (electric cords, clamps, etc.)		
ACT machine	2,500	2,500
TOTAL	**$21,100**	**$52,500**
Backup	21,100	50,000
TOTAL & BACKUP	**$42,200**	**$102,000**

include individuals whose background is nursing, respiratory therapy, perfusion, or medicine.

Core team members may be assigned: full-time to the ECLS program, rotating to other hospital duties when there are no ECLS patients, or assigned to other hospital programs such as nursing, respiratory therapy, or perfusion and rotating to ECLS on an established schedule. The former, full time ECLS specialist team is preferred.

The personnel cost depends on the scope of the program and the specific staffing model. ECMO is practiced in ICUs, and usually in two or more ICUs in any hospital. These ICUs serve different populations and have dedicated nursing teams. It is possible to consolidate ECMO activity in one pediatric ICU (for neonates, children and cardiac patients), or in one adult ICU (for medical and surgical patients) but most intensive care services prefer ECMO to be done in "their" unit rather than sending the ECMO patients to another unit. In addition, ECMO may be instituted in the emergency room, radiology, or during transports. For these reasons it is most economical to have a single central ECMO team to support the ECMO program wherever the patients are housed. This team is made up of a full time coordinator and enough specialists so that one is available 24/7 (6 FTEs total). The specialists can be full time on the ECMO team, or full time in other units (nursing, perfusion, respiratory therapy) but must be assigned only to the ECMO team when on duty for ECMO. This is the minimal

Table 35-2. Supplies (1 Year, 20 Cases)

Supply	Amount	Cost
Oxygenators	40 @ $800	$32,000
Pump disposables	40 @ $500	20,000
Tubing packs (includes venous bladder, heat exchanger, connectors, etc)	40 @ $500	20,000
Access cannulas	Range of sizes	40,000
ACT supplies		2,000
TOTAL		**$114,000**

size of the core team for a small program. The cost is the same whether the specialists are assigned to the central ECMO team or to another cost center which must be "back-filled" when specialists are on ECMO duty. The annual cost is the coordinator, $90,000, and the cost of the specialists, 5 x $70,000 or $350,000 per year. The assumptions are that the annual cost of individuals includes all related benefits and indirect costs. At the University of Michigan these costs are 35% more than the designated salary per year. Other assumptions are that the actual cost of specialists is $40 per hour, $320 per shift for an eight hour shift. The average specialist will work five shifts per week. Vacation and illness time is included in the annual salary. Therefore 6 FTEs are required to cover any activity with one person 24/7. The specialists may be paid from the ECMO budget, or from their home cost center, but the total cost is the same. This nearly half million dollar cost is not for taking care of patients; just supporting the program. The duties of the coordinator and these core team specialists are to manage the program, triage calls and patients, provide education and quality control, manage the monthly meetings and registry data, manage the budget, maintain supplies and equipment, run the training program, prepare and prime the circuit when needed (always an emergency), assist with cannulation and the first hours of ECMO, help with emergencies, make rounds 3-4 times daily on ECMO patients, assist with weaning and decannulation.

Before the new technology of safe simple circuits (ECMO I) (and still today in many ECMO centers) an ECMO specialist had to do the jobs listed above AND be at the bedside 24/7 to manage the circuit and the patient. The patient also required a bedside ICU nurse at a cost of $40 per hour or $1,360 per day, so the personnel cost was $2,720 per day per patient. The specialist was at the bedside, and not available to manage all the other duties of the in-house specialist described above. Therefore the program could manage only one patient at a time (the twenty patients per year in our hypothetical program). Managing more than one patient at a time required more team specialists, usually provided by a team of trained on-call specialists, or by adding to the full time team.

With the advent of ECMO II a different staffing system is possible. With appropriate training a group of nurses in each ICU can be trained and (internally) certified as ECMO nursing specialists. When there is an ECMO patient, one of the ECMO nursing specialists is assigned to that patient for each shift. This ECMO nurse specialist assumes all the responsibilities for bedside patient management: blood flow and gas exchange, monitor vascular access points, fix the circuit in the event of a device failure, measure the ACT and physiologic variables, manage ventilation, anticoagulation, blood products, fluid balance, CRRT, trips to the operating room or radiology and ECMO weaning. The inhouse core ECMO team specialist is available for supervision but is not responsible for minute to minute care of the patient. The additional cost of daily care is only the cost of educating and maintaining the ECMO nurse specialist team (one full week for annual training, $1600). This model allows managing two or more patients in each ICU at no additional cost to that ICU or to the core ECMO team. With this model the core team can manage an almost unlimited number of patients. With this model the cost of ECMO personnel is $440,000 per year plus the cost of educating and recertifying the ECMO nursing specialists (approximately $1,600 per nurse per year). Because the direct patient management is assumed by the ECMO nurse specialist, the background of the specialists on the core team can be nursing, perfusion, or respiratory therapy

Other costs

Other costs associated with an ECLS program include the cost of training personnel who will be treating ECMO patients (physicians,

ICU nurses, and respiratory therapists); the expenses of laboratory animal training; administrative costs (including quality assurance, record maintenance, office and equipment storage space, computers, telephones, parking); and the cost of patient followup. The cost of quality assurance and Joint Commission on Accreditation of Healthcare Organization (JCAHO) requirements are met in most centers by membership in ELSO, which provides detailed data comparing ECMO center performance to national and international benchmarks. The ECMO program will place additional requirements on other hospital departments, particularly nursing, respiratory therapy, pharmacy, radiology, blood bank, laboratory pathology, and rehabilitation. Whatever transport system the hospital uses for critically ill patients will be required to transport patients referred for ECMO and may become involved with on-ECMO transports, depending on the nature of the referral base.

With all these considerations, the actual cost of our hypothetical 20 case ECMO center is $600,000 per year (Table 35-3). The cost per case is $30,000 (Table 35-4.), although the combination of core team and ECMO nursing specialists will accommodate many more than 20 patients. With an average case run of 10 days, the cost per ECMO day is $3,000. This does not include all the other costs of the hospitalization. A reasonable estimate for other costs and overhead is $70,000 for an average 20 day stay. The typical average total cost is $100,000 per patient. Calculating the financial balance for each case

Table 35-3. ECLS: All Costs

	First Year	Annual
Equipment	$100,000	
Supplies	110,000	$110,000
Personnel Coordinator	90,000	90,000
Core Specialist/s/	350,000	350,000
Nurse Specialists Training (10)	16,000	8,000
Other		
Training		8,000
ELSO Membership	1,000	1,000
Travel, Education	10,000	10,000
Misc	5,000	5,000
TOTAL	**$682,000**	**$582,000**

includes referred patients who do not require ECMO, as discussed later.

Some private perfusion companies and one ECMO company (ECMO Advantage) will assume all care of an ECMO patient in an individual hospital throughout the ECMO run for a standardized fee. These companies will also provide instruction in cannulation and initial management. The company will instruct on site nurses and specialists during ECMO runs. The individual hospital can decide whether to use a contract service for all cases, or whether to take advantage of the training provided by the contractor to establish a hospital based ECMO program.

A hospital or HMO administrator looking at an annual cost of $600,000 for a 20-patient ECMO program might consider the expense excessive. ECLS is a complex technology that has a definite economy of scale and usage. Like organ transplantation, it is a good example of an activity that is usually limited to a few regionally based centers. Although it may not always be convenient for patients' families, and may be dissatisfying to the medical and nursing staff, most hospitals would be better off financially to refer all patients who require complicated intensive care to regional referral centers. However, there is another side to the ledger, discussed below.

Table 35-4. Estimated Annual Costs and Reimbursement of an ECLS Program. Assumptions: 40 patients admitted, 20 on ECLS, 20 Hospital days per patient

Costs	
Hospital Care[1]	$2,400,000
ECLS Program	600,000
Overhead (30%)	1,000,000
Total	$4,000,000
Cost Per Patient	$100,000
Reimbursement	
Annual Charges[2]	$10,000,000
Reimbursement (50%)	5,000,000
Reimbursement @ 50% per patient	125,000
Balance	
Overall	+ $1,000,000
Per Patient	+$25,000

[1]Estimated $3,000 per day total costs
[2]Typical charges $250,000 per patient

Charges and reimbursement

In the U.S., charges to patients and insurance carriers are itemized in detail based on UB 92 codes for hospital charges and on CPT codes (current procedural terminology) for physicians. These codes identify the names of specific charge items for hospitals (e.g., 24 hours in an ICU, use of a ventilator, supplying a bronchoscope, ECMO) or physicians (e.g., hourly care in an ICU, management of a ventilator, performing a bronchoscopy, cannulation for ECMO). The charges for each item are based on direct and indirect costs, plus a charge for anticipated bad debt, and a small profit margin. On average, the total charge is roughly three times the actual cost. The charges rendered by hospitals account for 80% of inpatient total costs and 20% of inpatient charges are rendered by physicians. The bills for these services are usually separate; in fact, there may be several hospital bills and additional invoices from several doctors for a single case. If all of the patient care is conducted in an insurance owned system (e.g., the Kaiser system), a single theoretical "bill" for all the patient care goes to the account holding the assets. All of this reimbursement is done in retrospect; that is, at the end of the case or the end of the year, the total expenses are tallied up, the amount of reimbursement is added up, and the balance is determined (the "margin"). In the U.S. system, it is possible to determine the total cost, the total charges, and the total reimbursement, along with the profit or loss, for each individual hospitalization although this is rarely done. More commonly, individual patient costs are estimated based on a series of assumptions and averages. Individual patient charges are accurately identified, but hospital accounting of reimbursement is usually based on some global income amount divided by some number of patients, or more commonly by identifying the classification of insurance carriers for a group of patients, calculating a payment-per-charge ratio, and multiplying the result by the number of patients. This common approach to the accounting of hospital finances seems bewildering and misleading to physicians who are responsible for administrating ECLS or other hospital programs. This type of approach to hospital accounting can identify whether the entire hospital made or lost money in a year, but is not useful when it comes to administrating a small program like an ECLS program. Hospital accountants can study the ECLS program, but without specific questions and help from the program administrator, the financial results may be deceptive.

To determine hospital and professional income for managing an ECMO program six simple questions must be answered: 1) What was the total number of patients referred for or admitted because of ECMO? 2) How many referred patients were turned away and why? 3) How many referred patients were admitted to the hospital? 4) How many of these patients were treated with ECMO? 5) For the patients admitted to the hospital, what was the total hospital bill for each patient? 6) What was the reimbursement for each patient? With the answers to these questions, the financial status of the ECMO program can be described.

Documentation of the number of referrals, turn-aways, transports, and actual admissions must be kept by the ECMO program. It is important to keep specific records on each of these categories, particularly turn-aways. If the overall analysis indicates that each case is profitable for the hospital, then the decision to increase the size of the program will depend on the number of referrals declined because of lack of ECMO facilities or lack of ICU beds. It is important to record the number of patients transferred for ECMO because all of these patients are counted as patients in the ECMO referral base. In a typical program, less than half of these patients will actually require ECMO, but all patients generate income, so the financial analysis of the ECMO program must include both the cost and the income related to patients who are not

treated with ECMO. Typical hospital charges associated with ECMO are shown in Table 35-5. To determine the actual hospital bill and true reimbursement for each individual patient, it is necessary to go to the hospital cashier's office with a list of patients, registration numbers, and specific hospital dates. Reimbursement takes 5-10 months, so the reimbursement side of this accounting must be updated a year or more after each patient is discharged. The hospital financial office will need the same list of names and dates to estimate reimbursement, but they will probably do it based on the mix of insurance carriers rather than the actual reimbursement figures.

Hospitals

In the U.S., the Federal and state governments use tax dollars to support health care for the elderly (Medicare), and the indigent (Medicaid and others). The federal government has developed a reimbursement system that applies to federally-supported health care. In this system, hospitals are paid a fixed fee for each patient admission based on diagnosis, not care provided. There are approximately 500 diagnosis-related groups (DRGs) codes ranging from acute respiratory failure to hysterectomy. The hospital is paid the same amount (with some modifiers) whether the patient is hospitalized for one day or one month. The payment per DRG is arbitrary and not based on actual data. For example, the highest paying DRG is tracheostomy, and one of the lowest is neonatal intensive care. The DRG code for ECMO is 003 and the reimbursement is one of the high-

Table 35-5. Typical Hospital Charges Related to ECLS

	Approx Cost
Day in ICU	$2,000
Ventilator/Day	$750
ECMO Setup	$4,500
ECMO/Day	$3,000

est value DRGs. The DRG system relates only to federally supported Medicare and Medicaid payment programs, but many private insurance carriers are using the federal DRG system for reimbursement as well.

Physicians

Physicians in the U.S. are paid for procedures according to a system called CPT. There are thousands of CPT codes, ranging from a simple history and physical to ligation of patent ductus arteriosus. Physicians decide how much they charge for each CPT, and insurance carriers decide how much they will pay per CPT. Medicare and Medicaid assign a payment value to each CPT based on a relative value scale, which attempts to assign payment according to complexity. If a new procedure does not have a CPT (e.g., extracorporeal liver support), there is a long, cumbersome method to establish a CPT. CPT codes related to ECMO are shown in Table 35-6.

ECMO is a good example of the principle that it costs money to make money. Although an ECMO program is very expensive for a relatively small number of patients, with a prudent approach to costs, and accounting done by the physician director or coordinator, almost all ECMO programs can generate a profit for the hospital and the individual physicians. For example, a small ECMO program generates 40 admissions per year, 20 actually go on ECMO. The charges for each patient are $250,000, or a total of $10 million. The cost of the ECMO program is $600,000. Physician charges for each

Table 35-6. Typical Professional Fees Related to ECLS

CPT Code		Charge
36822, 36810	ECLS cannulation	$3,000
33960	ECLS care, first 24 hours	$3,000
33961	ECLS care, subsequent 24 hours	$2,000
99291	Critical care/first hour	$300
99292	Critical care, subsequent care/hour	$250
99295	NICU care/initial hour	$300
99296	NICU care/subsequent/hour	$250
90996	Hemofiltration management/day	$300
99193	Institutional and first hour cardiopulmonary bypass	$700
99190	Pump oxygenator management/hour	$300

patient are approximately $50,000 per patient for $2 million per year. Even if the reimbursement for these charges is 50%, and hospital overhead costs are calculated at 30% above reimbursement, it is obvious that the ECMO program still generates a considerable profit for the hospital and the physicians (Table 35-4)

Intangible costs and benefits of ECMO

Although an ECMO program may be very profitable for a hospital, the intangible costs and benefits far outweigh the actual dollars. Needless to say, any institution considering instituting an ECMO program should consider the bottom line in the intangible category before proceeding to any direct financial analysis.

For the hospital or HMO, the primary intangible benefit is the level of sophistication and education of the hospital and resident staff in the ICUs involved with the ECMO program. Because of the complexity of the physiology, the difficulties with patient care, and the understanding of laboratory tests and interpretations required, the ICU staff achieves a high level of technical expertise. Although immeasurable, every ECMO center finds that the general care of ICU patients, particularly ventilator and shock patients, improves dramatically: ICU stays decrease; the need for blood gases, x-rays, and laboratory tests usually decreases; and there is improvement in the overall approach to anticoagulation, ventilator care, fluids, electrolyte management, and sedative and paralytic drugs. As care improves, the incidence of adverse events and lawsuits decreases, and the type of patients that can be accepted for care increases, thus increasing the overall referral population. Some programs such as neonatology, pediatrics, pediatric cardiology, and diagnostic radiology have measurable increases in patient activity. As the reputation of the hospital is enhanced, the best available resident applicants, nursing applicants, and other staff seek out these institutions. Valuable physicians remain, providing stability and leadership. Patient and family contacts from followup visits allow successful relationships to be established with referring physicians and hospitals, resulting in an increased number of referred patients. Assuming the institution is managed well, more patients are always a benefit rather than a cost.

Intangible liabilities to the institution inevitably come with increased numbers of more complex patients. Ancillary services such as laboratory, radiology, anesthesia, pharmacy, nutrition support, critical care nursing, and respiratory therapy will have to be increased. Blood bank, OR, housekeeping, ER, and transport will have new and unique challenges. Each patient represents a potential lawsuit. If the administrator views increased numbers and complexity of patients as a cost rather than a benefit, the ECLS program will bring only added expense.

For the staff and resident physicians, the intangible benefits are inherently obvious. The opportunity to actually save lives does not come along often in medical practice. ECLS offers that opportunity on a regular basis, and even if it only occurs 50% of the time it is intensely satisfying. ECLS is currently the state-of-the-art in high technology intensive care. Knowledge and understanding of the bioengineering and physiology involved brings all other aspects of critical care management to a higher level. Involvement with ECLS automatically brings online monitoring, oxygen kinetic physiologic monitoring, calorimetry and protein balance monitoring, hemofiltration, chronic neuromuscular blockade monitoring, advanced ventilator management techniques, and a variety of other intensive care procedures into focus. For academic physicians, the benefit of studying cardiac and pulmonary disease and the opportunity to work on the forefront of clinical life support research usually means a career in which laboratory research is in an adjuvant rather than a primary priority. This association with advanced technology in patient care that has a measurable and favorable endpoint leads

to overall physician satisfaction and results in recruitment and retention of the best doctors who have an interest in critical care. Financial income related to ECLS-referred patients is a minor benefit.

The costs to physicians are high, and should be considered carefully before establishing an ECLS program. ECLS patients are always acute emergencies and consume days to weeks at the bedside, without regard for the hour of the day, holidays, vacations, or family plans. Although physicians are accustomed to being on call, ECLS requires being available and often physically in the hospital every day and every week for extended periods. This applies, in some degree, to every physician involved with the program. Before beginning an ECLS program, an enthusiastic pediatric or adult intensivist must ascertain the commitment of surgeons, radiologists, cardiologists, and other physicians who might be needed on a moment's notice for an ECLS patient. For academic physicians, time spent at the bedside means time not spent at the laboratory bench.

Is it worth it?

Several years ago, a prominent physician responsible for health care in a small African country visited the University of Michigan ECMO program. After seeing a few patients, he commented that the cost of an ICU with an ECMO program designed for 20-30 patients was more than the entire public health budget for his country. If the worth of money spent for health care means the most good for the most people, then an ECLS program would not be prudent in this example. Health care funds might be better spent on education, birth control, water purification, or malaria prevention.

The answer to the value question of whether or not ECMO is worth the expense depends on the responder. To the patient or family, the opportunity for a return from acute, otherwise lethal illness to prolonged productive life is worth it regardless of the cost. If the survival rate were only 10%, or if the severe disability rate were 30%, efforts expended on an individual patient would not be worth the agony and expense imparted to the majority of dead or disabled patients and families. But with survival ranging from 50-90% and disability ranging from 5-15% to the individual patient the effort is definitely worth it if the chance of survival with conventional therapy is <50%.

For the physicians, the opportunity to salvage the dying patient is always worth the effort when the outcome is good. The question of value, however, must be individually answered by each physician involved, weighing hours at the bedside against hours not spent in other activities (e.g., office, laboratory, OR, time off).

For hospital staff, the value comes in the satisfaction of returning sick patients to a healthy and prolonged life. The demands on time and lifestyle imposed on the physicians by ECLS are not felt by most hospital staff who generally work on an hourly, salaried basis and work the same number of hours regardless of the activity. Although some hospital staff sees ECLS as merely extra intensive work, most of the staff, from the housekeepers to the ICU nurses, considers the balance to be positive. For the ECLS specialist team and coordinator, ECLS offers a new and usually exciting career opportunity, which brings new knowledge, extra satisfaction, and usually supplemental income.

For hospital administrators, the value of an ECLS program is measured in dollars, no matter how humanitarian the outlook of the administrator. As discussed in some detail above, a hospital administrator who regards an increase in patients as an asset will consider that the ECLS program is worth it while an administrator who considers additional patients a liability will not.

Similar reasoning applies to managers of insurance companies and HMOs. Prepaid insurance programs cater to younger working individuals. They avoid the liability of diseases of the elderly, but accept the liability of diseases of the young (trauma, obstetrical complications, newborn emergencies, and acute, lethal diseases such as severe respiratory failure). Although an acute lethal disease is unusual, it is always expensive, particularly when it is followed by chronic disability. Trauma care is much more of a problem for managed care companies than acute respiratory failure. Nonetheless, because each hospitalization is a liability relatively unrelated to income, any managed care or HMO administrator may view an ECLS program as a liability (or "the cost of doing business"). An HMO administrator who reads current literature may come to realize that the cost of ECMO-treated newborn patients is the same or less than similar patients treated with conventional ventilation; therefore, a newborn ECMO program might be considered an asset. Eventually, the same studies will be conducted on pediatric and adult cases, although the resulting analysis might not be as favorable.

Finally, the value to society depends on the characteristics of that society. For the small African nation with a very limited health care budget, it would not be financially sound to have an ECLS program, and for that matter an intensive care program for infants or adults. For a society like that of the U.K., decisions about programs like transplantation and ECLS are based on financial analysis. The National Health Service sponsored a prospective, randomized study of ECLS compared to conventional ventilator management in newborn infants, with the final endpoint being neurological and developmental status at age one. There were more than twice as many healthy survivors in the ECLS group; therefore, ECLS produced many more quality life years than conventional treatment.[2] In most other countries, whenever there is a good chance that a patient will return to a normal, healthy, productive life, almost any cost is justified, and the societal arguments become more scientific than financial.

References

1. Angus DC, Clermont G, Watson S, Linde-Zwirble WT, Clark RH, Roberts MS. Cost-effectiveness of inhaled nitric oxide in the treatment of neonatal respiratory failure in the United States. Pediatrics 2003; 124:1351-1360

2. Petrou S, Edwards L. Cost effectiveness analysis of neonatal extracorporeal membrane oxygenation based on four years results from the UK Collaborative ECMO trial. Arch Dis Child Fetal Neonatal Ed 2004; 89:F263-68

3. Van Litsenburg R, De Mos N, Edell D, Grivenwald C, Bohn DJ, Parshuram CS. Resource and health outcomes of paediatric extracorporeal membrane oxygenation. Arch Dis Child Fetal Neonatal Ed 2005; 90:F176-7

4. Walsh-Sukys MC, Bauer RE, Cornell DJ, Friedman HG, Stork EK, Hack M. Severe respiratory failure in neonates: Mortality and morbidity rates and neurodevelopmental outcome. J Pediatr 1994; 125:104-110.

5. Schumacher RE, Roloff DW, Chapman R, Snedecor S, Bartlett RH. Extracorporeal membrane oxygenation in term newborns. A prospective cost-benefit analysis. ASAIO J 1993; 39:873-879.

6. Mahle W, Forbess J, Kirshbom P, et al. Cost-utility analysis of salvage cardiac extracorporeal membrane oxygenation in children. J Thorac Cardiovasc Surg 2004; 129:1084-90

7. Schumacher, RE. Effect of Extracorporeal membrane oxygenation on the infant mortality rate. Pediatr Res 1991; 29:265A.

8. Wegman ME. Annual summary of vital statistics. Pediatrics 1991; 88:1081-1092.

9. Schumacher RE. ECMO: Will this therapy be as efficacious in the future? Ped Clin N Amer 1993; 40:1005-1022.

10. UK Collaborative ECMO Trial Group. UK collaborative randomized trial of neonatal extracorporeal membrane oxygenation. Lancet 1996; 348:75-82.

11. Peek GJ, Mugford M, Tiruvoipati R, Wilson A, et al. Efficacy and economic assessment of conventional ventilatory support versus extracorporeal membrane oxygenation for severe adult respiratory failure (CESAR): a multicentre randomized controlled trial. Lancet 2009; 374:1352-1363.

36

Regulatory and Legal Aspects of ECLS

Ronald B. Hirschl MD, Edward B. Goldman JD

Introduction

This chapter addresses regulatory and legal issues in the United States. In the US the federal agency "Food and Drug Administration, FDA" is responsible for sale of drugs and devices. FDA policies are the most restrictive of all developed countries, so the process for device certification by "CE Mark" in Europe (and other mechanisms elsewhere) follow similar guidelines but require only that the device is safe and effective for the stated purpose (pumping blood, for example rather than pumping blood to treat a specific disease). The discussion of legal issues is based on the US legal system, which is a combination of local, state, and federal policies and laws. The general principles are universal, but the specifics are different in every country where ECLS is practiced.

ECLS is a technique employing medical devices intended to provide prolonged cardiopulmonary support to patients with heart or lung failure.[1-3] The FDA does not review or approve medical procedures and cannot approve ECLS, but does regulate the medical devices used. These devices are regulated under authority first established by the U.S. Congress in 1938. In 1976, following several amendments to the Act of 1938 that authorized this empowerment, the FDA's authority was extended to regulate and ensure the safety and effectiveness of all medical devices sold in the U.S.

Subsequently, devices have been classified on the basis of the risk of illness or injury that could occur should the device fail and regulatory controls have been established to assure device safety and effectiveness. The classifications and controls have been implemented through an approval process that is founded on regulations pertaining to the 1976 Amendments to the Food, Drug and Cosmetics Act (FD&C) and the Safe Medical Devices Act (SMDA) of 1990.

The application and implications of the SMDA are diverse and complex. These include marketing, labeling, medical reporting, and off-label use. The applicable controls and regulations that have been put in place for the SMDA, or are in the process of being developed, are intended to result in the provision of safe and effective ECLS devices for medical use and the enhancement of patients' health status.

The legal process and legal aspects of the doctor-patient relationship, malpractice and defenses, and the probability of risk in this area will be discussed along with informed consent, followed by the rules of research. The chapter will then conclude with a discussion of the treatment process.

Summary of the statutory authority of the FDA for medical devices

In 1906, the U.S. Congress passed a Food and Drugs Act to prohibit interstate commerce in misbranded and adulterated foods, drinks, and drugs.[4] Devices were not included in this legislation. In 1938, Congress enacted the Federal FD&C Act that placed some therapeutic medical devices within FDA jurisdiction. Over the years, the FD&C Act was amended several times. Based on findings of device-related patient injuries in the Cooper Report of 1970, U.S. Congress passed the Medical Device Amendments of 1976 and extended the FDA's authority to ensure the safety and effectiveness of all medical devices sold in the U.S. Under the 1976 Amendments, the FDA was required to classify all devices into three classes; Class I, II, or III. In 1990, the FD&C Act was again amended to enhance the FDA's enforcement capability.[5] The current FDA Modernization Act (FDAMA) was passed in 1997 (Table 36-1).[6] This Act ordered the most wide-ranging reforms in FDA practices since 1938. It included measures to accelerate the review of devices and to regulate advertising of unapproved uses of approved devices. Finally, the Medical Device User Fee and Modernization Act (MDUFMA) of 2002 established medical device review fees to support the process for review of device applications. More importantly, the Act established performance goals for FDA device review, the ability for companies to use FDA–accredited persons to inspect qualified manufacturers, rules for the reprocessing of single-use devices, additional funds for post-market surveillance, and a means for using online labeling for devices. Finally, it dictated that panels reviewing devices for pre-market approval would include one or more pediatric experts, where appropriate, in order to develop safe and effective pediatric devices.[7]

Table 36-1. The content of the FDA Modernization Act of 1997. The entire act may be found at http://www.fda.gov/cder/guidance/105-115.htm.

Title II. Improving regulation of devices

Sec. 201. Investigational device exemptions

Sec. 202. Special review for certain devices

Sec. 203. Expanding humanitarian use of devices

Sec. 204. Device standards

Sec. 205. Scope of review; collaborative determinations of device data requirements

Sec. 206. Pre-market notification

Sec. 207. Evaluation of automatic class III designation

Sec. 208. Classification panels

Sec. 209. Certainty of review timeframes; collaborative review process

Sec. 210. Accreditation of persons for review of pre-market notification reports

Sec. 211. Device tracking

Sec. 212. Post-market surveillance

Sec. 213. Reports

Sec. 214. Practice of medicine

Sec. 215. Noninvasive blood glucose meter

Sec. 216. Use of data relating to pre-market approval; product development protocol

Sec. 217. Clarification of the number of required clinical investigations for approval

Table 36-2. The regulations from the amended FD&C Act which describe device classification. The entire FD&C act may be seen at http://www.fda.gov/opacom/laws/fdcact/fdctoc.htm.

SEC. 513. [360c] (a)(1) There are established the following classes of devices intended for human use:

(A) Class I, general controls—

    (i) A device for which the controls authorized by or under section 501, 502, 510, 516, 518, 519, or 520 or any combination of such sections are sufficient to provide reasonable assurance of the safety and effectiveness of the device.

    (ii) A device for which insufficient information exists to determine that the controls referred to in clause (i) are sufficient to provide reasonable assurance of the safety and effectiveness of the device or to establish special controls to provide such assurance, but because it—

        (I) is not purported or represented to be for a use in supporting or sustaining human life or for a use which is of substantial importance in preventing impairment of human health, and

        (II) does not present a potential unreasonable risk of illness or injury, is to be regulated by the controls referred to in clause (i).

(B) Class II, special controls—A device which cannot be classified as a class I device because the general controls by themselves are insufficient to provide reasonable assurance of the safety and effectiveness of the device, and for which there is sufficient information to establish special controls to provide such assurance, including the promulgation of performance standards, post-market surveillance, patient registries, development and dissemination of guidelines (including guidelines for the submission of clinical data in pre-market notification submissions in accordance with section 510(k)), recommendations, and other appropriate actions as the Secretary deems necessary to provide such assurance. For a device that is purported or represented to be for a use in supporting or sustaining human life, the Secretary shall examine and identify the special controls, if any, that are necessary to provide adequate assurance of safety and effectiveness and describe how such controls provide such assurance.

(C) Class III, pre-market approval—A device which because—

    (i) it

        (I) cannot be classified as a Class I device because insufficient information exists to determine that the application of general controls are sufficient to provide reasonable assurance of the safety and effectiveness of the device, and

        (II) cannot be classified as a Class II device because insufficient information exists to determine that the special controls described in subparagraph (B) would provide reasonable assurance of its safety and effectiveness, and

    (ii)

        (I) is purported or represented to be for a use in supporting or sustaining human life or for a use which is of substantial importance in preventing impairment of human health, or

        (II) presents a potential unreasonable risk of illness or injury, is to be subject, in accordance with section 515, to pre-market approval to provide reasonable assurance of its safety and effectiveness.

Device classification

All devices are assigned to one of three regulatory classes (Table 36-2). The classes are based on the level of control necessary to assure the safety and effectiveness of the device.

Class I devices

Class I devices require general controls. These are the baseline requirements of the FD&C Act that apply to all medical devices. Unless specifically exempted by regulation, Class I devices consist of those for which general regulatory controls are sufficient to provide reasonable assurance of safety and effectiveness. These devices are subject to the least regulatory control. They are not considered to present an unreasonable risk of illness or injury. General controls consist of device listing, registration of manufacturers, manufacturing devices in accordance with the Good Manufacturing Practices (GMP) regulation, labeling, and submission of a Premarket Notification [510(k)] prior to

marketing a device (Table 36-3). Approximately 93% of all Class I devices are exempt from the premarket notification process. A listing of exempt cardiopulmonary bypass (CPB) devices and their classification is provided on the FDA Web Site (www.fda.gov/).[8] Examples of Class I devices are accessory equipment such as a mounting bracket for an oxygenator or system priming equipment.[7] These devices have no contact with blood and are used in the bypass circuit to "support, adjoin, or connect components, or aid in the set-up of the extracorporeal line."

Class II devices

Class II devices are those that cannot be classified as Class I devices because the general controls by themselves are insufficient to provide reasonable assurance safety and effectiveness. Reasonable assurance for Class II devices can be obtained by applying special controls. Special controls may include mandatory performance standards, special labeling requirements, post-market surveillance, patient

Table 36-3. Regulations related to pre-market notification or 510(k) which is the most frequent method of device "clearance" and is specifically applied to those devices which are substantially equivalent to predicate devices and which are not of Class III.

510 (k) Each person who is required to register under this section and who proposes to begin the introduction or delivery for introduction into interstate commerce for commercial distribution of a device intended for human use shall, at least ninety days before making such introduction or delivery, report to the Secretary (in such form and manner as the Secretary shall by regulation prescribe)—

(1) the class in which the device is classified under section 513 or if such person determines that the device is not classified under such section, a statement of that determination and the basis for such person's determination that the device is or is not so classified, and

(2) action taken by such person to comply with requirements under section 514 or 515 which are applicable to the device.

SEC. 520. [360j] (a) Any requirement authorized by or under section 501, 502, 510, or 519 applicable to a device intended for human use shall apply to such device until the applicability of the requirement to the device has been changed by action taken under section 513, 514, or 515 or under subsection (g) of this section, and any requirement established by or under section 501, 502, 510, or 519 which is inconsistent with a requirement imposed on such device under section 514 or 515 or under subsection (g) of this section shall not apply to such device.

registries, or guidance documents. Examples of Class II devices include heat exchangers, blood tubing, pressure gauges, and monitors. Examples of FDA-cleared, ECLS Class II devices are provided in Table 36-4.

Class III devices

Class III devices usually support or sustain human life, are of substantial importance in preventing the impairment of human health, or present a potential, unreasonable risk of illness or injury. Class III devices require an in-depth assessment of safety and effectiveness and cannot be classified as Class I or II devices as the controls therein alone are insufficient to provide a reasonable assurance of safety and effectiveness. In general, the Class III devices are either new devices that are "not substantially equivalent" to any previously marketed device, or are devices in which failure would be catastrophic to patient health. They may undergo a pre-market approval (PMA) process in which in vitro, animal study, and/or clinical trial data are used to evaluate the device. This is in ad-dition to the general and special controls that are applied to Class I and Class II devices. The only exceptions to the PMA requirement are devices that were on the market in 1976 and were originally classified as Class III. To date, some of those devices, such as oxygenators, have been re-classified. These exceptions are reviewed under the 510(k) process. Examples of Class III devices include centrifugal pumps. Examples of devices approved by the FDA for ECLS are provided in Table 36-4.

As previously stated, pre-market notifications are also known as 510(k) applications. At least 90 days prior to first-time marketing of a device in the U.S., a pre-market notification must be submitted to the FDA. These applications provide enough information to demonstrate that the device is "substantially equivalent" to a predicate device. That is, one that is currently, legally marketed in the U.S. Unless a device is exempt, a pre-market notification is required when marketing the device for the first time or when there has been a substantial modification to the device. A change to the intended use, or population, or a significant design change may

Table 36-4. Frequently used ECLS devices and the device classification and whether clearance or approval for ECLS has been granted.

Device	Class	FDA approved for ECLS
Roller pump	II	none
Centrifugal pump	III	none
Blood tubing/cannula	II	Kendall infant VV catheter Origen cannula
Heat exchanger	II	Medtronic ECMOTHERM II Gish heat exchanger – HE-1
Oxygenator	II	Medtronic 600,800,1500
Bladder box	I	Zimmer
Reservoir	II	Gish ECMO bladder
S_vO_2 monitor	II	none
ACT monitor	II	none
Stopcock	II	none
Bubble detector	II	none

affect the safety and effectiveness and would require a 510(k). These 510(k) applications are "cleared" by the FDA if the device is found to be substantially equivalent to the predicate device. If a device is determined to be "not substantially equivalent" it is considered a Class III device and a pre-market approval must be obtained.

Regulatory approval process

One question that quickly arises is how manufacturers can distribute Class II and Class III devices for evaluation before they are approved for marketing since some devices may require clinical data for clearance or approval. Authorization to allow investigational devices to be tested on human subjects is required and may be obtained in the form of an Investigational Device Exemption (IDE). The IDE allows manufacturers to distribute devices to clinical investigators for use on human subjects. The FD&C Act authorizes the FDA to exempt these devices from certain requirements of the Act that would apply to devices in commercial distribution. FDA approval of the IDE is not required for "non-significant" risk devices, although Institutional Review Board (IRB) approval and adherence to IDE regulations is still necessary.

The process for FDA approval of a device is based on its classification. Class I devices follow the general controls described unless the devices were exempted from particular requirements before their intended marketing. Class II devices also follow a 510(k) clearance path, but require special controls. These may include performance standards, data based on in vitro, animal, and/or clinical studies, guidelines for 510(k) submissions, advisory panel evaluation, device labeling, post-market evaluation, and device tracking. Class III devices follow a PMA process that involves an in-depth review of the safety and effectiveness of the device, along with the general (Class I) and applicable special controls (Class II). Often, an advisory

committee consisting of persons with expertise related to the device under consideration is convened to provide independent review and to advise the FDA.

Regulatory processes for marketing ECLS devices

When the U.S. Congress passed the Medical Devices Amendments of 1976, numerous potential ECLS devices were already in use for cardiopulmonary bypass (CPB). Such devices were "grandfathered" in without formal clearance. This was done to establish baseline information for a cohort of CPB devices that could serve as predicate devices upon which subsequent CPB equipment could be evaluated. These devices are known as pre-amendment devices, and include those in commercial distribution prior to May 28, 1976. All devices introduced since that date must be approved prior to marketing by the FDA. Based on the SMDA, even those pre-amendment devices that are considered Class III must now be either reclassified or requested.

Issues with ECLS devices

Labeling of a device is based on the data provided from the manufacturer to the FDA. It includes details on the intended use, methods of use, contraindications, warnings, precautions, patient selection information, and a summary of clinical data. Especially pertinent to the use of CPB devices for ECLS is the duration of use labeling, which typically limits the use of CPB equipment to 6 hours. Generally, CPB devices are not, therefore, labeled for ECLS use.

Once 510(k) or PMA is obtained, device manufacturers may market the device. However, Medical Device Reporting regulations (21 CFR, Part 803) require that manufacturers report to the FDA all instances where marketed devices may have caused or contributed to a death or serious injury. This requirement also applies if a device has malfunctioned and death or serious injury would be likely to occur if the malfunction were to recur. All device users must provide to the manufacturer or the FDA information which suggests that a device has or may have contributed to serious injury or death. This information must be reported within 10 working days of a patient's injury or death. Such information is also summarized for the FDA by each device user on an annual basis. Finally, the FDA may require manufacturers to track a Class II or III device as part of routine post-market surveillance.

Implications of using an ECLS device off-label

The goal of the FD&C Act regulations is to oversee manufacturing, marketing, and sales of devices for specific uses. The focus of such regulations is not intended to, "limit or interfere with the authority of the health care practitioner to prescribe or administer any legally marketed device to a patient for any condition or disease within the legitimate health care practitioner-patient relationship." It is not illegal, therefore, to use devices in an "off-label" manner. It is, however, illegal for a manufacturer to promote an unapproved use of a legally marketed device. For example, a manufacturer may not label their device for ECLS use until the device has been approved for ECLS use. Physicians may also obtain devices that are not legally marketed for use in their practice by prescription via the custom device exclusion of the FD&C Act (Table 36-5). It is specified in the regulations, however, that such devices should not be generally available to, or generally used by, other physicians. This exclusion legally allows use of custom devices in a very limited fashion, and would generally not apply to devices used for ECLS.

The intent of the FDA is altruistic and worthy: provide patients and physicians with safe and effective devices. Clearly, a balance must be maintained between provision of needed devices to patient populations and appropri-

Table 36-5. The Custom Device Exclusion in the FD&C Act that details the capability of any physician to prescribe a device which is not commercially distributed for use by a manufacturer, is not generally used by other practitioners, and is to be used for a specific patient or in the practice of that physician/dentist.

Federal Food, Drug, and Cosmetic Act, as Amended, Chapter V; Subchapter A§520(b)(A)(I)(ii)(B)
Sections 514 and 515 do not apply to any device which, in order to comply with the order of an individual physician or dentist (or any other specially qualified person designated under regulations promulgated by the Secretary after an opportunity for an oral hearing) necessarily deviates from an otherwise applicable performance standard or requirement prescribed by or under section 515 if
(1) the device is not generally available in finished form for purchase or for dispensing upon prescription and is not offered through labeling or advertising by the manufacturer, importer, or distributor thereof for commercial distribution, and
(2) such device—
(A) (i) is intended for use by an individual patient named in such order of such physician or dentist (or other specially qualified person so designated) and is to be made in a specific form for such patient, or
(ii) is intended to meet the special needs of such physician or dentist (or other specially qualified person so designated) in the course of the professional practice of such physician or dentist (or other specially qualified person so designated), and
(B) is not generally available to or generally used by other physicians or dentists (or other specially qualified persons so designated).

ate regulation of such devices. The FDA has encouraged regulations that strike a healthy balance between these competing forces.

Is ECLS/ECMO FDA approved?

The simple answer to this commonly-asked question is "yes." That answer is satisfactory for most families, hospital staff, and IRBs. For those who wish a more detailed response, the answer requires a more detailed explanation: ECMO is a medical procedure and FDA is not involved with medical procedures, only the sale of drugs and devices by manufacturers. The drugs and devices used for ECMO are "FDA-approved." The devices are generally approved for use in extracorporeal circulation for six hours (based on the manufacturer's label). Using devices for a longer time is up to the physician who is directing the treatment. This is referred to as "off-label" use, which is sanctioned by all regulatory agencies and commonly practiced. For example, most of the drugs given to children are used off-label. When physicians use drugs and devices off-label they (not the manufacturer or FDA)assume responsibility for benefits and complications.

The legal process

Law is a system of social control. The symbol of justice holding a scale is appropriate for the legal system since the system is always trying to strike a balance of rights and responsibilities. For example, the First Amendment to the United States Constitution grants all citizens the right of free speech but does not allow one to yell "fire!" in a crowded theater.

Law is based on the notion that, in an adversary system, conflicts can be resolved in a way that is just and fair for both society and litigants. Because law is based on an adversary system, its rules differ substantially from health care. For example, an expert witness in the legal system is hired to advance the point of view of one side to a dispute, not to render an impartial opinion.

The legal system establishes guidelines for conduct within this adversary system. Inevitably, guidelines to be clear and predictable will by nature have an element of arbitrariness. For example, the rule in law called the statute of limitations states that a claim brought past a certain point of time is stale and cannot be heard in the courts. The period of time is set by the state legislatures and can vary from state to state. Thus, in one state an injured party may have two years to bring a lawsuit for malpractice, while in an adjacent state, an injured party may have three years.

When other routes fail, the legal system searches for truth and conflict resolution through litigation. Litigation occurs after the facts being disputed, and this provides opportunities to recount facts after the incident in question has occurred. Of course, this recreation of fact can create a "reality" far different from what really occurred. Decisions that are made in split seconds in the operating room can be examined two years after the fact over a matter of hours or days in the courtroom.

Indeed, the whole notion of "facts" is viewed differently by health care professionals and lawyers. Physicians are generally inductive, going from physical observation to conclusion, while lawyers are deductive, moving from general principles to conclusions. A general principle for lawyers may not be seen as fair in every case, but one that best balances the needs of society and individuals. A physician may conclude that a neonatal patient needs ECMO and would benefit from transfer to an ECMO center. After the fact, an attorney deducing from the general principle of "first do no harm" may, with the assistance of expert witnesses, conclude that the patient would have been better served by intensive care in the facility rather than risking deterioration during transfer.

The adversarial nature of the legal system, the "recreation of reality" problem, and the difference in definition of fact, are compounded by the problem of retroactivity. The legal system in civil law cases (disputes about property or injury) decides whether to award compensation only after the injury occurs. This allows the litigants to hire expert witnesses who reason backward and determine whether care was appropriate. Of course, hindsight is always 20/20 and, when reasoning backward, experts may often express an opinion that care should have been rendered in a different manner.

The system has specific rules of evidence and proof. The party claiming the right to compensation (the plaintiff) has the burden of proof and must present sufficient evidence to sustain a case before a trier of fact. In a civil case, the burden of proof is called "the preponderance of the evidence". The party with the burden of proof must prove a case by 51% certainty or better. This "preponderance" standard is used in civil law when compensation is what is at stake. In a criminal case, where life and liberty are at stake, the standard is "beyond a reasonable doubt", a much higher standard of proof. Therefore, in a civil case, the plaintiff can win by showing their case is slightly more likely than the defendant's, whereas in a criminal case, the state must prove beyond a reasonable doubt that the defendant is guilty.

Health care professionals are often not comfortable with the legal system's approach to reimbursement for injury. Typically, health care professionals seek certainty and want a system more akin to a mortality and morbidity conference. This creates tension between health care professionals and the legal system.

Individuals involved in the legal system should never lose sight of the fact that law is a process, and the procedural rules must be observed. Cases proceed in a specified fashion, and the parties engage in a sort of ritualized warfare out of which conflicts are resolved by a trier of fact. The aim of the system is both to resolve a conflict and to do so in a way that produces a just outcome.

With this background, the chapter will proceed to a specific discussion of malpractice issues.

Civil liability

The doctor-patient relationship

Health care professionals are responsible only for the care of their patients. The creation of the doctor-patient relationship is a contractual matter, although few health care professionals think of it in this way. Legally, what occurs is that a prospective patient asks whether a physician will provide care. The physician decides whether or not they wish to undertake this responsibility. If they do, they agree to provide care so long as the patient agrees to pay for the care and be a participant in the process. Either side can terminate the contract at any time except that the health care professional cannot terminate in a way which would cause injury to the patient. Termination that would cause injury is called "abandonment" as is defined as a physician discontinuing a relationship when it is reasonably likely that harm would occur. An extreme example of abandonment would be if a patient was started on ECMO and the physician then said, "I have decided that I am going to take a long weekend, and therefore, I am discontinuing ECMO." A physician may terminate doctor-patient relationship only in a way that does not harm the patient. The patient, however, can terminate the relationship at any time even if termination would cause injury to the patient. A typical example of termination by a patient is leaving a hospital against medical advice. Here, the patient is warned that leaving the hospital would be dangerous to their health, but the patient may decide to leave anyway. With competent adult patients, the physician need only document that the patient has refused medical advice. For minors where the parents want to refuse care, the physician can use the child abuse and neglect laws to treat the patient while the legal system resolves whether care should continue.

In an emergency, the doctor-patient relationship is created when the patient arrives at (or near) the emergency room. Any facility with an emergency room is legally bound to create a relationship with any patient having an emergency. Equally, when an ECMO unit accepts a patient in transfer, the unit and its staff have agreed to create a relationship.

Federal law via the Emergency Medical Treatment and Active Labor Act (EMTALA) requires a screening exam and subsequent stabilization for emergency patients seen at an emergency facility.[9] This means that any patient seen at an emergency department must receive an exam to determine if they have an emergency and if so, the nature and extent of the condition. Then, the patient must receive care designed to stabilize their condition regardless of their ability to pay for the care prior to transfer to another medical facility.

Once the doctor-patient relationship has been created, it is the obligation of the patient to provide the facts necessary for the doctor's diagnosis and treatment and to comply with the medical regimen. It is the responsibility of the physician to treat the patient in the same way that other similarly situated, reasonably prudent practitioners would. This is referred to in the legal system as the "standard of care" rule.

Malpractice

Malpractice simply means a claim by a patient that a medical professional has breached the standard of care, resulting in harm to the patient. It is no different than any other civil lawsuit for injury except that, in medical cases, it generally requires testimony from expert witnesses. A malpractice case could be brought against an architect for improper design of a structure resulting in injury, a lawyer for inappropriate legal advice resulting in injury,

or a physician for inappropriate diagnosis or treatment resulting in injury. The elements of malpractice are the existence of a doctor-patient relationship, duty, breach of duty, causation ("proximate cause"), and damages.

Duty means the obligation of the health care professional to provide treatment in the same manner as any other similarly situated, reasonably prudent practitioner. This means that treatment must be rendered according to commonly accepted norms in the profession. In areas involving advanced treatment such as ECMO, the physician's duty is to exhaust standard methods of treatment before proceeding to new approaches until the new approaches have been demonstrated to be as good as or better than existing modalities of treatment.

Breach of duty is a circumstance where the practitioner does not act in a reasonably prudent fashion. Together, duty and breach of duty are commonly referred to as "the standard of care". The standard of care can arise from general education and experience in the field (i.e., doing things the way that you were taught to do them), or it can arise from standards created by a governing body. For example, the American College of Obstetrics and Gynecology provides guidelines which describe standard ways to provide care.[10] Standards can also come from consensus development conferences and from state or federal law. For example, in some states, state legislators mandate how informed consent must be obtained for certain procedures. For example, the laws in Maine and Texas specify the elements of consent for specific procedures.[11,12]

Even if a standard of care may have been violated, this, in and of itself, will not necessarily allow a plaintiff to win a lawsuit. The plaintiff must also demonstrate that the violation resulted in an injury. These are the elements of "proximate cause" and "damages". To take an extreme example, air introduced into an IV system would constitute a violation of a standard of care. However, if the air was removed before damage occurred to the patient, there would be no viable malpractice case. If, however, air was introduced, and hypoxic brain injury resulted, all elements (relationship, duty, breach, proximate cause, and damage) of a claim would be present. The breach must be a cause of the injury.

Damages in a malpractice suit consist of economic damages and non-economic damages. Economic damages include hospital costs, lost wages, need for future health care, and costs of adaptive equipment. Non-economic damages are pain and suffering. Many states have, through tort reform, limited the amount of damages available to a plaintiff. For example, in many states, if a patient receives compensation for post-injury hospital care from an insurance company, the plaintiff cannot claim the cost of that care as damages. Similarly, in states with caps on non-economic damages, plaintiffs are limited to a specific dollar amount of recovery. For example, California, Michigan, and other states have a specific dollar cap on non-economic damages.[13]

Product liability

In product liability cases, claims can be brought not just against individuals, but also against equipment manufacturers. For example, if a catheter tip shears off in a patient, a claim may be brought against the physician for improper technique or against the company for improper design of the catheter. Product liability cases are brought against manufacturers on the theory that the manufacturer failed to take reasonably appropriate steps to make the product safe for its intended use. With ECMO, there may be claims against manufacturers for improper design of equipment. A claim might be made, for example, that setup of a system allowed lines to be damaged by friction, that fluids were not appropriately warmed, or that safeguards were not in place to prevent a flow of oxygen into the system, causing air embolism. In these cases, the claim would be made against the manufacturer. The manufacturer could argue

that the material was manufactured properly and was being used improperly by the end user. A manufacturer may argue that a piece of equipment was inappropriately modified by a hospital, or that it was used without following the appropriate maintenance standards. Typically, cases against manufacturers are brought for design and manufacturing defects.

Defenses

Once a plaintiff brings a suit, a defendant has an opportunity to raise both factual and legal defenses. Factual defenses might include claims that care was delivered appropriately; that patient was non-compliant; that a third party, such as a manufacturer or subsequent treating physician, was responsible; or that the plaintiff's claim is factually inaccurate. Legal defenses include the statute of limitations or other defenses provided by state or federal law. The statute of limitations sets a time within which a plaintiff must bring a suit or lose the right to bring that claim. These statutes are state specific. Generally, the statutes for adults require a claim to be brought within two or three years from the date of injury; however, statutes for children vary widely. In some states, children do not have to sue until after they become legal adults. In other states, children must sue by a specified time. For example, in Michigan a newborn has until age 10 to bring a claim.[14] In other states, if the injury results in damage so that the patient can never regain competency, claims can be brought at any time. If a suit is not brought within the relevant statute of limitations for the particular state where the injury occurred, then the claim cannot go forward regardless of how meritorious it is on its facts.

Another common defense is "comparative negligence". This means that the patient's negligence caused or contributed to the injury. The patient's negligence is then factored into the equation to determine how much compensation, if any, the patient can receive. For example, a physician may warn a patient not to operate heavy equipment for 48 hours post-surgery. If, during the 48 hours, the patient operates heavy equipment and is injured, the physician would be seen to have no negligence, while the patient would be seen to have full responsibility for his or her actions. This would result in a verdict of no cause of action for the plaintiff.

Application to ECMO

A claim could be brought in ECMO cases for improper diagnosis or treatment. An improper diagnosis claim could argue that the physician should have been aware of the existence of ECMO and its utility in a particular patient's case. An improper treatment claim could argue that a patient was placed on ECMO when there were contraindications such as intracranial hemorrhage. Cases could also be based on claims of improper maintenance of equipment, improper monitoring, improper follow-up, improper transfer, or any other deviation from the standard of care.

Probability of risk

Although there have been a few malpractice cases involving ECMO use in the U.S., the likelihood of a claim is not high so long as the equipment is well maintained, the staff is appropriately trained, ECMO equipment is used correctly, and patients are monitored appropriately. Currently, treatment, at least of neonates, is well established with generally accepted inclusion and exclusion criteria and generally accepted approaches for treatment.

Informed consent

The rule of informed consent states that health care professionals cannot conduct invasive procedures without prior consent of the patient. The patient must be competent to give or withhold consent. Patients may be unable to consent because of age or medical status. Patients under the legal age of majority cannot consent unless they are emancipated pursuant to state law. Typically, minors can be emancipated when they are married, in the armed services, or because a court has held that they can be responsible for their own actions. Adults are competent so long as they understand the nature and consequences of their actions. Adults may be incompetent if they are unconscious, developmentally disabled, psychotic, or unable to express an opinion about their care. If a patient is not competent, then a guardian needs to be appointed for the patient. The guardian then makes decisions on behalf of the patient. In ECMO cases involving children, parent(s) or a court appointed guardian would consent to treatment.

The rule of informed consent says that the nature of the proposed procedure, its significant risks, its possible benefits, and treatment alternatives need to be explained to the competent patient or guardian for the incompetent patient. A choice then needs to be made by the patient or guardian. It is the responsibility of the provider to explain options to the patient or guardian. The provider can, and should, indicate a professional opinion, but it is up to the patient to make the choice. If the patient makes a choice that the provider does not feel is appropriate, then the provider can look at options for ending the doctor-patient relationship without abandonment or attempt to demonstrate that the patient is not competent and suggest that a guardian be appointed.

In the event of a true life- or limb-threatening emergency, care can be provided without obtaining informed consent. However, this is a rare circumstance, and typically, there is sufficient time to have a discussion with a patient or guardian before therapy is initiated.

Competent adults can make choices which cannot be contested. However, in certain limited cases, if parents are making choices for their children that are felt by the health care providers to be inappropriate, cases can proceed to court for resolution. The most typical case is where a parent, for religious reasons, refuses a blood transfusion for the child. In this case, courts reason that since the child has not made a free election for the religion, the parents cannot put the child at risk. Accordingly, the courts appoint a guardian for the child and the guardian then can consent to a blood transfusion.[15]

Paying attention to informed consent is important for two reasons. First, it is necessary to avoid legal liability. Treatment in a non-emergency situation without consent constitutes an assault and battery for which the professional rendering the treatment can be held liable. Second, discussion of the procedure and its risks, benefits, and alternatives helps to create rapport between the treatment provider and patient. This rapport is important in establishing a good therapeutic relationship.

Informed consent is a process of information exchange. The results of the process should be charted in the medical record or on an informed consent document, but the critical part of the exercise is the exchange of information. The document is merely a memorial that the discussion took place and was understood by the patient. The document also shows the choice made by the patient.

The rules of research

Research occurs when health care professionals are interested in expanding the boundaries of knowledge. Research is a careful approach to proving or disproving a hypothesis through data obtained pursuant to a protocol. Rules for research funded by the U.S. government are set forth in Federal regulations written pursuant to the National Research Act of 1974 and the Federal Privacy Regulations.[16] The Federal Government rules are a reaction to past abuses where researchers conducted studies without consent from patients or against the best interest of the patients.[17] While this chapter cannot discuss the

Health and Human Services and the Food and Drug Administration rules or the privacy and security regulations in any detail, they are well explained in governmental websites.[18,19]

The rules for research require submission of protocols to institutional review boards for a review of the appropriateness of research before it can be carried out on human subjects. There are very specific rules for research involving minors. For example, the regulations require that researchers respect infants and children by protecting them from all but "minimal risk". Minimal risk is defined as the risks involved in provision of health care. Any research carrying more than minimal risk for children is allowed only if, there is an expectation of direct health-related benefit for the subject child, or if there is "a minor increase over minimal risk" with the possibility of generalized knowledge about the child's specific disease.[20] Creation of a database specifically for research purposes is also governed by the Federal rules of research and privacy regulations.

ECMO was initiated in the 1970 and 1980s and its role in improving the survival for neonatal respiratory failure was described by Bartlett et al.[21,22] Three randomized, controlled trials have been performed in this patient population and all have shown that ECMO significantly improves survival.[23-25] ECMO for neonatal respiratory failure became a commonly accepted modality, it is no longer subject to research rules, but rather is considered the standard of care for patients who meet the relevant eligibility criteria.

Legal implications as ECMO develops

As indications for ECMO develop, there is a question of how ECMO should be provided. National organizations such as the ELSO Registry publish documents serving as references for physicians. These documents suggest considerations for treatment. As data develop, the considerations for treatment become more concrete. However, there are always new modalities of treatment. Just as ECMO for neonates was originally experimental, new proposed treatments could be evaluated against ECMO for specific neonatal indications.

Data can be aggregated to allow for epidemiologic studies of the long-term results of ECMO. Of course, if the ELSO Registry data is used for research, it must be created in accordance with the HIPAA privacy regulations and the federal research rules and must be IRB approved. ELSO Registry data collection provides sufficient data that allows ECMO to be reviewed longitudinally. This demonstrates the efficiency of ECMO as well as its complications.

The standard of care is the level at which a competent physician is expected to practice. In newly developing areas of medicine such as ECMO there is no clearly defined standard of care until there is common agreement on how practice should occur. In the early phases of any new innovation in medicine the first approaches are seen by the legal system as research or "innovative care" and they do not establish a uniform standard of care by which practitioners may be judged. It is only after the medical profession agrees on how the procedure is to be performed that a standard of care by which practitioners can be measured emerges. In other words, having a group like ELSO suggest guidelines in this developing field does not mandate that all practitioners must strictly follow those guidelines. Instead, practitioners are in a continual quality improvement process designed to improve the field.

Conclusion

ECMO is a rapidly developing field so the standard of care is, in a real sense, a moving target. Patients are by definition critically ill, so intervention, assuming consent, is generally seen as preferable to non-intervention. Collection of data to show the efficacy of ECMO is important. Rapport with patients and families enhances trust and avoids claims of malpractice. Although this is a field dominated by critically ill patients and rapid advances in technology, the risk of lawsuit is low. Careful, prudent practice will minimize the risk of lawsuit while providing appropriate treatment for critically ill patients.

References

1. Hirschl RB. Extracorporeal Life Support. In: O'Neill JA, ed. *Pediatric Surgery* Chicago, IL: Year Book Medical Publishers, Inc.; 1998: page 89-102.
2. Bartlett R, Roloff DW, Custer J, Younger JG, Hirschl R. Extracorporeal life support: The University of Michigan experience. JAMA 2000; 283:904-908.
3. ELSO Registry. Ann Arbor, Michigan: Extracorporeal Life Organization; 2004.
4. Food and Drug Administration. Federal Food and Drugs Act of 1906 (The "Wiley" Act). Available at http://www.fda.gov/opa-com/laws/wileyact.htm. Accessed July 24, 2005.
5. Food and Drug Administration. Federal Food, Drug, and Cosmetic Act. Available at http://www.access.gpo.gov/uscode/title21/chapter9_.html. Accessed July 24, 2005.
6. Food and Drug Administration Modernization Act of 1997. Available at http://www.fda.gov/cder/guidance/105-115.htm. Accessed July 24, 2005.
7. Food and Drug Administration. Medical Device User Fee and Modernization Act of 2002. Available at http://www.fda.gov/oc/mdufma. Accessed July 24, 2005.
8. Food and Drug Administration. Title 21—Food and Drugs, Subchapter H-Medical Devices, Part 870 Cardiovascular Devices, Subpart E—Cardiovascular Surgical Devices [21CFR, Subpart E §870.4200(a)(b)]. Available at http://www.accessdata.fda.gov/scripts/cdrh/cfdocs/cfcfr/CFRSearch.cfm?CFRPart=870&showFR=1&subpartNode=21:8.0.1.1.21.5. Accessed July 24, 2005.
9. Federal Emergency Medical Treatment and Active Labor Act (EMTALA), 42 CFR, Parts 413, 482, and 489. Available at: www.emtala.com. Accessed May 27, 2005.
10. American College of Obstetrics and Gynecology. Available at: www.acog.org. Accessed May 27, 2005.
11. Texas law, Article 4590, the Medical Liability and Insurance Improvement Act.
12. Maine law, Title 24, Insurance Chapter 21, Maine Health Security Act Section 2905, Informed Consent to Health Care Treatment.
13. Pace NM, Zakaras L, Golinelli D. Capping Non-economic Awards in Medical Malpractice Trials. Santa Monica, California: Rand Corp.; 2004.
14. Michigan Compiled Laws, Annotated Section 600.5851(7).
15. Goldman EB, Oberman HA. Legal aspects of transfusion of Jehovah's Witnesses. Transfus Med Rev 1991; 5:263-270.
16. United States Department of Health and Human Services. Health Insurance Portability and Accountability Act of 1996 (HIPAA). HIPAA Privacy and Security Regulations, 45 CFR Section 164.512.
17. Levine R. Ethics and Regulation of Clinical Research. New Haven, Connecticut; Yale University Press: 1988.
18. United States Department of Health and Human Services. Health Insurance Portability and Accountability Act of 1996 (HIPAA). Available at: www.hhs.gov/ocr/hipaa. Accessed May 27, 2005.
19. United States Department of Health and Human Services. Office for Human Research Protections. Available at: www.hhs.gov/ohrp/. Accessed May 27, 2005.
20. Additional Protections for Children Involved as Subjects in Research; 45 CFR 46 Subpart D Section 46.406.
21. Bartlett RH, Andrews AF, Toomasian JM, Haiduc NJ, Gazzaniga AB. Extracorporeal membrane oxygenation for neonatal respiratory failure: forty-five cases. Surgery 1982; 92:425-433.
22. Kanto WP, Jr. A decade of experience with neonatal extracorporeal membrane oxygenation. J Pediatr 1994; 124:335-347.
23. Bartlett RH, Roloff DW, Cornell RG, Andrews AF, Dillon PW, Zwischenberger JB. Extracorporeal circulation in neonatal

respiratory failure: a prospective randomized study. Pediatrics 1985; 76:479-487.

24. O'Rourke PP, Crone RK, Vacanti JP, et al.
Extracorporeal membrane oxygenation and
conventional medical therapy in neonates
with persistent pulmonary hypertension of
the newborn: a prospective randomized
study. Pediatrics 1989; 84:957-963.

25. UK Collaborative ECMO Trial Group. UK
collaborative randomised trial of neonatal
extracorporeal membrane oxygenation.
Lancet 1996; 348:75-82.

37

ECMO Ethics in the Twenty-first Century

Tracy K. Koogler MD, John Lantos MD

Introduction

ECMO was first successfully developed for short term use in order to allow recovery of pulmonary function in neonates with single organ dysfunction. Neonates with chronic diseases and comorbidities, and older children, were initially not considered eligible.[1,2] As outcomes after ECMO improved, these initial restrictions were gradually relaxed. As other chapters in this volume indicate, ECMO is now used for numerous causes of respiratory failure in all age groups.[3] Many institutions now report success with ECMO in treating children with malignancies,[6,7] asthma,[8] trauma,[9,10] and rejection following heart and lung transplant.[11-14] ECMO is also used as a bridge to heart and lung transplant,[15,16] as postoperative support following complex heart surgery,[17,18] and repair of CDH.[19]

Evaluating the efficacy of ECMO is complex. Even as doctors get more comfortable using ECMO for a wide range of unstudied indications, advances in the non-ECMO medical management of respiratory failure, such as high frequency oscillators and inhaled nitric oxide, have improved outcomes as well, and have decreased the need to use ECMO for isolated respiratory failure.[4,5] As a result, the indications for ECMO are constantly shifting.

There are no recent prospective randomized trials comparing ECMO to state-of-the-art standard therapy in most clinical situations. Instead, evaluation of the efficacy of ECMO comes largely from clinical experience and from information reported to the ELSO Registry. Over 170 institutions register all ECMO cases in the ELSO Registry. This registry provides some guidance, but, in many situations there are only case reports of success with no comprehensive reporting of failures.

The lack of robust evidence from prospective trials may be inevitable. After all, ECMO was difficult to study even in neonates, and they are a more homogenous population. The evaluation of ECMO for older children and adults is complicated by the diversity of clinical indications and the small number of patients with each disease process who are candidates for ECMO. In this situation, it is often impractical to do randomized trials. Decisions concerning the necessity or potential benefits of ECMO will be individual decisions for physicians, patients, and families to make.

In the absence of evidence from clinical trials to guide decisions, clinicians must fall back on their own individualized assessment of the risks and benefits of ECMO in any particular clinical situation. Doctors who suggest ECMO must first determine whether to offer it at all, and then how long ECMO should be continued to give the failing organ sufficient time to recover or await a transplant. They must carefully consider issues of communication with patients and decide how to explain the current uncertainties about the utility of ECMO. Such situations raise a number of interesting and unique ethical dilemmas. We will discuss the process of informed consent and the ethical techniques that have been commonly used in other situations where an innovative treatment is proposed for a patient who lacks decision-making capacity.

Two Typical ECMO scenarios

There are two relatively distinct clinical scenarios in which ECMO is discussed in the PICU today. One involves a patient who is emergently transferred from an outside hospital with severe respiratory distress refractory to conventional medical therapies. Often, the doctors at the referring hospital have told the parents that only ECMO can save the patient's life. The patient usually arrives at the tertiary care institution with unstable vital signs. The ECMO team prepares to cannulate the patient as the intensivist attempts to achieve adequate oxygenation and ventilation with various therapeutic interventions. The intensivist or surgeon meets with the parents of a child (or the family/surrogate of an adult patient) and quickly explains the critical situation the patient is facing.

The second typical scenario of ECMO is one in which non-emergency ECMO use is considered part of a larger treatment plan. This situation may arise before a complex congenital heart surgery or during the evaluation of a patient with heart failure who is being placed on a transplant list. The patient with respiratory or circulatory failure whose response is not optimal to medical therapy may also be a candidate for early discussion. In many instances, these patients progress rapidly and often have only hours from admission to placement on ECMO. Ideally, if a surgeon or intensivist believes there is a reasonable chance the patient may need ECMO in the future, then early discussion, when the parties involved are calm and time is

not constrained, is ideal to present a realistic view of ECMO.

These two situations are similar in that both require careful consideration of the type of information given to patients or surrogates, and the type of cautions that should be included. They are different in that, in the first situation, it is virtually impossible to obtain informed consent or informed refusal. In the second, prior discussions make it possible for a patient or surrogate to think about the ECMO option before it becomes urgent.

Informed Consent

In both situations, it is important for the surrogate decision makers to understand the most serious side effects. These include death, intracranial bleeding, and life threatening circuit complications. It is crucial to inform parents (or other decision makers) that there are no guarantees that ECMO will be successful. The family should be told that use of ECMO involves a time-limited trial. They should be given an estimate of when efficacy will be reevaluated. This information can be put in a standard written format. This allows the family an opportunity to read it again at a later time when they are not hurried and emotionally distraught.

Given the recurrent nature of these situations, ECMO teams should develop a standardized informed consent form which could serve as a template for discussion about the risks and benefits (see model at end of chapter).

In most cases, informed consent for ECMO will come from a parent or a surrogate, because the patient is critically ill and unable to make decisions for themselves. There are two models for surrogate decision making - substituted judgment and best interests. Generally, substituted judgment - that is, trying to make the decision that the patient would have made, based upon what the proxies know about their values and preferences - is preferable if patients have been both cognitively intact and old enough to have developed and communicated their values. For younger children, or for patients who have never been competent, the best interest standard is more useful.

Best interest standard

Parents and legal surrogates of children (0-18 years of age) make decisions based on the best interest standard. This standard means that based on background, values, ethnicity, and family makeup, decisions are made which they believe are in the child's best interest. Parents have been given this right and responsibility, because it is inherent to child-rearing. Parents choose in what manner they raise their children (e.g., schools, religious practice, and home environment). A child's best interest is determined by a view of the child's situation in its entirety. The physician's role is to recommend therapies in the child's medical interest and allow the family to determine if the medical goals are compatible with the child's overall best interest.

Traditionally, physicians do not override the parental decisions unless not doing so will directly harm the child, or the parental decision will result in neglect. In such cases, court intervention is sought. One example of such an override based on the best interest standard, would be a child who is being raised as a Jehovah's Witness and requires a blood transfusion.

In the past, doctors have been reticent to seek court orders to override parental refusals of ECMO. There have been three reasons for this. First, survival after ECMO, though high, was far from certain. Second, the burdens of treatment imposed by ECMO were seen as extraordinary. Finally, the long-term sequelae of ECMO were not well quantified. Taken together, these led doctors to be cautious in their insistence upon ECMO if parents refused, and the need for ECMO seemed to be a reliable threshold at which the child's best interest could be deemed unclear, the indications for treatment ambiguous, and the long-term outcomes uncer-

tain. There may be some situations in which that is no longer the case. For example, the cumulative survival in the ELSO Registry for babies with meconium aspiration who receive ECMO is 94%. Such a survival rate may create a moral obligation for doctors to seek court approval to override parental refusals.

Substituted judgment

Adults who were once competent, but have become incompetent, often have well-known values regarding medical treatment. The best case scenario for substituted judgment is one in which a formerly competent adult has an advance directive. They may have designated a proxy decision maker using a durable power of attorney for healthcare (DPAH) or expressed specific treatment preferences in a living will. The DPAH is a legal document allowing a competent adult to authorize another person to make medical decisions on their behalf. The living will is a legal document that explicitly states certain preferences.

Even if neither a DPAH nor a living will exists, as is the case for many patients, a competent adult patient can still be asked who he or she would want to make medical decisions for him. This information should be recorded in the patient's medical record. If the patient has not designated a proxy, then the decision making process varies from state to state. Some states have laws that designate default decision makers. The lists are compiled in a hierarchical fashion, with spouse typically being first, adult children second, parents third, and friends or acquaintances designated last. The individual designated is expected to make decisions based on what the patient would do. Thus, this is referred to as "substituted judgment" rather than a "best interest" decision.

While a DPAH has the authority in most states to allow any decision the person could have made, the surrogate has some limitations on options when choosing life-prolonging therapies such as ECMO. A few states require proof of knowledge of prior patient wishes concerning withdrawal or withholding of life-prolonging therapies. If the physician believes that the surrogate in this situation is going against what the patient had previously requested for medical care, then the physician can challenge the decision. However, because of the high risk of ECMO, a physician should have very good cause to question the surrogate decision maker.

Emotions

Unlike other discussions physicians may have with families and surrogates, discussions surrounding ECMO are usually charged with emotion because of the critical nature of the situation. Therefore, despite realizing the risks and benefits of the procedure, many families will instruct the physician to do anything that might increase the risk for survival no matter how slight. The crisis situation often clouds rationality, and many never really hear or understand the potential long term sequelae or potential for death despite ECMO. Therefore, one must reiterate to families the potential consequences during subsequent conversations while their loved one is on ECMO, including daily updates about bleeding and infection risks, and the likelihood of a favorable outcome.

ECMO and futility

In some situations, doctors do not offer ECMO to a patient – or they suggest stopping ECMO that has already been initiated – because they think it will be futile. Assessments of futility can arise in three distinct situations: 1) situations in which doctors think ECMO will not work; 2) situations in which doctors think ECMO is inappropriate because of the patient's underlying condition; and 3) situations in which ECMO has been started but appears to be ineffective.

The first scenario, where doctors think ECMO will not work, rarely raises ethical dilemmas. Most families do not know to request or demand ECMO in the way they might know to request CPR. Instead, when doctors think ECMO is not indicated, they simply do not offer it. To the extent that dilemmas arise in this situation, they are usually intraprofessional disagreements among doctors about whether or not ECMO should be offered. Often, such disagreements arise in situations where ECMO use is most experimental or innovative. When ECMO is offered in these situations, it is crucial that parents understand that its use is nonstandard. In those situations, a different sort of informed consent might be necessary, highlighting the highly innovative nature of ECMO use.

In some situations, doctors deem ECMO inappropriate because of the patient's underlying condition. Many doctors, for example, think that ECMO is inappropriate for patients with Trisomy 13 or 18. In these cases, the decision to not offer ECMO is based upon a combination of two factors: the patient's poor prognosis for survival and the patient's poor prognosis for quality of life in the event of survival. Unfortunately, little is known about the efficacy of ECMO in these situations so the assessment of medical futility is somewhat speculative.

Finally, there are situations in which ECMO is initiated but is not producing the expected benefit. The medical facts in such situations are similar to those in which ECMO is not initially offered because of the patient's poor prognosis for survival. However, because they involve withdrawal, rather than the withholding, of ECMO, they are viewed differently. While lawyers and philosophers agree that withholding and withdrawing are legally and morally equivalent, doctors and families understand that emotionally they are not. In order to anticipate and address the special issues that arise with the withdrawal of ECMO, doctors should always include the idea of a "time-limited trial" as part of the initial consent process.

Defining time-limited trials

ECMO therapy should generally be offered as a time-limited trial and be described as such to all involved parties from the beginning. This is because outcomes with ECMO become worse as the duration of ECMO therapy increases. In this sense, ECMO is not like dialysis or mechanical ventilation – therapies that can, if necessary, be used for prolonged life-support.

In the early days of ECMO, there was a marked decline in survival after 2 weeks. More recent data suggests that, although the longer a patient is on ECMO, the lower the survival rate, many patients have stayed on for more than two weeks and have survived.[21,22] Thus, today, there is no easily definable time period after which ECMO should be considered futile. This time period will be based on the type of injury and the anticipated time course to healing. Data show that ECMO for cardiac failure after heart surgery continued beyond 3-5 days provides poor outcomes,[18,20] and ECMO beyond two weeks may not improve respiratory failure.[6]

Families should be told at the time of ECMO initiation that the likelihood of success will be periodically reevaluated. For each patient, doctors should try to state a time period after which ECMO might be considered futile. Parents should be informed that, after that time, if the patient is not improving, ECMO will be withdrawn. Such a discussion at the time of consent will help to prepare families for what is to come. To families, the patient may appear the same on day 1 of ECMO as on day 14, and they will not understand the need to remove the life-prolonging therapy. They may question why ECMO cannot continue indefinitely to give the patient every chance to get better.

The goal of such an approach is to avoid situations such as one described by Paris et al. who discuss a case in which parents request that ECMO be continued after the physicians believe the therapy is no longer beneficial. The patient had a pulmonary contusion and hemorrhage secondary to trauma.[23] The article discusses how physicians have no obligation to continue a therapy that will not improve the outcome for the patient but how that was not made clear to parents at the outset, leading to controversy. If ECMO is not improving the patient's health but is causing harm or merely prolonging the dying process, it is appropriate to discuss these complications with the family and withdraw ECMO before the time trial is completed.

Palliative care

Palliative care is essential when the patient is going to die despite having received ECMO. Preparation of the family for discontinuation of ECMO and discussions concerning what the family would like to do in preparation for removal of the circuit is crucial. Does the patient require religious ceremony such as baptism, last rites, or other religious blessings? Does the family want to be present during discontinuation of the circuit? Did the patient wish to be an organ or tissue donor? Do the parents wish to hold the child during removal from ECMO? Who should be in the room with the family? These questions must be considered, and reasonable requests should be granted, since, for most of these families, these may be the only decisions they truly make, while other decisions have been made by the physicians with family agreement.

Most infants can be placed in the parent's arms prior to clamping the circuit if there is planning for this, and it is explained that the circuit may alarm after the child is lowered into their arms. Allowing the parents to hold their baby prior to death, which, for some, may be the first time they have held their child, is critically important for the family. Older children and adults can have their hands held during discontinuation of ECMO. A palliative care team can also help the family in the coming months to deal with their loss and provide support.

Families whose children receive ECMO and survive with impairments are also likely to benefit from palliative care services. ECMO survivors are unlikely to be completely healthy. It is likely that the child will require some therapy, such as rehabilitation, supplemental oxygen, mechanical ventilation, or a feeding tube. They may also have seizures, developmental delay, cerebral palsy, or learning disabilities. Support from chaplains, social workers, and other specialists to determine the best way to take care of this special child and their family will minimize the trauma of this ICU experience. Unfortunately, most adult palliative care services are unable to provide these services; however, support services for the inevitable transitions for the adult patient and family are beneficial.

Conclusions

ECMO has proven effective in treating acute respiratory and cardiac failure. Failures as well as successes should be reported so that more information is available to physicians when determining which patients may or may not benefit from this therapy and which factors may indicate certain failure.

ECMO must be considered a time-limited trial, and physicians should administer it with the anticipation of a maximal length of trial. The time period should be relayed to the family and the medical team. The patient should be assessed daily to determine if the time period should be altered or other treatments considered such as transplant. If the time period expires and improvement is not seen, then it is the physician's ethical obligation to make the critical decision to remove ECMO, since it has failed to fulfill its goal.

Family support during this time of critical illness is crucial to help the family transition to caring for a family member with chronic medical issues or losing a family member. Palliative care teams, chaplains, and social workers may all be instrumental in achieving these goals.

If ECMO is unsuccessful, allowing the family some choices about the method of withdrawal of ECMO and the presence of family is imperative. As we continue to provide extraordinary therapies to save lives, we must also remember to provide extraordinary care when technological therapies fail and death is inevitable.

References

1. Bartlett RH, Gazzaniga AB, Toomasian J, Coran AG, Roloff D, Rucker R. Extracorporeal membrane oxygenation (ECMO) in neonatal respiratory failure. 100 cases. Ann Surg. 1986; 204:236-45.

2. Toomasian JM, Snedecor SM, Cornell RG, Cilley RE, Bartlett RH. National experience with extracorporeal membrane oxygenation for newborn respiratory failure. Data from 715 cases. ASAIO Trans. 1988; 34:140-7.

3. Conrad SA, Rycus PT, Dalton H. Extracorporeal life support registry report. ASAIO Journal. 2005; 51:4-10.

4. Hintz SR, Suttner DM, Sheehan AM, Rhine WD, Van Meurs KP. Decreased use of neonatal extracorporeal membrane oxygenation (ECMO): how new treatment modalities have affected ECMO utilization. Pediatrics. 2000; 106:1339-1343.

5. Hui TT, Danielson PD, Anderson KD, Stein JE. The impact of changing neonatal respiratory management on extracorporeal membrane oxygenation utilization. J Pediatr Surg. 2002; 37:703-705.

6. Masiakos PT, Islam S, Doody DP, Schnitzer JJ, Ryan DP. Extracorporeal membrane oxygenation for nonneonatal acute respiratory failure. Arch Surg. 1999; 134:375-379.

7. Linden V, Karlen J, Olsson M, et al. Successful extracorporeal membrane oxygenation in four children with malignant disease and severe Pneumocystis carinii pneumonia. Med Pediatr Oncol. 1999; 32:25-31.

8. MacDonnell KF, Moon HS, Sekar TS, Ahluwalia MP. Extracorporeal membrane oxygenator support in a case of severe status asthmaticus. Ann Thorac Surg 1981; 31:171-175.

9. Steiner RB, Adolph VR, Heaton JF, Bonis SL, Falterman KW, Arensman RM. Pediatric extracorporeal membrane oxygenation in posttraumatic respiratory failure. J Pediatr Surg 1991; 26:1011-1014.

10. Fortenberry JD, Meier AH, Pettignano R, Heard M, Chambliss CR, Wulkan M. Extracorporeal life support for posttraumatic acute respiratory distress syndrome at a children's medical center. J Pediatr Surg 2003; 38:1221-1226.

11. Hoffman TM, Spray TL, Gaynor JW, Clark BJ 3rd, Bridges ND. Survival after acute graft failure in pediatric thoracic organ transplant recipients. Pediatr Transplant 2000; 4:112-117.

12. Mitchell MB, Campbell DN, Bielefeld MR, Doremus T. Utility of extracorporeal membrane oxygenation for early graft failure following heart transplantation in infancy. J Heart Lung Transplant 2000; 19:834-839.

13. Dahlberg PS, Prekker ME, Herrington CS, Hertz MI, Park SJ. Medium-term results of extracorporeal membrane oxygenation for severe acute lung injury after lung transplantation. J Heart Lung Transplant 2004; 23:979-984.

14. Oto T, Rosenfeldt F, Rowland M, et al. Extracorporeal membrane oxygenation after lung transplantation: evolving technique improves outcomes. Ann Thorac Surg 2004; 78:1230-1235.

15. Levi D, Marelli D, Plunkett M, et al. Use of assist devices and ECMO to bridge pediatric patients with cardiomyopathy to transplantation. J Heart Lung Transplant 2002; 21:760-770.

16. Hopper AO, Pageau J, Job L, Heart J, Deming DD, Peverini RL. Extracorporeal membrane oxygenation for perioperative support in neonatal and pediatric cardiac transplantation. Artif Organs 1999; 23:1006-1009.

17. Kulik TJ, Moler FW, Palmisano JM, et al. Outcome-associated factors in pediatric patients treated with extracorporeal membrane oxygenator after cardiac surgery. Circulation. 1996; 94:II63-8.

18. Aharon AS, Drinkwater DC, Churchwell KB, et al. Extracorporeal membrane oxygenation in children after repair of congenital cardiac lesions. Ann Thorac Surg 2001; 72:2095-2101.

19. Heiss K, Manning P, Oldham KT, et al. Reversal of mortality for congenital diaphragmatic hernia with ECMO. Ann Surg 1989; 209:225-230.

20. Mehta U, Laks H, Sadeghi A, et al. Extracorporeal membrane oxygenation for cardiac support in pediatric patients. Am Surg 2000; 66:879-886.

21. Linden V, Palmer K, Reinhard J, et al.High survival in adult patients with acute respiratory distress syndrome treated by extracorporeal membrane oxygenation, minimal sedation, and pressure supported ventilation. Int Care Med 2000; 26:1630-1637.

22. Frenckner B, Palmer P, Linden V. Extracorporeal respiratory support and minimally invasive ventilation in severe ARDS. Minerva Anestesiol 2002; 68:381-386.

23. Paris JJ, Schreiber MD, Statter M, Arensman R, Siegler M. Beyond Autonomy — Physicians' Refusal To Use Life-Prolonging Extracorporeal Membrane Oxygenation. N Engl J Med 1993; 329:354-335.

Model Consent

I authorize _____and whomever he/she may designate as necessary to do a surgical procedure to place _____ on ECMO(extracorporeal membrane oxygenation).

I understand that ECMO is used to assist the heart and lungs when a patient is critically ill. Blood is removed from the body through the machine where oxygen is placed in the blood and carbon dioxide is removed similar to what happens in the lungs.

I understand that the patient will receive blood products while on ECMO. Blood products carry a very small risk of transmitting infections, such as hepatitis and HIV. There is also a risk that a patient can have a reaction to the blood product.

I understand that the risks of ECMO are infection, and bleeding which can be life-threatening. The bleeding can include bleeding in the brain, which can lead to permanent brain injury.

I understand that ECMO is usually a time limited trial, to allow the patient's lungs and/or heart to heal from surgery, infection, trauma, or other insult. I understand that at this time the physicians think the trial will be approximately_____. I understand the doctors will assess if ECMO is helping the patient heal or is it just prolonging the dying process at that time. If ECMO does not appear to be working according to the physicians at that time, ECMO may be stopped. ECMO may also be stopped earlier if there is significant bleeding, infection, or ECMO is not able to provide blood pressure support or oxygen to the patient appropriately.

ADDENDUM FOR INNOVATIVE ECMO USE IN UNUSUAL SITUATIONS:

I understand that ECMO has not been well-studied as a treatment for the problems that my child is now having. In these situations, it should be considered an innovative, unproven treatment. I also understand that my doctors think that it may offer the best chance to save my child's life since there are no treatments for his/her condition that have been proven to be effective.

Glossary

ACT	Activated Clotting Time
APTT	Activated Partial Thromboplastin Time
ARDS	Acute Respiratory Distress Syndrome
AVCOR	Arteriovenous Carbon Dioxide Removal
CPR	Cardiopulmonary Resuscitation
CPB	Cardiopulmonary Bypass
CRRT	Continuous Renal Replacement Therapy
CVP	Central Venous Pressure
DIC	Disseminated Intravascular Coagulation
ECCOR	Extracorporeal Carbon Dioxide Removal
ECLS	Extracorporeal Life Support
ECMO	Extracorporeal Membrane Oxygenation
VA	Venoarterial
VAV	Venoarteriovenous
VV	Venovenous
VVA	Venovenoarterial
ECMO I	ECMO using traditional roller pumps and silicon membrane oxygenators
ECMO II	ECMO using Mendler-designed centrifugal pumps and polymethylpentene hollow-fiber oxygenators
ECPR	Extracorporeal Cardiopulmonary Resuscitation
ELSO	Extracorporeal Life Support Organization
FiO$_2$	Fractional Inspired Oxygen Concentration
HFOV	High Frequency Oscillatory Ventilation
ICU	Intensive Care Unit
IPPV	Intermittent Positive-Pressure Ventilation
MAP	Mean Arterial Pressure, or Mean Airway Pressure
NICU	Neonatal Intensive Care Unit
NIV	Non-invasive Ventilation
PCO$_2$	Partial pressure of carbon dioxide
PO$_2$	Partial pressure of oxygen
PEEP	Positive End-Expiratory Pressure
PICU	Pediatric Intensive Care Unit
PIP	Peak Inspiratory Pressure
Pplat	Plateau Inspiratory Pressure
PT	Prothombin Time
RPM	Revolutions Per Minute
SvO$_2$	Mixed venous oxygen saturation
VAD	Ventricular Assist Device
LVAD	Left Ventricular Assist Device
RVAD	Right Ventricular Assist Device
BiVAD	BiVentricular Assist Device